Lecture Notes in Computer Science 8529

Commenced Publication in 1973
Founding and Former Series Editors:
Gerhard Goos, Juris Hartmanis, and Jan van Leeuwen

Vincent G. Duffy (Ed.)

Digital Human Modeling

Applications in Health, Safety, Ergonomics and Risk Management

5th International Conference, DHM 2014
Held as Part of HCI International 2014
Heraklion, Crete, Greece, June 22-27, 2014
Proceedings

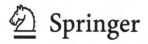 Springer

Volume Editor

Vincent G. Duffy
Purdue University
School of Industrial Engineering
West Lafayette, IN 47907, USA
E-mail: duffy@purdue.edu

ISSN 0302-9743   e-ISSN 1611-3349
ISBN 978-3-319-07724-6   e-ISBN 978-3-319-07725-3
DOI 10.1007/978-3-319-07725-3
Springer Cham Heidelberg New York Dordrecht London

Library of Congress Control Number: 2014940291

LNCS Sublibrary: SL 3 – Information Systems and Application, incl. Internet/Web
and HCI

Typesetting: Camera-ready by author, data conversion by Scientific Publishing Services, Chennai, India

Printed on acid-free paper

Springer is part of Springer Science+Business Media (www.springer.com)

Foreword

The 16th International Conference on Human–Computer Interaction, HCI International 2014, was held in Heraklion, Crete, Greece, during June 22–27, 2014, incorporating 14 conferences/thematic areas:

Thematic areas:

- Human–Computer Interaction
- Human Interface and the Management of Information

Affiliated conferences:

- 11th International Conference on Engineering Psychology and Cognitive Ergonomics
- 8th International Conference on Universal Access in Human–Computer Interaction
- 6th International Conference on Virtual, Augmented and Mixed Reality
- 6th International Conference on Cross-Cultural Design
- 6th International Conference on Social Computing and Social Media
- 8th International Conference on Augmented Cognition
- 5th International Conference on Digital Human Modeling and Applications in Health, Safety, Ergonomics and Risk Management
- Third International Conference on Design, User Experience and Usability
- Second International Conference on Distributed, Ambient and Pervasive Interactions
- Second International Conference on Human Aspects of Information Security, Privacy and Trust
- First International Conference on HCI in Business
- First International Conference on Learning and Collaboration Technologies

A total of 4,766 individuals from academia, research institutes, industry, and governmental agencies from 78 countries submitted contributions, and 1,476 papers and 225 posters were included in the proceedings. These papers address the latest research and development efforts and highlight the human aspects of design and use of computing systems. The papers thoroughly cover the entire field of human–computer interaction, addressing major advances in knowledge and effective use of computers in a variety of application areas.

This volume, edited by Vincent G. Duffy, contains papers focusing on the thematic area of Digital Human Modeling and Applications in Health, Safety, Ergonomics and Risk Management, addressing the following major topics:

- Modelling posture and motion
- Anthropometry, design and ergonomics

- Ergonomics and human modelling in work and everyday life environments
- Advances in Healthcare
- Rehabilitation applications
- Risk, safety and emergency

The remaining volumes of the HCI International 2014 proceedings are:

- Volume 1, LNCS 8510, Human–Computer Interaction: HCI Theories, Methods and Tools (Part I), edited by Masaaki Kurosu
- Volume 2, LNCS 8511, Human–Computer Interaction: Advanced Interaction Modalities and Techniques (Part II), edited by Masaaki Kurosu
- Volume 3, LNCS 8512, Human–Computer Interaction: Applications and Services (Part III), edited by Masaaki Kurosu
- Volume 4, LNCS 8513, Universal Access in Human–Computer Interaction: Design and Development Methods for Universal Access (Part I), edited by Constantine Stephanidis and Margherita Antona
- Volume 5, LNCS 8514, Universal Access in Human–Computer Interaction: Universal Access to Information and Knowledge (Part II), edited by Constantine Stephanidisand MargheritaAntona
- Volume 6, LNCS 8515, Universal Access in Human–Computer Interaction: Aging and Assistive Environments (Part III), edited by Constantine Stephanidis and Margherita Antona
- Volume 7, LNCS 8516, Universal Access in Human–Computer Interaction: Design for All and Accessibility Practice (Part IV), edited by Constantine Stephanidis and Margherita Antona
- Volume 8, LNCS 8517, Design, User Experience, and Usability: Theories, Methods and Tools for Designing the User Experience (Part I), edited by Aaron Marcus
- Volume 9, LNCS 8518, Design, User Experience, and Usability: User Experience Design for Diverse Interaction Platforms and Environments (Part II), edited by Aaron Marcus
- Volume 10, LNCS 8519, Design, User Experience, and Usability: User Experience Design for Everyday Life Applications and Services (Part III), edited by Aaron Marcus
- Volume 11, LNCS 8520, Design, User Experience, and Usability: User Experience Design Practice (Part IV), edited by Aaron Marcus
- Volume 12, LNCS 8521, Human Interface and the Management of Information: Information and Knowledge Design and Evaluation (Part I), edited by Sakae Yamamoto
- Volume 13, LNCS 8522, Human Interface and the Management of Information: Information and Knowledge in Applications and Services (Part II), edited by Sakae Yamamoto
- Volume 14, LNCS 8523, Learning and Collaboration Technologies: Designing and Developing Novel Learning Experiences (Part I), edited by Panayiotis Zaphiris and Andri Ioannou

- Volume 15, LNCS 8524, Learning and Collaboration Technologies: Technology-rich Environments for Learning and Collaboration (Part II), edited by Panayiotis Zaphiris and Andri Ioannou
- Volume 16, LNCS 8525, Virtual, Augmented and Mixed Reality: Designing and Developing Virtual and Augmented Environments (Part I), edited by Randall Shumaker and Stephanie Lackey
- Volume 17, LNCS 8526, Virtual, Augmented and Mixed Reality: Applications of Virtual and Augmented Reality (Part II), edited by Randall Shumaker and Stephanie Lackey
- Volume 18, LNCS 8527, HCI in Business, edited by Fiona Fui-Hoon Nah
- Volume 19, LNCS 8528, Cross-Cultural Design, edited by P.L. Patrick Rau
- Volume 21, LNCS 8530, Distributed, Ambient, and Pervasive Interactions, edited by Norbert Streitz and Panos Markopoulos
- Volume 22, LNCS 8531, Social Computing and Social Media, edited by Gabriele Meiselwitz
- Volume 23, LNAI 8532, Engineering Psychology and Cognitive Ergonomics, edited by Don Harris
- Volume 24, LNCS 8533, Human Aspects of Information Security, Privacy and Trust, edited by Theo Tryfonas and Ioannis Askoxylakis
- Volume 25, LNAI 8534, Foundations of Augmented Cognition, edited by Dylan D. Schmorrow and Cali M. Fidopiastis
- Volume 26, CCIS 434, HCI International 2014 Posters Proceedings (Part I), edited by Constantine Stephanidis
- Volume 27, CCIS 435, HCI International 2014 Posters Proceedings (Part II), edited by Constantine Stephanidis

I would like to thank the Program Chairs and the members of the Program Boards of all affiliated conferences and thematic areas, listed below, for their contribution to the highest scientific quality and the overall success of the HCI International 2014 Conference.

This conference could not have been possible without the continuous support and advice of the founding chair and conference scientific advisor, Prof. Gavriel Salvendy, as well as the dedicated work and outstanding efforts of the communications chair and editor of *HCI International News*, Dr. Abbas Moallem.

I would also like to thank for their contribution towards the smooth organization of the HCI International 2014 Conference the members of the Human–Computer Interaction Laboratory of ICS-FORTH, and in particular George Paparoulis, Maria Pitsoulaki, Maria Bouhli, and George Kapnas.

April 2014

Constantine Stephanidis
General Chair, HCI International 2014

Organization

Human–Computer Interaction

Program Chair: Masaaki Kurosu, Japan

Jose Abdelnour-Nocera, UK
Sebastiano Bagnara, Italy
Simone Barbosa, Brazil
Adriana Betiol, Brazil
Simone Borsci, UK
Henry Duh, Australia
Xiaowen Fang, USA
Vicki Hanson, UK
Wonil Hwang, Korea
Minna Isomursu, Finland
Yong Gu Ji, Korea
Anirudha Joshi, India
Esther Jun, USA
Kyungdoh Kim, Korea

Heidi Krömker, Germany
Chen Ling, USA
Chang S. Nam, USA
Naoko Okuizumi, Japan
Philippe Palanque, France
Ling Rothrock, USA
Naoki Sakakibara, Japan
Dominique Scapin, France
Guangfeng Song, USA
Sanjay Tripathi, India
Chui Yin Wong, Malaysia
Toshiki Yamaoka, Japan
Kazuhiko Yamazaki, Japan
Ryoji Yoshitake, Japan

Human Interface and the Management of Information

Program Chair: Sakae Yamamoto, Japan

Alan Chan, Hong Kong
Denis A. Coelho, Portugal
Linda Elliott, USA
Shin'ichi Fukuzumi, Japan
Michitaka Hirose, Japan
Makoto Itoh, Japan
Yen-Yu Kang, Taiwan
Koji Kimita, Japan
Daiji Kobayashi, Japan

Hiroyuki Miki, Japan
Shogo Nishida, Japan
Robert Proctor, USA
Youngho Rhee, Korea
Ryosuke Saga, Japan
Katsunori Shimohara, Japan
Kim-Phuong Vu, USA
Tomio Watanabe, Japan

Engineering Psychology and Cognitive Ergonomics

Program Chair: Don Harris, UK

Guy Andre Boy, USA
Shan Fu, P.R. China
Hung-Sying Jing, Taiwan
Wen-Chin Li, Taiwan
Mark Neerincx, The Netherlands
Jan Noyes, UK
Paul Salmon, Australia

Axel Schulte, Germany
Siraj Shaikh, UK
Sarah Sharples, UK
Anthony Smoker, UK
Neville Stanton, UK
Alex Stedmon, UK
Andrew Thatcher, South Africa

Universal Access in Human–Computer Interaction

**Program Chairs: Constantine Stephanidis, Greece,
and Margherita Antona, Greece**

Julio Abascal, Spain
Gisela Susanne Bahr, USA
João Barroso, Portugal
Margrit Betke, USA
Anthony Brooks, Denmark
Christian Bühler, Germany
Stefan Carmien, Spain
Hua Dong, P.R. China
Carlos Duarte, Portugal
Pier Luigi Emiliani, Italy
Qin Gao, P.R. China
Andrina Granić, Croatia
Andreas Holzinger, Austria
Josette Jones, USA
Simeon Keates, UK

Georgios Kouroupetroglou, Greece
Patrick Langdon, UK
Barbara Leporini, Italy
Eugene Loos, The Netherlands
Ana Isabel Paraguay, Brazil
Helen Petrie, UK
Michael Pieper, Germany
Enrico Pontelli, USA
Jaime Sanchez, Chile
Alberto Sanna, Italy
Anthony Savidis, Greece
Christian Stary, Austria
Hirotada Ueda, Japan
Gerhard Weber, Germany
Harald Weber, Germany

Virtual, Augmented and Mixed Reality

**Program Chairs: Randall Shumaker, USA,
and Stephanie Lackey, USA**

Roland Blach, Germany
Sheryl Brahnam, USA
Juan Cendan, USA
Jessie Chen, USA
Panagiotis D. Kaklis, UK

Hirokazu Kato, Japan
Denis Laurendeau, Canada
Fotis Liarokapis, UK
Michael Macedonia, USA
Gordon Mair, UK

Jose San Martin, Spain
Tabitha Peck, USA
Christian Sandor, Australia

Christopher Stapleton, USA
Gregory Welch, USA

Cross-Cultural Design

Program Chair: P.L. Patrick Rau, P.R. China

Yee-Yin Choong, USA
Paul Fu, USA
Zhiyong Fu, P.R. China
Pin-Chao Liao, P.R. China
Dyi-Yih Michael Lin, Taiwan
Rungtai Lin, Taiwan
Ta-Ping (Robert) Lu, Taiwan
Liang Ma, P.R. China
Alexander Mädche, Germany

Sheau-Farn Max Liang, Taiwan
Katsuhiko Ogawa, Japan
Tom Plocher, USA
Huatong Sun, USA
Emil Tso, P.R. China
Hsiu-Ping Yueh, Taiwan
Liang (Leon) Zeng, USA
Jia Zhou, P.R. China

Online Communities and Social Media

Program Chair: Gabriele Meiselwitz, USA

Leonelo Almeida, Brazil
Chee Siang Ang, UK
Aneesha Bakharia, Australia
Ania Bobrowicz, UK
James Braman, USA
Farzin Deravi, UK
Carsten Kleiner, Germany
Niki Lambropoulos, Greece
Soo Ling Lim, UK

Anthony Norcio, USA
Portia Pusey, USA
Panote Siriaraya, UK
Stefan Stieglitz, Germany
Giovanni Vincenti, USA
Yuanqiong (Kathy) Wang, USA
June Wei, USA
Brian Wentz, USA

Augmented Cognition

Program Chairs: Dylan D. Schmorrow, USA,
and Cali M. Fidopiastis, USA

Ahmed Abdelkhalek, USA
Robert Atkinson, USA
Monique Beaudoin, USA
John Blitch, USA
Alenka Brown, USA

Rosario Cannavò, Italy
Joseph Cohn, USA
Andrew J. Cowell, USA
Martha Crosby, USA
Wai-Tat Fu, USA

Rodolphe Gentili, USA
Frederick Gregory, USA
Michael W. Hail, USA
Monte Hancock, USA
Fei Hu, USA
Ion Juvina, USA
Joe Keebler, USA
Philip Mangos, USA
Rao Mannepalli, USA
David Martinez, USA
Yvonne R. Masakowski, USA
Santosh Mathan, USA
Ranjeev Mittu, USA

Keith Niall, USA
Tatana Olson, USA
Debra Patton, USA
June Pilcher, USA
Robinson Pino, USA
Tiffany Poeppelman, USA
Victoria Romero, USA
Amela Sadagic, USA
Anna Skinner, USA
Ann Speed, USA
Robert Sottilare, USA
Peter Walker, USA

Digital Human Modeling and Applications in Health, Safety, Ergonomics and Risk Management

Program Chair: Vincent G. Duffy, USA

Giuseppe Andreoni, Italy
Daniel Carruth, USA
Elsbeth De Korte, The Netherlands
Afzal A. Godil, USA
Ravindra Goonetilleke, Hong Kong
Noriaki Kuwahara, Japan
Kang Li, USA
Zhizhong Li, P.R. China

Tim Marler, USA
Jianwei Niu, P.R. China
Michelle Robertson, USA
Matthias Rötting, Germany
Mao-Jiun Wang, Taiwan
Xuguang Wang, France
James Yang, USA

Design, User Experience, and Usability

Program Chair: Aaron Marcus, USA

Sisira Adikari, Australia
Claire Ancient, USA
Arne Berger, Germany
Jamie Blustein, Canada
Ana Boa-Ventura, USA
Jan Brejcha, Czech Republic
Lorenzo Cantoni, Switzerland
Marc Fabri, UK
Luciane Maria Fadel, Brazil
Tricia Flanagan, Hong Kong
Jorge Frascara, Mexico

Federico Gobbo, Italy
Emilie Gould, USA
Rüdiger Heimgärtner, Germany
Brigitte Herrmann, Germany
Steffen Hess, Germany
Nouf Khashman, Canada
Fabiola Guillermina Noël, Mexico
Francisco Rebelo, Portugal
Kerem Rızvanoğlu, Turkey
Marcelo Soares, Brazil
Carla Spinillo, Brazil

Distributed, Ambient and Pervasive Interactions

**Program Chairs: Norbert Streitz, Germany,
and Panos Markopoulos, The Netherlands**

Juan Carlos Augusto, UK
Jose Bravo, Spain
Adrian Cheok, UK
Boris de Ruyter, The Netherlands
Anind Dey, USA
Dimitris Grammenos, Greece
Nuno Guimaraes, Portugal
Achilles Kameas, Greece
Javed Vassilis Khan, The Netherlands
Shin'ichi Konomi, Japan
Carsten Magerkurth, Switzerland

Ingrid Mulder, The Netherlands
Anton Nijholt, The Netherlands
Fabio Paternó, Italy
Carsten Röcker, Germany
Teresa Romao, Portugal
Albert Ali Salah, Turkey
Manfred Tscheligi, Austria
Reiner Wichert, Germany
Woontack Woo, Korea
Xenophon Zabulis, Greece

Human Aspects of Information Security, Privacy and Trust

**Program Chairs: Theo Tryfonas, UK,
and Ioannis Askoxylakis, Greece**

Claudio Agostino Ardagna, Italy
Zinaida Benenson, Germany
Daniele Catteddu, Italy
Raoul Chiesa, Italy
Bryan Cline, USA
Sadie Creese, UK
Jorge Cuellar, Germany
Marc Dacier, USA
Dieter Gollmann, Germany
Kirstie Hawkey, Canada
Jaap-Henk Hoepman, The Netherlands
Cagatay Karabat, Turkey
Angelos Keromytis, USA
Ayako Komatsu, Japan
Ronald Leenes, The Netherlands
Javier Lopez, Spain
Steve Marsh, Canada

Gregorio Martinez, Spain
Emilio Mordini, Italy
Yuko Murayama, Japan
Masakatsu Nishigaki, Japan
Aljosa Pasic, Spain
Milan Petković, The Netherlands
Joachim Posegga, Germany
Jean-Jacques Quisquater, Belgium
Damien Sauveron, France
George Spanoudakis, UK
Kerry-Lynn Thomson, South Africa
Julien Touzeau, France
Theo Tryfonas, UK
João Vilela, Portugal
Claire Vishik, UK
Melanie Volkamer, Germany

HCI in Business

Program Chair: Fiona Fui-Hoon Nah, USA

Andreas Auinger, Austria
Michel Avital, Denmark
Traci Carte, USA
Hock Chuan Chan, Singapore
Constantinos Coursaris, USA
Soussan Djamasbi, USA
Brenda Eschenbrenner, USA
Nobuyuki Fukawa, USA
Khaled Hassanein, Canada
Milena Head, Canada
Susanna (Shuk Ying) Ho, Australia
Jack Zhenhui Jiang, Singapore
Jinwoo Kim, Korea
Zoonky Lee, Korea
Honglei Li, UK
Nicholas Lockwood, USA
Eleanor T. Loiacono, USA
Mei Lu, USA

Scott McCoy, USA
Brian Mennecke, USA
Robin Poston, USA
Lingyun Qiu, P.R. China
Rene Riedl, Austria
Matti Rossi, Finland
April Savoy, USA
Shu Schiller, USA
Hong Sheng, USA
Choon Ling Sia, Hong Kong
Chee-Wee Tan, Denmark
Chuan Hoo Tan, Hong Kong
Noam Tractinsky, Israel
Horst Treiblmaier, Austria
Virpi Tuunainen, Finland
Dezhi Wu, USA
I-Chin Wu, Taiwan

Learning and Collaboration Technologies

Program Chairs: Panayiotis Zaphiris, Cyprus, and Andri Ioannou, Cyprus

Ruthi Aladjem, Israel
Abdulaziz Aldaej, UK
John M. Carroll, USA
Maka Eradze, Estonia
Mikhail Fominykh, Norway
Denis Gillet, Switzerland
Mustafa Murat Inceoglu, Turkey
Pernilla Josefsson, Sweden
Marie Joubert, UK
Sauli Kiviranta, Finland
Tomaž Klobučar, Slovenia
Elena Kyza, Cyprus
Maarten de Laat, The Netherlands
David Lamas, Estonia

Edmund Laugasson, Estonia
Ana Loureiro, Portugal
Katherine Maillet, France
Nadia Pantidi, UK
Antigoni Parmaxi, Cyprus
Borzoo Pourabdollahian, Italy
Janet C. Read, UK
Christophe Reffay, France
Nicos Souleles, Cyprus
Ana Luísa Torres, Portugal
Stefan Trausan-Matu, Romania
Aimilia Tzanavari, Cyprus
Johnny Yuen, Hong Kong
Carmen Zahn, Switzerland

External Reviewers

Ilia Adami, Greece
Iosif Klironomos, Greece
Maria Korozi, Greece
Vassilis Kouroumalis, Greece

Asterios Leonidis, Greece
George Margetis, Greece
Stavroula Ntoa, Greece
Nikolaos Partarakis, Greece

HCI International 2015

The 15th International Conference on Human–Computer Interaction, HCI International 2015, will be held jointly with the affiliated conferences in Los Angeles, CA, USA, in the Westin Bonaventure Hotel, August 2–7, 2015. It will cover a broad spectrum of themes related to HCI, including theoretical issues, methods, tools, processes, and case studies in HCI design, as well as novel interaction techniques, interfaces, and applications. The proceedings will be published by Springer. More information will be available on the conference website: http://www.hcii2015.org/

General Chair
Professor Constantine Stephanidis
University of Crete and ICS-FORTH
Heraklion, Crete, Greece
E-mail: cs@ics.forth.gr

Table of Contents

Modelling Posture and Motion

Anthropometry, Design and Ergonomics

Ergonomics and Human Modelling in Work and Everyday Life Environments

Advances in Healthcare

Rehabilitation Applications

Risk, Safety and Emergency

Modelling Posture and Motion

Human Energy Expenditure Models: Beyond State-of-the-Art Commercialized Embedded Algorithms

Ricard Delgado-Gonzalo[1], Philippe Renevey[1], Enric M. Calvo[1], Josep Solà[1], Cees Lanting[2], Mattia Bertschi[1], and Mathieu Lemay[1]

[1] CSEM, Signal Processing, Neuchâtel, Switzerland
{ricard.delgadogonzalo,philippe.renevey,enric.muntanecalvo,
josepsolaicaros,mattia.bertschi,mathieu.lemay}@csem.ch
[2] CSEM, Marketing & Business Development, Neuchâtel, Switzerland
cees.lanting@csem.ch

Abstract. In the present study, we propose three new energy expenditure (EE) methods and evaluate their accuracy against state-of-the-art EE estimation commercialized devices. To this end, we used several sensors on 8 subjects to simultaneously record acceleration forces from wrist-located sensors and bio-potentials estimated from chest-located ECG devices. These subjects followed a protocol that included a wide range of intensities in a given set of activities, ranging from sedentary to vigorous. The results of the proposed human EE models were compared to indirect calorimetry EE estimated values (kcal/kg/h). The speed-based, heart rate-based and hybrid-based models are characterized by an RMSE of 1.22 ± 0.34 kcal/min, 1.53 ± 0.48 kcal/min and 1.03 ± 0.35 kcal/min, respectively. Based on the presented results, the proposed models provide a significant improvement over the state-of-the-art.

Keywords: energy expenditure, walking/running speed, human model, physical activity monitoring.

1 Introduction

The rapidly increasing prevalence of overweight and obesity is a worldwide health problem. Due to the associated serious medical conditions, it is estimated that obesity already accounts for up to 7% of healthcare costs in EU. Moreover, this value increases when considering the costs to wider economy associated with low productivity lost output and premature health problems [1]. At the simplest level, obesity results from a disturbed energy balance that reaches equilibrium only in an obese state. This situation occurs when energy intake is high and EE (physical activity) is low. Despite advances in dietary, exercise-based, behavioral, pharmacological and bariatric surgical approaches, lifestyle intervention remains the cornerstone of the prevention and treatment of obesity [2]. EE measurements are important indicators to consider for the estimation of spontaneous physical activity, as well as energy intake when body weight is stable (i.e., when EE equals energy intake).

V. G. Duffy (Ed.): DHM 2014, LNCS 8529, pp. 3–14, 2014.

Numerous laboratory methods can be used to estimate whole-body EE at rest and during exercise such as detailed activity/food diary [3], isotopic measurements [4], and direct and indirect calorimetry methods [5]. These methods have advantages and drawbacks that make them more appropriate in one situation or another, but, because of their cost, technical difficulties, or infrastructure, none of them is suitable for daily-life EE monitoring. To overcome this issue, other methods, based on approaches such as pedometry, actigraphy or electrocardiography have been proposed. These methods use human kinetic models based on diverse parameters; namely step counts, heart rate (HR), speed, weight, sex, etc. The resulting EE estimation of such models might be sufficient for several applications. However, most of them are characterized by biased and inaccurate instantaneous EE values and necessitate specific calibration protocols.

Recent studies have presented new approaches which combined long-term wearable miniaturized sensors and activity-specific EE models [6-7]. These approaches first classify the physical activity of the subject, and then apply an activity-specific EE model. However, the evaluation of these models is not clear or is poorly documented. Moreover, the EE model inputs vary from activity class, through subject's anthropometric parameters and subject's fitness indicators, to precise calibration values and HR [8-9]. A clear overall picture of the accuracy of such EE models is therefore required.

In the present study, we propose three different human activity-specific EE models and evaluate their accuracy. These models range from two simple models based on (i) the subject's estimated speed and anthropometric parameters (speed-based model), (ii) instantaneous fitness parameters (HR-based model), or a (iii) multimodal model using estimated speed, anthropometric parameters and fitness parameters (hybrid-based model). The performance of these three models is evaluated with respect to gold standards (treadmill speed and body energy expenditure estimated from indirect calorimetry) and compared to published human EE models embedded in commercial devices.

2   Method

The following section describes the database and the protocol used in this study. It also describes the different proposed human speed and EE models. Finally, it contains the evaluation procedure and the statistical tools used to quantify the performance of the proposed models and to compare them against commercialized EE monitors.

2.1   Database and Protocol

In order to develop various human EE models, acceleration forces from CSEM's proprietary wrist-located sensors and bio-potentials estimated from chest-located dry electrodes were recorded simultaneously over 8 healthy male subjects. The distribution of the subjects' anthropometric parameters is shown in **Error! Reference source not found.**. The subjects followed a standardized protocol that included a wide set of activities, ranging from sedentary to vigorous, recorded in laboratory settings.

More precisely, it consisted in three 3-minute phases of resting (lying down, standing up and sitting) and 3-minute walking/running phases (from 0.5 m/s to exhaustion; with steps of 0.5 m/s).

In order to validate both the human EE models and their human walking/running speed sub-models, gold standard measurements were simultaneously recorded, namely the speed values labelled v_{ref} obtained from a treadmill (Technogym's Excite® Med), the HR values labelled HR obtained from an ambulatory ECG monitoring device, and the EE values labeled PMETAMAX obtained from a Cortex's METAMAX® 3B device (accuracy of ±2.1% MET or kcal/kg/h) using an embedded indirect calorimetry approach. An Actigraph's GT1M® device is also measuring the EE simultaneously.

Before recording each subject, the oxygen (O2), carbon dioxide (CO2) analyzers and the atmospheric pressure and air volume sensors were calibrated using a medical grade calibration gas with known concentrations and known total volume. The air of the room was also taken into account in the indirect calorimetry computation.

Table 1. Subjects' anthropometric parameters

Characteristic	$\mu \pm \sigma$ (N = 8)	Range
Age [years]	35.95 ± 6.74	27 - 46
Height [m]	1.82 ± 0.07	1.72 - 1.95
Weight [kg]	75.88 ± 6.35	65 - 87

2.2 Activity Classification and Human Speed Estimation

In this study, the 3D accelerometer signals (x-, y- and z-axis) are used for two purposes: classification of activity and estimation of the speed. Firstly, these 3D signals are used to classify each subject's physical activity for every sample. In the context of this study, the considered classes of activities are: resting (subdivided in lying down, standing and sitting postures), walking, and running. The resulting activity-specific episodes were used to train an activity-specific human speed model based on common anthropometric parameters (i.e., weight, height and sex) and biomechanics principles. The proposed human EE models are finally trained by the resulting speed estimates (defined as $\hat{v}$) and the identified activity-specific episodes.

2.3 Human Energy Expenditure Models

Speed-Based Model: SPE^{2}AR. As previously mentioned, each timestamp (sampling frequency of 0.9 second) is first classified in one of the following categories: resting, walking or running. Then, a multi-linear regression is performed for each category taking into account the speed and anthropomorphic parameters. The resulting model is denoted as SPE^{2}AR (Speed-based Piece-wise Energy Estimation using AntRopomorphics). Formally, the regression model can be written as:

$$P_{\text{SPE}^2\text{AR}} = \begin{cases} \alpha_{\text{rest}}\, v + \beta_{\text{rest}}\, w + \gamma_{\text{rest}}\, h + \delta_{\text{rest}}, & \text{if resting} \\ \alpha_{\text{walk}}\, v + \beta_{\text{walk}}\, w + \gamma_{\text{walk}}\, h + \delta_{\text{walk}}, & \text{if walking} \\ \alpha_{\text{run}}\, v + \beta_{\text{run}}\, w + \gamma_{\text{run}}\, h + \delta_{\text{run}}, & \text{if running} \end{cases} \qquad (1)$$

where v is the speed in km/h, w is the weight in kg and h is the height in cm.

HR-Based Model: HEET. A multi-linear regression is performed for each category using instantaneous HR values. These instantaneous HR values are obtained from applying an embedded R-wave detection algorithm to ECG signals. The resulting model is denoted as HEET (HR-based Energy EstimaTion). Formally, the regression model can be written as:

$$P_{HEET} = \begin{cases} \alpha_{\text{rest}} HR + \beta_{\text{rest}}, & \text{if resting} \\ \alpha_{\text{active}} HR + \beta_{\text{active}}, & \text{if active} \end{cases}, \qquad (2)$$

where HR is the instantaneous HR in min^{-1}.

Hybrid-Based Model: QI^{2}Hybrid. Our multimodal hybrid model combines both previous models into a single expression with the addition of two quality indicators labelled as $p_{\text{SPE}^2\text{AR}}$ and p_{HEET} (speed and HR values). Once both models have been properly calibrated, QI^{2}Hybrid (Quality Indicator Hybrid) model can be written as:

$$P_{\text{QI}^2\text{Hybrid}} = p_{\text{SPE}^2\text{AR}} P_{\text{SPE}^2\text{AR}} + p_{\text{HEET}} P_{\text{HEET}}, \qquad (3)$$

where $p_{\text{SPE}^2\text{AR}}$ is the probability of $P_{\text{SPE}^2\text{AR}}$ producing a better estimate than P_{HEET} and p_{HEET} is the probability of P_{HEET} providing a better estimate than $P_{\text{SPE}^2\text{AR}}$. Note that the relation $p_{\text{SPE}^2\text{AR}} = 1 - P_{\text{HEET}}$ always holds. These quality indicators are defined as

$$p_{\text{SPE}^2\text{AR}} = 1 - Q_{\text{HR}} \frac{\text{RMSE}_{\text{SPE}^2\text{AR}}}{\text{RMSE}_{\text{HEET}} + \text{RMSE}_{\text{SPE}^2\text{AR}}} \qquad (4)$$

and

$$p_{\text{HEET}} = 1 - p_{\text{SPE}^2\text{AR}}, \qquad (5)$$

where $0 \le Q_{\text{HR}} \le 1$ is a value that informs about the quality of the current estimation of the HR value, and $\text{RMSE}_{\text{HEET}}$ and $\text{RMSE}_{\text{SPE}^2\text{AR}}$ are the root mean squared errors of the HEET and SPE^{2}AR models, respectively. Note that in the extreme case, when $Q_{\text{HR}} = 0$, the estimation of the EE is completely based on SPE^{2}AR model:

$$P_{\text{Hybrid}} = P_{\text{SPE}^2\text{AR}}. \qquad (6)$$

Analogously, when $Q_{\text{HR}} = 1$ the estimation of EE is based on the convex combination of both methods relative to their performance:

$$P_{Hybrid} = \frac{\text{RMSE}_{\text{HEET}}}{\text{RMSE}_{\text{HEET}} + \text{RMSE}_{\text{SPE}^2\text{AR}}} P_{\text{SPE}^2\text{AR}} + \frac{\text{RMSE}_{\text{SPE}^2\text{AR}}}{\text{RMSE}_{\text{HEET}} + \text{RMSE}_{\text{SPE}^2\text{AR}}} P_{\text{HEET}}. \qquad (7)$$

Note that all EE models are expressed in MET or in kcal/kg/h.

Statistical Analysis. In order to deal with the limited number of subjects (N=8) in the database, a leave-one-out cross validation procedure is applied to the entire database in order to fit the EE models and to evaluate their respective performance with respect to the ground truth values (METAMAX® 3B values). That is, the parameters of each model are estimated using N-1 subjects and validated against the remaining one, and this procedure is iterated for each subject. The two quality indicators p_{SPE^2AR} and p_{HEET} are obtained in the same manner. Concerning SPE²AR, the coefficient of determination (R^2) distribution equals 0.96 ± 0.02, whereas for HEET and QI²Hybrid models, the R^2 distributions equal 0.92 ± 0.05 and 0.96 ± 0.02.

For the evaluation of the performance over the entire database of the proposed models, three performance indicators are defined: the distribution of the absolute and relative errors and the distribution of the RMSE. These distributions are characterized by their mean μ and standard deviation σ. In order to compare our results with other studies, MET values are converted into kcal/min. Table 2 defines these three performance indicators.

Table 2. Description of the performance indicators

Performance indicator	Equation
Absolute energy error [kcal]	$\left|E_{METAMAX} - \hat{E}\right|$
Relative energy error [%]	$\left|E_{METAMAX} - \hat{E}\right|/E_{MetaMax}$
Root mean squared error (RMSE) [kcal/min]	$w \times \sqrt{\dfrac{\int \left|P_{METAMAX} - \hat{P}\right|^2}{\Delta t}}$

Here, $E_{METAMAX}$ is the total energy measured by METAMAX® 3B, which equals $w \times \int P_{METAMAX}\, dt$. $\hat{E}$ is the total energy estimated by the proposed models, which equals $w \times \int \hat{P}\, dt$. RMSE provides insight on the instantaneous error, while absolute and relative energy errors show how the errors accumulate over time. When these errors are accumulated over the entire recording sessions, they are referred as total EE errors.

Comparison with Commercialized EE Estimates. The comparison against commercial estimates is based on a limited set of published academic studies. Only the Actigraph's GT1M provided real-time EE estimates that could be simultaneously acquired during the recordings. To provide a fair comparison, we contrast the published measures against appropriate test conditions within our protocol (e.g. walking episodes compared to low intensity activities).

3   Results

3.1   Performance of the Three Proposed Models

The overall performance of the activity-specific speed model is characterized by an RMSE distribution of 0.114 ± 0.063 km/h. The performance of the proposed activity-specific EE models (SPE2AR, HEET and QI2Hybrid models) is shown in Table 4 in terms of absolute, relative and RMS errors.

Table 3. Performance of activity-specific EE models

EE model	Total EE absolute error distribution ($\mu\pm\sigma$)	Total EE relative error distribution ($\mu\pm\sigma$)	RMSE distribution ($\mu\pm\sigma$)
SPE^2AR	17.91 ± 9.32 kcal	$5.52\ \% \pm 2.21\ \%$	1.22 ± 0.34 kcal/min
HEET	18.80 ± 9.40 kcal	$6.17\ \% \pm 3.08\ \%$	1.53 ± 0.48 kcal/min
$QI^2Hybrid$	14.57 ± 8.47 kcal	$4.45\ \% \pm 2.30\ \%$	1.03 ± 0.35 kcal/min

Fig.1 displays an example of the evolution of EE during the execution of the different tasks included in the experimental protocol. The EE evolution of each model is compared to the ground truth EE values measured by METAMAX® 3B. Panels A and B represent the estimated EE values from SPE^2AR, HEET and $QI^2Hybrid$ models, respectively. Resting (lying down, standing and sitting postures), walking and running episodes are alternately displayed in gray and white areas. In this case, the subject starts to run at the 21:50.6 minute which is 50.6 sec after starting the 2 m/s step.

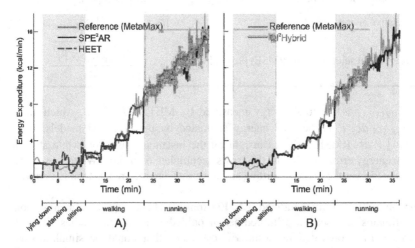

Fig. 1. Evolution of estimated EE values (in kcal/min) and ground truth values of a subject over the entire protocol. Panel A displays the results from SPE^2AR and HEET, while panel B display the results from $QI^2Hybrid$.

Fig 2 displays the absolute error distribution of QI2Hybrid with respect to the activity class for the same subject (see Fig. 1 B). The resting-, walking- and running-specific error distributions are characterized by mean and standard deviation values of -0.20 ± 0.41 kcal/min, 0.17 ± 0.77 kcal/min and -0.03 ± 0.91 kcal/min, respectively. The first two distributions are bimodal and significantly biased. Moreover, the error distribution during running is characterized by unbiased values ($p<0.05$).

These statistical results are obtained using a Krustal-Wallis one-way analysis of variance between the estimated and ground truth EE values for each class of activities (resting, running and walking).

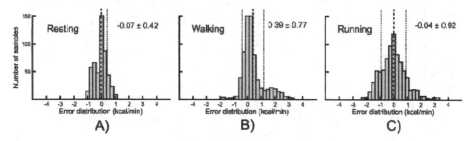

Fig. 2. Example of QI²Hybrid error distributions with respect to activity (resting in panel A, walking in panel B and running in panel C). The results correspond to the one showed in Fig. 1 B.

The distribution of EE errors with respect to each 3-minute phases obtained with QI²Hybrid over the entire database is showed in Fig. 3. Resting (lying down, standing and sitting postures), walking and running episodes are alternately displayed in gray and white areas. The subject-dependent walking-to-running transition zone is also displayed. As for the error distributions showed in Fig. 2, the overall distributions associated with resting and walking activities are significantly biased. Moreover, the overall distributions associated with running activities are characterized by unbiased values ($p<0.05$). These statistical results are also obtained using a Krustal-Wallis one-way analysis of variance between the estimated and ground truth EE values for each class of activities (resting, running and walking).

3.2 Commercial off-the-Shelf EE Monitoring Devices

The performance of typical off-the-shelf EE monitoring devices is not necessarily accurate (particularly the instantaneous value) but suffices for several applications. Despite their low complexity, the estimation algorithms are proprietary or unpublished. Moreover, the results displayed by the graphic user interface of these devices remain difficult to interpret (e.g., EE per epoch or activity). The following section presents an overview of some available systems, compares, if possible, their performance with our proposed appropriate model. This evaluation is divided into the following methodologies: pedometry, actigraphy, electrocardiography and photoplethysmography.

Pedometry. Used originally by sports and physical fitness enthusiasts, pedometers are now becoming popular as an everyday exercise measurer and motivator. They record how many steps a subject has walked during that day. Some pedometers will also erroneously record movements other than walking, such as bending to tie one's shoes, or road bumps incurred while riding a vehicle. Because the length of each person's step varies, an informal calibration, performed by the user, is required if presentation of the distance covered in km is desired (odometer).

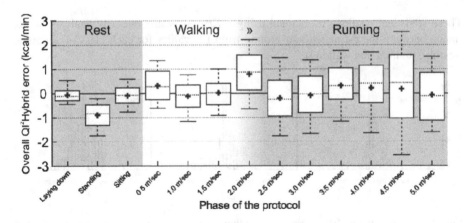

Fig. 3. QI2Hybrid EE performance with respect to specific tasks on the entire database. Resting, walking, running and walking/running transition zones are also displayed in alternate grey and white areas. Each distribution shows the mean (bold cross), the median (dotted line), the 25th and 75th percentile (lower and upper bounds of the box) and the minimum and maximum (lower and upper lines) values.

In Table 4, we present a comparison of the performances of the SPE2AR model and a standard pedometer against the same ground truth. For a fair comparison, the statistics of our methods are restricted over low-intensity exercise, that is, similar conditions in which the other method was tested.

Table 4. Comparison with a pedometry-based device for low-intensity exercises

EE Model	RMSE
Walk4Life Elite	5.0 kcal/6min [8]
SPE^{2}AR	**4.62 ± 1.76 kcal/6min**

Actigraphy. Actigraphy is a non-invasive method of monitoring human rest/activity cycles. A small actigraph unit is worn by a person to measure gross motor activity. The unit continually records the movements it undergoes. Information on body position can be combined with motion data to increase accuracy. Movement is not directly related to metabolism, since movement type and conditions influence the estimation, and movement based methods cannot generally describe reliably the intensity of physical activity. Additionally, activity counts are defined differently by each sensor's manufacturer (i.e., Actigraph counts, and the equations derived from them, are not directly comparable to Actical or Actiheart counts). In Table 5, we present a comparison, in terms of relative energy, of SPE2AR with several commercial actigraphy-based solutions against the same ground truth.

Table 5. Comparison with actigraphy-based devices

EE Model	Total EE relative error distribution ($\mu\pm\sigma$)
Actigraph GT1M - Harris-Benedict (N=16)	26.8 % [9]
Actical (N=19)	17.8 % [9]
IDEEA (N=18)	17.5 % [9]
Directlife (N=19)	13.6 % [9]
Fitbit (N=16)	28.7 % [9]
SPE^{2}AR	**5.52 % ± 2.17 %**

In Table 6, we present a comparison, in terms of absolute and relative energy, of SPE^{2}AR with an GT1M device by Actigraph over the proposed protocol.

Table 6. Comparison with Actigraph GT1M for our experimental protocol

EE Model	Total EE absolute error distribution ($\mu\pm\sigma$)	Total EE relative error distribution ($\mu\pm\sigma$)
Actigraph GT1M - Work energy theorem	110.45 ± 49.50 kcal	35.60 % ± 16.51 %
Actigraph GT1M - Vector magnitude	127.85 ± 49.43 kcal	40.99 % ± 14.68 %
SPE^{2}AR	**17.91 ± 9.32 kcal**	**5.52 % ± 2.17 %**

Electrocardiography. Electrocardiography (ECG) is a bio-potential technique aiming at monitoring electrical activity of the heart and constitutes the gold standard technique to monitor HR. When the ECG monitoring systems are wearable, they are specifically referred as Holter systems. A large variety of alternative devices which monitor averaged HR values (one HR value over a specific time window) or heartbeat intervals based on bio-potential measurements exists. Their bio-potential sensors are based on gel, dry or textile electrode principles. There is also a family of strapless/wireless devices that temporally estimates fingertip bio-potentials using sensors embedded into watches (including Health Touch Plus by Timex, Vital by MIO and SmartHealth by Salutron).

In Table 7, we present a comparison, in terms of absolute energy, of HEET, QI^{2}Hybrid and two commercialized HR-monitoring devices. For a fair comparison, the statistics of our methods are restricted over low-intensity exercises, that is, similar conditions in which the other methods were tested. It is important to mention that the database used in Erdogan study [10] was dedicated to overweight and obese subjects during low-intensity exercises.

Table 7. Comparison with electrocardiography-based devices for low-intensity exercises

EE Model	Total EE absolute error distribution ($\mu \pm \sigma$)
Polar S810i^{TM} (N=43)	0.5 ± 0.5 kcal/min [10]
SenseWear Pro Armband ^{TM} (N=43)	~2.5 ± 1.1 kcal/min [10]
HEET	**0.85 ± 0.41 kcal/min**
Hybrid	**0.72 ± 0.31 kcal/min**

Photoplethysmography. Photoplethysmography is an optical technology aiming at measuring tissue light propagation changes during cardiac cycle. In the daily activity monitoring context, the measurement of volumetric changes of microvascular bed of tissue due to blood flow is the target. This measure brings information on arterial pulsatility content. Wearable HR monitoring devices using this technology are already available on the market (including Nonin's Onyx 2, MIO's Alpha and Basis products). Unfortunately, to our knowledge, no peer-reviewed studies exist on the EE estimation performance based on this technology.

4   Discussion

4.1   Performance and Validation

The present study demonstrates that SPE2AR provides already an accurate estimate of EE with an average of 1.22 kcal/min across all activities and subjects. Since the model is based on two complementary modes (walking vs. running), the system produces an artifact when the subjects switch from one mode to the other. We can observe this interphase around the minute 22 within Fig. 1 A.

We observe that HEET provides an overall performance of 1.53 kcal/min (see Fig. 1 A), which is slightly worse than the one offered by SPE2AR. However, HEET does not experience any artifact in the interphase between the walking to running modes. The accuracy of the HR-based model might be explained by the fact that the HR values are estimated for every time stamp using a small amount of previous detected R-waves instead of using global averages. Moreover, we also observe the well-known phenomenon that the HR-based model has a bigger relative error for low HR. This can be noticed in the resting phases within Fig. 1 A (lying down, standing up and sitting).

Finally, the combination of both methods (QI2Hybrid) still exhibits a small jump at interphase between the running and walking phases. However, this discontinuity is mostly smoothed out by the contribution of the HR-based model (see Fig. 1 B). Moreover, the hybrid method provides a more robust estimation of the energy consumption for low values of HR (see lying down, standing up and sitting categories within Fig. 1 B). This is due to the fact that the speed-based method regularizes the variability introduced by the HR-based method. In Fig. 3, we can observe the behavior of the error distribution for the different tasks comprised in the protocol. It can be shown that the dispersion of the error increases as the activity becomes more vigorous. This is due to increase in the variance of the estimate of our method as well as the METAMAX® 3B (see Fig. 1 for a typical example). In particular, we observe this phenomenon in the width of the distributions shown in Fig. 2. The distribution in the resting category exhibits a sharp peak at zero, but it contains a second mode due to the poor estimation of the energy while standing (see Fig. 3). The error distribution becomes broader in the walking category, and a new secondary mode can be observed which corresponds to the transition towards running (see 2.0 m/sec in Fig. 3). Finally, the error distribution in the running category exhibits a Gaussian appearance with the largest support.

All three EE models have shown to adjust properly to the subjects of the database, being the mean coefficients of determination R^2 0.96, 0.92 and 0.96. Moreover, the standard deviations of these coefficients are quite low (0.02, 0.05 and 0.05). This indicates that our statistical models are robust to the change of the training data.

4.2   Models versus Commercialized Devices

In view of these preliminary but promising results, it suggest that the proposed models, specially the one combining all source of information, seem accurate at low, moderate and high activity levels. In particular, the accuracy of our speed-based method has shown to be comparable to the one reported by Walk4Life for low-activity levels (see Table 4), and to improve by an order of magnitude most of the commercial solutions based on actigraphy (see Table 6). For a fair comparison, we also used an actigraphy-based method as control within out protocol (see Table 7). The results were in concordance with the ones reported by the referred study [9] (see Table 6).

As discussed, the HR-based method seems accurate even during stationary physical activities (see Fig. 1 A). Moreover, the accuracy of our methods using HR information have shown to be comparable to the ones reported by the state-of-the-art methods based on ECG (see Table 8).

Finally, the hybrid model consistently compensates for the deficiencies of the two models individually, producing a lower error estimate (absolute energy, relative error and RMSE) and a comparable standard deviation. Our EE estimation models embedded into wrist-located devices would produce EE estimate performance at the state-of-the-art level in an accurate, non-obtrusive, daily integrated, inconspicuous manner.

Conclusion. Based on the presented results, it is concluded that there is high potential to improve the performance of the off-the-shelf commercialized devices (in terms of energy expenditure estimation) by using one of the proposed models. The model selection should be dictated by the implemented type of embedded sensors such as 3D accelerometers, GPS (providing gold standard speed values), and/or dry electrodes.

Acknowledgements. This study was possible by grants from the FP7 EU project PEGASO (FP7-ICT-2013.5.1), and the Wilsdorf Foundation. The authors would also like to thanks all CSEM's collaborators who were involved in the design and development of the wrist-located device and the respective algorithms.

References

1. World Health Organization: Prevention and control of noncommunicable diseases in the European region: A Progress Report, pp. 1–65 (2013)
2. Jensen, M.D., Ryan, D.H., Apovian, C.M., Ard, J.D., Comuzzie, A.G., Donato, K.A., Hu, F.B., Hubbard, V.S., Jakicic, J.M., Kushner, R.F., Loria, C.M., Millen, B.E., Nonas, C.A., Pi-Sunyer, F.X., Stevens, J., Stevens, V.J., Wadden, T.A., Wolfe, B.M., Yanovski, S.Z.: 2013 AHA/ACC/TOS Guideline for the management of overweight and obesity in adults: A report of the American College of Cardiology/American Heart Association Task Force on Practice Guidelines and The Obesity Society (2013) doi: 10.1161
3. Yamamura, C., Tanaka, S., Futami, J., Oka, J., Ishikawa-Takata, K., Kashiwazaki, H.: Activity diary method for predicting energy expenditure as evaluated by a whole-body indirect human calorimeter. J. Nutr. Sci. Vitaminol. 49(4), 262–269 (2003)
4. Stroud, M.A., Coward, W.A., Sawyer, M.B.: Measurements of Energy Expenditure Using Isotope-labelled Water ($^2H_2^{18}O$) During an Arctic Expedition. Eur. J. Appl. Occup. Physiol.~67(4), 375--379 (1993)
5. Levine, J.A.: Measurement of energy expenditure. Public Health Nutrition. 8(7A), 1123–1132 (2005)
6. Bonomi, A.G., Plasqui, G., Goris, A.H.C., Westerterp, K.R.: Improving assessment of daily energy expenditure by identifying types of physical activity with single accelerometer. J. Appl. Physiol. 107(3), 655–661 (2009)
7. Rumo, M., Amft, O., Tröster, G., Mäder, U.: A stepwise validation of a wearable validation of a wearable system for estimating energy expenditure in field-based research. Physiol. Meas. 32(12), 1983–2001 (2011)
8. Van Hees, V.T., Ekelung, U.: Novel daily energy expenditure estimation by using objective activity type classification: Where do we go from here? J. Appl. Physiol. 107(3), 639–640 (2009)
9. Charlot, K., Cornolo, J., Borne, R., Brugniaux, J.V., Richalet, J.-P., Chapelot, D., Pichon, A.: Improvement of energy expenditure prediction from heart rate during running. Physiol. Meas. 35(2), 253–266 (2014)
10. Nielson, R., Vehrs, P.R., Fellingham, G.W., Hager, R., Prusak, K.A.: Step counts and energy expenditure as estimated by pedometry during treadmill walking at different stride frequencies. J. Phys. Act. Health. 8(7), 1004–1013 (2011)
11. Dannecker, K.L., Sazonov, N.A., Melanson, E.L., Sazonov, E.S., Browning, R.C.: A comparison of energy expenditure estimation of several physical activity monitors. Med. Sci. Sports Exerc. 45(11), 2105–2112 (2013)
12. Ergogan, A., Cetin, C., Karatosun, H., Baydar, M.L.: Accuracy of the Polar S810i™ heart rate monitor and the Sensewear Pro Armband™ to estimate energy expenditure of indoor rowing exercise in overweight and obese individuals. J. Sports Sci. Med. 9, 508–516 (2010)

Human Skeleton Extraction of Depth Images Using the Polygon Evolution

Huan Du[1], Jian Wang[1,2,*], Xue-xia Zhong[3,1], Ying He[1] and Lin Mei[1]

[1] Cyber Physical System R&D Center,
The Third Research Institute of Ministry of Public Security, Shanghai 201204, P. R. China
`huan_du@163.com, wjconan@ieee.org x, 489331003@qq.com, 13524514531@126.com`

[2] School of Electronic Information and Electrical Engineering, Shanghai Jiao Tong University, Shanghai 200240, P. R. China
`wjconan@ieee.org`

[3] School of Communication and Information Engineering, Shanghai University, Shanghai 200072, China
`zhongxuexia2013@163.com`

Abstract. This paper proposes a novel skeleton extraction approach in the depth image based on the polygon evolution. The external contour of person is firstly extracted from the depth image and evolved to a external polygon using a polygon evolution method. Subsequently, the depth histogram is used to extract internal self-occlusion body parts, and contours of these parts are evolved to internal polygons. In external and internal polygons, skeleton points are extracted under different criterias respectively. Finally, all skeleton points are linked to a complete skeleton. Experimental results on a variety of postures demonstrate the robustness and reasonability of our skeleton extraction approach.

Keywords: skeleton extraction, depth image, polygon evolution, external polygon, internal polygon.

1 Introduction

As a natural means of activity allowing complex information to be conveyed, human motion has been one of the most popular research hotspots, and its applications have cover a variety of fields, such as human-machine interaction, security surveillance, content-based retrieval, sports training, virtual reality, etc. In order to analyze motion in an image serial or a video, human motion usually need to be separated into combination of a series of movements of body parts.

For tracking human full-body pose in real-time, a person must wear cumbersome markers or special suits with a large number of sensors in order to provide position signal of skeletons and joints to camera-based motion capture systems. In a past decade, unmarked human pose estimation methods[1, 2] and improved approaches

---

* Corresponding author.

V. G. Duffy (Ed.): DHM 2014, LNCS 8529, pp. 15–23, 2014.

with multiple cameras[3, 4] have attracted more attention as a research focus in computer vision. However, tracking complex human movements under a general environment is still a great challenge due to the sensitivity of the image to illumination variation and body occlusions.

Having a substantial immunity to lighting conditions and variations in visual appearance, novel depth cameras develop rapidly based on recent technological advances in very recent years. Such camera allows acquiring dense scans of a scene for constructing depth images, which gives a easy way to obtain three-dimensional model in real-time. Regarded as a prominent representative of depth camera, Microsoft Kinect incorporates several advanced sensing hardware, i.e. a depth sensor, a color camera, and a four-microphone array, for providing various perception capabilities on full-body 3D motion capture, facial recognition, and voice recognition[5]. With help of the depth camera, many researchers have proposed different algorithms to address pose estimation and human motion capture from depth images[6]. For a given body part, e.g. head, its six degrees of freedom (DOF) of motion could be recover from a sequence of depth images[7]. Combining local optimization with global retrieval techniques, a data-driven hybrid strategy speeds up pose estimation procedure for real-time tracking full-body motions[8].

In order to obtain a well-connected skeleton, a connectivity criterion was proposed to generates a connected Euclidean skeleton[9]. Based on a set of point pairs along the object boundary, basic idea of the criterion is to determine whether a given pixel is a skeleton point independently. Based on a graph-based representation of the depth data used to measure geodesic distances between body parts that are invariant to body movement, a skeleton body model can be fitted by detecting anatomical landmarks in the 3D data and fitting for obtaining human full-body pose estimation[10]. By executing graph contraction and surface clustering iteratively under given constraints, a curve skeleton of a 3D shape may be extracted with the correct topological structure[11]. Without a large number of marked-based motion capture data for training, human skeletons are extracted from depth images based on the symmetry of skeletons to object boundaries which are identified with different types[12]. In order to gain the skeleton with a simplest possible structure that provides a best possible reconstruction of a given shape, skeleton pruning as a trade-off between skeleton simplicity and shape reconstruction error is cast[13]. Another skeleton pruning method uses contour partitioning to obtain skeletons which do not have spurious branches[14]. Based on a learned boundary edge function, the kinematic skeleton is extracted by computing a set of motion boundaries which correspond to all possible articulations of the 3D object[15].

As the essential for general shape representation, a skeletonization algorithm must be able to extracted accurate skeleton, be robust to noise, occlusion, position translation and rotation transformation. For precise motion analysis, a connected skeleton has to preserve topological and hierarchical properties of human body[9]. Unfortunately, most state-of-the-art methods cannot overcome these problem with low computational complexity.

Using polygon evolution, this paper proposes a novel skeleton extraction method to extract external skeleton and internal self-occlusion skeleton. The criterion of skeleton extraction in polygons can remove redundant branches in skeleton model, and preserve original anatomical topology. The remain of this paper is organized as follows. Section 2 describes the proposed skeleton extraction approach in detail. Experimental results are presented in Section 3, and conclusions are given in Section 4.

2   The Proposed Approach

The procedure of the proposed approach is shown in Fig. 1. It contains four stages: (1) external polygon generation, (2) internal polygon generation, (3) skeleton extraction, and (4) skeleton linking. In the following sections, we introduce these stages respectively.

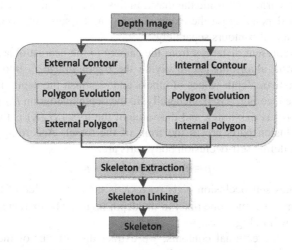

Fig. 1. The procedure of the proposed approach

2.1   External Polygon Generation

In the depth image, each player is randomly assigned an index number by Kinect[16]. We use this index number to obtain the mask depth image I_d of each player (see Fig. 2 (b)) and extract the contour of this mask as the external contour of the player C_e (see Fig. 2 (c)). Due to the external contour C_e is closed, we evolve it to a external polygon P_e (see Fig. 2 (d)) using the Douglas-Peucker(DP) algorithm in[17].

Specifically, partial contours of player's limbs sometimes may be inside the mask. In order to ensure the accuracy of extracted skeleton, we should add these contours to the external polygon. Firstly, we use Canny edge detector[18] to extract edges in the mask depth image. Then using the DP algorithm to evolve these edges. We reserve edges which are evolved to approximate vertical lines and add these lines L_e to the external polygon P_e. The final external polygon P_e is shown in Fig. 2 (f).

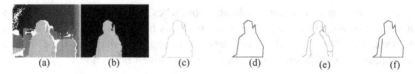

Fig. 2. The procedure of extracting the external polygon. (a) the original depth image; (b) the mask depth image; (c) the external contour; (d) the polygon of the external contour; (e) the Canny edge detector; (f) the external polygon.

2.2 Internal Polygon Generation

Because of the complicacy of human postures, there may appear self-occlusion situation that player's arms are inside the mask. In this case, we can not extract skeleton in these parts just depending on the external polygon. To solve this problem, we need extract these internal contours separately.

Depth data represent distances from the camera to the nearest object, we use Pyramid segmentation algorithm[19] to divide the depth image I_d into uniform depth blocks. Then statistic depth values of blocks and establish the depth histogram H_d for the depth image (see Fig. 3 (b)). Generally, in the depth histogram H_d, the value of the background $H_d(0)$ is maximum and the value of the torsel $H_d(K)$ is the second maximum. Self-occlusion parts are in the front of the torsel. According to these priori knowledge, we define self-occlusion body parts are:

$$p \in \aleph, \; if \; Depth(p) > K \tag{1}$$

where $\aleph$ denotes self-occlusion body parts, K is the depth value of the torsel in the depth histogram, p denotes one pixel in the depth image. The extracted self-occlusion body part is shown in Fig. 3 (c).

Similarity as the external contours, we extract the contour of the self-occlusion body part (see Fig. 3 (d)) and evolve it to an internal polygon P_i using the DP algorithm. The internal polygon P_i is shown in Fig. 3 (e).

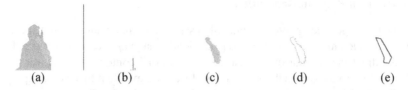

Fig. 3. The procedure of extracting the internal polygon. (a) the segmented depth image; (b) the depth histogram; (c) the self-occlusion body part; (d) the internal contour; (e) the internal polygon.

2.3 Skeleton Extraction

The central axis of contours is usually known as skeleton. To simplify the extraction process, we extract skeleton in evolutive polygons rather than in contours.

To guarantee the property that the skeleton is symmetrical to the polygon, we use the criterion proposed in[12] to compute the skeleton:

$$
\begin{cases}
D^2(q_1,p) - D^2(q_2,p) \le \max\left(\|x_1 - x_2\|, \|y_1 - y_2\|\right) \\
D(p,q_0) \le D(q_1,q_2)
\end{cases}
\tag{2}
$$

where p is a given point inside the polygon, q_1 and q_2 are two closest edge points to p which are on two different edges of the polygon (q_1 and q_2 are called generating points of p in the rest of paper), q_0 is the midpoint of line $\overline{q_1 q_2}$, $D(\bullet)$ denotes the Euclidean distance, (x_1, y_1) and (x_2, y_2) are the coordinates of q_1 and q_2 respectively.

Usually, if p satisfies the Eq.2, we regard p as a skeleton point. However, this criterion just can ensure the symmetry of the skeleton with respect to polygons, and can not suppress noise and remove spurious skeleton branches. In this case, we increase constraint strategies to external and internal polygons respectively.

In the external polygon P_e, if two generating points of p are all on edges of the polygon, the point which satisfies both Eq.2 and Eq.3 is a skeleton point:

$$
\begin{cases}
D\left(\overline{q_1}, \overline{q_2}\right) > T_1 \\
L_1 \cap L_2 = \varnothing
\end{cases}
, \; if \; q_1 \in P_e, q_2 \in P_e
\tag{3}
$$

where L_1 and L_2 are edges which q_1 and q_2 are on respectively. If q_1 is a vertex of the external polygon P_e, $\overline{q_1}$ denotes the vertex q_1. If q_1 is not a vertex of the external polygon P_e, $\overline{q_1}$ denotes the edge L_1. $\overline{q_2}$ is similar to $\overline{q_1}$. T_1 is a parameter to suppress spurious skeleton points. Under the constraint of Eq.3, excess skeleton points which may be generated by adjacent edges can be suppressed in the external polygon.

If a generating point of p is on the line L_e, the point which satisfies both Eq.2 and Eq.4 is a skeleton point:

$$
p \in Square\,[L_1, L_2], \; if \; q_1 \in L_e \, \| \, q_2 \in L_e
\tag{4}
$$

where $Square[L_1, L_2]$ denotes a convex quadrilateral with edges L_1 and L_2.

The illustration of extracted skeleton points in the external polygon is shown in Fig. 4 (a).

In the internal polygon P_i, the point which satisfies both Eq.2 and Eq.5 is a skeleton point:

$$
\begin{cases}
D\left(\overline{q_1}, \overline{q_2}\right) > T_2 \\
\alpha < angle\left(L_1, L_2\right) < \beta, \; if \; L_1 \cap L_2 \neq \varnothing
\end{cases}
\tag{5}
$$

where $angle(\bullet)$ denotes the angle between two lines. T_2, α and β are parameters to suppress spurious skeleton points. Under the constraint of Eq.5, we can guarantee generating points of selected skeleton points are at the suitable distance, not too close nor too far.

The illustration of extracted skeleton points in the internal polygon is shown in Fig. 4 (b).

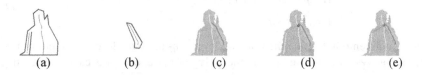

(a)   (b)   (c)   (d)   (e)

Fig. 4. The illustration of skeleton extraction and linking. (a) the external skeleton; (b) the internal skeleton; (c) external and internal skeletons in the depth image; (d) the shoulder center in the depth image; (e) the complete skeleton.

2.4   Skeleton Linking

In skeleton points, some points are close to each other. We firstly perform point linking to group them into skeleton lines. As shown in Fig. 4 (c), yellow lines are external skeletons generating by the external polygon, blue lines are internal skeletons generating by the internal polygon.

To generate a complete skeleton, we need to connect upper limbs and the torsel. The shoulder center $P_{s\text{-}c}$ (see the red point in Fig.4 (d)) is the most accurate point in the skeleton tracing by Kinect. According to the relative position with $P_{s\text{-}c}$, we judge each skeleton line is left upper limb, right upper limb or their overlap and link them with the shoulder center $P_{s\text{-}c}$. The complete skeleton is shown in Fig. 4 (e).

3   Experiments and Comparison

We implement our approach using C++. It takes about 1.8 seconds to process one single frame without code optimization on regular desktop with AMD core 4 3.8GHz CPU and 4GB RAM.

In order to evaluate the skeleton extraction performance of our approach, we extract skeletons from depth images of humans with different postures. Specially, we divide postures into three categories of face-on standing postures, lateral standing postures and sitting postures. And then compare our approach with Kinect[5] and Shen's approach[13].The implementation code of Shen's approach can be downloaded from http://wei-shen.weebly.com/publications.html.

Fig. 5 and Fig. 6 show skeletons of face-on and lateral standing postures respectively. Fig. 7 shows skeletons of sitting postures. As a skeleton pruning method, Shen's approach can obtain reasonable skeletons based on external contours for face-on standing postures as shown in Fig. 5 (c). However, for lateral standing postures and sitting postures, there are large structural changes in skeletons due to the particularity of postures in Fig. 6 (c) and Fig. 7 (c). In general, Shen's approach can generate simplified skeleton based on external contours but can not gain self-occlusion internal skeleton. Generally, for outsize body movement, Kinect's skeleton tracking can

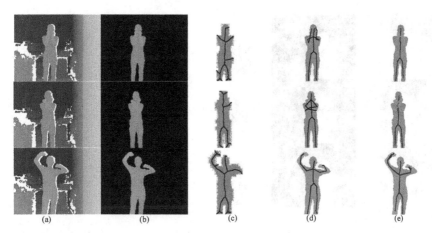

Fig. 5. Face-on standing postures. (a) original depth images; (b) mask depth images; (c) Shen's approach ; (d) Kinect's skeleton; (e) our approach.

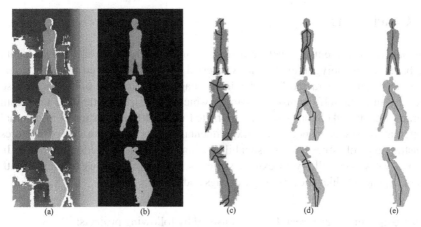

Fig. 6. Lateral standing postures. (a) original depth images; (b) mask depth images; (c) Shen's approach ; (d) Kinect's skeleton; (e) our approach.

obtain accurate skeleton results such as the 1st and 3rd in Fig. 5 (d). In the case of occlusion, Kinect sometimes estimates accurate skeleton positions of occluded body parts such as 1st in Fig. 6 (d). But in most cases, estimated skeleton results are not particularly accurate (see the 2nd in Fig. 5 (d), the 2nd and 3rd in Fig. 6 (d)). For sitting postures, results of Kinect's skeleton tracking are inaccurate due to there is no sit mode (see Fig. 7 (d)). Compared with Shen's approach and Kinect, our approach not merely can obtain simplicity external skeleton without excess spurious branches but also can gain reasonable internal skeleton no matter in face-on standing postures (see Fig. 5 (e)), lateral standing postures (see Fig. 6 (e)) or sitting postures (see Fig. 7 (e)).

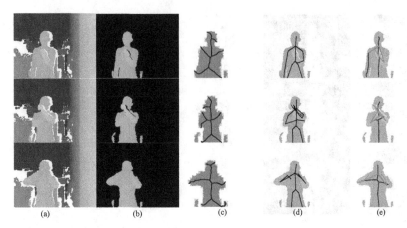

Fig. 7. Sitting postures. (a) original depth images; (b) mask depth images; (c) Shen's approach ; (d) Kinect's skeleton; (e) our approach.

4   Conclusions

In this paper, we present a novel human skeleton extraction approach in the depth image based on the polygon evolution. A external polygon is evolved from the external contour which is extracted form the depth image. Then internal polygons are also evolved by internal self-occlusion contours which are extracted through the depth histogram. Besides, skeleton points are extracted under different criterias in external and internal polygons respectively. Experimental results on a variety of postures demonstrate the robustness and reasonability of our skeleton extraction approach. In our future work, we will try to extract skeleton from depth images of human with different appendants like packsacks, hand bags and so on.

Acknowledgement. Our research was sponsored by following projects:

- National High-tech R&D Program of China ("863 Program") (No. 2013AA014603);
- National Science and Technology Support Projects of China (No. 2012BAH07B01);
- Program of Science and Technology Commission of Shanghai Municipality (No. 12510701900, No. 13ZR1410400, No. 12DZ0512100);
- 2012 IoT Program of Ministry of Industry and Information Technology of China;
- Program of Third Research Institute of the Ministry of Public Security (No.C13348).

References

1. Urtasun, R., Darrell, T.: Sparse probabilistic regression for activity-independent human pose inference. In: Proceedings of IEEE Conference on Computer Vision and Pattern Recognition (2008)
2. Jaeggli, T., Koller-Meier, E., Gool, L.V.: Learning generative models for multi-activity body pose estimation. International Journal of Computer Vision 83(2), 121–134 (2009)
3. Kehl, R., Gool, L.: Markerless tracking of complex human motions from multiple views. Computer Vision and Image Understanding 104(2), 190–209 (2006)
4. Bandouch, J., Engstler, F., Beetz, M.: Accurate human motion capture using an ergonomics-based anthropometric human model. In: Proceedings of V Conference on Articulated Motion and Deformable Objects Andratx, Mallorca, Spain (2008)
5. Zhang, Z.: Microsoft Kinect sensor and its effect. IEEE Multimedia 19(2), 4–10 (2012)
6. Kohli, P., Shotton, J.: Key developments in human pose estimation for Kinect. In: Consumer Depth Cameras for Computer Vision, pp. 63–70. Springer, London (2013)
7. Kondori, F.A., Yousefi, S., Li, H., et al.: 3D head pose estimation using the Kinect. In: Proceedings of International Conference on Wireless Communications and Signal Processing, Nanjing, China, pp. 1–4 (2011)
8. Baak, A., Müller, M., Bharaj, G., et al.: A data-driven approach for real-time full body pose reconstruction from a depth camera. In: Proceedings of IEEE International Conference on Computer Vision, Barcelona, Spain, pp. 1092–1099. IEEE (2011)
9. Choi, W.-P., Lam, K.-M., Siu, W.-C.: Extraction of the Euclidean skeleton based on a connectivity criterion. Pattern Recognition 36, 721–729 (2003)
10. Schwarz, L.A., Mkhitaryan, A., Mateus, D., et al.: Human skeleton tracking from depth data using geodesic distances and optical flow. Image and Vision Computing 30, 217–226 (2012)
11. Jiang, W., Xu, K., Cheng, Z.-Q., et al.: Curve skeleton extraction by coupled graph contraction and surface clustering. Graphical Models 75(3), 137–148 (2013)
12. Shen, W., Xiao, S., Jiang, N., et al.: Unsupervised human skeleton extraction from Kinect depth images. In: Proceedings of the 4th International Conference on Internet Multimedia Computing and Service, Wuhan, China, pp. 66–69 (2012)
13. Shen, W., Bai, X., Yang, X., et al.: Skeleton pruning as trade-off between skeleton simplicity and reconstruction error. Science China Information Sciences 56(4), 1–14 (2013)
14. Bai, X., Latecki, L.J., Liu, W.Y.: Skeleton Pruning by Contour Partitioning with Discrete Curve Evolution. IEEE Transactions on Pattern Analysis and Machine Intelligence 29(3), 449–462 (2007)
15. Benhabiles, H., Lavoue, G., Vandeborre, J., et al.: Kinematic skeleton extraction based on motion boundaries for 3D dynamic meshes. In: Proceedings of Eurographics Workshop on 3D Object Retrieval, Cagliari, Italy, pp. 71–76 (2012)
16. Leyvand, T., Meekhof, C., Wei, Y.-C., et al.: Kinect Identity: Technology and Experience. Computer 44(4), 94–96 (2011)
17. Douglas, D.H., Peucker, T.K.: Algorithms for the reduction of the number of points required to represent a line or its caricature. The Canadian Cartographer 10(2), 112–122 (1973)
18. Canny, J.: A computational approach to edge detection. IEEE Transactions on Pattern Analysis and Machine Intelligence 8(6), 679–698 (1986)
19. Antonisses, H.J.: Image segmentation in pyramids. Computer Graphics and Image Processing 19, 367–383 (1982)

Biomechanics Investigation of Skillful Technician in Spray-up Fabrication Method

Converting Tacit Knowledge to Explicit Knowledge in the Fiber Reinforced Plastics Molding

Tetsuo Kikuchi[1,2,*], Yuichiro Tani[2], Yuka Takai[3], Akihiko Goto[3], and Hiroyuki Hamada[2]

[1] Toyugiken Co., Ltd. Minamiashigara-shi, Kanagwa, Japan
tetuo-kikuchi@toyugiken.co.jp
[2] Department of Advanced Fibro-Science, Kyoto Institute of Technology, Kyoto, Japan
hhamada@kit.ac.jp
[3] Osaka Sangyo University, Osaka, Japan
{takai,gotoh}@ise.osaka-sandai.ac.jp

Abstract. Spray up fabrication has been used for forming composite structures since ancient times as it can be performed as long as the mold, skills, and materials are available. Hence highly specialized control technique and the tradition of skill are required to ensure the consistent stability of product quality. In this study, the authors thus conducted a motion analysis experiment using hand lay-up fabrication experts as subjects. The experiment, seemingly a new and only attempt in Japan, quantified techniques that are not visibly apparent and considered to be tacit knowledge. The dimension stability of samples was measured, and their relationships with the motions of experts were also evaluated. It was also suggested that highly specialized control techniques, the appropriate training of non-experts, and technical tradition are possible.

Keywords: Spray up fabrication, Dimension stability, Motion analysis, Composites, Explicit knowledge.

1 Introduction

In Spray up fabrication work, the characteristics of the composite material will be usually the same regardless of which forming method is used as long as the reinforced substrate, reinforcement morphology, matrix resin, and volume content of reinforcing material are the same. Composite materials, particularly fiber reinforced plastics (FRP) made of fibers and resins, are basically formed by impregnating fibers with resin, i.e., replacing the air contained in fibers with resin. With the spray up technique, rollers are used to impregnate reinforced fibers with resin. Consequently, the impregnation method is expected to contribute to changes in the properties of the interface formed. To review the effects of different roller use in the spray up technique on the mechanical properties of the composite structure, an experiment was

V. G. Duffy (Ed.): DHM 2014, LNCS 8529, pp. 24–34, 2014.
© Springer International Publishing Switzerland 2014

conducted to analyze the process of work and investigate the relationships with mechanical strength and dimension stability of the structures built in craftsmen (experts, intermediates, and non-experts) specializing in making bathtubs using the spray up technique, who were asked to create FRP structures.

2   Methodology

2.1   Subjects

In this study, two people were tested: an expert spray up craftsman (male, 42 years old, 19-year work career) and a non-expert (male, 37 years old, 1-year work career). The biological data of the subjects is shown in table 1. Both subjects were right handed, and didn't have physical handicaps or a disease that restricted their work. The purpose and method of this study were explained in advance to the subjects. Their consent to participate was obtained.

Table 1. Biological data of subjects

Subject	Age	Years experience	Height (cm)	Weight (kg)	Dominant- hand
Expert	42	19	162	65	right
Non-expert	37	1	166	70	right

2.2   Measurement Techniques

Motion analysis and eye movement measuring were done from start to finish for the entire work process. The experiment was performed under the same circumstances as their usual workplace so that the subjects could work as normal. Moreover, instructions—except restrictions for measurement—were omitted so that the subjects could work at their own pace. In addition, three-dimensional motion and eye movements were measured separately.

2.3   Analysis Objective

The object of the analysis was to evaluate the work done for fabricated composites using the spray up method. The size of the mold was 1820 mm high and 910 mm wide. A blue rectangle (1250 mm x 800 mm) was drawn on the 1 square meter spray region. In addition, in this experiment, it was presupposed that the process of degassing (pressing down with a roller after completely spraying on the resin and the roving) would not be done. Since the surface smoothness and thickness distribution vary greatly through control of a roller, in this research only spray up skills were evaluated.

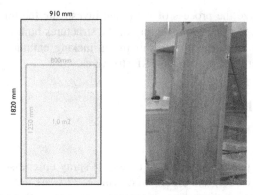

Fig. 1. Mold used in this study (1820mm high, 910 mm wide)

2.4   Spray up Method

The spray up machine that was used was made in Japan. The quantities and conditions of the spray up method were:

Amount of resin sprayed on	:	2044 [g/min]
Amount of glass fiber sprayed on	:	1080 [g/min]
Spread angle of resin	:	200 mm / 500 mm

Here, the glass fiber was in a continuation filament cut into 4 or 25 mm strands, and then sprayed on. As a base material, glass roving was used, as well as isophthalic unsaturated polyester resin.

2.5   Three-Dimensional Motion Measurement

Three-dimensional motion measurement was performed using an optical real-time motion capturing system (Fig.2), the MAC 3D System (manufactured by Motion Analysis Corporation). Before measurements were taken, in order to acquire the three-dimensional coordinates of markers, an L-shaped frame (with infrared markers attached) was shot and the calibration of the shooting range was performed using a T-shaped wand (with two infrared markers attached).

A total of 19 infrared reflective markers were attached to the subjects' bodies. Similarly, three markers were attached to the tool. The position of each marker was captured with six cameras (manufactured by Motion Analysis Corporation), and the three-dimensional position data of all the markers was synchronously downloaded to a PC (sampling rate: 120 Hz). Moreover, the data from one digital video camera was also simultaneously synchronized. Here, the x axis was defined as perpendicular to the spray direction. The y axis was defined as the spray direction and the z axis was defined as the height. For data processing, the coordinate data from the 19 markers attached to each joint was obtained using EvaRT Ver. 5.0.4 software (manufactured by Motion Analysis Corporation).

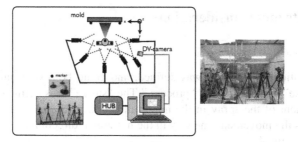

Fig. 2. Motion analysis system

2.6   Eye Movement Measurement

Eye movement measurement was performed using TalkEyeII (manufactured by Takei Scientific Instruments Co., Ltd.) for analyzing eye movement. A goggle-like apparatus was worn by the subjects. The subjects' point of view was captured with the camera from the center of both eyes, and two cameras detected the point of view. The sampling rate was 30 Hz. Moreover, a digital video camera was used to record the motion of objects. Cameras were arranged so that the motion could be captured clearly. The eye movement measurement system and the experimental area are shown in Fig.3.

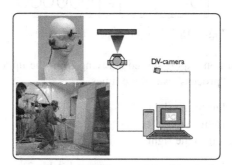

Fig. 3. Eye movement measurement system

2.7   Dimensional Stability

To compare the dimensional stability of the expert and non-expert, the surface coarseness of the plane of the acquired molded product was measured. A micrometer was used for measuring thickness. All samples (1250 mm x 800 mm) obtained in the experiment were cut and divided into 16 sections. Moreover, the thickness of the cross section of each area was measured every 10 mm. About 1,110 data points were obtained per subject.

3   Results and Considerations

3.1   Process Analysis

First, each motion under work was defined, and could be divide into two motions: first the "stroke" and second the "process." The "stroke" was defined as the reciprocating movement of the spray in the height direction of the mold and the "process" was defined as the movement one way in the horizontal direction of the mold by repetitive "strokes" (Fig.4).

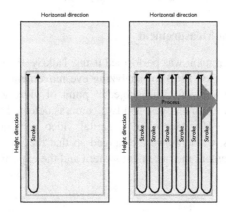

Fig. 4. Definition of "stroke" and "process"

Both the expert and non-expert started spraying from the upper left. For both, the number of times of the "process" was three times.

- Process 1: From the left to the right
- Process 2: From the right to the left
- Process 3: From the left to the right

The number of "strokes" in each process is compared (table 2).

Table 2. The number of strokes

	Expert	Non-expert
Process 1	7	6
Process 2	7	5
Process 3	6	9

In process 1 and 2, the expert took seven strokes. On the other hand, the non-expert took five and six strokes. In process 3, the expert took six strokes, and the non-expert took nine. The number of strokes made by the non-expert in each process varied although the number of strokes made by the expert was consistent.

Next, the mean work time of the stroke in each process was compared (Fig.5). The mean work time of the expert and non-expert shortened with the increase in process. The expert's mean work time was short by 19.5%. On the other hand, the non-expert was short by no less than 31.5%. That is, the spray per stroke gradually became faster.

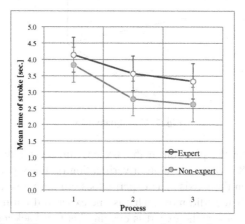

Fig. 5. The mean work time per stroke for each process

3.2   Motion Analysis

The operations at the time of the spraying by the expert and non-expert were compared. Attention was paid to the motion (toe tips, knee and greater trochanter) of the lower half of the body. The difference in motion was especially noted (Fig.6).

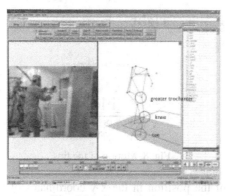

Fig. 6. Motion analysis

Here, the x axis is defined as the direction perpendicular to the spray. The y axis is defined as the spray direction. And the z axis is defined as the height direction (Fig.7).

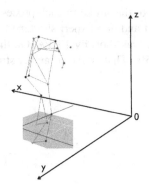

Fig. 7. Coordinate axes

First, the change in the position in the x-y coordinates for the toe tips (foot) is shown in Fig.8. Fig.8 shows the duration verification on the x-y axis of the toe tips. The mold is placed on the x axis. The expert's toes did not move at all. On the other hand, the non-expert's toes did move. That is, the expert did not move his foot at the time of spray up. Moreover, the expert is opening his foot back and forth. However, the non-expert was not doing this.

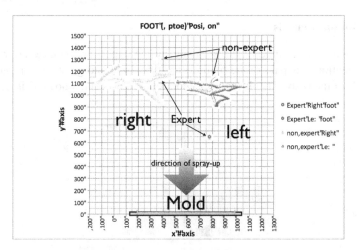

Fig. 8. Motion of toe tips

Next, the change of the position in the x-y coordinates of the knees is shown in Fig.9. The expert's knees almost do not move, but the non-expert's knees move in the direction of the x and y axis. Although about 150 mm displacement is seen in y-axis direction for the expert's knee, there is no displacement in the x-axis direction. On the other hand, the knees of the non-expert were displaced by about 600 mm in the x-axis direction with the displacement of his toe tips.

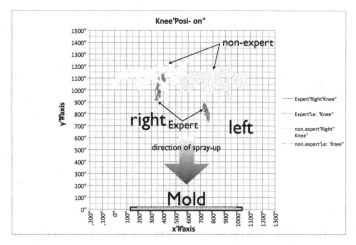

Fig. 9. Motion of knees

Next, the change in the position of the x-y coordinates of the greater trochanter is shown in Fig.10. When the motions along the direction of the y axis of the expert and the non-expert were compared, it turned out that the motion of the non-expert is about 50 mm less. Therefore, with the expert, being on tiptoes serves as a reference point for a series of motions. On the other hand, with the non-expert, it turns out that the greater trochanter is a reference point for a series of motions. Furthermore, to better understand the series of motions, the "crookedness expansion movements" of the expert and non-expert were compared.

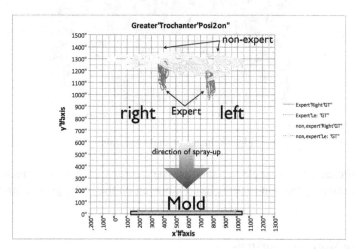

Fig. 10. Motion of greater trochanter

Next, the angle variations between the knee, greater trochanter and shoulder (right side) are shown in Fig.11.

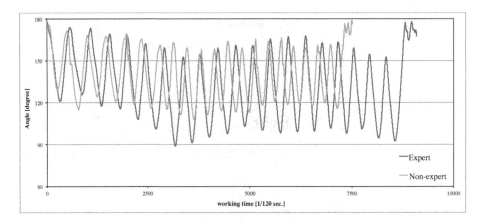

Fig. 11. Angle between the knee, greater trochanter and shoulder (right side)

The expert had a wide angle variation (wide arc) and it turns out that this is the stable angle variation. Moreover, it is clear that the expert is further "crooked" by about 20 degrees, and it turns out that the "crookedness expansion movement" for each stroke by the expert was performed smoothly. That is, the expert is performing the "crookedness expansion movement" efficiently while on tiptoes. An image of an angle variation is shown in Fig.12.

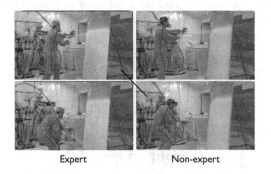

Expert   Non-expert

Fig. 12. Image of angle variation

The difference in the angle variation can be clearly seen from this figure. Moreover, the motion of the non-expert placed a burden on the body, preventing a smooth motion.

3.3   Eye Movement Analysis

A comparison of the points of view of the expert and non-expert is shown in Fig.13. The expert's point of view was stable and the path of the point of view matches the path of the stroke. On the other hand, it is clear that the non-expert's eye movement is not smooth.

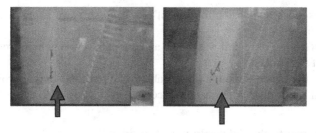

Fig. 13. Comparison of points of view (left: expert, right: non-expert)

3.4 Dimensional Stability

The dimensional stability (thickness distribution) of the expert and non-expert are shown in Fig. 14. The classification by color in the figure is every 1.0 mm.

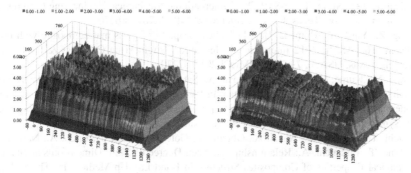

Fig. 14. Comparison of thickness distribution (left: expert, right: non-expert)

The expert's average thickness was 3.52 mm and the coefficient of variation (CV) value was 11.4%. On the other hand, the average thickness for the non-expert was 2.47 mm and the CV value was 16.2%. As the theoretical thickness of this study was 3.50 mm, the non-expert's thickness distribution was thin and the CV value was also large. The CV value of the horizontal cross-sectional thickness for the non-expert was especially high. This thickness came from overlapping strokes or an inconsistent speed. Moreover, the ends of the horizontal sections were extremely thin.

The thickness distribution of the superior extremity and the lower end shows that the expert had precise thickness control. Therefore, the expert's loss of spray also decreased. In addition, to refine the spray up method, there needs to be a consistent coefficient of variation of less than 10%. Improving the spray up technology would substantially contribute to dimensional stability and reduced waste.

4 Conclusions

Analysis of the spray up method revealed the following:

1. The "crookedness expansion movement" was efficient because it was performed on tiptoes.

2. The "crookedness expansion movement" for each stroke was performed smoothly by the expert.
3. The expert's point of regard was stable and the path of the point of regard matched the path of the stroke.
4. Moreover, the expert's motion data is able to be fed to a spray up robot, resulting in minimal errors during fabrication of composite.

Acknowledgements. Special thanks to KIT members.

References

1. Kikuchi, T., Koyanagi, T., Hamada, H., Nakai, A., Takai, Y., Goto, A., Fujii, Y., Narita, C., Endo, A., Koshino, T.: Biomechanics investigation of skillful technician in hand lay up fabrication method. In: The ASME 2012 International Mechanical Engineering Congress & Exposition, Houston, Texas, USA, p. 288 (2012) IMECE2012-86270
2. Zhang, Z., Yang, Y., Hamada, H.: Mechanical property of glass mat composite with open hole. In: The ASME 2012 International Mechanical Engineering Congress & Exposition, Houston, Texas, USA, p. 79 (2012) IMECE2012-87270
3. Shirato, M., Kume, M., Ohnishi, A., Nakai, A., Sato, H., Maki, M., Yoshida, T.: Analysis of daubing motion in the clay wall craftsman: Influence on several kinds of clay with different fermentation period on the daubing motion properties. In: Symposium on Sports Engineering: Symposium on Human Dynamics 2007, Japan, pp. 254–257 (2007)
4. Kikuchi, T., Hamada, H., Nakai, A., Ohtani, A., Goto, A., Takai, Y., Endo, A., Narita, C., Koshino, T., Fudauchi, A.: Relationships between Degree of Skill, Dimension stability and Mechanical Properties of Composites Structure in Hand Lay-Up Method. In: The 19th International Conference on Composite Materials, Montreal, Canada, pp. 8034–8042 (2013)
5. Kikuchi, T., Fudauchi, A., Koshino, T., Narita, C., Endo, A., Hamada, H.: Mechanical Property of CFRP by carbon Spray up method. In: The ASME 2013 International Mechanical Engineering Congress & Exposition, San Diego, California, USA, p. 63 (2013) IMECE2013-64144

Study on Three Dimensions Body Reconstruction and Measurement by Using Kinect

Qi Luo

College of Sports Engineering and Information Technology,
Wuhan Sports University,430079, China
emeinstitute@126.com

Abstract. A point cloud is a set of data points in some coordinate system. Point clouds may be created by Three Dimensions scanners. These devices measure in an automatic way a large number of points on the surface of an object, and often output a point cloud as a data file. The point cloud represents the set of points that the device has measured. Using Microsoft Kinect to obtain the depth body data and get the depth image. In this paper, the function and the depth scanning principle of the Microsoft Kinect has been researched. The concept of Point cloud has been also introduced. Point cloud data processing has been proposed in the paper. First, the depth data obtained by Kinect are transformed into the form of Three Dimensions point cloud to store and visualize. And then, make rejections, filtering, and simplification for point cloud. Finally In the process of simplification, we take the advantage of the minimum distance method and the angular deviation method, an improved self-adapting method of simplification was introduced in the paper.

1   Introduction

The appearance of the non-contact Three Dimensions body scanner has made it to be true. Presently, non-contact Three Dimensions body scanning technology is not very advanced in our country. Non-contact Three Dimensions body scanner from foreign country is so large and expensive that many costume manufacturers cannot afford it. Meanwhile, using traditional Three Dimensions body scanner to obtain the characteristic data of the body surface is very complicated. Therefore, exploring the small volume, high precision and low cost Three Dimensions body scanner has comprehensive value in research and prospect for application. In this thesis, a scheme of Three Dimensions body scanning system based on Microsoft Kinect has been proposed.

Using Microsoft Kinect to obtain the depth body data and get the depth image. In this paper, the function and the depth scanning principle of the Microsoft Kinect has been researched. the concept of Point cloud has been also introduced.

Point cloud data processing has been proposed in the paper. First, the depth data obtained by Kinect are transformed into the form of Three Dimensions point cloud to store and visualize. And then, make rejections, filtering, and simplification for point cloud. Finally In the process of simplification, we take the advantage of the minimum

V. G. Duffy (Ed.): DHM 2014, LNCS 8529, pp. 35–42, 2014.

distance method and the angular deviation method, an improved self-adapting method of simplification was introduced in the paper.

2   Kinect

Kinect is a line of motion sensing input devices by Microsoft for Xbox 360 and Xbox One video game consoles and Windows PCs. Based around a webcam-style add-on peripheral, it enables users to control and interact with their console/computer without the need for a game controller, through a natural user interface using gestures and spoken commands. The first-generation Kinect was first introduced in November 2010 in an attempt to broaden Xbox 360's audience beyond its typical gamer base. A version for Windows was released on February 1, 2012[1]. Kinect competes with several motion controllers on other home consoles, such as Wii Remote Plus for Wii, PlayStation Move/PlayStation Eye for PlayStation 3, and PlayStation Camera for PlayStation 4. Kinect for Xbox 360 see Figure 1

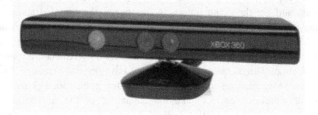

Fig. 1. Kinect for Xbox 360

Kinect builds on software technology developed internally by Rare, a subsidiary of Microsoft Game Studios owned by Microsoft, and on range camera technology by Israeli developer PrimeSense, which developed a system that can interpret specific gestures, making completely hands-free control of electronic devices possible by using an infrared projector and camera and a special microchip to track the movement of objects and individuals in three dimensions. This Three Dimensions scanner system called Light Coding employs a variant of image-based Three Dimensions reconstruction.

Kinect sensor is a horizontal bar connected to a small base with a motorized pivot and is designed to be positioned lengthwise above or below the video display. The device features an "RGB camera, depth sensor and multi-array microphone running proprietary software", which provide full-body Three Dimensions motion capture, facial recognition and voice recognition capabilities. At launch, voice recognition was only made available in Japan, United Kingdom, Canada and United States. Mainland Europe received the feature later in spring 2011. Currently voice recognition is supported in Australia, Canada, France, Germany, Ireland, Italy, Japan, Mexico, New Zealand, United Kingdom and United States. Kinect sensor's microphone array enables Xbox 360 to conduct acoustic source localization and ambient noise suppression, allowing for things such as headset-free party chat over Xbox Live.

The depth sensor consists of an infrared laser projector combined with a monochrome CMOS sensor, which captures video data in Three Dimensions under any ambient light conditions. The sensing range of the depth sensor is adjustable, and Kinect software is capable of automatically calibrating the sensor based on game play and the player's physical environment, accommodating for the presence of furniture or other obstacles.

Described by Microsoft personnel as the primary innovation of Kinect, the software technology enables advanced gesture recognition, facial recognition and voice recognition. According to information supplied to retailers, Kinect is capable of simultaneously tracking up to six people, including two active players for motion analysis with a feature extraction of 20 joints per player. However, Prime Sense has stated that the number of people the device can "see" (but not process as players) is only limited by how many will fit in the field-of-view of the camera.

This infrared image shows the laser grid Kinect uses to calculate depth .The depth map is visualized here using color gradients from white (near) to blue (far)Reverse engineering has determined that the Kinect's various sensors output video at a frame rate of ~9 Hz to 30 Hz depending on resolution. The default RGB video stream uses 8-bit VGA resolution (640 × 480 pixels) with a Bayer color filter, but the hardware is capable of resolutions up to 1280x1024 (at a lower frame rate) and other colour formats such as UYVY. The monochrome depth sensing video stream is in VGA resolution (640 × 480 pixels) with 11-bit depth, which provides 2,048 levels of sensitivity. The Kinect can also stream the view from its IR camera directly (i.e.: before it has been converting into a depth map) as 640x480 video, or 1280x1024 at a lower frame rate. The Kinect sensor has a practical ranging limit of 1.2–3.5 m (3.9–11.5 ft) distance when used with the Xbox software. The area required to play Kinect is roughly 6 m2, although the sensor can maintain tracking through an extended range of approximately 0.7–6 m (2.3–19.7 ft). The sensor has an angular field of view of 57° horizontally and 43° vertically, while the motorized pivot is capable of tilting the sensor up to 27° either up or down. The horizontal field of the Kinect sensor at the minimum viewing distance of ~0.8 m (2.6 ft) is therefore ~87 cm (34 in), and the vertical field is ~63 cm (25 in), resulting in a resolution of just over 1.3 mm (0.051 in) per pixel. The microphone array features four microphone capsules and operates with each channel processing 16-bit audio at a sampling rate of 16 kHz.

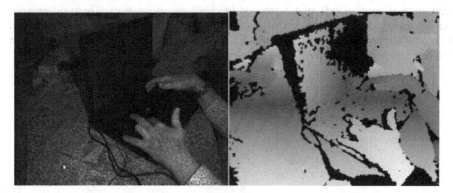

Fig. 2. The laser grid Kinect uses to calculate depth and The depth map is visualized here using color gradients from white (near) to blue (far)

Because the Kinect sensor's motorized tilt mechanism requires more power than the Xbox 360's USB ports can supply, the device makes use of a proprietary connector combining USB communication with additional power. Redesigned Xbox 360 S models include a special AUX port for accommodating the connector, while older models require a special power supply cable (included with the sensor) that splits the connection into separate USB and power connections; power is supplied from the mains by way of an AC adapter.

3   Point Cloud

A point cloud is a set of data points in some coordinate system. In a three-dimensional coordinate system, these points are usually defined by X, Y, and Z coordinates, and often are intended to represent the external surface of an object.

Point clouds may be created by Three Dimensions scanners. These devices measure in an automatic way a large number of points on the surface of an object, and often output a point cloud as a data file. The point cloud represents the set of points that the device has measured.

As the result of a Three Dimensions scanning process point clouds are used for many purposes, including to create Three Dimensions CAD models for manufactured parts, metrology/quality inspection, and a multitude of visualization, animation, rendering and mass customization applications.

While point clouds can be directly rendered and inspected, usually point clouds themselves are generally not directly usable in most Three Dimensions applications, and therefore are usually converted to polygon mesh or triangle mesh models, NURBS surface models, or CAD models through a process commonly referred to as surface reconstruction.

There are many techniques for converting a point cloud to a Three Dimensions surface. Some approaches, like Delaunay triangulation, alpha shapes, and ball pivoting, build a network of triangles over the existing vertices of the point cloud, while other approaches convert the point cloud into a volumetric distance field and reconstruct the implicit surface so defined through a marching cubes algorithm.

One application in which point clouds are directly usable is industrial metrology or inspection. The point cloud of a manufactured part can be aligned to a CAD model (or even another point cloud), and compared to check for differences. These differences can be displayed as color maps that give a visual indicator of the deviation between the manufactured part and the CAD model. Geometric dimensions and tolerances can also be extracted directly from the point cloud. Please see the figure

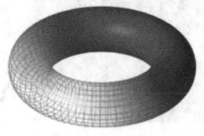

Fig. 3. A point cloud image of a torus

Point clouds can also be used to represent volumetric data used for example in medical imaging. Using point clouds multi-sampling and data compression are achieved.

In geographic information system, point clouds are one of the sources to make digital elevation model of the terrain. The point clouds are also employed in order to generate Three Dimensions model of urban environment, e.g.

4   Depth Image Processing by Kinect

Kinect is different from all other input devices, because it provides a third dimension. It does this using an infrared emitter and camera. Unlike other Kinect SDKs such as OpenNI, or libfreenect, the Microsoft SDK does not provide raw access to the IR stream. Instead, the Kinect SDK processes the IR data returned by the infrared camera to produce a depth image

The IR or depth camera has a field of view just like any other camera. The field of view of Kinect islimited, as illustrated in Figure 4. The original purpose of Kinect was to play video games within the confines of game room or living room space. Kinect's normal depth vision ranges from around two and a half feet (800mm) to just over 13 feet (4000mm). However, a recommended usage range is 3 feet to 12 feet as the reliability of the depth values degrade at the edges of the field of view.

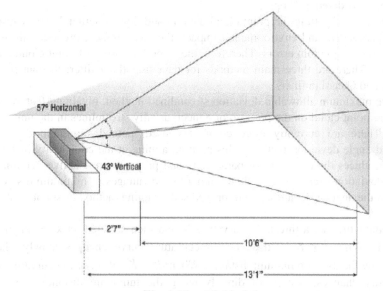

Fig. 4. Kinect field of view

Like any camera, the field of view of the depth camera is pyramid shaped. Objects farther away from the camera have a greater lateral range than objects nearer to Kinect. This means that height and width pixel dimensions, such as 640×480, do not correspond with a physical location in the camera's field of view. The depth value of each pixel, however, does map to a physical distance in the field of view. Each pixel represented in a depth frame is 16 bits, making the BytesPerPixel property of each frame a value of two. The depth value of each pixel is only 13 of the 16 bits, as shown in Figure 5.

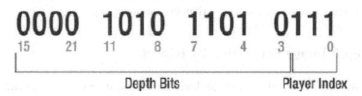

Fig. 5. Layout of the depth bits

5   Point Cloud Data Processing

When obtaining the point cloud data, because of the large data, it is prone to errors. Hope is also known as distortion point, most due to the changes in the surrounding environment parameters and produces the equipment. First, identifying and removing the "jump point" is the first step performing point cloud data processing. In the same row or column of data, if the distance of a point from its neighboring point is big, this point can be considered as "hops".

In the process of getting the point cloud data, in addition to outliers' error caused by device parameters and environmental impact, the measurement process will also inevitably produce random errors. Therefore, the smoothing work of point cloud data is necessary. There are three main methods for data smoothing filter: median filter, mean filter and Gaussian filter.

Adaptive maximum allowable deviation streamlined method, obtaining features of the acquired point cloud on the purpose of Kinect, usually streamlines in the unit of a direction. There are currently more commonly used method--minimum distance method and angle deviation method. This section, aiming at the complexity of body surface, introduces the curvature of parameters and proposes an adaptive maximum allowable deviation streamlined method, taking the advantages of minimum distance method and the angular deviation, an improved self-adapting method of simplification as follows:

The method first set a threshold curvature K and then selected an x to calculate curvature k. When $k < K$, this section curvature curve changes slowly, then streamlines by the use of minimum distance; When $k > K$, this section curvature of curve rapidly changes, instead of directly using the minimum distance. So two parameters-- angle threshold θ_{min} and chord high threshold h_{min} --should be set to streamline data threshold. The smaller the value of θ_{min} , the higher the precision of the reconstruction model, generally ranging between 0 -15 . It can also select good

$\theta_{\min}$ value according to the actual situation to test. $h_{\min}$ is determined by the formula :

$$h_{\min} = \mu \frac{N_b}{N_a} \sin \theta_{\min} \qquad (1)$$

where u is the normal value of the distance between adjacent points, N_a the number of former streamline point, and N_b the number of latter streamline point.

Algorithm steps are as follows:

1) Given a threshold curvature K and step length x.

2) The curvature k data points per segment is calculated in accordance with sub-step x .

3) According to the curvature segment k of data points, if $k < K$, then set a minimum distance threshold $d_{\min}$.

4) From the first point of data points in one direction in order to find the distance between two adjacent d.

5) If $d < d_{\min}$, then the latter point has been deleted, whereas retention, till the last point of data points , determining whether this step is the last step length. If so, end ; if not, read the next step curvature.

6) If $k > K$, then given a threshold angle $\theta_{\min}$ and calculate the chord high threshold $h_{\min}$.

7) From the start point of data points select three adjacent points p_1, p_2, p_3 , If the last point of the segment is p_3 , go to step 9). Otherwise, calculate the angle between $p_1 p_2$ and $p_2 p_3$, chord height $h = p_1 p_2 \sin \theta$.

8) If $h < h_{\min}$, then delete the point p_2 , and shift p_2 back forward. Let $p_2 = p_3 p_3 = p_4$, go to step 7) , or delete the point p_2 if $\theta < \theta_{\min}$, shifting the poin p_2 back forward. Let $p_2 = p_3 p_3 = p_4$, go to step 7), otherwise keep the point p_2 , the point p_1 shift back forward, $p_1 = p_2, p_2 = p_3, p_3 = p_4$ go to step 7).

9) Determine whether this step is the last step length. If so, end ; if not, read the next step curvature.

6   Conclusion

Using Microsoft Kinect to obtain the depth body data and get the depth image. In this paper, the function and the depth scanning principle of the Microsoft Kinect has been researched. the concept of Point cloud has been also introduced. Point cloud data processing has been proposed in the paper. First, the depth data obtained by Kinect are transformed into the form of Three Dimensions point cloud to store and visualize.

And then, make rejections, filtering, and simplification for point cloud. Finally In the process of simplification, we take the advantage of the minimum distance method and the angular deviation method, an improved self-adapting method of simplification was introduced in the paper.

References

1. http://latimesblogs.latimes.com/technology/2009/06/microsofte3.html
2. Fujimoto, M., Kariya, K.: An improved method for digitized data reduction using an angle parameter. Measurement 12(2), 113–122 (1993)
3. Martin, R.R., Stroud, I.A., Marshall, A.D.: Data reduction for reverse engineering. RECCAD, Deliverable Document 1 COPERNICUS project, No 1068. Computer and Automation Institute of Hungarian Academy of Science (January 1996)
4. Veron, P., Léon, J.C.: Static polyhedron simplification using error measurements. Computer- Aided Design 29(4), 287–298 (1997)
5. Song, S.: Research on 3D body reconstruction and measurement techniques based on Kinect. Donghua University Master Dissertation 30, 31 (2013)

Comparison of Gait Analysis by the Way of Semi-structured Interviews

Masaru Ohgiri[1], Katsuma Yamada[1], Hisanori Yuminaga[2], Noriyuki Kida[1], and Hiroyuki Hamada[1]

[1] Kyoto Institute of Technology, Graduate School of Science and Technology, Kyoto, Japan
summersoniclove@yahoo.co.jp, haagen-kattsu@nike.eonet.ne.jp, {hhamada,kida}@kit.ac.jp
[2] Department of Physical Therapy, Kansai Vocational College of Medicine, Osaka, Japan
yuminaga@kansai.ac.jp

Abstract. In this study, we showed a video with five samples of patients walking to three practicing Physical Therapists. We used a one-on-one semi-structured interview to investigate how the Physical Therapists would predict problems and plan treatment programs based on what they observed in the video, and then we analyzed the results. We obtained qualitative data from interviews and charted them as quantitative data for analysis, which is a new approach for motion observation.

Keywords: Posture Prediction and Analysis, semi-structured interview, gait analysis, physical therapy.

1 Introduction

According to article 2 of the law governing physical and occupational therapists, physical therapy is defined as, "To carry out treatment or regular exercise for a person with physical disabilities to restore basic motion ability, and to apply physical approaches such as electrostimulation, massage and thermal treatment." As mentioned in the law, physical therapists (hereinafter referred as PT) are required to improve the basic motion ability of their patients. Analysis and observation of basic motion is very important in clinical practice to comprehend the status of a patient in a limited amount of time. According to Usuda 1), exercise and motion analysis in the clinical practice of physical therapy plays the central role in evaluation and treatment, which is conducted by the PT. In general, qualitative analysis of motion patterns is performed. Based on the observed phenomenon, the PT infers the cause of exercise and motion dysfunctions through top-down thinking. According to Fukui 2), physical therapy is recognized as an applied science. The best way to become a good PT is to show strong interest in restoration and support of a patient while conducting motion analysis and accruing empirical value.

V. G. Duffy (Ed.): DHM 2014, LNCS 8529, pp. 43–54, 2014.
© Springer International Publishing Switzerland 2014

However, under the present circumstances, the ability and method of motion observation varies depending on the PT. The approach to treatments derived from motion observation also differs. Thus, it is said that the therapeutic effect also differs depending on the accuracy of motion observation. For this reason, physical therapy is hardly considered a therapeutic action with scientific elements when it comes to assigning medical fees. The lack of standardization of motion observation methods has led to confusion among physical therapy students in clinical practices. In order to solve these problems, we will review the process of standardizing motion observation in physical therapy. Practical evidence-based physical therapy (EBPT) enhances the scientific validity of motion observation in physical therapy and is useful in educating students who aspire to become PT.

Suzuki 3) argues that it is important to not just observe patients but to comprehend "the order in which (the joints) move", "correlation of articular movement" and "displacement of joint angles per each motion." It is obvious that keen observation of motion is important, but there are many gray areas that are difficult to convey to the PT or PT training school students with less clinical experience. However there are some PTs with superior observation ability. They are generally referred to as skilled PTs with effective therapeutic abilities, and they can deduce the problem immediately upon observing the motion of a patient in clinical practice. An inexperienced PT with less experience in clinical practice who has a difficult time deducing problems from observing the motion of patients can receive guidance from a skilled PT and then offer effective treatments for patients. Every PT goes through this at some point. While recognizing the presence of skilled PTs, Bonkohara 4) reported that a PT's years of experience had no effect on their ability to observe and comprehend joint angle status per each phase of a walking patient. MacGinly 5) et al also reported that there is no connection between the experience and basic observation ability of PT.

The purpose of this study is to improve motion observation techniques for PTs and to establish the scientific validity of motion observation. We accumulated objective data based on a PT's motion observation in clinical practice using the qualitative research method of interviews and surveys. Then, we compared and discussed the factors involved in motion observation capability.

2   Method

2.1   Subjects

Of the three PTs who participated in this study; two are working at general hospitals and one is a teacher at a PT vocational training school. They are all practicing PTs and have six to eleven years clinical experience (the average years of experience is 8.6 years). Property of Subjects is shown in Table 1. Since this study is intended to accumulate the objective data from the thinking process of general PTs when it comes to observing motion, we selected the above mentioned PTs for the study with reference to the study of Yamada 6), et al. We verbally explained the purpose of the study and obtained their informal consent to cooperate with our research.

Table 1. Property of Subjects

PT ID	Place of Work	Age	Gender	Years of Experience
1	General hospital	27	Female	6 years
2	General hospital	33	Male	9 years
3	PT vocational training school	40	Male	11 years

2.2   Models for Walking Video

The people in the walking video are actual patients. At the time of recording, rehabilitation was conducted at our hospital. We asked five patients who could walk safely during the video shooting to cooperate in this experiment. The name and duration of the diseases afflicting the model patients are shown in Table 2. Since our hospital has only an orthopedic surgery section, we selected patients with many opportunities to be treated in a clinic, such as patients with osteoarthritis or postoperative patients that have had surgery on their cervical region or lower limbs. Upon fully explaining the purpose of the study to the patients and obtaining their informal consent for cooperation in our research, we shot the video of the patients walking while taking into consideration the safety and stamina of the patients. The video recording was conducted in the rehabilitation room of our hospital. We set up the digital video camera (Nikon) at fixed points and recorded each patient walking along a 4-meter path twice. The filming was done from the front, back and side of the patient.

Table 2. Models for Walking Video

ID	Name of Disease	Age	Gender	Duration of Disease
1	spondylosis deformans	52	male	2 months
2	osteoarthritis	75	male	14 years
3	ossification of posterior longitudinal ligament	66	male	1 year
4	femoral diaphyseal fracture	40	male	9 months
5	knee joint intraarticular fracture	64	female	3 months

2.3   Collection of Data

The three participating PTs observed the video of patients walking, and then were each interviewed by a PT who is the head author of this paper with eight years of clinical experience as a PT. Since this study was designed to research the thinking process of PTs from observing action to planning a treatment program, we did not disclose any information about the patients' diagnoses or their course of rehabilitation beforehand in order to conduct the research in a non-biased way. Each of the PTs was able to watch the videos twice from the front and side angles. To avoid having the order of the videos affect the thinking process of the PTs, the interviewer randomly determined the order in which the videos were played.

The interview survey of the PTs was conducted by using a semi-structured interview technique. We performed interviews for about 10-15 minutes per subject. The interview time per PT is shown in Table 3. The semi-structured interview is a method to roughly determine questions in advance and ask more detailed questions during the flow of a casual conversation. This method allows us to obtain unadulterated answers to questions and carry out our investigation in a short time. In order to bring out the thinking process of the PT as much as possible, we applied a semi-structured interview technique rather than a structured interview that asks prepared questions without changing their orders. In a semi-structured interview, we are allowed to add questions according to the flow of a conversation.

In the interview, we asked the PTs, "By observing this video, what action do you focus on and how do you approach treatment?" We had the PTs reply as specifically as possible and added more questions based on the flow of the conversations such as, "Is there any other point that concerned you?" The conversation during the interview was recorded with the consent of the subjects. When identifiable personal information was stated during recording, we eliminated that part. The head author transcribed the conversations related to the physiotherapeutic thinking process.

Table 3. Interview time

		Time(min.sec)		
ID	Name of Disease	PT1	PT2	PT3
1	spondylosis deformans	14.13	10.38	11.33
2	osteoarthritis	13.24	12.30	17.29
3	ossification of posterior longitudinal ligament	14.13	11.20	14.02
4	femoral diaphyseal fracture	13.47	12.30	7.59
5	knee joint intraarticular fracture	10.31	8.50	12.13
	Total	66.80	55.48	63.16

2.4   Categorization

We labeled the speech data obtained in the interviews. Labeling was conducted for basically 1.Region, 2.Walking phase, 3.Physical function. When multiple regions or body functions were mentioned, we corresponded appropriately and labeled these statements in higher categories. For instance, the speech data referring to "the alignment of initial stance also shows strong abduction-external rotation of hip joint" consist of hip joint (1.region), initial stance (2.walking phase) and alignment

Table 4. List of Analyzed Category from Speech Data : Region x Time

				time							the others
				swing phase			stance phase				
				total swing	initial swing	terminal swing	total stance	initial stance	mid stance	terminal stance	
region	Upper limbs	entire upper limbs	26	2			3	1			
		head and neck	1								6
		scapular arch	2								8
		shoulder joints	2	1			1		1		
		finger									6
	Trunk	trunk	7	3	1		4	1	5	2	83
	Pelvis	pelvis	6	2		1	1			1	20
	Lower limbs	entire lower limbs	5	5			7			1	24
		hip joints	6	10			23	6	12	6	86
		knee joints	5	8		4	14	6	3	10	65
		ankle joints	7				3			12	26
	the others			6	2		18	1	13	9	116

(3.physical function). It was defined as a single meaning unit (hip joint, initial stance, alignment). Another case that stated "the output of the gluteus medius is weak for the swinging left leg" was defined as a single meaning unit (hip joints, swing phase, muscle). We classified single meaning units according to similarity and divided them into groups. Then we categorized each group based on similarities among the groups. For categories formed through the extraction process mentioned above, we charted three patterns: 1.region x 2 walking phase, 1.region x 3. physical function, 2. walking phase x 3. physical function. Then, we calculated the number of meaning units in each group (Table 4, 5, 6).

Table 5. List of Analyzed Category from Speech Data : Function x Region

		region											the others
		Upper limbs					Trunk	Pelvis	Lower limbs				
		entire upper limbs	head and neck	scapular arch	shoulder joints	finger	trunk	pelvis	entire lower limbs	hip joints	knee joints	ankle joints	
		26	1	2	2		7		5	6	5	7	
function	muscle		2				22	1	10	41	23	3	
	range of motion						8	6	17	8	4		
	sensory								2				
	reflex					6	2					2	
	clonus											2	
	spasticity						2					2	
	skin						2						
	motion direction			3	1		33	17		47	39	20	
	alignment		4	4	1		14	5	2	20	25	1	2
	clearance			1					8	1	3	1	
	falling tendency												4
	safety								1				
	stability						2	1	2	6	1		3
	grounding status										2	1	5
	total stance time									1			9
	timing										2	1	
	training						1		5	5	5		
	weighted center						9		7	1			5
	motion progression							1		1			
	separability						3						
	inertia force												2
	the others	6				1	1		2	2	1	4	135

Table 6. List of Analyzed Category from Speech Data : Function x Time

		time							the others
		swing phase			stance phase				
		total swing	initial swing	terminal swing	total stance	initial stance	mid stance	terminal stance	
		4	2		6		4	2	
function	muscle	3			8	2			89
	range of motion	3		1	3		1		35
	sensory								2
	reflex								10
	clonus								2
	spasticity								4
	skin								2
	motion direction	13	3	1	24	3	18	25	73
	alignment	4		3	9	7	1	3	51
	clearance	7					1		6
	falling tendency	1			2		1		
	safety	1							
	stability				4	1	1		9
	grounding status				7				1
	total stance time				2		2	5	1
	timing								3
	training								16
	weighted center				1	1	5		15
	motion progression								2
	separability								3
	inertia force							2	
	the others	5			8	1	1	3	177

3   Results

First, we focused on the track of the marker attached to the handle of the pounding brush. The total speech time of the three subject PTs was 185 minutes (15 cases x several min. per each case), and the average speech time per person was 61.7 minutes (12.3 min. per each case). From speech content related to the physiotherapeutic thinking process, we extracted 716 meaning units for analysis. And we eventually categorized three main categories and eight sub-categories. Hereinafter, in this document, we indicate speech content with 「」, meaning unit with 【】, sub-category with < >, main category with ≪≫, and a lower category than sub-category with [].

There were three main categories: ≪region≫, ≪time≫, ≪function≫. The ≪region≫ category indicated the physical parts that the PTs mentioned related to motion observation. Furthermore, the main category of ≪region≫ was divided into four sub-categories: < upper limbs >, < trunk >, < pelvis >, < lower limbs >. These four sub-categories were also divided into eleven lower-categories: [entire upper limbs], [head and neck], [scapular arch], [shoulder joints], [finger], [trunk], [pelvis], [entire lower limbs], [hip joints], [knee joints], [ankle joints]. The ≪time≫ category was limited to the speech contents referring to the walking phase observed by the PTs. ≪Time≫ was divided into two main categories: < swing phase > and < stance phase >. These two categories were divided into seven categories: [total swing], [initial swing], [terminal swing], [total stance], [initial stance], [mid stance] and [terminal stance]. The speech content referring to physical functions was categorized as ≪function≫. The main category of ≪function≫ was divided into two sub-categories: < anatomical physiological function > and < mobility function >. These two sub-categories were divided into 21 lower categories: [muscle], [range of motion], [sensory], [reflex], [clonus], [spasticity], [skin], [motion direction], [alignment], [clearance], [falling tendency], [safety], [stability], [grounding status], [total stance time], [timing], [training], [weighted center], [motion progression], [separability], [inertia force].

3.1   Region

There were 551 meanings units referring to <<region>> among the 716 total meaning units. In the subcategories, 354 meaning units arose for <lower limbs>, the most of all subcategories. Next was 106 meaning units for <trunk>. The least-mentioned subcategory was <pelvis> with 31 units. In the lower category level of <<region>>, 149 meaning units were extracted for [hip joints], which got the most mentions. Next was 115 units for [knee joint]. The least mentioned lower category was [shoulder joints] with 5 units.

As for the meaning units on the PT level, 164 meaning units arose for PT1, 138 for PT2, and 251 units for PT3 (Table 7). On the PT level, the meaning units referring to <lower limbs> got the most mentions. On an individual basis, PT2 made more mention of [trunk] and [knee joints] than [hip joint]. The results for PT1 and PT2 were different.

Table 7. Total Number of Meaning Units for Region (Per PT)

	PT1	PT2	PT3
Upper limbs	14	20	26
Trunk	26	33	47
Pelvis	12	9	10
Entire lower limbs	14	9	19
Hip joint	56	20	73
Knee joints	35	32	48
Ankle joints	7	13	28

3.2   Time

Of the 716 total meaning units, 215 referred to <<time>>. In the sub-categories, there were 164 meaning units for <stance phase> and 51 units for <swing phase>. In the lower category level of <<time>>, there were 74 meaning units for [total stance], which got the most mentions. Next was 41 units for [total swing]. And the least mentioned categories were 5 units for [initial swing] and [terminal swing], respectively.

On the PT level, 81 meaning units arose for PT1, 40 units for PT2 and 94 units for PT3 (Table 8). The meaning units referring to [total stance] got the most mentions on the PT level as well. For individual analysis, 32 meaning units referred to <swing phase> arose for PT3, which was more than the 8 units for PT1 and 11 units for PT2.

Table 8. Total Number of Meaning Units for Time (Per PT)

	PT1	PT2	PT3
Total swing	8	6	27
Initial swing	0	5	0
Terminal swing	0	0	5
Total stance	26	7	41
Initial stance	3	4	8
Mid stance	29	3	3
Terminal stance	15	15	10

3.3   Function

Of the 716 total meaning units, 503 referred to <<function>>. In the sub-categories, <mobility function> received the most mentions, 338, followed by 165 for <anatomical physiological function>. In the lower categories for <<function>>, the meaning units for [motion detection] had the most mentions, at 160, Next was 102 meaning units for [muscle]. The least mentioned categories were [sense], [clonus] and [inertia force] with 2 meaning units.

On the PT level, 166 meaning units arose for PT1, 117 units for PT2 and 220 units for PT3 (Table 9). <Physical function> got the most mentions on PT level as well. On an individual basis, PT3 mentioned [muscle] more than [motion direction], which showed the different tendency when compared to PT1 and PT2.

Table 9. Total Number of Meaning Units for Function (Per PT)

	PT1	PT2	PT3
Muscle	17	18	67
Motion range of joints	15	14	14
Reflex	0	0	10
Motion direction	64	48	48
Alignment	23	15	40
Clearance	6	1	7
Weighted center	9	9	4

3.4   Correlation between Region and Time

Of the 716 total meaning units. 166 referred to <<region>> and <<time>>. The distribution of all meaning units is shown in table 10. In the sub-categories, the meaning units referring to <lower limbs> x<stance phase> counted for 103, which got the most mentions. The meaning units referring to <pelvis>x<stance phase>, or <upper limbs>x<swing phase> were the least mentioned, accounting for 2-3 mentions.

On the PT level, 63 meaning units arose for PT1, 30 units for PT2 and 73 units for PT3. The results were similar in that the meaning units referring to <lower limbs>x<stance phase> were mentioned most on the PT level as well. Also the meaning units referring to <pelvis>x<swing phase>, and <upper limbs>x<stance phase> were least mentioned. On an individual basis, 27 meaning units arose for <upper limbs>x<swing phase> and <lower limbs>x <swing phase> for PT3, which was more than the 7 for PT1 and 9 for PT2.

Table 10. Total Number of Meaning Units Referring to Region and Time

	Swing phase	Stance phase
Upper limbs	3	6
Trunk	4	12
Pelvis	9	2
Lower limbs	27	103

3.5   Correlation between Region and Function

Of the 716 total meaning units, 473 referred to <<region>> and <<function>>. Distribution of all meaning units is shown in table 11. In the sub-categories, the meaning units referring to <lower limbs>x<mobility function> got the most mentions with 208. The meaning units referring to <upper limbs>x<anatomical physiological function>

and <pelvis>x<anatomical physiological function> got the fewest mentions with 8 and 7, respectively.

On the PT level, 150 meaning units arose for PT1, 114 units for PT2 and 209 units for PT3. The meaning units referring to <lower limbs>x<mobility function> got the most mentions on the PT level as well. Only a few meaning units referred to <upper limbs>x<anatomical physiological function> and <pelvis>x<anatomical physiological function>.

Table 11. Total Number of Meaning Units Referring to Region and Function

	Anatomical physiological function	Mobility function
Upper limbs	8	14
Trunk	36	62
Pelvis	7	24
Lower limbs	114	208

3.6   Correlation between Time and Function

Of the 716 total meaning units, 179 meaning units referred to <<time>> and <<function>>. Distribution of all meaning units is shown in table 12. In the sub-categories, <stance phase>x<mobility function> got the most mentions with 125. The least mentioned subcategory, with 7 meaning units, was <swing phase>x<anatomical physiological function>.

On the PT level, 74 meaning units arose for PT1, 31 units for PT2 and 74 units for PT3. Similarly, high distribution was observed for <stance phase>x<mobility function>. On an individual basis, 23 meaning units arose for <swing phase>x<anatomical physiological function> and <swing phase>x<mobility function> for PT3, which was more than the 8 units for PT1 and 9 units for PT2.

Table 12. Total Number of Meaning Units Referring to Time and Function

	Anatomical physiological function	Mobility function
Swing phase	7	33
Stance phase	14	125

4   Discussion

In this study, we showed a video with five samples of patients walking to three practicing PTs. We used a one-on-one semi-structured interview to investigate how the PTs would predict problems and plan treatment programs based on what they observed in the video, and then we analyzed the results. The categories that arose, the number of meaning units and their distribution are discussed below.

The interview lasted 55 to 66 minutes for all five cases. No significant time difference was observed in each PT, even considering that the interview investigator had adjusted time. However, PT1 subjected 226 of the 716 total meaning units to analysis, compared with, 182 for PT2 and 306 for PT3. Significant differences were observed from PT to PT. Moreover, in the category <<region>> and subcategory [hip joints], 149 meaning units, the most in all categories, arose. 56 meaning units arose for PT1, 20 units for PT2 and 73 units. That figure for PT3 was almost a majority. Significant differences were observed from PT to PT. We continued to consider the category of [hip joint], which got the most meaning units from PT3.

Looking at the correlation between region x time for [hip joints] per PT, the distribution for PT1 was 1 for [swing], 9 for [stance], 3 for [initial stance], 11 for [mid stance], and 2 for [terminal stance]. The distribution for PT2 was 2 for [stance], 1 for [initial stance] and 2 for [terminal stance]. Neither PT mentioned [swing] and [mid stance], which are in the lower category of [hip joints]. The distribution for PT3 was 9 for [swing], 12 for [stance], 2 for [initial stance], 1 for [mid stance], 2 for [terminal stance]. In comparison with the other two PTs, the meaning units extracted for [swing] were decidedly more. For [swing], PT3 had 9 meaning units, while PT1 had only 1 and PT2 had none. Some of the comments referring to [swing] included, "What I am concerned about is that the flexion of hip joint hardly seems troubled when swinging out the right leg." or "If a patient can smoothly swing out his left leg, he can sustain his left lower limb by left hip joint adduction". The PT carefully observed not only [stance], [initial stance], [terminal stance] of [hip joint], but also [swing]. This indicates that their scope of observation had widened.

Looking at the correlation of region x function for [hip joint] per PT, the distribution for PT1 showed 7 for [muscle], 9 for [range of motion], 25 for [motion direction], 6 for [alignment], 1 for [clearance], 5 for [training] and 1 for [motion progression]. For PT2, there were 6 for [muscle], 4 for [range of motion], 7 for [motion direction], 1 for [alignment] and 1 for [weighted center]. No meaning units referred to [clearance], [training], [motion progression] in the lower category of [hip joint]. PT3 mentioned 28 for [muscle], 4 for [range of motion], 2 for [sensory], 15 for [motion direction], 13 for [alignment] and 5 for [stability]. In comparison with the other two PTs, he had more meaning units concerning [muscle], [motion direction] and [alignment].

Seven lower categories -- [initial stance], [initial stance], [terminal stance], [muscle], [range of motion], [alignment], [motion direction] -- were mentioned by all three PTs. When observing the motion of the hip joint, these seven categories mentioned have high objectivity as observation viewpoints. Each PT carefully observed [stance], requiring more resistance ability in walking motion compared to [swing], the activity of [muscle] around the hip joint such as the gluteus maximus muscle and the gluteus medius, flexion and extension of the hip joint, and [range of motion] and [motion direction] including internal/external rotation, adduction and abduction.

In the lower categories, no commonalities were observed among the three PTs. The meaning unit referring to [training] arose for PT1. Comments included, "Conduct training to change the motion from flexion to extension of hip joint", and "Incorporate training for one-leg support such as bridge motion by one leg". For the treatment program, she selected [training] as a necessary method upon considering [muscle] or [motion direction] of the [hip joint]. Meaning units referring to [stability] and [sense] arose for PT3. Sample comment for [stability] were, "The stability of hip joint is low" and "Take an approach to stabilize hip joint" These statements indicated that they were observing joint stability based on their observation of [hip joint] muscles, [motion direction] and [alignment]. Sample comments related to [sensory] included, "Sensory of hip joint is low" and "It is important to be conscious of hip joint". These statements indicated that they were conducting motion observation for [sensory] upon considering the [muscle] of [hip joint], [range of motion], [motion direction] and [alignment].

5   Conclusion

Since the distribution of meaning units in these categories resulted from interviews of PTs about their thinking processes after observing patients walking, the appearances of the main categories such as <<region>> and <<function>> were predictable. Moreover, the patients who participated in this study have in total one case of hip joint disease (femoral diaphyseal fracture), 2 cases of knee-joint disease (osteoarthritis, knee-joint intraarticular fracture) and 2 cases of (ossification of posterior longitudinal ligament, spondylosis deformans), it was predictable that the meaning units referring to [hip joint], [knee joints] and [trunk] occupied the top ranks in the lower category of <<region>>. However, evaluating the distribution of meaning units in this category using charts is a novel approach. The quantitative research for motion observation has been scattered to some extent, and no study was found to capture qualitative data as quantitative data when it comes to motion observation analysis. Therefore, we obtained qualitative data from interviews and charted them as quantitative data for analysis, which is a new approach for motion observation.

Commonality in the low categories per each PT was clarified through charts. The charts also revealed the low categories with less commonality such as [training] for PT1, and [stability], [sense], [swing] for PT3. In the study of Brunnekreef 7), et al, they showed video of 30 patients with orthopedic disease to 10 PTs with different years of experience and had them fill in the structured form for walking analysis. Then they analyzed the intra-class and interobserver reliability, reporting that it was affected to a certain extent according to the clinical experience of the observer. This study also suggested the thinking process during motion observation differed according to years of experience. By increasing the scientific validity of this research, feedback was facilitated to confirm or compare with others during motion observation. With increasing scientific validity and facilitated feedback, this chart is useful for training inexperienced PTs or vocational training school students in motion observation.

The limitations of this study include the number of subjects, 3, and their years of experience, from 6 to 11. Also five people participated as walking models, so it is hard to draw out generalizations. We therefore, will increase the number of PT subjects and walking models in future studies, considering these steps necessary to increase scientific validity. Although the result of this study is insufficient, there was no study to chart qualitative data as quantitative data from motion observation for comparison and analysis. We believe the result of this study helps comprehend the thinking process of PTs during motion observation.

References

1. Shigeru, U., Eiki, T.: Scientific Verification of Exercise and Motion Analysis in Clinical. Physical Therapy 31(8), 483–488 (2004)
2. Tsutomu, F.: Clinical Movement Analysis and Kinetic Chain. Physical Therapy 36(8), 472–474 (2009)
3. Toshiaki, S., Takashi, N.: Motion Observation / Motion Analysis. Journal of Kansai Physical Therapy 3, 33–39 (2003)
4. Shuzou, B., Sumiko, Y.: Reliability and Accuracy of Observational Gait Analysis. Physical Therapy 23(6), 742–752 (2008)
5. MaGinly, J.L., Glodie, P.A., et al.: Accuracy and reliability of observational gait analysis data: Judgments of push-off in gait after stroke. Phys.Ther. 83, 146–160 (2003)
6. Yoichi, Y., Hitoshi, M.: Training Issues Arising from Physical Therapists' Self-recognition: A Survey of Physical Therapists Working in Medical Institutions. Physical Therapy 27(4), 385–389 (2012)
7. Brunnekreef, J.J., van Uden, C.J., et al.: Reliability of video-taped observational gait analysis in patients with orthopedic impairment. BMC Musculoskeletal Disorders 6(17), 1–9 (2005)

Motion Analysis of the Pounding Technique Used for the Second Lining in the Fabrication of Traditional Japanese Hanging Scrolls

Yasuhiro Oka[1,*], Akihiko Goto[2], Yuka Takai[2], Chieko Narita[3], and Hiroyuki Hamada[3]

[1] Oka Bokkodo Co., Ltd, East Asian art conservation, Kyoto, Japan
okayas@mac.com
[2] Osaka Sangyo University, Faculty of Design technology, Osaka, Japan
{gotoh,takai}@ise.osaka-sandai.ac.jp
[3] Kyoto Institute of Technology, Graduate School of Science and Technology, Kyoto, Japan
{hhamada10294,soy155apf}@gmail.com

Abstract. This study focuses on the technique used to adhere the second lining in the fabrication of traditional Japanese hanging scrolls, or *kakejiku*. We analyzed the motions of both expert and non-expert artisans during the adhesion process, using optical and infrared motion captures. We then conducted a peel test from both samples, and used the results of this test to correlate the motion of the artisan with the adhesive strength of the second lining.

Keywords: scrolls, secondary lining, pounding brush, motion analysis.

1 Introduction

Hanging scrolls are a traditional Japanese ornamental art, which can include paintings and calligraphy. Distinct from Western picture frames, scrolls have the unique ability to be unrolled and hung on a wall or in an alcove when displayed, and rolled up in a box for storage. Figure 1 shows an image of a hanging scroll on display in an alcove. This method has been recognized as a superior way to preserve paintings and calligraphy, because the works of art are better protected from light and air.

To allow each scroll to hang straight when displayed and roll smoothly for storage, four layers of paper, called "lining papers," are adhered with starch paste to the back of the scroll. The lining papers are typically numbered with the first lining paper pasted closest to the artwork, followed by the second, third, and final lining papers. In production, each lining paper is adhered to the back of a hanging scroll in a process called "pounding," with each step named with the layer of paper being adhered. This study focuses on the pounding of second lining.

The adhesive used for each layer of lining paper is made by heating wheat starch. The paste used for the first lining paper has strong adhesive properties, and is made by cooling the paste right after heating. For the second and subsequent layers, a

---

* Corresponding author.

V. G. Duffy (Ed.): DHM 2014, LNCS 8529, pp. 55–65, 2014.

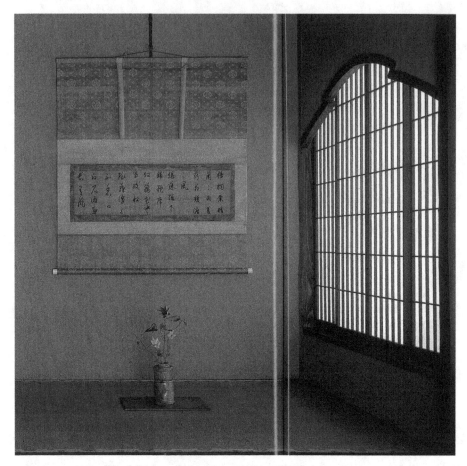

Fig. 1. Image of a hanging scroll on display in an alcove

special adhesive, known as aged paste is used. The aged paste is kept in a cool dark place, allowing the adhesive properties of the aged paste's to become weaker. Scroll makers then use a traditional technique of pounding the surface of each lining paper with a special "pounding brush" to provide better adhesion. The pounding brush has bristles made of hemp-palm fibers, and typically weighs about 460 grams. One such brush is shown in Figure 2.

After dilution, aged paste is applied to the second lining paper, which is then placed carefully on the back of the first lining paper. Care is taken to prevent any wrinkles from appearing. Once the second lining paper is in place, the surface of the paper is pounded with the bristles of the pounding brush.

During pounding, the bristles of hemp-palm make holes in the surface of the second-ary lining paper, penetrating to the first lining paper layer. This process allows the mul-berry paper fibers contained in the first lining paper to rise. These plant fibers tangle together with the fibers of the second lining paper, enhancing adhesion property of the aged paste. This adhesion mechanism is shown in the schematic diagram in Figure 3.

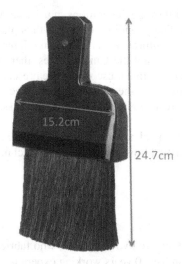

Fig. 2. Image and measurement of a pounding brush

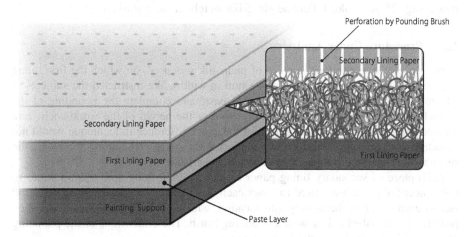

Fig. 3. Diagram of the adhesion mechanism between the first lining paper and secondary lining paper

If too much power is used during pounding, the bristles of the brush penetrate even the first lining paper and reach the art work beneath. In the worst case, it opens very small holes in the art work. However, using too little power out of caution, will not obtain the desired adhesive effect.

It is a simple operation to pound the surface of a lining paper with a brush, but to pass down the proper technique and control is a very difficult task. As with other traditional techniques, this technique has been passed down only through the observation of expert craftsmen.

Moreover, this pounding technique is considered indispensable for repairing valuable paintings or works declared to be cultural assets. A hanging scroll, which has been preserved and repaired through generations, must continue to remain a hanging scroll through many repairs. The pounding technique thus plays a pivotal role in protecting and restoring valuable cultural assets. As many Japanese and East Asian hanging scrolls are now in Europe and the United States, there has been a need to teach this technique in order to ensure that these works are preserved.

In this study, we analyzed the pounding technique of an expert and a non-expert and observed the correct traditional technique, passed down from craftsman to craftsman.

We also conducted a peel test on pounded samples of second lining paper from each craftsman and verified how proper pounding technique influences adhesiveness.

2   Method

2.1   Subjects

The subjects for this study are two craftsmen, who fabricate and repair hanging scrolls. The "expert" technician has 20 years working experience, (age 38 years, 171cm height, 72kg weight, male, right-handed), and the "non-expert" has four years working experience, (age 25 years old, 170cm height, 54kg weight, male, right-handed).

2.2   Procedure Under Analysis

In the place of a work of art, a piece of plain silk was used, on which the first lining was completed, (700mm in length x 400mm in width). We instructed the subjects to adhere the second lining paper using aged paste and complete the pounding of the second lining. If the weight or shape of a tool or the height of the workbench were diriated from normal, then comparison of the exact difference in technique would not be detected accurately. Therefore, we conducted the study in the workshop where the subjects work, using the same equipment and materials.

Each piece of secondary lining paper is about 150mm long and 700mm wide, so three pieces of paper were used to cover each sample. The subjects applied paste and placed each paper in the appropriate location, with no signs of wrinkles. They then pounded as described below with a pounding brush. The dimensions of the pounding brush used in this study are shown in Figure 2.

Both subjects started pounding from the right near side, gradually moving the brush away from their body until they reached the far side. They continued pounding evenly, progressing to the left side, and then slowly moving back to the right side. The track of the brush movement is shown in the schematic diagram in Figure 4.

To cover the entire surface shown in gray in Figure 4, the craftsmen pounded from the near right corner to the near left corner in the course indicated by the solid line ①, completing the first process. While pounding in the opposite direction, as indicated by the dotted line ②, each subject returned to the starting location. Finally, as represented by line ③, they pounded in the same direction as ①, finishing in the near left corner. Thus, they completed the pounding technique for the second lining in one and a half circuits of the paper.

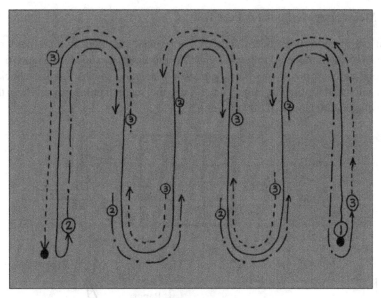

Fig. 4. Diagram of the progession of the pounding brush

2.3   Measuring Conditions for Motion Analysis

The poundings executed by the subjects were recorded by two digital cameras. One real-time optical motion capture system (MAC 3D SYSTEM, Motion Analysis Corporation) and six infrared cameras (Raptor-H, Motion Analysis Corporation) were used. For behavior analysis, infrared reflective markers were attached on both shoulders, elbows, and wrists of the subjects, and on the handle of the pounding brush. The sampling rate was set at 120Hz. The subjects applied aged paste to the second lining paper on the pasting board, placing it carefully on the samples prepared with the first lining paper. The samples were then pounded to enhance the adhesion of the paste. We measured the movements during pounding using the attached markers, as shown in Figure 5.

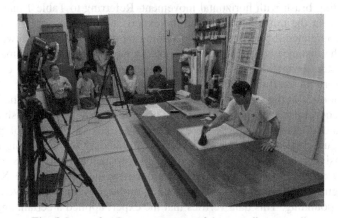

Fig. 5. Image for the measurement of the pounding process

2.4   Measuring Methods for Peel Test

We cut out three vertical pieces and three horizontal pieces from three parts of each sample, with each piece 20 mm wide and 200 mm long, as shown in Figure 6. 10mm at the end of each piece was then dipped in water and pinched in the chuck of an Instron universal testing machine, set to peel the second lining paper from the silk sample at a peeling speed of 300 mm/min.

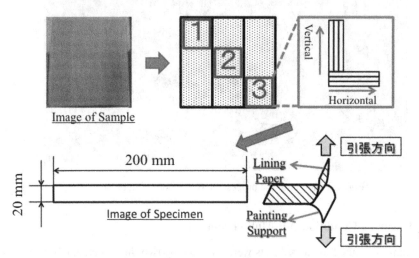

Fig. 6. Procedure of the peeling test

2.5   Results and Discussion

First, we focused on the track of the marker attached to the handle of the pounding brush. We extracted the track of the marker for one row of pounding for both craftsmen, as shown in Figure 7. While the non-expert seemed to proceed by simply moving the pounding brush up and down, the expert combined the vertical movement of the pounding brush with horizontal movement. Referring to Table 1 and Figure 7, the difference in the movement between the expert and the non-expert can be seen. The expert completed the second lining pounding more quickly and in fewer pounds. Measuring the distance between pounded spots by the movement of the markers, we verified that the expert had wider spacing. This result suggests that the expert conducted the work more efficiently than the non-expert.

We then looked at the track of the markers attached to the handle of the brush using an X-Y coordinate grid. This allows us to observe the track of the brush handle as seen from above. As in Figure 7, we extracted the track of one row of pounding, shown in Figure 8. We found that the expert was pounding while rotating the brush handle extensively, where the non-expert did not show such extensive movement.

We also extracted one row of movements done by the expert in the X-Z plane, shown in Figure 9. This corresponds to the track of the movement observed from the front during pounding. This data verifies that the expert applied a certain angle to the brush while pounding.

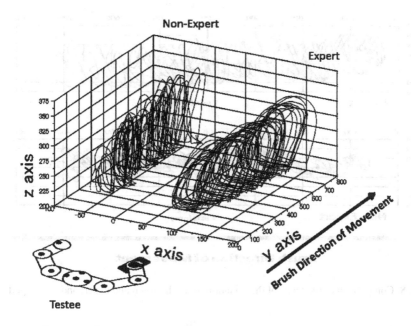

Fig. 7. Comparison of brush movement between the expert and non-expert

Table 1. Comparison of "working time", "pound number", and "interval of pound" between expert and non-expert

	Working Time (sec)	Pound Number	Interval of Pound (mm)
Expert	451	1120	25.1±9.9
Non-Expert	603	1358	18.0±9.0

The reason that the expert tilted the brush while pounding has to do with the shape of the trimmed bristles of the brush. In the manufacturing process, the bristles of the pounding brush are tied by a paper band a few centimeters from the tip of the brush and trimmed. When opening the paper band for regular work, the bristles are curved, as shown in the diagram in Figure 10. This curved shape makes it ideal to incline the brush and pound at an angle, instead of swinging the brush down perpendicular to the surface.

By using the brush at an angle, the craftsman is able to take advantage of the large surface area of the bristles, preventing the brush from hitting the paper's surface more strongly than necessary. This is one aspect of the traditional technique that is explicitly shared with non-experts. As the track in Figure 9 shows, the expert practiced this behavior to reduce the risk of bristles passing through the first lining paper to the silk beneath.

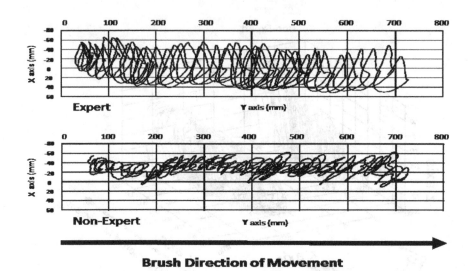

Fig. 8. Comparison of the locus of the pounding brush between and expert and non-expert

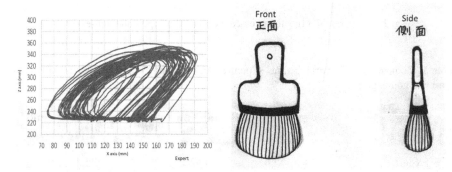

Fig. 9. Expert's locus of the pounding brush shape

Fig. 10. Diagram of the pounding brush bristle

Figure 11 shows the movement of the markers attached to the brush handle in the non-expert's work. It suggests that the non-expert was also attempting to apply a certain angle to the brush at the time of pounding. However, the angle was so shallow that the brush was almost in the upright position. The data also suggests that the angle of pounding was not constant. In order for a scroll to hang straight, the adhesion must be even across the back of the scroll. This reveals a significant difference in the pounding techniques between the two craftsmen.

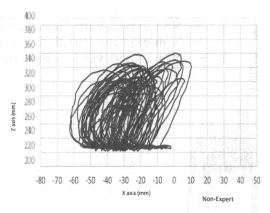

Fig. 11. Non-expert's locus of the pounding brush (X-Z)

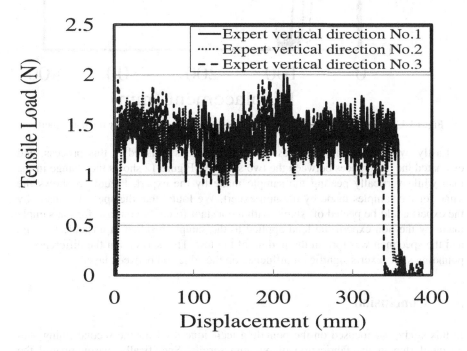

Fig. 12. Change in the load while vertically peeling the sample made by the expert

Comparing figures 9 and 11, it is obvious that there were differences in the angle of the brush during pounding. The expert tilted the brush to a greater degree, which enabled him to pound a larger area than the non-expert each pound.

As the results in Table 1 suggested, this increase in surface area leads the expert's shorter work time and fewer pounds. Similarly, the increased surface area of each pound caused by pounding at an angle would contribute to the expert's wider distance between pounding spots compared to the non-expert.

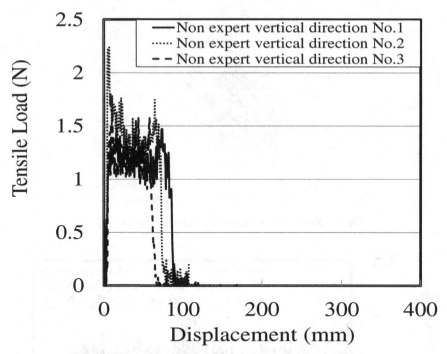

Fig. 13. Change in the load while vertically peeling the sample made by the non-expert

Lastly, we conducted a peel test on the specimens finished in this process, and evaluated the differences between the two samples. Figure 12 shows the change in the load while vertically peeling the sample made by the expert. Figure 13 shows the same for the samples made by the non-expert. We found that the specimen made by the expert could be peeled off stably with a constant force. In contrast, for the sample made by the non-expert, the load applied to the sample resulted in unstable peeling, and the specimen was torn in the middle of the test. This shows that the difference in pounding skills exerts significant influence on the adhesion between layers.

3   Conclusion

In this study, we focused on the pounding technique used for the second lining—an essential step in the fabrication of hanging scrolls. Specifically, we compared the pounding technique performed by an expert craftsman and a non-expert. As a result, we found that the expert was practicing the traditional method of pounding the brush at an angle, which has been passed down through the ages. This element was not clearly observed in the non-expert's technique. The peel test revealed an obvious difference in the adhesion status of the samples taken. The sample made by the expert could be peeled off with stable force, and adhesion was less uneven when compared to the sample made by the non-expert.

Our behavior analysis revealed that correct pounding technique is strongly correlated with stronger adhesion.

References

1. Nishikawa, K.: Science of Japanese Painting Frame – Special Research "Scientific Research for Preservation and Restoration of Japanese Hanging Scroll". National Research Institute for Cultural Properties, Tokyo (1977)
2. Hayakawa, N., Kigawa, R., Kawanobe, W., Higuchi, H., Oka, Y., Oka, I.: Basic Research of "Aged Paste" (Furunori) –Traditional Japanese Restoration Material – by GPC and HPLC for Organic Acid Analysis. Science for Conservation 41, 15–28 (2002)
3. Hayakawa, N., Kimijima, T., Kusunoki, K., Oka, Y.: The Adhesive Effect of Uchibake (Beating Brush) in Japanese Paper Conservation. Science for Conservation 43, 9–16 (2004)

Analysis of Expert Skills on Handheld Grinding Work for Metallographic Sample

Takuya Sugimoto[1,*], Hisanori Yuminaga[2], and Akihiko Goto[3]

[1] KOYO Netsuren Corporation, Kyoto, Japan
t-sugi@koyo-kinzoku.com
[2] Kansai Vocational College of Medicine, Osaka, Japan
yuminaga@kansai.ac.jp
[3] Osaka Sangyo University, Osaka, Japan
gotoh@ise.osaka-sandai.ac.jp

Abstract. Most common heat treatment process for hardening ferrous alloy is known as carburizing. The quality assurance of carburizing process requires metallographic analysis of case depth, retained austenite, intergranular oxidation, and carbide network by means of metallographic sample. Metallographic preparation consists of sectioning, mounting, plane grinding, polishing to mirror surface, and etching. It is difficult for non-expert to prepare metallographic sample with global mirror surface because preparation skill needs long time experience in this field. There is no study on expert skills in preparation of metallographic samples. In this study, the difference of handheld plane grinding motion of metallographic specimen between expert and non-expert execution was analyzed. For this clarification, an electromyogram (EMG) of the muscle activities between expert and non-expert were investigated. As a result of investigation, we found the clear difference in the muscle activities of triceps, flexor digitorum superficialis, and abductor pollicis brevis between expert and other subjects.

Keywords: grinding, polishing, emg, metallographic preparation.

1 Introduction

Carburizing increases strength and wear resistance by diffusing carbon into the surface of the steel creating a substantially lesser hardness in the core. This treatment is applied to low carbon steels after machining. Usually one or more test specimens used for quality assurance accompany with the heat treatment lot. The quality assurance of carburizing process requires metallographic analysis of case depth, retained austenite, intergranular oxidation, and carbide network with an optical microscope at x 100-1000 magnification by means of the metallographic mounted sample made by the above test specimen.

The preparation process of such metallographic mounted sample is very important for the quality assurance of carburizing process. If the sample edge rounded during the preparation, accurate microstructural information needed for subsurface inspection

---

* Corresponding author.

V. G. Duffy (Ed.): DHM 2014, LNCS 8529, pp. 66–77, 2014.

cannot be obtained. Then, it leads the wasting time and money because the re-preparation of metallographic sample is required.

Fig. 1 shows the preparation process of metallographic sample. First, a section is cut perpendicularly from the surface measurement location of the specimen. Second, the obtained specimen was hot-mounted with epoxy resin and then ground by SiC coarse papers with hand to acquire plane surface. Step-wise grinding was then performed in order to produce a flat surface, followed by refined abrasive polishing, to obtain a mirror finish surface by semi-automated polishing machine.

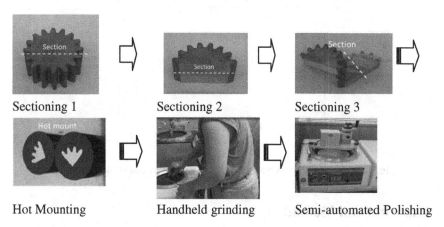

Sectioning 1   Sectioning 2   Sectioning 3

Hot Mounting   Handheld grinding   Semi-automated Polishing

Fig. 1. Preparation process for metallographic sample

The process for the grinding and polishing process is standardized [1]. Polishing techniques for the thermal spray coating is analyzed [2]. Many techniques for polishing process of metallographic process is contained in the technical documents [3-4]. However, most studies have not focused on the expert skills of grinding and polishing process. In fact, the surface finish of metallographic sample differs between expert and non-expert preparation. The resulting measurements of the surface roughness for ground surfaces are shown in Figure 2. Measurements were performed by Surface measurement equipment (Tokyo seimitsu, SJ-301). Rt is Sum of height of the largest profile peak height Rp and the largest profile valley Rv within an evaluation length. The mean of Rt on each gear teeth by the expert was better than that by the non-expert 1, non-expert 2, and beginner. The deviation of Rt by the expert was also better than that by the non-expert 1, non-expert 2, and beginner.

The ground surfaces of the specimen prepared by the expert were more horizontal and more uniform in roughness, making them more ideal. This quantitatively verified the expert's superior grinding technique, although his skill has been well known to his colleagues for some time.

For the efficient transfer of the skills from expert to non-expert, it is necessary to compare and clarify the difference between the expert and non-expert execution. Comparison of the motion between expert and non-expert is commonly used for the development program for beginner and non-expert.

In this study, we compared and analyzed the differences in hand-held grinding motion and muscular activity for all subjects during the grinding procedure. Motion during the grinding process was measured by electromyography (EMG), and the EMG activity of the upper limb on the dominant arm holding the abrasive was recorded. We then evaluated the differences in grinding motion and muscular activity using the data collected. We hope that this study's results will serve as a useful educational reference for the technical development of metallography technicians.

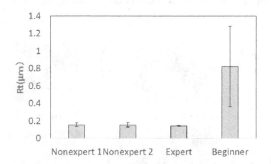

Fig. 2. Surface roughness on final surface finish between subjects

2   Experimental Method

2.1   Subjects

Subjects were 4 males having 20 (Expert), 5(Non-expert 1), 2(Non-expert 2), and 0 (Beginner) year experience in handheld grinding operations respectively.

2.2   Samples to be Ground

Carburized gears for an aircraft component part which is made of 9310 Steel NiCr–Mo alloy (AMS6265) were used as the sample to be ground and polished. These gears were normalized, tempered, carburized, hardened, subzero cooled, and final tempered in the same heat treatment lot. After heat treatment, the specimens were cut into quarters of a gear consisting of four teeth, then hot mounted with epoxy (Durofast, Struers, an epoxy resin with high content of mineral and glass filler).

2.3   Grinding Machine

One grinding machine (Refine Tec Ltd, STO-228B) was used for the experiment. This machine has one rotating table. This grinding machine is usually used for the preparation of metallographic specimens by the subjects. The grit P120 SiC abrasive which was usually used for plane grinding process of carburized gear sample was used for the experiment.

2.4   Motion Analysis Method

To analyze each technician's technique, each subject grasped a specimen for metallographic examination and pressed it down on a rotating disk (300rpm) to grind the surface of the specimen. The activity of the upper limb on the subject's dominant side, which operated the grinder, was recorded from a side view using a digital video camera (HC-V520M, Panasonic) for analysis. In order to measure actual motions and muscle activities during the grinding process, we carried out the recording in synchronization with the EMG and behavior measurements.

2.5   Electromyographic Measurement System

Electromyography analysis was conducted using an EMG multi-channel telemeter system WEB-1000 (NIHON KOHDEN CORPORATION). The sampling frequency rate was fixed at 1000Hz and the data loaded into computer via A/D converter for analysis. In order to evaluate the relationship between hand and upper limb while holding a metallographic sample, we attached EMG markers at eight positions: on the middle fibers of the deltoid (D), the pectoralis major (PM), the biceps brachii (BB), the triceps brachii (T), the extensor carpi radialis brevis (ECRB), the flexor digitorum superficialis (FDS), the abductor pollicis brevis (APB), and the 1st dorsales interossei muscles (1/D) as shown in figure 3. The grinding motion, conducted in 5 seconds for three times, was subject to EMG waveform analysis.

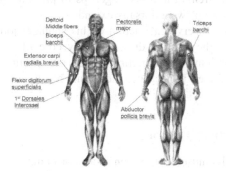

Fig. 3. The measured muscle

2.6   Data Analysis

Average Rectified Value of EMG (mVsec) during the three plane grinding motions for 5 seconds was calculated. The above mean value (mVsec) was divided by the EMG value (mVsec) corresponding to each muscle during the rest on each subject.

3   Results

3.1   Characteristics in Motions

During the expert technician's session, the movements of the elbow joint, figure joints and maniphalanx were hardly seen against the rotational force of the disc while he was grinding the specimen under the rotational load of the grinding disc. Slight adduction and abduction on the shoulder joints was observed, but his upper limb was generally stabilized. His hand and maniphalanx were in the functional positions of the intrinsic muscles. He grasped the metallographic specimen at four points, using his thumb, index finger, middle finger and ring finger to press down on the rotating disk. As to the details of each finger position when holding the specimen, the CM joint on thumb was in the palmar abduction position, the MP and IP joints were extended, the MP joint on the index finger was flexed, the PIP joint was slightly flexed, and DIP joint was extended. The MP joint of the middle finger was slightly extended, and the PIP and DIP joints were slightly flexed.

For non-expert subject 1, we observed adduction and abduction on the shoulder joint. His elbow joint flexed and fluctuated widely. As he put strength into his fingertips to press the specimen against the rotating disk, his finger joints were dorsally extended.

For non-expert subject 2, we observed only abduction on the shoulder joint. When he pressed down the specimen on the rotating disk, his body core tilted and his elbow joint flexed. As he put strength into his fingertips to press the specimen against the rotating disk, his finger joints were dorsally extended.

For the beginner, we observed abduction on his shoulder joint. When he pressed down the specimen on the rotating disk, his body core tilted and his elbow joint flexed. As he put strength into his fingertips to press the specimen against the rotating disk, his elbow and finger joints fluctuated, and his finger joints were dorsally extended.

3.2   The Muscle Activity Pattern

Figure 4 shows the EMG muscle activity on each subject during grinding motion.

Deltoid. We observed an increase in D muscular activity for non-expert 1, which was sustained throughout the trial. Non-expert 2 showed a slight increasing and decreasing pattern, although his rate of increase in muscular activity was lower than non-expert 1. The muscular activity of the expert showed a constant pattern, which was lower than other subjects. The beginner showed a constant muscular activity pattern, but it tended to increase slightly more than the expert's did.

Pectoralis Major. All subjects except the beginner displayed a constant pattern without increase in activity. The beginner showed a constant pattern.

Biceps Brachii. Non-expert 1 showed a constant pattern. Non-expert 2 showed an unstable pattern with high activity. The expert showed a stable pattern without increase in activity. The beginner displayed a pattern with high activity similar to non-expert 2.

Triceps Brachii. Non-expert 1 displayed an unstable pattern with increases in activity. Non-expert 2 showed a pattern with decreasing activity in the first half, and increasing activity in the last half. The expert showed a constantly active pattern. The beginner showed no increase in activity.

Extensor Carpi Radialis Brevis. Non-expert 1 showed a constant pattern of high activity. Non-expert 2 showed a decrease in activity in the first half, an increase in activity in the middle, and a final decrease at the end of the trial. The expert showed a stable pattern without increase in activity. The beginner showed a constantly increasing pattern, similar to that displayed by non-expert 2.

Flexor Digitorum Superficialis. Non-expert 1 showed a constant pattern. Non-expert 2 showed a gradually increasing pattern but without significant increase in activity. The expert showed a stable and constant pattern. The beginner displayed a pattern of slight increases, but not to the same extent as the other subjects.

1st Dorales Interossei Muscle. Non-expert 1 showed an unstable pattern in muscular activity, which fluctuated slightly. Non-expert 2 showed a decrease in activity in the first half, an increase in activity in the middle, and a final decrease at the end of the trial. The expert showed a stable pattern without significant increase in activity. The beginner showed a constantly active pattern without significant increase in activity.

Abductor Pollicis Brevis. Non-expert 1 showed a pattern with increasing activity at the beginning of operation and decreasing activity during operation. Non-expert 2 showed a constant pattern without increase in activity. The expert showed a significant increase in activity at the beginning of operation, and then a decrease in activity. The increase in activity was higher for the expert than for other subjects. The beginner's pattern decreased at first and then stabilized.

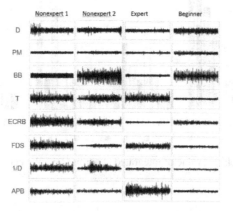

Fig. 4. The EMG during Grinding motion

3.3   Muscle Activity Relative Value

In order to calculate the amount of muscular activity during grinding, we assumed an EMG integrated value of each muscle at rest in a sitting position as 100%. The measurements described below are relative to this baseline, and are calculated using the EMG readings for each subject to allow us to compare the amount of muscular activity more easily. (Figure 5).

In non-expert 1, we observed the following levels of muscular activity. 119% for D, 158% for PM, 309% for BB, 1002% for T, 881% for ECRB, 1099% for FDS, 1479% for 1/D, and 1296% for APB. Non-expert 1 also showed a slightly increase in muscle activity for the D, PM and BB. However, he showed a significant increase in muscular activity for the T, ECRB, FDS, 1/D, and APB.

In non-expert 2, we observed the following levels of muscular activity. 232% for D, 237% for PM, 371% for BB, 666% for T, 331% for ECRB, 479% for FDS, 719% for 1/D, and 270% for APB. He showed a tendency towards increased activity in each muscle when compared to his resting state, especially for the T and 1/D.

In the expert technician, we observed the following levels of muscular activity. 113% for D, 111% for PM, 121% for BB, 419% for T, 132% for ECRB, 1083% for FDS, 330% for 1/D, and 1240% for APB. Compared to other subjects, the expert displayed less muscular activity for the D, PM, BB and ECRB. More significant increases in activity were observed for the FDS and APB. We also observed a tendency towards increased activity for the T, but it was less than the increases shown for the FDS and APB.

The beginner displayed the following levels of muscular activity. 174% for D, 200% for PM, 312% for BB, 203% for T, 343% for ECRB, 414% for FDS, 704% for 1/D and 340% for APB. Only the 1/D muscle showed an increase in activity, and the increased activity levels of other muscles were generally lower than other subjects.

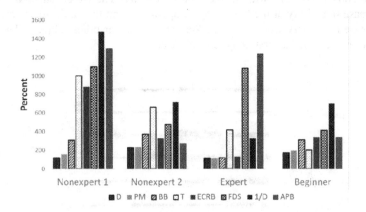

Fig. 5. The relative value of integrated electromyography between subjects

3.4 The Average EMG during Grinding Motion

The muscular activity of each subject was observed for the duration of the grinding operation. The data was normalized with the time axis at 100% and smoothed for comparison analysis as shown in Figure 6.

Deltoid. The data for the expert was more consistent, and shows a significantly low value compared to the other subjects. Both non-experts 1 and 2 showed unstable activity, which did not indicate a consistent value.

Pectoralis Major. All subjects exhibited similar values. However, the values for the expert and non-expert 1 were more stable and consistent than the values for non-expert 2 and the beginner.

Biceps Brachii. The expert's readings showed a constant and stable level of activity, which was significantly lower than other subjects'. Non-expert 1 and the beginner showed more activity in comparison with the expert, while non-expert 2 showed inconstant and unstable levels.

Triceps Brachii. The expert displayed a consistent and stable level of activity. Non-expert 1 has similar data to the expert, while non-expert 2 had a more inconsistent and unstable level of activity. The beginner had the lowest level of activity.

Extensor Carpi Radialis Brevis. The expert showed a constant and significantly low level of activity. The beginner showed a tendency towards increase compared to the expert. Non-expert 1 showed inconstant and unstable activity. Non-expert 2 showed a significant increase in activity compared to other subjects.

Flexor Digitorum Superficialis. The expert showed a stable and increased level of activity compared to the non-experts and the beginner. Non-expert 1 showed a greater increase in activity than other subjects.

Interossei Dorsales Muscle. The expert showed a low level of activity, as did the beginner. Non-expert 1 showed a high level of activity. Non-expert 2 was unstable, shifting from low to high levels of activity.

Abductor Pollicis Brevis. The expert showed a significant increase in activity compared to other subjects. He showed an increase in activity at the beginning of operation and a slight decrease just before the end of operation. The other subjects showed similarly low rates, but unlike the expert, they showed a more constant level of activity.

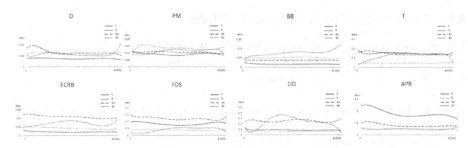

Fig. 6. The average EMG on each muscle during Grinding motion

Based on the analysis of the expert, we observed a constant increase in activity for the T, FDS and APB. The other muscles sustained constant activity without any significant increase. In contrast, non-expert 1 showed a difference in muscular activity patterns for the BB, D, T, ECRB, FDS and 1/D. He showed unstable activity patterns for the D, BB, ECRB, FDS and 1/D, while the expert showed a constant pattern in these muscles' activities. Although non-expert 1 showed no significant increase in activity for the APB, the expert showed a significant increase in activity, totally opposite the result from non-expert 1.

Non-expert 2 showed a slightly increasing tendency in muscle activity for the T, ECRB, FDS and 1/D. He showed a significant increase in activity for the BB, but no increase in activity for the APB. These results were also different from the expert. The BB and T, which provide for elbow joint movement, moved simultaneously. The muscles related to the finger joints and maniphalanx showed changes in activity different to the expert's pattern. The beginner showed an increase in muscular activity of the D and BB. This pattern was not observed for the expert.

As the results shows, the muscle activities of elbow joints, finger joints and maniphalanx of the expert showed a reciprocal relationship of agonist muscle and antagonist muscle. The data verified that his muscular activity pattern included no simultaneous activity resembling that observed in the other subjects. The activity patterns observed in other subjects differed significantly from that of the expert. The muscular activity of the expert for the BB and APB showed a definite difference compared to the other subjects.

4   Discussions

Compared to the other subjects, the expert's patterns displayed certain significant characteristics. The characteristics observed involved the T functioning as the extension muscle of the elbow joints, the FDS functioning to manipulate the finger joints and maniphalanx, and the abductor pollicis brevis influencing the maniphalanx. Those muscles related to the maniphalanx, elbow joints and finger joints were well coordinated, with balanced activity of the agonist muscle and antagonist muscle. Similarly to the T, the APB showed an increase in activity. We suggest that the muscular activity of the T increased so strongly because the expert strongly grasped the specimen to stabilize it and press it down on the rotating disk.With regards to the ECRB and FDS, the activity of the ECRB decreased, but the activity of the FDS increased. It is suggested that these muscles provide a strong grasp of the specimen and stabilize the subject's grip. These muscles also work to stabilize the finger joints in volar flexion. Grasping an object mainly uses the intrinsic muscles, including the interossei and lumbricales. When more strength is required, extrinsic muscles provide further stability for the maniphalanx. The result suggests that the FDS showed more activity when strong force was required to press the specimen down on the rotating disc.

To press the specimen effectively, the finger joints are set in the volar flexion position to activate the intrinsic muscles. This is known as Tenodesis grasp. Therefore, we observed increases in the activity patterns of the volar flexion muscles of the finger joints, including the flexor digitorum superficialis, and decreases in the muscular activity patterns for the finger joints and dorsal extension muscles, including the ECRB. This reciprocal relationship can be acknowledged for the 1/D and APB. Since the 1/D affects the MP joints in flexion position and the PIP and DIP joints in extension position, we expected an increase in the activity patterns in this study, but activity actually decreased, contrary to our expectations. This suggests that the thumb functions more than the index finger when grasping a specimen. While pressing the specimen down on the grinding disk, both muscles were activated. However, it was presumed that the expert took advantage of the thumb to stabilize and pressed down strongly. The 1/D functions in regular grasping motions, which accounts for the increase in 1/D activity observed for other subjects, but the expert took advantage of the function of APB to provide a more effective grasp. One more difference observed was that the expert showed no function of the BB compared to other subjects. This was greatly different from the other subjects. Since the other subjects held the scapulohumeral joints in the abduction position, when their upper limb was pulled in the abduction direction by the rotating force of the grinding disc, they attempted to use the BB to hold their elbow joints in the flexion position.

Moreover, the expert showed a low activity rate for deltoid-related shoulder joints in comparison with the other subjects. This suggests that the expert pressed the specimen down on the grinding disc using only his elbow joints, finger joints and maniphalanx, without fixing his shoulder joints. In comparison, the coordination in agonist and antagonist muscles observed in the expert was not detected in the other subjects. The upper limbs are generally stabilized by the function of the proximal shoulder joints. However, the other subjects used their deltoid muscles to fix their shoulder joints. This action was not observed in the expert. Also, the expert showed no significant increase in activity compared to his resting state. This result suggests that the expert applied pressure by effectively controlling the muscles affecting his elbow, finger joints, and maniphalanx without fixing his shoulder joints. However, the other subjects displayed simultaneous action of agonist muscle and antagonist muscle, coupled with a decrease in muscular activity, which strongly opposes the behavior exhibited by the expert.

Moreover, the expert kept his body core upright and maintained the position of his upper limb adequately. The other subjects were more strongly affected by the rotating force of the grinding disc, and so failed to keep their upper limbs stable, which caused their body core and elbow joints to be in flexion positions. This evidence suggests that the expert relaxed the tension of his shoulder to a certain extent, and pressed down the abrasive without using excessive force. In contrast, the other subjects opened their sides, and could not effectively transfer adequate force to the abrasive. Thus, no coordination in muscular activity was observed in other subjects.

The expert showed a greater amount of muscular activity in the T, FDS, and APB compared to other muscles. This result suggests an increase in muscular activity. The different correlation between each joint observed in the expert was not detected in the muscular activity of the other subjects. This suggests that the non-experts maintained an effective grinding position, but they ineffectively pressed down the specimen with brute force, lacking either sufficient function to press down or effective function of the anterior upper limb muscles. This evidence verifies that the expert effectively pressed down the specimen on the rotating disk in accordance with the rotating movement. This behavior led to the difference in the muscular activity pattern and amount of action seen. An educational reference for the training of beginner and non-expert technicians is under preparation. Thanks to this study, we added the useful instruction of, "shoulder down and extend elbow joints," to the training materials.

We investigated about the feature of "Grinding" motion and work disorder by using surface electromyography. In this study, we investigated the feature of the "Grinding" motion by using a metallographic sample with different of its surface.

The muscular function is different by the muscular shape and the muscle contraction property. In this study, it is showed two muscle activity types of muscles activity increased with motion and continuous muscle activity patterns with "Grinding". It is showed coordinated muscle patterns with "Grinding". The features of expert's body movement during "Grinding" are upright trunk to forward keeping his upper arm extension position and intrinsic position of hand. But Non-experts' body movement during "Grinding" are trunk was round back, elbow flexion and fingers flexed.

Deltoid is a prime mover for nearly all movements of the shoulder. The deltoid also plays an important role in stabilizing the shoulder. It is a powerful abductor. Pectoralis Major is a powerful chest muscle responsible for movements in front of the body, such as pushing, reaching, throwing et al. This feature maintains the leverage of the different fibers in the various positions possible in the shoulder. Biceps Brachii is fusiform shape and multijoint function limit its mechanical advantage compared with powerhouse synergists other muscle, which have pinnate fiber muscles. Triceps is a strongest function it is extension of elbow joint, which is accomplished by all fibers of the muscle. Extensor Carpi Radialis Brevis works closely to extend the wrist. This muscle also radially deviates the wrist. Flexor Digitrum Superficialis is particularly strong in this function when the wrist is fixation and fingers flexion. 1st Dorsal Interosseous and Abdunctor Pollicis Brevis works MP joint flexion, PIP joint and DIP joint extension when take a pinch material.

5   Conclusions

In this study, we examined the muscular activity of technicians when grinding specimens for metallographic testing. The results revealed significant differences between subjects in increases in muscular activity for the T, FDS, and APB, and in the amount of muscular activity for other muscles. These results verify that the T, FDS, and APB are likely connected with the grinding action. When comparing the expert's muscular activity with that of other subjects, we found no noticeable difference in activity for the T, FDS and APB.

References

1. ASTM International, Standard Guide for Preparation of Metallographic Specimens, E3 - 2011 (2011)
2. Smith, M.F.: A Comparison of Techniques for the metallographic Preparation of Thermal Sprayed Samples. Journal of Thermal Spray Technology, 287–294 (1993)
3. Vander, G.F.: Metallography: Principles and Practices. ASM International (1984)
4. Samuels, L.E.: Metallographic Polishing by Mechanical Methods. ASM International (2003)

Caregiver`s Gaze and Field of View Presumption Method During Bath Care in the Elderly Facility

Akiyoshi Yamamoto[1], Noriyuki Kida[2], Akihiko Goto[3], Tomoko Ota[4],
Tatsunori Azuma[1], Syuji Yamamoto[1], Henry Barrameda Jr[1]

[1] Super Court Co., Ltd, Osaka, Japan
yamamoto@city-estate.co.jp,
{azuma,osakajyokoen,henrybarramedajr}@supercourt.co.jp
[2] Kyoto Institute of Technology, Kyoto, Japan
kida@kit.ac.jp
[3] Osaka Sangyo University, Osaka, Japan
gotoh@ise.osaka-sandai.ac.jp
[4] Chuo Business Group, Osaka, Japan
tomoko.ota@k.vodafone.ne.jp

Abstract. Reduced mental fatigue and ease of mind on caregivers are crucial in order to deliver safe bath care assistance in the elderly facility. In this paper, we present an experiment quantifying the eye gaze and field of view of the caregiver while performing bath care assistance. First, we used optical motion analyzing apparatus, head mounted gaze measuring apparatus, motion sensor (applied to 5 points: wrist, waist, neck, head and ankle in sequence) and compared data. Subjects imitated the motions of bathing assistance in a laboratory. Second, we clarified the validity of data by studying simultaneously recorded multiple people's data taken under role play settings (caregiver role and care receiver role) in an actual bathroom setting. The findings of the study are highly relevant in outlining a safe and secure bathing assistance related to reducing the mental burden on caregivers as well as giving them "ease of mind" while performing bath care.

Keywords: caregiver, elderly facility, bath care assistance, presumption method, blind spot, motion capture.

1 Research Background and Problem Identification

1.1 Nursing Care for the Elderly

Japan faces a critical need for nursing care as its elderly population continues to grow along with the rise of the number of elderly people who are bedridden, suffering from dementia, and of those requiring extended care. According to the 2013 White Paper on the Aging Society, 29.67 million people, or 23.2% of the entire Japanese population of 127.76 million, are senior citizens over the age of 65. That number is well above the 7% threshold that defines a country as an aging society. Furthermore, a very high 11.8% of the population is over the age of 75.

V. G. Duffy (Ed.): DHM/HCII2014, LNCS 8529, pp. 78–87, 2014.
© Springer International Publishing Switzerland 2014

The aging of society has increased demand for nursing care, with 5.49 million people as of October 2012 qualifying for some type of care in their daily life. This pressing social need necessitated specialized care in the nursing business. In 1987, the Certified Social Workers and Certified Care Workers Act was enacted to provide and maintain quality nursing care, giving specialized nursing care providers with national certification.

This also had the effect of directing the spotlight on the overwhelming challenges of the families dealing with nursing care for their elderly, and a growing call for socialized nursing care led to the enactment of the long-term care insurance program in 2000, giving recipients a choice in the type of nursing care they receive. The first article of the long-term care act advocates for socially supported quality welfare services that recognize the right to a dignified life for all individuals. It states that" The purposes of this Act are to improve health and medical care and to enhance the welfare of citizens. With regard to people who are under condition of need for long-term care due to disease, etc., as a result of physical or emotional changes caused by aging, and who require care such as for bathing, bodily waste elimination, meals, etc., and require the functional training, nursing, management of medical treatment, and other medical care, these purposes are to be accomplished by establishing a long-term care insurance system based on the principle of the cooperation of citizens, solidarity, and determining necessary matters concerning related insurance benefits, etc., in order to provide benefits pertaining to necessary health and medical services and public aid services so that these people are able to maintain dignity and an independent daily life routine according to each person's own level of abilities."

1.2   Bathing Assistance: Its Background and Issues

Bathing is indispensable for both hygiene and as part of Activities of Daily Living (ADL). It encourages blood circulation and promotes higher metabolism. It also relaxes the muscles, helps prevent bedsores and infections, regulates bowel movements and supports other such functions of the body. For many elderly people suffering from anxiety and tension, bathing is an important time for them to relax. It has the added mental benefit for the elderly, who consider bathing one of life's pleasures. Furthermore, cleansing the body of dirt and odors helps strengthen interpersonal relationships and encourages active social engagement. Bathing is thereby an extremely significant way to assist in the daily lives of the elderly, and in order to realize quality welfare service, effective bathing assistance is a necessity.

Bathing has many benefits -- physiological, mental and social. And yet, it can be risky, fraught with such dangers as falling and drowning. The external causes of bathing accidents include exposure to the cold while dressing/undressing, the warm temperature in the bathtub or bathroom, and the hydrostatic pressure within the bathtub are considered to have a negative impact on the bodies of the elderly. In many cases, the elderly tend to suffer from multiple complications, such as high blood pressure and diabetes, as well as arteriosclerotic changes and a deteriorating autonomic nervous system response. Therefore, some of the internal causes of bathing accidents can be attributed to changes in blood pressure, dehydration and blood coagulation.

These physiological changes expose the elderly to a higher risk of cardiac arrest, cerebrovascular disorder, dizziness and cataleptic attacks. A complex mix of these factors heightens the risk of falling and injury, drowning and even death. Delivering quality bathing assistance depends on overcoming variety of issues.

Assisting with bathing is extremely hard work and has been an issue at welfare facilities for the elderly. There have been numerous reports published about the level of burden incurred while performing tasks during bath care assistance (Fujimura, 1995). One of them (Nagata, 1999) involves a survey of caregivers who work in the nation's 969 special nursing home for the elderly. According to the survey, the most physically taxing aspect of care is bathing assistance, followed by diaper change and transfers. The burden incurred by bathing assistance is threefold: physiological, physical and mental. The high temperature in the bathroom is demanding on the caregiver's body, and it causes physiological challenges. According to a study by Kawahara and his team (2010), caregivers showed high cortisol levels -- a benchmark for stress-response -- after assisting with bathing, linking the activity with high physiological stress.

The high stress level in handling a lot of transfers from one place to another or changing position like transferring from the wheelchair to the bathtub and back, as well as supporting the elderly in an upright position while he or she dresses or undresses in a high-temperature bathroom can be compared to working in an assembly-line style work environment.. These are all tough on the back. Bathing assistance in a nursing care facility with a large bath involves not only horizontal, but lots of vertical movements that impact and stress the musculoskeletal structure, which in turn invites fatigue. Also, with the progressive bathing system most widely used in care facilities, caregivers end up with five manual transfers of an elderly from one location to another, including the move from the bedroom to the bathroom, which again causes stress to the caregiver.

Because bathroom floors could be slippery and may trigger a fall, constant vigilance can cause mental stress to caregivers. According to a survey by Nagata (1999), 18% of the caregivers cited "fear of a fall" as their biggest mental stress while assisting with bathing. Furthermore, the survey revealed that bathing assistance is the most conducive to feeling negative about nursing care (Kawahara 2010).

As detailed above, bathing assistance is extremely taxing work and is believed to be one of the main reasons why some people leave the job. The turnover rate for care jobs was 18.7% in 2008, which is high compared against the industry's rate of 14.6%. With regards to active job-opening ratios, the number declined to 1.34 in September 2009, after peaking at 2.53 in December 2008. To this day, the ratio continues hovering above 1 -- a big issue to consider in delivering quality care.

1.3   Research Trends in Bathing Assistance

To tackle the above-mentioned problems, fundamental and practical research is being done, with some of the research showing promise of mitigating the physical toll of bathing on the elderly. For instance, Kanda (1991) published the results of his research involving the physiological burdens of bathing in the winter and in the summer. Nagahiro's research (2006) on the impact of bathroom temperatures on the circulatory system of healthy elderly people shows temperature levels that promote lower blood pressure after bathing.

On the other hand, numerous studies conducted in the areas of sanitary engineering and structural engineering have contributed to the development of comfortable clothing and structural improvements in buildings to reduce the physiological impact of care-giving on care workers.

In terms of dealing with the physical stress, caregivers are provided with ergonomic and biomechanic suggestions and nursing equipment that help reduce back strain. For instance, when comparing the efficiency between the use of a mechanical lift and a manual lift when transferring a fully dependent care receiver to a wheelchair, a Tomioka study (2008) showed that the mechanical lift reduced the work time considerably after a period of training and that the mechanical lift was effective in reducing the caregivers' back strain. Furthermore, after analyzing the burden on the back by studying the angle of the upper body and the results of electromyogram, the Tomioka report (2007) showed that using the mechanical lift to get in and out of the bathtub reduced the caregiver's forward-leaning posture and strain on the muscles -- all of which contributed to an overall reduction in work-related stress. The report also pointed to increased back strain that comes from bending forward when the caregiver has to wash a care receiver or help her dress/undress while she remains seated, or when adjusting the footrest on the wheel chair.

1.4   Identifying the Problem

There's been a lot of research done for the purpose of lessening the physiological and physical burdens for both the caregivers and the care receivers, many of them outlining specific nursing techniques and new policies. However, when it comes to easing the mental burdens, basic research doesn't go far enough, and there are as yet no solutions.

Bathing assistance is more prone to accidents, the caregiver must be on constant alert, especially when dealing with elderly with dementia, who often move and act in unpredictable ways. Creating a safe way to offer bathing assistance that can prevent falls or drowning accidents is in a way reducing mental stress. This could achieve "peace of mind," and make quality nursing care a reality.

We have identified the main issue in our research as reducing the caregivers' mental stress by preventing accidents, such as falls and drowning.

2   Preventing Accidents during Bathing Assistance

2.1   Causes of Falls: Care Receivers' Physical Issues

Kawamura (2003) pointed out that medical incidents surrounding nursing care mostly involve falls. Not just limited to bathing time, falling accidents by elderly people can severely interfere with their health, for instance forcing them to be bedridden. A large number of studies have been conducted on the link between fitness levels and falling accidents of an elderly person. Accident-prevention programs based on those findings have been shown to be effective.

Falls can be caused by many factors: old age, disease, loss of muscle strength and deterioration of other physical functions of the care receiver. Therefore, to prevent a fall, the report said that one must assess the risks care receivers are exposed to and design a preventative program.

2.2   Causes of Falls: Environmental Factors

The causes of falls are not limited to declining physical functions of the care receivers: steps, slippery floors, footwear and poor lighting are also culpable. These are referred to as environmental factors and can be addressed to prevent falls. Ergonomic research -- through the quantitative studying of the positioning, line of vision and visual field of train conductors, automobile drivers and other people who work in dangerous environments -- has done much to contribute to safety policies. The study has led to the development of a technology that can detect vehicles within a blind spot by anticipating when a vehicle in the opposite lane enters into a driver's blind spot. Blind spots occur where the driver cannot see an object that also does not show up in the rearview and side view mirrors. The larger the vehicle, the larger the blind spot. Accidents are more likely to happen when the driver fails to see objects in the blind spot. By warning the driver of a vehicle within the blind spot, the driver can reduce his chances of getting into an accident.

On the other hand, nursing care takes place where people, labor, machines and the environment come together harmoniously. It is an extremely difficult line of work where caregivers have to respond to sudden and unexpected actions of the care receivers with flexibility. Furthermore, chronic staff shortages at care sites mean caregivers do not have the luxury to foster harmony between the people and their environment, and the environment is not set up to take better care of the caregivers themselves; blind spots are everywhere. With regards to research on blind spots in care sites, most are focused on positioning video cameras in places that reduce these blind spots. In the area of care giving, it is hoped that the technological development is based on ergonomics, promoting independent living and normalization, general respect and respect toward basic human rights, self-actualization and other crucial principles of welfare. Therefore, research on blind spots -- such as one that involves the use of video cameras -- must take into consideration the rights of the caregivers before launching into quantifying blind spots that occur daily in the care line of work.

Research into quantifying blind spots has just begun. Quantifying blind spots during bathing assistance, or ideas on where and how caregivers and receivers can position themselves to minimize those blind spots -- these are all areas for potential growth.

2.3   Predicting and Safeguarding against Falls

Elderly people, who form the majority of care receivers, suffer from a deterioration of various physical and mental functions. Therefore they require assistance to bath safely and with peace of mind. That means caregivers have to be able to predict a care receiver's set of risks and improve on their ability and judgment to draw information from multiple sources and act accordingly. In other words, when it comes to preventing bathing accidents from happening, it is imperative that caregivers are able to sense the receiver's mood, and assess the local environment. This also means that caregivers need the skill to sense danger and be able to act on it accordingly.

It is said that our sense of danger is grasped mainly through our vision -- more than 80% out of all five of our senses. When caregivers and receivers come together during a bath and the caregiver uses her vision to sense danger, the caregiver should either consciously or subconsciously know where he or she is looking to perceive that danger and turn that into data of sorts. But there has yet to be an objective evaluation of visually extracted information at care sites. Plus, it isn't clear where a caregiver should look and what to look for in order to effectively sense danger. To predict a fall during a bath requires a superior level of observation, judgment and then on top of that, the ability to handle it with flexibility. These types of skills are not acquired in a short amount of time; it requires years of experience and learning.

Also, caregivers try not to interfere with the activities of the care receivers as much as they can to encourage their independence. At care sites, the idea of "monitoring" is of paramount significance. Even when monitoring during bathing assistance, where the caregiver should look (for danger signs) has not yet been quantified. It has been a nursing technique acquired mostly through intuition and experience.

2.4   Solving Problems

This research recommends that in order to prevent a fall during a bath, a practical system be instituted whereby neither a caregiver's gaze nor the care receiver end up in a blind spot. For that to happen, the caregiver's and care receiver's location in the bathroom or changing room has to be recorded in a timed series. As for the caregivers, tracking their gaze in a timed series can help quantify blind spots, potentially even turning the caregiver's monitoring skill into data.

3   Predicting Positions and Field of Vision

3.1   Motion Capture

With respect to measuring physical exercise and positional information, the most commonly used system is the DLT motion-capture system, which primarily uses visual data. In a motion-capture system, an optical motion measuring apparatus is used, and multiple infrared cameras are used to measure the three-dimensional coordinate of a marker. This system is capable of accurately measuring a three-dimensional coordinate and is extremely expensive, but its use is limited to water-free locations.

For compiling eye-gaze data, an eye-gaze tracking device that uses pupil corneal reflection technique is mounted on the head. This technique can accurately track the eye gaze, but the device is extremely expensive and raises some privacy issues as it records the image of the care receiver taking a bath.

The use of motion-capture systems and head-mounted eye-gaze tracking devices can be problematic and difficult to justify. They are large and intrusive, and raise privacy issues.

3.2   Estimating by Using Motion Sensors

In recent years, accelerometers and GPS sensors have become standard features in mobile phones. In much the same way, motion sensors such as accelerometers, gyro sensors and geomagnetic sensors have become compact and affordable due to the MEMS technology. Motion sensors, which are attached to different parts of the body, can read bodily rotations and translational motion in a simple and unrestricted way. Because it doesn't require video images to capture positioning, eye-gaze and visual field data, the technique is highly anticipated, even from a privacy standpoint.

Since data retrieved from motion sensors are accelerated, posture data, which is an important element in measuring physical exercise, can be attained by the conversion of the angular velocity's integration operator or the gravitational acceleration.

However, when taking the angular velocity through integral value calculation, drift errors contained in the power output of gyro sensors compound and lower the accuracy of the outcome the longer the measuring process. Furthermore, converting from gravitational acceleration doesn't provide information on direction, and with passing time, the acceleration sensor reads the dynamic acceleration as error. The gyro sensor's drift error can be corrected in a number of suggested methods -- gyro sensors, accelerometers, algorithms that predict roll, pitch and yaw angles from geomagnetism sensors, as well as algorithms that predict quaternions.

Therefore, we suggest instituting a system by which the caregiver's gaze can be quantified at an actual bathing site. The goal is to reduce the mental burdens at care sites by delivering a safe way to assist with bathing and creating "peace of mind." This system has the ability to quantify assisting skills and blind spots, and monitor activity while assisting with bathing. It can also evaluate staff assignments objectively. In order to make this system a reality, what is necessary as part of basic research is the verification of the accuracy of positioning, gaze and field of view data acquired through motion sensors.

4   Suggested Systems

4.1   System Outline

This is a system that uses motion sensors to estimate position and visual field data. Calculating the caregiver and the care receiver's position within 10cm of accuracy in the bathroom, then making an estimate of the caregiver's field of view data in the direction that the caregiver is facing (front) is thought to be helpful for the caregiver. Position estimation by motion sensor is not new. However, methods for estimating visual fields have yet to be tested and are considered something of a novelty. By dispensing with the use of videos in the process, the system makes no privacy breaches, making it a strong candidate for use in welfare care studies, psychology, ergonomic and other areas of research. Furthermore, the skills caregivers apply during bathing -- assisting and monitoring -- have always been ambiguous. Quantifying those skills from gaze data offers an unprecedented viewpoint. This research is being used for system development intended as feedback to care sites and has a practical application: reducing mental burden is effective in improving the work environment of care sites.

Using this system will more clearly reveal the difference in bathing assistance and monitoring skills between veteran caregivers and novice caregivers. The system can eventually develop into one that supports skill development and offers assessments that can help with monitoring skills to better assist with bathing. The existence of blind spots in bathing assistance work has been made clear, paving the way for smarter staff appointments. Clarifying policies that promote safe bathing assistance by observing the location and movements of the caregivers and care receivers also contributes to the safe management of care welfare facilities.

4.2   Basic Experiment

The experiment aimed at clarifying the reliability and validity of motion-sensor data -- as it is conducted as an experiment in a laboratory -- based on the three-dimensional coordinate data derived from optical motion measurement equipment. It was conducted on general subjects at a laboratory. In the experiment, four sets of infrared cameras (Raptor-H, Hawk-I, made by Motion Analysis Corp.) and a real-time optical motion capture system (MAC 3D System made by Motion Analysis Corp.) were used to collect three-dimensional data from four reflective marker points mounted on to the subjects' heads (Fig.1). As for the motion sensors, small sensors (Fig.2, LP-WS1201, Logical Product) consisting of a 3-axis accelerometer, a 3-axis angular velocity sensor, a 3-axis geomagnetism sensor and a GPS sensor were fixed to the subjects' heads and the data was collected at 1000Hz. The subjects were allowed to walk around and look around (Fig.3). By integrating the motion-sensor data, the subjects' body position and orientation were computed. And then their location, base and field of view information were estimated (Fig.4). As a result, movements and body orientations that are prone to estimation errors as well as places to attach motion sensors that produce the least amount of estimation errors have been made clear.

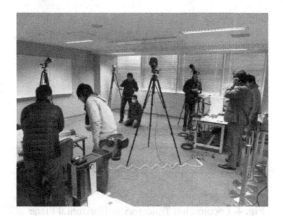

Fig. 1. Experiment in a laboratory setting

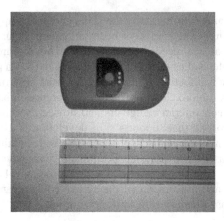

Fig. 2. Logical Product LP-WS1201 Wireless Motion Sensor

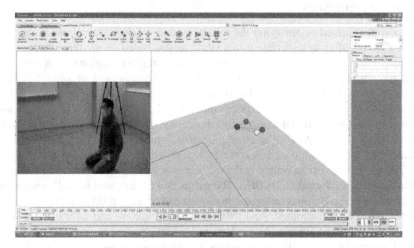

Fig. 3. Motion Capture Configuration Screen

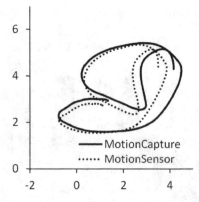

Fig. 4. Locomotion Trajectory in Horizontal Plane

5   Conclusion

Reduced mental fatigue and ease of mind on caregivers are crucial in order to deliver safe bath care assistance in the elderly facility. In this paper, we presented an experiment quantifying the eye gaze and field of view of the caregiver while performing bath care assistance. We used optical motion analyzing apparatus, head mounted gaze measuring apparatus, motion sensor and compared data. Subjects imitated the motions of bathing assistance in a laboratory. As a result, movements and body orientations that are prone to estimation errors as well as places to attach motion sensors that produce the least amount of estimation errors have been made clear. The findings of the study would be highly relevant in outlining a safe and secure bathing assistance related to reducing the mental burden on caregivers as well as giving them "ease of mind" while performing bath care.

References

1. Fujimura, T.: Roujin Ho-mu ni okeru Kaigo Sagyou no Mondaiten to Youtsuu Taisaku. Roudou no Kagaku 509, 13–16 (1995) (in Japanese)
2. Nagata, H.: Tokubetsu Yougo Roujin Ho-mu de no Kaigo Roudou no Jittai Chousa to kongo no Kourei Kaigo Roudou no Kentou. Roudou Kagaku 75, 459–469 (1999) (in Japanese)
3. Kawahara, Y.: Current State of Bathing Care and Necessity of New equipment for Bathing Care Institution. J. Human and Living Environment. 171, 23–30 (2010)
4. Kanda, K.: Koureisha no Touki to Kaki ni okeru Nyuuyoku Kankyou to Nyuuyokuji no Seiriteki Futan ni Kansuru Chousa. Bull. Inst. Public Health 40, 388–390 (1991)
5. Nagahiro, C.: Effects of Room Temperature on Circulatory Dynamics During Bathing in the Elderly. Japanese Journal of Public Health 533, 178–186 (2006)
6. Tomioka, K.: Low Back Load and Satisfaction Rating of Caregivers and Care Receivers in Bathing Assistance Given in a Nursing Home for the Elderly Practicing Individual Care. San Ei Shi 49, 54–58 (2007) (in Japanese)
7. Tomioka, K.: Low Back Pain among Care Workers Working at Newly-built Nursing Homes for the Aged. San Ei Shi 50, 86–91 (2008) (in Japanese)
8. Kawamura, H.: Hiyari Hatto: 11,000 Jirei ni yoru Era- mappu Kanzenbon. Igaku shoin, 88–91 (2003) (in Japanese)

Anthropometry, Design and Ergonomics

Research on the Continuous Descent Approach (CDA) Operational Error of Pilot Base on Cloud Model and Uncertainty Theory

Yang Gao and Yanchen Hou

The safety of civil aviation, Research Institute of Civil Aviation Safety, China
{437571079,1301333590}@qq.com

Abstract. Through the Cloud model and uncertainty theory research on Continuous Descent Approach (CDA) procedures is a simple and rapid method. This paper analyzed aircraft's required time of arrival (RTA) in CDA process with the Cloud model, meanwhile the six operational errors of pilot were defined. From uncertainty theory, the probability distribution of the CDA operational error of pilot will be faintly determined. Although data for CDA operating experience are sparse in China, further research will continue.

Keywords: Continuous Descent Approach, Cloud model, required time of arrival, operational error, uncertainty theory.

1 Introduction

As an important part of the Next Generation Air Transportation System (NextGen), CDA procedures can be effective at reducing aircraft noise in the airports, meanwhile, results of the experiments of economic and environmental benefits indicate that the CDA provides fuel burn and emissions impact reductions. Although CDA are beneficial for reducing aircraft noise and fuel savings, related uncertainties to these operations can cause terminal area capacity to be reduced. For this reason, CDA arrival routes have only been operated during low-density traffic operations.

Continuous Descent Final Approach (CDFA) is the name of CDA in China, but it was still in the stage of theoretical research. Civil Aviation Administration of China (CAAC) issued advisory circular about CDFA, and put forward the concepts about it. CDFA is a significant technology for civil aviation of China in future.

With the conventional aircraft approach, an aircraft would be given clearance by Air Traffic Control from the bottom level of the holding stack (normally an altitude of 6000 or 7000 feet) to descend to an altitude of typically 3000 feet. The aircraft would then fly level for several miles before intersecting the final 3 degree glide path to the runway. During this period of level flight, the pilot would need to apply additional engine power to maintain constant speed. [1]

In contrast to a conventional approach, when a CDA procedure is flown the aircraft stays higher for longer, descending continuously from the level of the bottom of the stack (or higher if possible) and avoiding any level segments of flight prior to

V. G. Duffy (Ed.): DHM 2014, LNCS 8529, pp. 91–100, 2014.

intercepting the 3 degree glide path. A continuous descent requires significantly less engine thrust than prolonged level flight. As illustrated in Figure1, because the aircraft flying a CDA is higher above the ground for a longer period of time, the noise impact on the ground is reduced in certain areas under the approach path. [1]

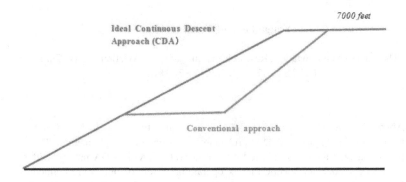

Fig. 1. Comparison between a CDA and a conventional approach

2   Research Model

2.1   The Cloud Model

Cloud model is proposed by Deyi Li who is a member of the Chinese Academy of Engineering to represent the uncertainty transition between qualitative concept and quantitative description in 1995.

Researcher establish a cloud model about the arrival routes of CDA, based on a lot of flight trajectory survey data. Because of the characters of fuzziness and randomness, the required time of arrival (RTA) could be described by a cloud model. From the model, the number of sample set will be increasing and the persuasion of data will be enhancing.

2.2   The Normal Cloud Model

Suppose U is a domain of definition expressed by precise value, in the quantity concept C corresponding to U, there be a stable tended random number to a random element x in the domain of definition, which is defined as follows:

$$\mu : U \rightarrow [0,1]$$

$$\forall x \in U, x \rightarrow \mu(x)$$

The distribution of x in the domain of definition is called C(X), x is called a cloud drops, and C(X) is combined by many Cloud drops.

Cloud model has three digital characteristics: Expected value (Ex), Entropy (En) and Hyper-Entropy (He), which will integrate the fuzziness and randomness of spatial concepts in unified way. Expected value (Ex) is the center value of concept in the domain of definition, and it's the representative value of the qualitative concept. Entropy (En) is the measuring of the fuzziness of qualitative concept, reflects the numerical range which can be accepted by this concept in the domain of definition, and reflect the uncertain margin of the qualitative concept. The bigger the entropy is, the bigger numerical range can be accepted by the concept. Hype Entropy（He） reflects the dispersion of the cloud drops. The bigger the Hyper Entropy is, the bigger of its dispersion and the randomness of degree of membership.

Backward cloud generator (BCG) is a generator between quantitative values and qualitative concept, which is a mapping mode about backward cloud. A certain number of data be translated into the cloud's digital character C (Ex En, He) which is model as follows. (figue2)

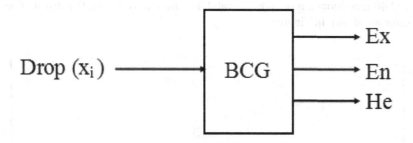

Fig. 2. Backward cloud generator

2.3　Backward Cloud Generator Procedure Code

The input of the backward cloud generator is the quantitative value of N cloud drops Xi, and the output is three digital characteristics Ex, En, He. The backward cloud generator BCG in details is:

INPUT:
Cloud drops $x_i (i = 1, 2, ..., n)$

OUTPUT:
Three digital characteristics Ex, En, He

Algorithm:

(1) Calculate: $Ex = \dfrac{1}{n} \sum\limits_{i=1}^{n} x_i$

(2) Calculate: $En = \sqrt{\dfrac{\pi}{2}} \times \dfrac{1}{n} \sum\limits_{i=1}^{n} |x_i - Ex|$

(3) Calculate: $He = \sqrt{\dfrac{1}{n-1}\sum_{i=1}^{n}(x_i - Ex)^2 - En^2}$

To calculate the errors of required time, system uses four-dimensional (4D) trajectories, which are generated for the estimated times of arrival (ETAs) for both aircraft. Through a lot of experiments calculate each aircraft's required time of arrival (RTA), which a large proportion of RTA be caused by the operational error of pilot.

From the experiments of Federal Aviation Administration (FAA), we know system can calculate each aircraft's required time of arrival with a ground-based sequencer and scheduler. The aircraft's time error and final approach speed would be received through the experiment of FAA. Same aircraft type is the first condition of experiment and the trajectory be selected for the 3°-CDA arrival routes.

Through the data of FAA, we know the 4,000 assigned RTA errors (100-aircraft streams and 40 repetitions), however, the valid data have only 3,960. The distribution of RTA error are shown in Figure3.

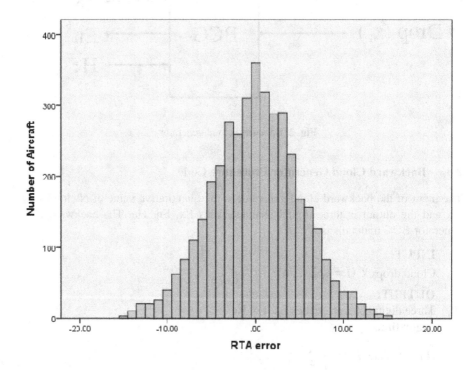

Fig. 3. The distribution of RTA error

Each aircraft of RTA error can be viewed as a cloud drop in the model, which can constitute a trend of error. According to the parameter of model, the figure of cloud model will be established by the matlab, and the procedure code of cloud model as follow.

```
%generate a cloud model(Ex=0.04,En=4.912,He=0.519,n=3960)
Ex = 0.04;
En =4.912;
n = 3960;
cloud_drop=1:n;
u=1:n;
for i=1: n
    cloud_drop(i)=0;
    u(i)=0;
end
He =0.569;
    for i=1: n
        Enn = normrnd(En,He);
        cloud_drop(i) = normrnd(Ex,abs(Enn));
        u(i)=exp(-(cloud_drop(i)-Ex)^2/(2*Enn^2));
    end
    plot(cloud_drop,u,'r.');
    xlabel('RAT error');
    ylabel('Certainty');
```

2.4   The Cloud Model of RTA Error

The trend of cloud model (Ex=0.04, En=4.912, He=0.519, n=3960) is shown in Figure 4.There is an obvious differences between the figure of cloud model and the veritably distribution of RTA error. The histogram of RTA error is only used as a statistical result, those errors would represent just one specific of an aircraft, but the figure of cloud model is a likely trend for the future development. Because the ability of cloud model, we can estimate the trend of RTA error when the aircraft to reach large numbers.

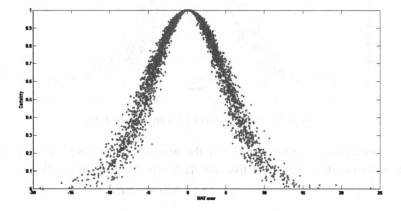

Fig. 4. The cloud model of RTA error (N=3960)

Nowadays, the capacity of terminal airspace increasing is a necessary trend, for example, Tianjin International Airport's aircraft movements reach the number of 100,151 in 2013. To reply the increasing the capacity requirement of terminal airspace, large sample analysis will be used in future study for the RTA error in CDA. The cloud model of RTA error when the number of sample attain10, 000 or50, 000.The model is shown in Figure 5 and Figure 6

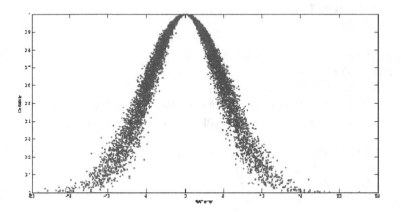

Fig. 5. The cloud model of RTA error (N=10000)

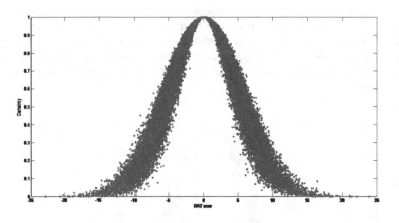

Fig. 6. The cloud model of RTA error (N=50000)

There are a group of cloud drops△X in the dimensional domain U, which is a contribution degree△C for the qualitative concept A, which is defined as follows:

$$\Delta C \approx \mu_A(x) * \Delta x / \sqrt{2\pi} En$$

Obviously, contribution degree C is a relevant concept about all the element in the dimensional domain the equation C is

$$C = \frac{\int_{-\infty}^{+\infty} \mu_T(x)\,dx}{\sqrt{2\pi}En}$$

For

$$\frac{1}{\sqrt{2\pi}En} \int_{Ex-3En}^{Ex+3En} \mu_T(x)\,dx = 99.74\%$$

Therefore, all the cloud drops about the qualitative concept included in the interval [Ex-3En, Ex+3En].

2.5   The Risk Layer of RTA Error

According to calculation we know, the percentage of interval [Ex-0.67En, Ex+0.67En] is 53.11% in all the cloud drops, and the percentage of contribution degree about qualitative concept of the interval is 50%, cloud drops in the interval be known as the core of interval. Similarly, the percentage of interval [Ex-En, Ex+ En] is 73.46% in all the cloud drops, and the percentage of contribution degree about qualitative concept of the interval is 68.26%, cloud drops in the interval be called basic interval. The percentage of interval [Ex-2En, Ex- En] U [Ex+ En, Ex+2En] is 22.50%, but the percentage of contribution degree about qualitative concept of the interval is 27.18%, cloud drops in the interval be called outside the range. Meanwhile, the percentage of interval [Ex-3En, Ex-2En] U [Ex+2En, Ex+3En] is 4.04%, but the percentage of contribution degree about qualitative concept of the interval is 4.3%, cloud drops in the interval be called outside the weak range.

According to the theory of cloud scale, a cloud model can be divided into four intervals, the core of interval, basic interval, outside the range and outside the weak range. Because the different of distribution, there is a huge difference that the contribution degree of the four intervals. About the RTA error when operating the process of CDA, we can build four layers, absolute safety layer, basic safety layer, slight danger layer and danger layer. In the course of studies, where absolute safety layer is the core of interval, basic safety layer is basic interval, slight danger layer is outside the range and danger layer is outside the weak range, respectively.

Table 1. The risk layer of RTA error

Layer	Interval	RTA Error (s)
Absolute Safety Layer	[Ex-0.67En, Ex+0.67En]	[-3.25,3.33]
Basic Safety Layer	[Ex-En, Ex+ En]	[-4.86,4.96]
Slight Danger Layer	[Ex-2En, Ex- En] U [Ex+ En, Ex+2En]	[-9.78,-4.87]U[4.97,9.87]
Danger Layer	[Ex-3En, Ex-2En] U [Ex+2En, Ex+3En]	[-14.69,-9.79]U[9.88,14.779]

As is shown in Table 1, the critical value of RTA error is - 9.79 seconds, which is a spacing buffer. The buffer can ensure the safety of the process of CDA, it is significant that research operational error of pilot. From the study of cloud model we know that RTA error is an inevitable trend in CDA process, the uncertain RTA error factor may affect precise aircraft spacing at the runway and increase the risk of accident.

3   Research on Operational Error of Pilot

3.1   Operational Error of Pilot

Operational error of pilot is a very significant element in RTA error, this is one reason why reducing the operation of pilot is so important in the process of CDA. Research on possible cause of pilot operational can against inadvertent operation, this type of error can occur for various reasons, such as a pilot accidentally bumps a control when intending to CDA process, or accidentally actuates one control when intending to actuate a different control.

The operational error of pilot in CDA process can be divided into the following categories

- Lack of training
- Fatigue of pilot
- Data entry error
- Slippage Resistance of control
- Habit of pilot
- Communicative disorders

1. Lack of training. The process of CDA is a complex operation for a pilot who lack of specialty training. For ensure the safety of CDA, the pilot need to undertake training activities before execute the process of CDA.
2. Fatigue of pilot. The reason of pilot fatigue has many aspects. Sleep-deprived, disease, and work overload are all included. The research shows that the fatigue will cause such problems as sight, hearing and attention decrease, respond time extension and operation error increase in the CDA process.
3. Data entry error. Because a variety of environments, use conditions, and other factors, pilot may input error data in the CDA process, these abnormal operations will influence the accuracy of CDA process and the safety of approach.
4. Slippage Resistance of control. The physical design and materials used for controls can reduce the likelihood of finger and hand slippage. However, a pilot is likely to slip out of the hand in CDA process.
5. Habit of pilot. Each pilot has its own operating habits, for example, CDA process should be operated by both left-handed and right-handed pilots. If the controls designed to be not operated with left-handed pilot, the probability of making mistakes will be increase a threshold.
6. Communicative disorders. Pilots and controllers were asked to speculate the accuracy meaning of each other, because of the reason of language, information and different meaning, some pilots may be given a wrong meaning in the CDA process.

3.2   Research Prospect of Uncertainty Theory

Uncertainty theory was founded by Liu and refined by Liu. Nowadays the uncertainty theory has become a branch of mathematics for modeling human uncertainty.

First, in order to acquire the data of operational error, we have to invite some domain experts to evaluate their error rate that each human error will occur. Since human beings usually overrate human error, the error rate may have much larger variance than the real frequency. However, the result of uncertainty theory still reflect the situation of the CDA operational error of pilot.

Second, according to the score that domain experts grade on the basis of experience, Set up ξ is an uncertain variables, $\Phi(x; \theta_1, \theta_2...\theta_n)$ is a form of uncertain distribution, $\theta_1, \theta_2...\theta_n$ is a series of unknown parameter. The data is $(x_1, \alpha_1), (x_2, \alpha_2), \cdots, (x_n, \alpha_n)$ from the domain experts, the x, it's going to be the harm extent of the CDA operational error of pilot, the α, it's going to be the probability of operation, then

$$\hat{a} = \left\{ 3 \left[\frac{\alpha_1 + \alpha_2}{2} x_1 + \sum_{i=2}^{n-1} \frac{\alpha_{i+1} - \alpha_{i-1}}{2} x_i + (1 - \frac{\alpha_{n-1} + \alpha_n}{2} x_n) \right] \right\}^{-\frac{1}{2}}$$

Third, because of the expert's data is $(x_1, \alpha_1), (x_2, \alpha_2), \cdots, (x_n, \alpha_n)$, $\hat{a}$ is the result of computational formula. Similarly, the numeric of $\hat{b}$ could be calculated. The density of operational error of pilot probability formula, then

$$\Phi(x; a, b) = \hat{a} x + \hat{b}$$

Because of the lack of CDA operating experience in China, it is difficult to find the suitable expert to assess the six operational errors of pilot and obtain accurate data, so we unable to get basic data for uncertainty theory in short period of time. Further research will continue.

4   Conclusion

The computed result of the CDA operational error of pilot is an important part of the research about human factor. It's still show great reference significance in the layer of air traffic management. As a process of human-computer interaction (HCI), the operation of pilot is a core direction in the study of civil aviation safety.

References

1. Basic Principles of the Continuous Descent Approach (CDA) for the Non-Aviation Community, Environmental Research and Consultancy Department Civil Aviation Authority, GAO
2. Chen, X., Liu, B.: Existence and Uniqueness Theorem for Uncertain Differential equations. Fuzzy Optimization and Decision Making 9, 69–81 (2010)

3. Davison Reynolds, H.J., Reynolds, T.G., John Hansman, R.: Human Factors implications of Continuous Descent Approach Procedures For Noise Abatement. In: Air Traffic Control, Europe Air Traffic Management R&D Seminar, Baltimore, USA, June 27-30, pp. 1–3 (2005)

4. Cao, B., Li, D., Qin, K., Chen, G., Liu, Y., Han, P.: An Uncertain Control Framework of Cloud Model. In: Yu, J., Greco, S., Lingras, P., Wang, G., Skowron, A. (eds.) RSKT 2010. LNCS (LNAI), vol. 6401, pp. 618–625. Springer, Heidelberg (2010)

5. Weitz, L.A., Hurtado, J.E., Bussink, F.J.L.: Increasing Runway Capacity for Continuous Descent Approaches Through Airborne Precision Spacing. In: AIAA Guidance, Navigation, and Control Conference and Exhibit, pp. 15–18 (2005)

6. Clarke, J.P.B., Ho, N.T., Ren, L., et al.: Continuous descent approach: Design and flight test for Louisville International Airport. Journal of Aircraft 41(5), 1054–1066 (2004)

7. No, A.C.: 20-175. This advisory circular (AC) provides guidance for the installation and airworthiness approval of flight deck system control (2011)

8. Yan-bin, S., An, Z., Xian-jun, G., et al.: Cloud model and its application in effectiveness evaluation. In: 15th Annual Conference Proceedings, International Conference on Management Science and Engineering, ICMSE 2008, pp. 250–255. IEEE (2008)

9. Barmore, B.E., Abbott, T.S., Capron, W.R., et al.: Simulation results for airborne precision spacing along continuous descent arrivals. Perspective 22, 27 (2008)

10. Deyi, L., Yi, D.: Uncertainty in artificial intelligence. National Defence Industry Press (2005)

Study on the Evaluation of Automotive Seat Comfort during Prolonged Simulated Driving

Xianxue Li[1], Li Ding[1], Qianxiang Zhou[1], Huimin Hu[2], and Chaoyi Zhao[2]

[1] Key Laboratory for Biomechanics and Mechanobiology of Ministry of Education, School of Biological Science and Medical Engineering, Beihang University, Beijing, China
li36101120@126.com, ding1971316@buaa.edu.cn, zqxg@buaa.edu.cn
[2] China National Institute of Standardization, Beijing, China
huhm@cnis.gov.cn, zhaochy@cnis.gov.cn

Abstract. Prolonged driving can affect driver's lumbar and neck such as low back pain and cervical spondylosis. The purpose of this study is to clarify the relationship between drivers' comfort and their physiological parameters, the seat pressure distribution during prolonged driving in order to evaluate the comfort of different automotive seats. The experiment was performed on two actual automobiles. Six male drivers, aged 20 to 24 years participated in the simulated driving experiment in which the drivers sat in the car and simulated the driving movements in 2 hours. Electromyography (EMG), seat pressure distribution and oxygen saturation were measured during the experiment with subjective questionnaire. According to the results, MPF, MF, Pm and longitudinal pressure integral (PL) are high significant with the subjective comfort, otherwise the oxygen saturation was almost constant during the whole experiment which has little significance. Therefore from the study we can see the most sensitive part to feel discomfort during prolonged driving and the relationship between discomfort and physiological parameters was also clarified which can be used to find which automotive seat is more comfortable.

Keywords: automotive, seat comfort, electromyography, pressure distribution.

1 Introduction

In common parlance comfort may refer to both comfort and discomfort. But speaking precisely the item 'comfort' is associated with feelings of relaxation, well-being and aesthetics. While 'comfort' is connected with the aspects of 'favor', the item 'discomfort' characterizes the aspects of 'suffering'. Discomfort is associated with biomechanical factors that produce feelings of pain, numbness and stiffness.[1]

Time to spend on driving is increasing as the automotive becomes more and more popular. The comfort of automobile driving is one of the most important factors for consumers to assess the performance of automobile, it's related to the automobile's natural vibration performance and the driving environment, driver's physiological and Psychological status. However, prolonged driving can affect driver's lumbar and neck

V.G. Duffy (Ed.): DHM 2014, LNCS 8529, pp. 101–111, 2014.

such as low back pain and cervical spondylosis. So it's important to find how to evaluate the comfort during prolonged driving in order to choose a more comfortable vehicle, especially for the automotive seat.

For car manufacturers, seating comfort is becoming more and more important in distinguishing themselves from their competitors. There is a simultaneous demand for shorter development times and more comfortable seats. Comfort in automobile seats is a multidimensional and complex problem. Many current sophisticated measuring tools were consulted, but it is unclear on which factors one should concentrate attention when measuring comfort.

The previous study mainly concentrate on the subjective survey, sitting posture analysis, pressure distribution, performance analysis and electromyography. Otherwise, simulation method is also used to evaluate the comfort of automotive seat which is more convenient and timesaving. The subjective survey is commonly used and is relatively reliably which because it doesn't need special measurement instrument and it's visual and easy to operate. However, it requires the experimenter to be professional and the results is hard to be quantified. Pellettiere, Parakkat [2] developed objective methods for determining and predicting human comfort in operation and prototype U.S. Air Force crew seat cushions and found some factors, such as muscular fatigue levels, that are suspected of being significant contributors of discomfort during seated long-term flight. Andreoni, Santambrogio [3] present a multi-factor method for the analysis of sitting posture and the resulting interactions of the car driver body with the cushion and the backrest. Kolich [4] demonstrates the viability of employing a neural network for the purpose of predicting subjective perceptions of automobile seat comfort. This study suggests that subjective perceptions of automobile seat comfort can be predicted using a neural network. Grujicic, Pandurangan [5] study the seating comfort for passenger-vehicle occupants using a finite element model which includes seat-cushion and soft-tissue material.

The purpose of this study is to clarify the relationship between drivers' comfort and their physiological parameters, the seat pressure distribution during prolonged driving in order to evaluate the comfort of different automotive seats.

2   Method

Experiment Design. The experiment was performed on two actual automobiles, automobile A is Chevrolet LOVA and automobile B is Volkswagen Santana. Six male drivers, aged 20 to 24 years participated in the simulated driving experiment in which the drivers sat in the car and simulated the driving movements in 2 hours (Fig.1). The subjects could adjust the automobile seat and tilt steering wheel initially but were not allowed to make readjustments thereafter. Electromyography (EMG), seat pressure distribution and oxygen saturation were measured during the experiment with subjective questionnaire.

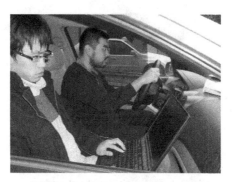

Fig. 1. Simulated driving posture

Subjective Survey. It was decided to concentrate on physical discomfort of drivers rather than on mental discomfort in this study. Subjective surveys on comfort of several body parts (such as neck, shoulders, back, lumbar, thighs and buttocks) were conducted twice: ten minutes after the beginning of the experiment and ten minutes before the ending of the experiment. Discomfort in whole body is also included. Depending on the degree of discomfort, the test items were classified into seven levels from "very comfort" to "very discomfort" which were "very comfort", "comfort", "a little comfort", "feel nothing" , "a little discomfort", "discomfort" and "very discomfort". Each level was accredited with different points ranging from 7 (very comfort) to 0 (very discomfort).

Electromyography. The instrument used in this experiment is MP150 (Fig.2), and the recording software is Acqknowledge 3.8.1.

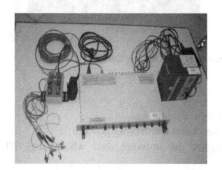
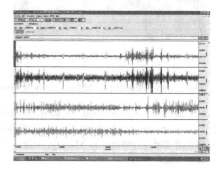

Fig. 2. EMG test device and measurement output screen

EMG (electromyography) was continuously monitored from 4 muscle sites during the 120-minute simulated driving with bipolar surface electrodes through a 50–200 Hz band-pass filter. Sampling rate was 1000Hz. Each electrode in a pair was set 5 cm apart from each other. Two pairs of surface EMG electrodes (Ag/AgCl electrodes) were, after abrasion and cleaning of the skin with alcohol, bilaterally attached to the skin over: the left and right latissimus dorsi (L1 level) and the left and right trapezius muscles. (Fig.3)

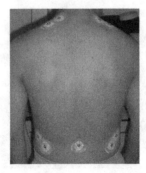

Fig. 3. Location sites of the electrodes

Pressure Distribution. The pressure distribution appears to be one of the most objective measure comprising with the clearest association with the subjective ratings.

During the experiment the subject-cushion and subject-backrest seat pressure distribution was measured with two sensor sheets (Pliance X. System, Germany-Novel Electronics, Germany) (Fig.4) and it was measured only once, ten minutes after the beginning of the experiment.

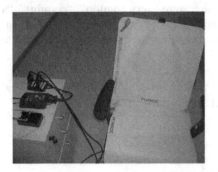 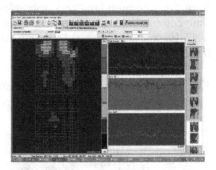

Fig. 4. Pliance X. System and measurement output screen

The experimental procedure is as follows:

1. Fix the sensor sheets on the seat cushion and backrest;
2. Let the participant sit on the sensor sheets and keep the driving posture;
3. When the pressure is steady, start to acquire the pressure data which lasts 20 seconds.

Oxygen Saturation. Regional blood oxygen saturation of right foot thumb in the lower extremities was measured every 20 minutes with clop-on oximeter (Fig.5).

Data Analysis. The root-mean-square (RMS), mean power frequency (MPF) and medium frequency (MF) of the EMG signal for each muscle measured were calculated. The contact area, maximum pressure (Pm) and longitudinal pressure integral (P_L) of pressure distribution for each automotive were got. The correction between these parameters with the subjective results was also studied to find their relationship.

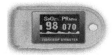

Fig. 5. Oximeter

3 Results and Dopiscussion

3.1 Subjective Survey

The subjective questionnaire showed that the first three discomforting parts are lumbar, thigh and the neck. From the results, we can see that after prolonged driving the lumbar will be affected most significantly which is due to there is no support for the lumbar. Figure 6 shows the comfort rating of lumbar before and after the driving experiment for automobile A and B. It shows that the lumbar comfort decreased significantly for both automobile A and B. However, there is no significant difference between automobile A and B which automobile B is a little more comfort after the driving experiment than automobile A. From figure 7, we can see that automobile B is more comfort overall than A both before and after the experiment.

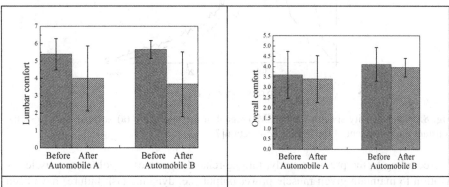

Fig. 6. Lumbar comfort rating before and after the experiment for automobile A and B	**Fig. 7.** Overall comfort rating before and after the experiment for automobile A and B

3.2 Electromyography

The EMG root-mean-square (RMS), median frequency (MF) and mean power frequency (MPF) are analyzed to find the correction of these parameters with subjective ratings.

RMS is calculated through (1)

$$RMS = \sqrt{\frac{1}{n}\sum_{i=1}^{n} s_i^2} \qquad (1)$$

Where S_i is the EMG signal.

MF is calculated through (2)

$$\int_0^{MF} PSD(f)\,df = \int_{MF}^0 PSD(f)\,df = \frac{\int_0^\infty PSD(f)\,df}{2} \tag{2}$$

Where PSD is the power spectral density.

MPF is calculated through (3)

$$MPF = \frac{\int_{-\infty}^{+\infty} \omega F(\omega)\,d\omega}{\int_{-\infty}^{+\infty} F(\omega)\,d\omega} \tag{3}$$

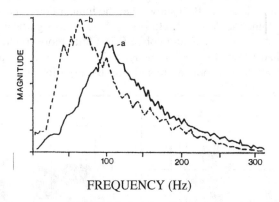

FREQUENCY (Hz)

Fig. 8. Power density spectra of the EMG signal at the beginning (a) and the end (b) of the constant force segment of the muscle contraction[7]

According to the previous study, fatigue-related decreases in voluntary muscle activation to maintain given muscle power output (i.e. dynamic task failure) have been exclusively assessed by the measurement of the EMG signal during maximal voluntary isometric contractions[6]. The EMG MF is an effective parameter for measuring changes in EMG waveform that are associated with metabolic correlates to fatigue (Fig. 8)[7]. Because the MF is a spectral estimate of a stochastic signal, it was necessary to monitor this parameter only during isometric, constant-force contractions (i.e. during lifting of some weight) when conditions of EMG signal stationarity could be satisfied.[8] Generally, the MF will shift to the lower frequency while the relevant muscle becomes fatigued[9-11]. The overall decrease in the initial value of the MF for each test contraction was used as an indication of whether localized physiological fatigue was present. The RMS, MF and MPF were calculated using a program developed by MATLAB.

Figure 9 and figure 10 shows the change in the mean normalized RMS of the EMG for each automobile tested in lumbar and shoulder. The RMS measures were normalized

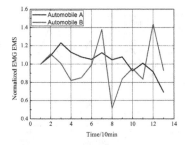

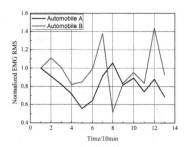

Fig. 9. Normalized RMS value of EMG for lumbar

Fig. 10. Normalized RMS value of EMG for shoulder

to the baseline value as level 1. The results of figure 9 and 10 both demonstrate that automobile A was associated with the greatest decrease in RMS, whereas automobile B showed slight decrease in RMS activity during the two hour driving period. The results mean that automobile A is easier to make drivers fatigued than automobile B which is consistent with subjective ratings.

Figure 11 and figure 13 show that the MF and MPF of people in automobile A decrease during the simulated driving experiment which showed the driver felt uncomfortable with fatigue.

Figure 12 and figure 14 show that the MF and MPF of people in automobile B slightly increase during the simulated driving experiment which show the driver didn't get fatigued. It's not sure to conclude that people can become comfortable during the prolonged driving, however based on the variation of MF and MPF automobile A is easier to make people uncomfortable than automobile B. Meanwhile, the MF of latissimus dorsi decreased faster than the trapezius muscles which meant the lumbar was easier to get fatigued or uncomfortable than the shoulder during the prolonged simulated driving, and this did also match with the subjective feelings. The MPF of automobile A decreased larger than automobile B which meant automobile A was easier to make the driver fatigued than automobile B.

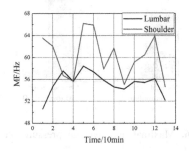

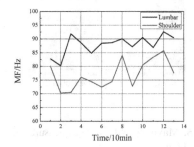

Fig. 11. MF along with time for automobile A

Fig. 12. MF along with time for automobile B

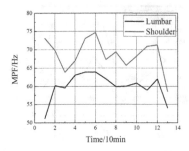
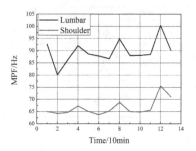

Fig. 13. MPF along with time for automobile A   **Fig. 14.** MPF along with time for automobile B

3.3   Pressure Distribution

According to figure 15 and figure 16, the maximal pressure of automobile 2 is higher than automobile A, otherwise the average pressure of automobile A and B is similar. The maximal pressure on seat cushion is 10kPa for automobile A and 12kPa for automobile B. The maximal pressure on backrest is about 5kPa for automobile A and 6kPa for automobile B. The results mean that the hardness of automobile B's seat cushion and backrest is larger than automobile A's. Since the soft interface will be easier to make people fatigue than hard interface, so automobile B will make people feel more uncomfortable than automobile A during prolonged driving.

Pm is calculated through (4)

$$P_m = \max(P_1, P_2, \ldots \ldots P_N) \tag{4}$$

Where N is the number of sensors in the sensor sheets.

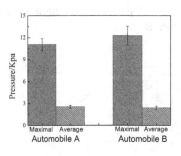
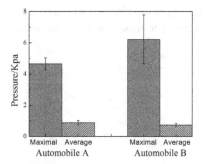

Fig. 15. Maximal and average pressure on seat cushion

Fig. 16. Maximal and average pressure on backrest

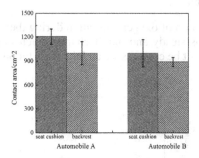

Fig. 17. Driver-seat contact area

Figure 17 shows the driver-seat interface contact area for automobile A and B. The results demonstrate that automobile A's contact area is larger than automobile B which means automobile is softer than automobile. So during prolonged driving, automobile A is easier to make people fatigued.

According to figure 18 and figure 19, the longitudinal pressure integral (P_L) of automobile A and B is similar with each other. However the maximal pressure of automobile B appears earlier which is near to the truck than automobile A. In figure 18, the proximal thigh of automobile B will bear larger pressure and compress the nerve and vascular which will make people fatigue.

P_L is calculated through (5)

$$P_L(x_i) = \sum_{j=1}^{N} P(x_i, y_j) \bullet \Delta L_j \tag{5}$$

Where $P(x_i, y_j)$ is the pressure in site (x_i, y_j).

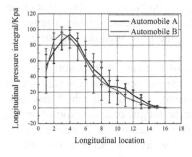

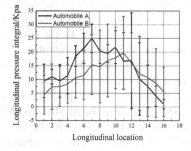

Fig. 18. Longitudinal pressure integral on seat cushion

Fig. 19. Longitudinal pressure integral on backrest

3.4   Oxygen Saturation

Figure 20 shows the variation of oxygen saturation during the prolonged driving which the oxygen saturation was steady and didn't change much in the whole time. That's perhaps the vascular doesn't be compressed and the toe's blood is sufficient.

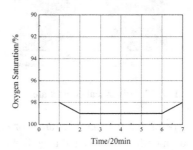

Fig. 20. Oxygen saturation along with time

4   Conclusion

Subjective ratings, EMG, sitting pressure distribution and oxygen saturation were measured to evaluate the comfort of two kinds of automobiles. Subjective ratings of the lumbar are sensitive to the driving comfort. By comparing the variation of MPF and MF with the subjective ratings, the decrease of MPF and MF can indicate the fatigue of drivers or discomfort. The maximal pressure, average pressure, contact area and longitudinal pressure integral were analyzed, maximal pressure is relate to the hardness of seat cushion and backrest. According to previous study, driver will be easier to get fatigued with soft seat cushion during prolonged driving and hard seat cushion will make driver more comfort. From the results, automobile B's seat cushion is harder than automobile A, so we can conclude that automobile B can be more comfort than automobile A which is in accordance with the subjective ratings. The longitudinal pressure integral is relate to the feeling of numbness from thigh that larger longitudinal pressure integral will easier to make driver fell uncomfortable. The results of oxygen saturation show that it is constant during the prolonged driving, so in this experiment this index is not suitable.

Overall, MPF and MF of EMG, Pm and P_L of pressure distribution are high significant with the subjective comfort, otherwise the oxygen saturation was almost constant during the whole prolonged simulated driving experiment which has little significance. The decrease of MPF and MF indicate the fatigue or discomfort of driver, large Pm and PL are in favor of the comfort of driver. Based on the objective results, automobile A is more comfortable than automobile B which is in accordance with the subjective results. Therefore from the study we can see the most sensitive body part to feel discomfort during prolonged driving and the relationship between discomfort and physiological parameters was also clarified which can be used to find which automotive seat is more comfortable.

Acknowledgment. This work is supported by the ergonomics laboratory of China National Institute of Standardization.

References

1. Zenk, R., et al.: Predicting Overall Seating Discomfort Based on Body Area Ratings. SAE International (2007)
2. Pellettiere, J., et al.: The Effects of Ejection Seat Cushion Design on Physical Fatigue and Cognitive Performance, p. 37 (2006)
3. Andreoni, G., et al.: Method for the analysis of posture and interface pressure of car drivers. Applied Ergonomics 33(6), 511–522 (2002)
4. Kolich, M.: Predicting automobile seat comfort using a neural network. International Journal of Industrial Ergonomics 33(4), 285–293 (2004)
5. Grujicic, M., et al.: Seat-cushion and soft-tissue material modeling and a finite element investigation of the seating comfort for passenger-vehicle occupants. Materials & Design 30(10), 4273–4285 (2009)
6. González-Izal, M., et al.: EMG spectral indices and muscle power fatigue during dynamic contractions. Journal of Electromyography and Kinesiology 20(2), 233–240 (2010)
7. De Luca, C.J.: Myoelectrical manifestations of localized muscular fatigue in humans. Crit. Rev. Biomed. Eng. 11(4), 251–279 (1984)
8. Sheridan, T.B., et al.: Physiological and Psychological Evaluations of Driver Fatigue During Long Term Driving. SAE International (1991)
9. Cao, Y., Hu, Y.: Analysis of surface electromyography of back muscle fatigue on sitting and standing position. Chin. J. Ind. Hyg. Occup. Dis. 24(12) (2006)
10. Liang, H., et al.: A monitoring study of electromyography median frequency on fatigue of elector spinalis in drivers working. Chin. J. Ind. Hyg. Occup. Dis. 20(6) (2002)
11. Pi, X., et al.: Methods applied to muscle fatigue assessment using surface myoelectric signals. J. Biomed. Eng. 23(1) (2006)

Simulation on Thermal Control System
of the Extravehicular Spacesuit

Tanqiu Li[1], Jing Zhang[2], Xiugan Yuan[1], and Li Ding[2,*]

[1] School of Aeronautic Science and Engineering, Beihang University,
No.37 XueYuan Road, HaiDian District, Beijing 100191, China
bj_tqli@sohu.com, yuanxg@buaa.edu.cn
[2] School of Biological Science and Medical Engineering, Beihang University,
No.37 XueYuan Road, HaiDian District, Beijing 100191, China
zhangjing@be.buaa.edu.cn, ding1971316@buaa.edu.cn

Abstract. The extravehicular (EVA) spacesuit is the life support system for astronauts in the extravehicular activity and help the astronauts perform the assembling of large space vehicle and maintenance. The thermal control system is one of the most important functions for extravehicular spacesuit, and it's directly related to the thermal protection structure and active temperature control, especially to the human body heat load. In this study, a human-suit thermal control model was built and the effect of human heat load, outside thermal environment and their composition effect to the thermal control system was analyzed. The extravehicular spacesuit prototyping system was used to validate the model. The results show as the follows.(1) It's reasonable to set 3 percent of the chiller flow as the lowest gear of thermal control system which can maintain the inside suit thermal comfort during low temperature and low metabolism situation. (2) The thermal control system's response will be faster if the temperature gear is higher. (3) It is not significantly affected to the temperature response of cooling input if the human metabolism rate is below 500W. (4) Thermal control model's validation and evaluation by dry thermal manikin is receivable. Overall, the human-suit thermal control model can be used to improve the design of extravehicular spacesuit's thermal protection system.

Keywords: spacesuit, thermal control, human body heat load.

1 Introduction

The extravehicular (EVA) spacesuit is basic protection and support system for astronauts' extravehicular working performance and is the core equipment system for the construction and maintenance of the large space facility. Thermal protection and vacuum pressure protection are the core functions of the EVA spacesuit. After nearly half a century of technological development, spacesuit thermal control system has become the active / passive integrated, ventilation / liquid-cooled mixed and liquid

---

* Corresponding author.

V.G. Duffy (Ed.): DHM 2014, LNCS 8529, pp. 112–123, 2014.
© Springer International Publishing Switzerland 2014

cooling dominated form [1-2], but there is still much room for improvement of the comfort and economy of the thermal control system [3-5]. For the thermal comfort evaluation of the EVA spacesuit, Yifen Qiu et al has done simulating calculation for the 'space environment - spacesuit – human' system. However, they simply put the spacesuit into two parts, EVA spacesuit and liquid-cooled suit, lacking more specific analysis on the internal structure of the spacesuit. SINDA, the U.S. spacesuit portable life support system simulation software, uses 41 notes' human thermal model and the spacesuit model to combine the spacesuit' thermal control device model and human heat transfer model, and then through computer simulation methods, it guides the costume design[6-7]. However, the current structure division of spacesuit of the software is relatively simple [8-9]. In order to meet the overall thermal design requirements and applications of the EVA spacesuit thermal control system, this paper did system-level simulation analysis and experimental research on the spacesuit's all levels of thermal control and dynamic thermal response of mutual restraint.

2   The Composition of the Spacesuit Thermal Control System and Thermal Model

From outside to inside, all levels of the EVA spacesuit's protective structures are vacuum shield insulation layer, pressure suit layer, comfortable layer, ventilation layer, liquid-cooled suit layer and underwear layer (Figure 1). While temperature, heat flux and other physical parameters exhibit distributed features in the actual process, considering that the inside of EVA spacesuit system is closed ventilation system, the temperature is largely homogenized, so this paper tries to build dynamics model and analyze the system using lumped parameter method. That is each layer considered as a lumped node, and each node representing all the physical properties and structural properties, thermal parameters of the certain layer, without considering the temperature distribution differences on each spatial location.

According to the general design and testability considerations, this paper takes the vacuum shield insulation layer, pressure suit layer and comfortable layer as a total

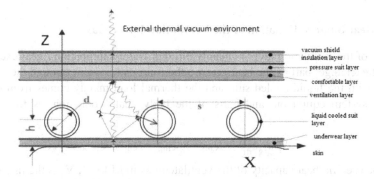

Fig. 1. The composition of the spacesuit thermal control system and thermal model

protective layer, so the thermal control system can be simplified into three layers which are protection layer, ventilation layer and liquid-cooled layer (considering the underwear and human skin together as thermal load model). The heat balance equations of all levels are as follows.

2.1 Thermal Equation of State of the Outer Protective Layer

The temperature variation of the thermal protective layer depends on the heat capacity and the heat flux which is accepted, reflected by the protective layer and penetrates through it. The thermal equation of state is as formula (1).

$$C_{sp} M_{sp} \frac{dT_{sp}}{dt} = Q_r - Q_e + Q_{leak} \tag{1}$$

C_{sp} represents the integrated heat capacity of the EVA spacesuit outer protective layer, and the unit is kJ/kgK; M_{sp} is the total mass of outer protective layer, in kg; T_{sp} is the average temperature, in °C. Q_e is the external heat flux absorbed by the outer surface, in W; Q_r is the neat flux the outer surface radiates to the external space, in W, and its value as the formula (2).

$$Q_r = A_{sp} \, \varepsilon \, \sigma \, T_a^4 \tag{2}$$

A_{sp} is the superficial area of the outer surface of EVA spacesuit, and the unit is m²; T_a is the surface temperature of the outer protective layer, in K; ε is the material emissivity of the outer layer; σ is the Boltzmann constant. Q_{leak} is the leakage bustling flow of the EVA spacesuit, in W; its value is as follows.

$$Q_{leak} = k_{eq}(T_g - T_a) \tag{3}$$

k_{eq} is the equivalent heat transfer coefficient of thermal protective layer, and the unit is W/m2°C; T_g is the average gas temperature of the EVA spacesuit ventilation layer, in K.

According to the formula (1), (2) &(3), and assuming that the system temperature change having the same overall trends, we can get the temperature conversion relations of the outer casing, as the formula (4).

$$C_{sp} M_{sp} \frac{dT_o}{dt} = -Q_e + A_{sp}\varepsilon\sigma T_o^4 + k_{eq}(T_g - T_o) \tag{4}$$

2.2 Heat Balance Equation of the Ventilation Layer Gas

Airflow of the ventilation layer is mainly through water sublimation / heat exchanger for heat exchange; part of the heat get into the fluid path system through the heat exchange with the liquid-cooled suit, and the thermal load mainly comes from the life support system equipment and parts of the body heat production, as formula (5) shows.

$$C_g V_g \, \rho_g \frac{dT_g}{dt} = Q_{plss} + Q_{mg} - Q_{lg} - Q_{leak} - Q_{gs} \tag{5}$$

C_g is the specific heat capacity of the ventilated gas in kJ/kg°C; V_g is the internal volume of the spacesuit, in m³; ρ_g is the internal gas density, in kg/ m3; T_g of the average temperature of the ventilation layer gas, in ℃; Q_{plss} is the heat production rate of the built-in life support system (excluding the part liquid-cooled pumps taken), in W; Q_{lg} is the heat exchanging rate between the ventilation layer and liquid-cooled layer, in W; Q_{leak} is heat leakage rate of the system (leakage of heat per unit time), in W; Q_{mg} is the heat exchanging rate between the ventilation air and the bod, in W; its value is as follows.

$$Q_{mg} = hA_m \ (T_w - T_g) \tag{6}$$

h is the heat exchanging coefficient and the unit is W/m2℃; A_m is the surface area of the human body, in m2; TW is the average temperature of the liquid-cooled ventilation layer interface, in ℃; Q_{gs} is the cooling rate of the cold water source of the water sublimator to the gas (the heat taken from the air road per unit time), in W, and its value is as follows.

$$Q_{gs} = c_g m_g \Delta T_{sp} = c_g m_g \ (T_{go} - T_{gs}) \tag{7}$$

m_g is the ventilation gas flow rate, and the unit is kg/s; C_g is the specific heat of the ventilation gas, in kJ/kg℃; T_{go} is the inlet temperature of the ventilation air, in ℃; T_{gs} is the outlet air temperature of the water sublimator, in ℃.

Combining the formula (5), (6) and (7), we get the heat balance equation of the ventilation layer gas.

$$C_g V_g \rho_g \frac{dT_g}{dt} = Q_{plss} + hA_m(T_w - T_g) - k_{eq}A_{sp}(T_g - T_a) - C_g M_g(T_{go} - T_{gs}) - Q_{lg} \tag{8}$$

2.3   Liquid Thermal Power Equation of the Liquid Circuit

The heat exchange between the fluid within the fluid circuit and the external part includes those from the human body, the ventilation layer, the fluid path inside the device heat rate and the internal device of the fluid path. Finally, the heat from the fluid path is discharged into the space by cold source / heat exchanger, without considering the radiative heat exchange between the wall of the tubes in liquid cooling suit and the inner wall of the pressure suit (due to the relatively small temperature difference). The liquid thermal power equation of the liquid circuit is as follows.

$$C_w M_w \frac{dT_{wa}}{dt} = Q_{ml} + Q_p + Q_{lg} - Q_{ls} \tag{9}$$

C_w is the specific heat of water, in kJ/kg℃; M_w is the total mass of the liquid fluid loop, in kg; Twa is the average water temperature of the liquid cooling suit, in ℃; Q_p is the heat generation rate of the liquid cooling circuit, in W; Q_{ml} is the heat exchange rate of liquid cooling system with the human body, in W, which is as follows.

$$Q_{ml} = K_w(T_s - T_i) \tag{10}$$

Q_{lg} is the heat exchange rate between the liquid-cooled layer and the ventilation layer, ignoring the thermal resistance of the liquid cooling tubes, and the unit is W. Its value is as follows.

$$Q_{lg} = h_x \pi \, dL(T_w - T_{wa}) \tag{11}$$

h_x is the natural convection heat exchange coefficient for the ventilation layer and the liquid-cooled tube, in W/m2°C; d is the diameter of the liquid-cooled tube, in m; L is the total length of the liquid-cooled pipeline, in m. Q_{ls} is the heat exchange rate of the liquid-cooled suit via the sublimation's cold source, in W, and its value is as follows.

$$Q_{ls} = C_w M_w (T_o - T_{ws}) \tag{12}$$

T_o represents the outlet temperature of the liquid-cooled suit, in °C; T_{ws} is the outlet water temperature of the sublimation, in °C.

Combining (9) - (12), we get formula (13).

$$C_w M_w \frac{dT_{wa}}{dt} = K_w (T_s - T_i) - C_w M_w (T_o - T_{ws}) + Q_p + h_x \pi \, dL(T_w - T_{wa}) \tag{13}$$

In summary, the EVA spacesuit thermal control system can be described synthetically by formula (4), (8) and (13).

3   Parameters Affecting the Life Support System

In the EVA spacesuit life support system, adjustment device of the cold source and valve controller are key links of the thermal control. The following analysis shows the relevant characteristics in the above formulas.

3.1   Water Sublimator

Water sublimator is simultaneously a cold source and heat exchanger of the system, as well as the main pathway to control the heat exchange of the active temperature control system with the external space. Analysis and testing show that the outlet gas temperature and outlet water temperature is stable on the whole for the water sublimation device with full cooling capacity and efficiency. This paper regards T_{gs} and T_{ws} in the formula (7) and (11) as constants (little change were found of the value in testing).

3.2   Temperature Adjustment Device

As shows in figure 2, the active temperature control system, the shunt flow ratio inflowing the water sublimation can be regulated by setting the thermostatic valve at different stalls; the ratio is denoted as k_n (n corresponds to the 0,1,2,3,4,5 stall separately). Relationship of the temperatures is as follows.

$$T_o - T_i = \frac{k_n(T_i - T_{ls})}{1 - k_n} \tag{14}$$

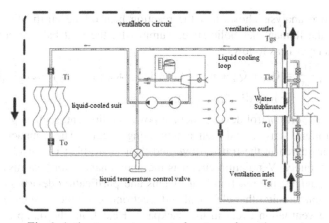

Fig. 2. Active temperature control system schematics

In the formula (13), T_{wa} can be represented by the average temperature at the outlet and inlet.

$$T_{wa} = \frac{T_i + T_o}{2} \tag{15}$$

So, the liquid thermal power equation of the liquid circuit-formula (13) - is further expressed as (16).

$$\frac{C_w M_w}{(1-K_n)} \frac{dT_i}{dt} = K_w(T_s - T_i) + Q_p + Q_{lg} - \frac{C_w M_w}{1-K_n} K_n(T_o - T_i) \tag{16}$$

For the ventilation circuit, the ventilating air flow is fixed and non-adjustable; the temperature relationship can be expressed as (17).

$$T_{go} - T_{gs} = 2(T_g - T_{gs}) \tag{17}$$

Q_{plss}, the built-in heat production rate of life support system, generally consists of fans, pumps and its controllers, sensors and its conditioning circuit, and purification device. Under working condition, in addition to the purification device producing reaction heat, the rest devices produce fixed heat according to their device power; we set it as Q_d. LiOH is widely used to absorb CO_2 and the reaction equation is as follows.

$$2LiOH + CO_2 = Li_2CO_3 + H_2O$$

This reaction is an exothermic reaction, producing heat and water vapor. The reaction heat is 158 J/mol; the clean tank heat balance equation can be expressed as (18).

$$c_g \rho_g V_p \frac{dT_g}{dt} = c_g M_g(T_{go} - T_g) + Q_m \, \beta \, F \, \rho_{co_2}^0 \tag{18}$$

Vp is the gas volume of the purification tank; Qm is the heat from human body; β is the apparatus for the purification of the void coefficient and F is a parameter associated with the purification contact area in the purification apparatus. ρ_{co2}^0 is the outlet concentration of CO2 gas of the purification tank.

The above analysis shows that the reaction heat of the purification apparatus is related to the human metabolic state. Summarily, the heat balance equation of the ventilation layer is as follows.

$$c_g \, \rho_g \, V_p \frac{dT_g}{dt} = Q_m + Q_d + hA_m\left(T_w - T_g\right) - k_{eq}\left(T_g - T_a\right) - 2C_gM_g\left(T_g - T_{go}\right) -$$
$$h_x \, \pi \, dL(T_w - T_{wa}) \tag{19}$$

Other life support control devices include power equipment, such as pumps, fans and their controllers, sensors and their conditioning circuits. Their impact on the power cycle is considered in the traffic flow, and their heat effect is considered with other devices separately. Ventilation circuit is the main channel for heat dissipation of the protection devices; the reaction heat of fans and purification device are directly into the ventilation circuit; other electrical and electronic equipment exchange heat mainly through the ventilation cycle in the backpack. Heat from the pump are directly included in the liquid loop load. As closed to the cold source of the water sublimation, part of the life support system equipment can directly heat, but since it is a very small part of the overall, it is not considered when analyzing the whole system.

4   Dynamics Model of the Thermal Control System

Human heat regulation model is necessary for the simulation of human-uniform-environment whole system. Dual-node model by Gagge is prior in the process of parameters collection in human heat regulation model. Both dynamic model of the thermal control system and simulation model applied the same dummies experiment. This section introduces the simulation model by combining the equation of (4), (16), (19) and the structure of spacesuit thermal control system and flow parameters. CO_2 injection was applied in simulation of heat condition in human metabolism.

4.1   Model of Warm Body Mummy

Dynamic characteristics of extravehicular spacesuit are closely related with its response to heat fluctuation. Equations above and human heat regulation model provide the feasibility for analysis of human-uniform-environment characterization. This paper focuses on the spacesuit heat control feature and the corresponding authentication method investigation. The investigation of heat feature experiments was conducted by simulation heat load and mummy experiments. Mummy heat load model, including heat section, liquid cooling section and ventilation section, was summarized by the following equation.

$$C_mM_m \frac{dT}{dt} = Q_m - Q_{ml} - Q_{mg} \tag{20}$$

Where C_m, M_m and Q_m are specific heat capacity, total mass and simulation metabolism heat of mummies, respectively. Heat load equation can be rewritten with equation (6) and (10).

$$C_mM_m \frac{dT}{dt} = Q_m - K_w(T_s - T_i) - hA_m(T_w - T_g) \tag{21}$$

4.2   Heat Control System Parameters

Several parameters are related to the above model. A ccording to the test, extravehicular spacesuit solar absorption spectrum α_s=0.2, emissivityε=0.85, typical ventilation flow is 150-170 L/min, liquid ventilation is about 50 L, circle flow is 100-120 kg/h, total mass of circle flow is 2.5-3 kg, temperature of ventilation outlet is 6-8 ℃.

5   Result and Analysis of System Feature and Simulation

This section mainly discusses the sensitivity of heat control system response to environment, heat load, and control variables. Matlab 7 was applied to simulation different environment in simulation.

5.1   Low Temperature Simulation

Cryogenic condition is the process of spacesuit transforming from airlock to cryogenic condition. According to the preparation of spacesuit in transition process and temperature condition in airlock, initial temperature in and out of spacesuit was set as 20℃, and the stalls of temperature controller was set as 0 stage (K_n=0.1, i.e. Cooling flow was 10% of the total cooling flow), initial metabolism of warm body mummy was 100 W, fans and pumps in life support system and purification device reaction heat was 17 W, which was corresponding to the 100 W metabolism. Figure 3 was the inlet temperature Ti of the cooling liquid, average temperature of ventilation Tg and temperature of the out surface were compared with the experiment result, external heat temperature was set as 100 K.

The simulation results reveal that the temperature of spacesuit out surface drops rapidly due to the external dark environment. Besides, the significant temperature difference promotes the heat leak, and hence, the temperature of internal of spacesuit and mummy drops. Under the condition given above, the temperature of internal of spacesuit and mummy drops 5 ℃ in 30 min, which can feel by people obviously. Apparently, the temperature then cannot support the comfortable environment.

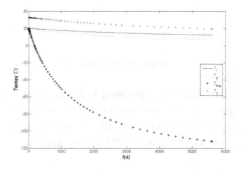

Fig. 3. Metabolism 100 W feature at the range from 100 K to homoeothermy

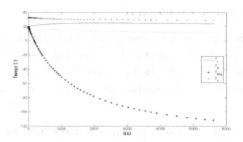

Fig. 4. Temperature of in/out spacesuit behavior under the condition of 100 W metabolism

Heat radiation including the heat leaking from the insulation layer (external heat exchange behavior refers to the heat radiation under cold background) and liquid cooling system. Depress the liquid cooling system heat radiation is a feasible method to achieve comfortable heat balance. Liquid flow can be controlled by valve so that the heat radiation is depressed. Figure 4 reveals the simulation result under the condition of 3% total circle flow. It can be seen that the temperature in the spacesuit can be sustained and the cooling flow decreases 7%. Therefore, basic heat balance can be supported by decreasing liquid cooling flow, and the heat exchange then decreases about 100 W.

Actually, under the given condition (kn= 0.1), comfortable environment can be achieved by increasing body metabolism. Figure 5 reveal the simulation result of 200 W metabolism. Internal temperature by then can be sustained (air temperature stable, warm body mummy temperature increases, and the liquid cooling temperature at inlet increases). Obviously, under the 100 W metabolism condition, heat leak was less than 100 W, which was agree with the method of decreasing liquid cooling flow.

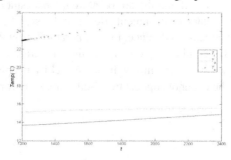

Fig. 5. Simulation result of temperature behavior under 200 W metabolism

Figure 6 reveal that the internal temperature behavior when metabolism increased to 400 W (k_n= 0.1). Figure 7 is the simulation result of internal temperature under the low temperature metabolism (k_n= 0.1). Simulation metabolism varies from 100 W (20 min)-200 W (20 min)-400 W (80 min) - 250 W (30 min), and internal temperature changes accordingly.

Above simulation results reveals that liquid flow set as 3% is reasonable, and internal temperature and comfortable environment can be achieved under this condition.

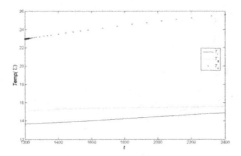

Fig. 6. Simulation result of temperature behavior under 400 W metabolism

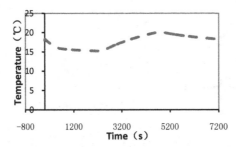

Fig. 7. Simulation result of internal temperature under the low temperature metabolism

5.2   Average Out Heat Flow Heat Simulation

As introduced in above heat balance experiment result, spacesuit under the condition of external heat radiation, heat leak is about 30 W, which is the most close to the orbit extravehicular condition. Figure 8 shows the temperature behavior with 400 W simulation metabolism under different flow condition. It can be seen that temperature controller switches to 1 stage (k_n= 0.2), internal temperature can be controlled well. The simulation results also shows that when the controller switches to higher stage, heat control system respond more rapidly. This is mainly attributed to the heat inertia of liquid circle. The bigger the liquid flow mass is, the more heat exchange is. The liquid cooling response time is about 3~8 min, air temperature in ventilation circle changes more rapidly due to the low heat capacity.

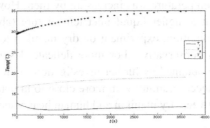

Fig. 8. 400 W metabolism of 1 stage (kn=0.2) under average temperature condition

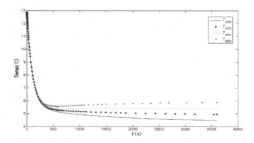

Fig. 9. Effect of different metabolism on liquid inlet temperature when flow parameter kn=0.6

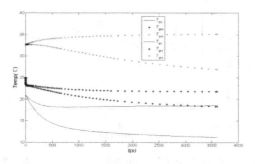

Fig. 10. Comparison of simulation heat exchange parameter and mummy heat radiation control

Figure 9 shows different simulation metabolism effect on spacesuit under the same flow (k_n= 0.6). The results reveal that different metabolism affect inlet temperature little when the metabolism bellows 500 W. It because that under the same flow, cooling source heat radiation almost reaches stability (when k_n= 0.5 and metabolism reaches 500 W, temperature controls stable). When metabolism changes, astronaut needs to adjust controller valve frequently so that comfortable heat environment can be obtained.

Figure 10 compares the experiment heat exchange parameter (Kwr≈25) and warm body mummy heat radiation parameter (Kwr≈15). It can be seen that the inlet liquid temperature dropped about 11 ℃ when the warm body mummy reached heat balance, and its average temperature was increasing by then. However, human body can reaches heat balance at a higher liquid inlet temperature (about 19 ℃). Therefore, comparing with real condition, experiment on dry manikin to simulate the spacesuit heat control system is conservative. For more delicate design, more closed to real condition result can be obtained by further investigation in the following two aspects: (1) develop more advanced mummy with more close to human to be test on; (2) find out the relationship between dry manikin and human heat response experiment.

6   Conclusion

This paper carried out warm body mummy test and external temperature heat control by applying the spacesuit prototype thermal control system under vacuum condition. The results show simulation analysis is highly agreed with experiment data, which possess high engineering value in system solution design and analysis.

Acknowledgment. This project is supported by the National Natural Science Foundation of China, Grant No. 51175021 & the National Science and Technology Support Program of China, Grant No.2014BAK01B05.

References

1. Nyberg, K.L., Diller, K.R., Wissler, E.H.: Analysis of LCG thermal performance and control. SAE972321
2. Kissen, A.T., et al.: Evalation of a water-cooled helmet liner. Aerospace Medical Research Laboratory Wright-Patterson Air Force Base, 11 (1994)
3. Barer, A.S.E.: Medical prodlems. Acta Astronautica, 23 (1991)
4. Waligora, J.M., Horrigan, D.J.: Metabolism & Pheat dissipation during Apollo EVA periods. In: Johnston, R.S., Dietlein, L.F., Berry, C.A. (eds.) Biomedical Results of Apollo, NASA SP-368 (1975)
5. Waligora, J.M., Horrigan, D.J.: Metabolic cost of extravehicular activities. In: Johnston, R.S., Dietlein, L.F. (eds.) Biomedical Results from Skylab,NASA SP-377 (1977)
6. Szeleinyi, E.: Contributions to thermal physiology. Pergaman (1981)
7. Lawrence, H.R.: Control of thermal balance by a liquid circulating garment base on a mathematical representation of the thermore-gulatory system. NASA TMX- 58190, 10 (1976)
8. Ruel, S., Margiott, V.: EMU thermal modifications for the cold EVA environments on the hubble space telescope servicing mission. In: AIAA 94-4623,AIAA Space Programs and Technologies Conference, September 27-29, (1994), Huntsville AL
9. Williams, J.L., Copeland, R.J.: Advanced extravehicular protective system study. NASA CR 114832

Calibration of Online Situation Awareness Assessment Systems Using Virtual Reality

Sebastien Mamessier, Daniel Dreyer, and Matthias Oberhauser

Airbus Group Innovations, Ottobrunn, Germany,
Creative Concept and Design Center,
Ottobrunn, Germany

Abstract. In an attempt to predict and prevent accident situations in complex socio-technical systems, one needs to be able to model and simulate concepts such as situation awareness (SA) and processes responsible for maintaining it. This is particularly true in the case of online support systems and adaptive displays which cannot rely on SA measurement techniques based on freeze probe techniques. This work investigates the state of the art in computational models of situation awareness and proposes a method to calibrate and evaluate such models using virtual reality human-in-the-loop experiments. This work introduces a new methodology to evaluate and calibrate online SA assessment systems taking advantage of the flexibility and reconfigurable power of virtual reality environments. This technology provides the experimenter with full control on the scenarios, cockpit types and interfaces. It also allows testing of off-nominal situations such as the loss of an instrument and more severe failures. Moreover, eye tracking capabilities provide an accurate way of registering monitoring events and feed SA assessment models with realistic data.

Keywords: situation awareness, mental models, virtual reality.

1 Introduction

In complex socio-technical environments such as modern aircraft cockpits, accidents still occur because of poorly designed human-integrated systems. Situation awareness of the pilot is often degraded by abnormally high workload or pilots' faulty mental models of the autoflight systems. Operators have to maintain an accurate representation of the situation supported by a good knowledge of the system's dynamics. Therefore, dangerous situations often occur when the complexity of the system or unexpected workload compromises the operator's situation awareness [31]. In order to improve the automation's design or develop situation awareness-centered support systems [8], we need a methodology to evaluate the impact of design changes on SA as well as good indicators of SA for online assessment. The introduction of SA in the design loop assumes the development of SA assessment methods. However, SA is an abstract concept and its realization depends on many inputs such as the operator's mental

V.G. Duffy (Ed.): DHM 2014, LNCS 8529, pp. 124–135, 2014.

model, the current workload and general monitoring and anticipating efforts. Methodologies such as SAGAT [9] provide a substantial help to measure SA and evaluate socio-technical systems. However most of these methods rely on "freezes" during simulations which makes them irrelevant to the design of online support systems. One needs computational models for the online assessment of SA based on live measurements to allow the existence of intelligent systems aiming to maintain and restore the operator's SA in real-time circumstances. This work introduces a methodology to evaluate and calibrate online SA assessment systems using virtual reality (VR) environments. VR cockpits can be modified easily and instruments hidden by the experimenter. Moreover, VR enables quick reconfiguration of the cockpit elements and can therefore be used to evaluate adaptive displays aimed to maintain or restore SA of the pilot.

2 Background

2.1 Situation Awareness

In 1988, Sarter and Woods introduced the concept of situation awareness without the support of an accurate definition [31]. In 1995, Endsley [7] gave a formal definition and broke down SA into three different levels : perception (L1), comprehension (L2) and anticipation (L3). Endsley's theory is widely accepted across different fields of application such as aviation and nuclear safety as a critical concept to understand accidents and dangerous situations. Dekker et al. discussed the usefulness of what they call a *folk model* [3] : a consensual abstraction that hides the real phenomena. Whether SA is more an abstract product or a fundamental process is still discussed among human factor experts. Nevertheless, SA remains of great importance for safety [32] and methods for measuring SA have led to operational results.

Methodologies for measuring SA includes the Situation Awareness Global Assessment Technique (SAGAT) developed by Endsley [6,9] in which situation awareness is believed to be measurable by freezing a task [6] and simply querying the operator's understanding of the situation. SAGAT is a well validated method and is widely used to evaluate interfaces, and validate design changes such as new displays. Therefore it is often used in the design phase of the product lifecycle. However its intrusive nature prevents SAGAT from supporting the assessment of SA in real time circumstances. Other potential measurement techniques are described by Endsley in [8] involve psychophysiological metrics such as eye tracking data. They are described as appealing since unobtrusive and continuously available - thus suitable for live SA assessment - but are indirect and require a huge amount of calibration. Moreover the link between processes believed to maintain SA and SA remains unclear. Rare examples show that eye tracking can nevertheless give precious hints about the operator's situation awareness [28,33]. Ratwani et al. trained a statistical model of SA capable of significantly predicting operators' ability to detect conflicting situations involving UAVs from eye-tracking data [28].

2.2   SA-Based adaptive interfaces

Safety critical concepts like SA should not only benefit to the design phase of complex systems. Indeed, testing and validation is limited to a finite set of scenarios and struggle at handling unexpected situations. Approaches such as Work Domain Analysis and Ecological Interface Design [35] strive for event-independent design and are therefore helpful to extend the effectiveness of a design to off-nominal situations. Nevertheless, static interfaces are inherently limited since they don't capture the specific features of a situation.

Adaptive interfaces can change the position and saliency of different instruments during the operation. Changes can be driven by users' preferences, experience, fatigue, current task demands [30] or any other factors measurable by the system. Dehais et al. developed adaptive displays deploying cognitive countermeasures to prevent perseveration syndrome [2] and used performance-based validation metrics. Letsu and Ntuen [21] designed an adaptive interface for the DURESS II system [34].

Generally speaking, adaptive displays are the front-end of support systems that we believe should help maintain and restore situation awareness. Therefore there is a crucial need for online situation awareness computational models.

2.3   Computational Models of SA Lack Validation

Several computational models of situation awareness were developed around human models. Hoeey et al. modeled and predicted situation awareness of a human performance model of a pilot in [12]. Their model included models of visual attention, perception and working memory but is limited to SA of discrete *Situational Elements*. Moreover, Hoeey et al. don't consider the impact of mental models, known to be one of the main factors responsible for maintaing SA [8]. Mc Carley et al. created an heuristic model for general SA accounting for attention and workload [27]. This model was also used to predict the impact of dynamic SA display supports. However, SA is modeled as a unidimensional quantity which limits the adaptability power of the dynamic support interface. SAMPLE [36] is a fully integrated situation awareness prediction system of pilots involved in air combat. SAMPLE uses an extensive human model accounting for information processing and decision making. A Kalman filter is used to predict the pilot's estimate of continuous state variables and the pilot's knowledge of scenarios is represented as a bayesian network. Hanson et al. proposed to use SAMPLE as an online intelligent agent evaluating the pilot's situation assessment [11]. However, SAMPLE does not benefit from online measurements such as eye tracking data but is only based on assumed monitoring patterns. In the field of interface design for nuclear plant operators, Lee and Seong [20] proposed a comprehensive model of SA including the effects of working memory decay, discrete mental models and instrument saliency. Mamessier et al. enhanced a computational human performance model [10] with situation awareness and mental model capabilities [25,23] including mental models of continuous and discrete dynamics. The model used in [25,24] generates a multivariate belief function representing the current situation awareness of the operator.

However few of these approaches use live measurements of the pilot's behavior to provide the model with realistic and online data. Furthermore many of these methods serve as an evaluation system for complex human-integrated designs but were not validated as such.

3 Evaluation and Calibration of Online SA Assessment Systems

Non-intrusive SA assessment systems with real-time constraints inherently rely on indirect measures of SA and therefore on an underlying model integrating them into a quantitative indicator of situation awareness. Therefore, such computational models of SA should be evaluated and calibrated.

3.1 Requirements

There are several factors that should be covered by any online SA assessment system. Jones et al. [14] analyzed 262 errors in 143 flight incidents. Around 50% of errors were caused by failures to observe data or detect important clues. 15% were related to incorrect mental models, the rest being distributed between unavailable data (13%), forgotten data (8.5%), misinterpretation (8.7%) and other causes. Therefore computational models aiming to predict losses of SA and develop countermeasures should try to model and capture the operator's attention, data collection and account for mental models. Otherwise such models might overlook substantial evidence of loss of situation awareness.

3.2 Process Indices

Since non-intrusive SA assessment systems with real-time contraints cannot afford to query the pilot about his immediate knowledge, they rely on indirect measures. Psychophysiological measurement such as eye tracking methods are often referred to as *Process indices* as they don't directly measure SA but some of the processes contributing to the development of SA. Depending on the models and technology available, useful process indices could include recording of actual pilot actions, eye-tracking data, workload-related physiological measure, verbal communication between pilots. However, demonstrating which process indices are better for online SA assessment is not the main focus of this work. [29] emphasizes on their disadvantages, indirect nature and practical issues. The conclusion made in Salmon et al.'s extensive review of SA measurement methods [29] confirms SAGAT as as the most accurate and objective approach and overlooks methods based on process indices. The main idea behind this work is that we can evaluate online SA assessment systems by comparing their outputs with SAGAT objective measurements in a experimental setup. Instead of comparing *Process indices* and SAGAT as it was done in [29,8], we aim to use SAGAT as a widely recognized and validated SA measurement method to evaluate and calibrate indirect and model-based online SA assessments systems.

3.3 SA and Virtual Reality

As listed above in the requirements, a SA assessment system should account for diverse processes such as attention/perception, mental models, workload and working memory decay. In order to evaluate and calibrate such complex models, one needs a flexible and reconfigurable environment providing the capability of decoupling the impact of influential factors. For instance, hiding instruments temporarily disconnects the perception loop to focus on the impact of mental models, normalizing the instruments' saliency enables the experimenter to limit the influence of design-dependent factors. Physical simulators are very constraining, onerous and too static to satisfy the needs of such an experiment.

On the other hand, virtual reality environments have many advantages. The assessment of SA within virtual environments was already theoretically discussed in the late nineties [5]. Consequently, the original ideas of assessing SA in VR were picked up again by Matthews et al. [26] for the analysis of night vision goggles during dismounted soldier simulations. After each simulated night mission, the soldiers completed the Mission Awareness Rating Scale (MARS), an instrument designed to assess the subjective SA and workload experienced during a given mission. Laptaned [19] used tools like VRSAGAT, VRSARM and VRSART [15,16,17] in order to set SA, immersion, presence and performance in relation to each other. His research indicates a correlations between immersion and presence, and presence with SA. Horsch et al. [13] used Virtual Environments to test Urban Search and Rescue Robots. Their experiments showed no significant differences in SA and performance during several elementary tasks (e.g. slalom) between a virtual world and an experiment in reality. Recently, Dreyer et al. [4] conducted experiments in a Virtual Reality Flight Simulation and used NASA-TLX and SART questionnaires in order to assess workload and SA in different cockpit layouts.

4   Virtual Reality Experiment

A VR engine can load 3D models of aircraft cockpit as well as of a nuclear plant control room. The experiment presented here uses a VR aircraft cockpit and simulates flight scenarios involving a pilot. Since modern cockpits are considered as highly-sophisticated and complex human-integrated systems, we believe that the approach conveyed in this work can fit other domains as well as far as SA assessment systems are concerned.

4.1 The Virtual Reality Flight Simulator

The virtual reality environment used in this work is similar to the virtual reality flight simulator (VRFS) presented by Dreyer et al. [4]. This system is based on a consumer flight simulator that is extended in order to get VR capabilities. The actual position and orientation of the user's head is gathered via a head-tracking system and the viewpoint in the flight simulation software is adjusted accordingly [1]. With a three-dimensional cockpit geometry and a realistic outside view, both provided by the flight simulator, and a state of the art head mounted display (HMD) a highly immersive experience is provided. In addition, stereoscopic vision is achieved by slightly changing the camera positions for the right eye and the left eye. The use of hardware elements in the virtual reality flight simulator - e.g a throttle quadrant and a flight stick - creates a so called mixed mockup. To monitor the pilots' gaze behavior, an eye tracking system is part of the experimental setup. Commonly eye-tracking systems consist of an eye and a field camera. As the pilots eye is obscured the eye camera has to be mounted inside the HMD. To cover individual anatomic variations the camera position can be moved along a circular rail to fit most test persons [22]. Instead of a physical field camera, the visual content provided by the flight simulator must be used and is provided by a second synchronized instance of the flight simulator. Figure 1 shows the architecture of the virtual flight simulator adapted for the current evaluation.

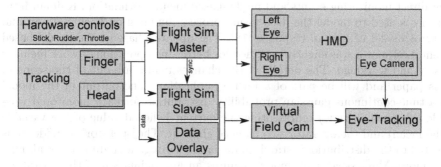

Fig. 1. Architecture of the Virtual Reality Flight Simulator

4.2   Methodology

As mentioned in 3.2, this work aims to use the well validated SAGAT method to assess the validity of online SA Assessment models and calibrate them. Depending on the assessment system, additional psychophysiological sensing capabilities may be required. We used eye-tracking information and live knowledge of the operator's actions as an online data stream to feed the model being evaluated. An example of both pilot view and experimenter view enhanced with eye-tracking sensing in shown in Figure 2. In parallel, the model makes an online assessment/prediction of the operator's situation awareness based on live data that we compare against direct and objective measurement using SAGAT-like questionnaires. To this end, the simulation is frozen at random times and instruments are hidden from the subject. The pilot is asked to describe his current knowledge of the situation, including important state variables and his/her degree of confidence. Fine calibration of the model with respect to mental models for example can be made by hiding instruments during a short period of time without freezing the simulation.

The exact scenario and methodology depends on the model being evaluated. We believe that VR provides the experimenter with an increased flexibility enabling easier decoupling of influential variables. The analysis will be generally carried out by comparing the predictions issued by the online SA assessment system fed with live data and the SAGAT results.

4.3   Example of Calibration

Online SA Assessment Model. As a proof of concept, we chose to roughly calibrate the model of SA proposed by Mamessier and Feigh [23,24] and used in the simulation of human-automation interaction in cockpit operations. This model focuses on the importance of modeling pilots' mental models of continuous and discrete dynamics of the aircraft. Situation awareness of continuous state variables such as *altitude* or *airspeed* is modeled as the result of merging direct monitoring events and model-based mental estimation. Kalman filter theory is used to model the data fusion process, building on Kleinman optimal control model of human response [18]. The update phase of the model-based mental estimator was slightly modified for better incorporation of work memory decay and workload. The details of the changes mades are out of the scope of this paper and will be part of a future publication. The output of the model is a time-continuous gaussian probability distribution for each monitored variable (airspeed,altitude) representing the current believed value of the variable (the mean) and the operator's confidence about it. The operator's confidence is related to the distribution's standard deviation through a credible interval. Furthermore, Mamessier et al. model requires an approximation of the operator's mental model. We used the very simple mental model of altitude kinematics provided in [23] to fit our scenario needs. Moreover, a workload indicator between 0 and 1 was heuristically assumed from the pilot's activity and plugged into the model. Three parameters have to be calibrated representing respectively the impact of workload on memory decay rate, on the Kalman gain, and the credible interval.

Scenario. A standard instrument landing system (ILS) approach with a 3° glide slope (GS) angle is chosen for this scenario. The flight starts at an altitude of $10200ft$ with the GS and the Localizer (LOC) already caught and centered, meaning the aircraft is perfectly on track. The autopilot is in the approach mode, roll and pitch of the aircraft are controlled by the autopilot. Besides the monitoring of the autopilot's flightpath the pilot has to manually control the airspeed using the throttle lever. To simulate different levels of workload, new airspeed clearances are verbally communicated to the pilot every 60s. The pilot uses a Head-Up-Display (HUD) similar to the one studied by Dreyer in [4] and represented in Figure 2. Freezing times are generated by a gaussian incremental process with inter-freeze times sampled from $\mathcal{N}(30s, 100s^2)$ to prevent the subject to anticipate the freezing schedule.

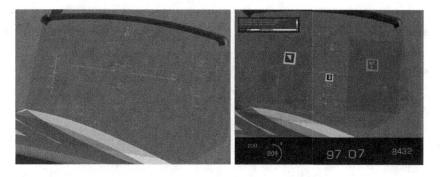

Fig. 2. Pilot and experimenter view

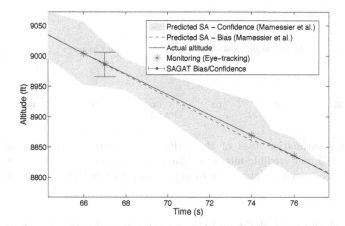

Fig. 3. Predicted Situation Awareness of the altitude (blue) based on the detection of online monitoring events (red stars) compared against SAGAT answers (red bars and dots)

Example of Calibration Data. Figure 3 shows an example of output of the SA online assessment system inspired from Mamessier et al., replacing simulated monitoring patterns with realistic monitoring events obtained with eye-tracking data. The black line is the actual altitude of the aircraft. The red stars represent the very times at which the pilot checked the altimeter and red bars stand for the SAGAT freezes results. The bar's length represents the pilot's confidence about his answer and the red dot his belief of the altitude. The dotted blue line is the predicted pilot's altitude belief and the light blue area the predicted credible interval.

The C-credibility interval of the gaussian bayesian belief of variable x_i is $I_{C\%} = [x^i \pm \sqrt{2}\sigma^i erf^{-1}(\frac{C}{100})]$ [25]. It means that the operator is C % sure that the actual value is within I_C. In order to compare the subject's SAGAT results about confidence and credible intervals predicted by the model, we need to pick a value for C. This value can be calibrated by aligning the smallest I_C predicted

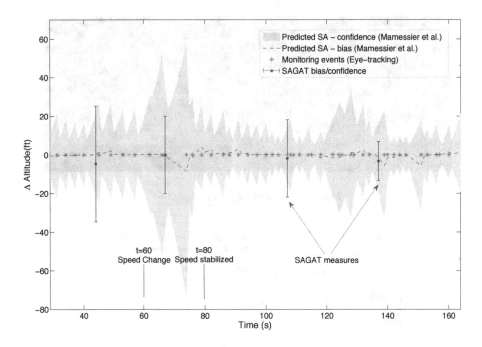

Fig. 4. Pilot's estimation bias of the altitude, recentered on the actual altitude ($\Delta Altitude = 0$) and credible intervals obtained by feeding Mamessier et al.'s model with online eye-tracking data (monitoring events) and compared against SAGAT queries

by the model along the flight and the subject's best confidence across SAGAT freezes. In this example, we found that $C = 85\%$ led to a good calibration.

Figure 4 represents both online predicted and SAGAT-measured situation awareness of the pilot recentered on the actual aircraft altitude. Workload peaks and predicted consequences on the operator's SA can be observed between 60 and 80s, 120s and 140s where the pilot had to change and stabilize the airspeed. The actual (SAGAT) and predicted pilot's bias (difference between believed altitude and actual altitude) is close to zero most of the time due to a high monitoring frequency. We observe a short increase in the absolute predicted bias around 70s due to the temporary absence of monitoring and the change of speed. Indeed, vertical speed slightly increased due to the speed change making the operator's mental model inaccurate until more monitoring finally allows the pilot to adapt.

5   Conclusion

Due to the increasing complexity of socio-technological systems, operators' situation awareness has become a critical concept for safety. Using SA measurement methods like SAGAT in the design loop of such systems is crucial to improve human-automation interaction. However non-intrusive online SA assessment is needed to cope with unpredictable situations through live support systems such as adaptive displays. To that end, we introduced a methodology based on the well validated SAGAT method and on the reconfigurable power of virtual reality to evaluate and calibrate online SA assessment systems and models based on SA process indices measurements. Mamessier et al. model was used as an example and was connected to a virtual reality flight simulator and eye-tracking system. Our experimental setup turned out to be very flexible and already provided many promising insights to extend and improve online SA assessment models. Based on this example, future work will include a full-scale statistical analysis and calibration of a SA online assessment model with professional pilots. Moreover, adaptive displays based on calibrated SA assessment models can be evaluated with the same experimental setup using the flexibility of virtual reality.

References

1. Aslandere, T.I.: Interaction Methods in a Generic Virtual Reality Flight Simulator. Master's thesis, Technische Universitat Munchen (2013)
2. Dehais, F., Tessier, C., Christophe, L., Reuzeau, F.: The perseveration syndrome in the pilots activity: Guidelines and cognitive countermeasures. In: Palanque, P., Vanderdonckt, J., Winckler, M. (eds.) HESSD 2009. LNCS, vol. 5962, pp. 68–80. Springer, Heidelberg (2010)
3. Dekker, S., Hollnagel, E.: Human factors and folk models. Cognition, Technology & Work 6(2), 79–86 (2004)
4. Dreyer, D., Bandow, D., Oberhauser, M.: Hud symbology evaluation in a virtual reality flight simulation. Paper submitted to HCI Aero 2014, Silicon Valley, USA (2014)
5. Ehrlich, J., Knerr, B., Lampton, D., McDonald, D.: Team situational awareness training in virtual environments: Potential capabilities and research issues. Tech. rep., U.S. Army Research Institute for the Behavioral and Social Sciences (1997)
6. Endsley, M.R.: Measurement of situation awareness in dynamic systems. Human Factors: The Journal of the Human Factors and Ergonomics Society 37(1), 65–84 (1995)
7. Endsley, M.R.: Toward a theory of situation awareness in dynamic systems. Human Factors: The Journal of the Human Factors and Ergonomics Society 37(1), 32–64 (1995)
8. Endsley, M.R.: Designing for situation awareness: An approach to user-centered design. Taylor & Francis, US (2003)
9. Endsley, M.: Situation awareness global assessment technique (sagat). In: Proceedings of the IEEE 1988 National Aerospace and Electronics Conference, NAECON 1988, pp. 789–795. IEEE (1988)
10. Feigh, K.M., Gelman, G., Mamessier, S., Pritchett, A.R.: Simulating first-principles models of situated human performance. IEEE Transactions on System Man and Cybernetics: Part A (submitted June 2012)
11. Hanson, M.L., Sullivan, O., Harper, K.A.: On-line situation assessment for unmanned air vehicles. In: FLAIRS Conference, pp. 44–48 (2001)
12. Hooey, B.L., Gore, B.F., Wickens, C.D., Scott-Nash, S., Socash, C., Salud, E., Foyle, D.C.: Modeling pilot situation awareness. In: Human Modelling in Assisted Transportation, pp. 207–213. Springer, Heidelberg (2011)

13. Horsch, C., Smets, N., Neerincx, M., Cuijpers, R.: Comparing performance and situation awareness in usar unit tasks in a virtual and real environment. In: Proceedings of the 10th International ISCRAM Conference, Baden-Baden, Germany, pp. 556–560 (2013)
14. Jones, D.G., Endsley, M.R.: Sources of situation awareness errors in aviation. Aviation, Space, and Environmental Medicine (1996)
15. Kalawsky, R.: New methodologies and techniques for evaluating user performance in advanced 3d virtual interfaces. IEEE Colloquium Digest 98/43 (1998)
16. Kalawsky, R.: Vruse - a computerised diagnostic tool for usability evaluation of virtual/synthetic environment systems. Applied Ergonomics 30, 11–25 (1999)
17. Kalawsky, R., Bee, S., Nee, S.: Human factors evaluation techniques to aid understanding of virtual interfaces. BT Technology Journal 17(1), 128–141 (1999)
18. Kleinman, D., Baron, S., Levison, W.: An optimal control model of human response part i: Theory and validation. Automatica 6(3), 357–369 (1970)
19. Laptaned, U.: Situation awareness in virtual environments: A theoretical model and investigation with different interface designs. In: Proceedings of the 9th IASTED International Conference Computers and Advanced Technology in Education, Lima, Peru, pp. 277–283 (2006)
20. Lee, H.C., Seong, P.H.: A computational model for evaluating the effects of attention, memory, and mental models on situation assessment of nuclear power plant operators. Reliability Engineering & System Safety 94(11), 1796–1805 (2009)
21. Letsu-Dake, E., Ntuen, C.A.: A case study of experimental evaluation of adaptive interfaces. International Journal of Industrial Ergonomics 40(1), 34–40 (2010)
22. Liesecke, S.: Eye-Tracking in Virtual Reality. Master's thesis, Universitt der Bundeswehr Munchen (2013)
23. Mamessier, S.: A computational approach to situation awareness and mental models in aviation. Master's thesis, Georgia Institute of Technology (2013)
24. Mamessier, S., Feigh, K.: Simulating the impact of mental models on human automation interaction in aviation. In: Duffy, V.G. (ed.) DHM/HCII 2013, Part I. LNCS, vol. 8025, pp. 61–69. Springer, Heidelberg (2013)
25. Mamessier, S., Feigh, K.: A computational approach to situation awareness and mental models for continuous dynamics in aviation. IEEE Transactions on Human-Machine Systems, (2014) (Under review)
26. Matthews, M., Beal, S., Pleban, R.: Situation awareness in a virtual environment: Description of a subjective assessment scale. Tech. rep. U.S. Army Research Institute for the Behavioral and Social Sciences (2002)
27. McCarley, J.S., Wickens, C.D., Goh, J., Horrey, W.J.: A computational model of attention/situation awareness. In: Proceedings of the Human Factors and Ergonomics Society Annual Meeting, vol. 46, pp. 1669–1673. SAGE Publications (2002)
28. Ratwani, R.M., McCurry, J.M., Trafton, J.G.: Single operator, multiple robots: An eye movement based theoretic model of operator situation awareness. In: 2010 5th ACM/IEEE International Conference on Human-Robot Interaction (HRI), pp. 235–242. IEEE (2010)
29. Salmon, P., Stanton, N., Walker, G., Green, D.: Situation awareness measurement: A review of applicability for c4i environments. Applied Ergonomics 37(2), 225–238 (2006)
30. Sarter, N.: Coping with complexity through adaptive interface design. In: Jacko, J.A. (ed.) Human-Computer Interaction, Part III, HCII 2007. LNCS, vol. 4552, pp. 493–498. Springer, Heidelberg (2007)
31. Sarter, N.B., Woods, D.D.: Situation awareness: A critical but ill-defined phenomenon. The International Journal of Aviation Psychology 1(1), 45–57 (1991)

32. Stanton, N.A., Chambers, P., Piggott, J.: Situational awareness and safety. Safety Science 39(3), 189–204 (2001)

33. Tien, G., Atkins, M.S., Zheng, B., Swindells, C.: Measuring situation awareness of surgeons in laparoscopic training. In: Proceedings of the 2010 Symposium on Eye-Tracking Research & Applications, pp. 149–152. ACM (2010)

34. Vicente, K., Pawlak, W.: Cognitive work analysis for the duress ii system. Cognitive Engineering Laboratory, Department of Industrial Engineering, Toronto, Canada CEL, pp. 94–93. University of Toronto (1994)

35. Vicente, K.: Cognitive work analysis: Toward safe, productive, and healthy computer-based work. Lawrence Erlbaum (1999)

36. Zacharias, G.L., Miao, A.X., Illgen, C., Yara, J.M., Siouris, G.M.: Sample: Situation awareness model for pilot-in-the-loop evaluation. Final Report R 95192 (1996)

A Digital Human Model for Performance-Based Design

Tim Marler[1], Steve Beck[1], Uday Verma[1], Ross Johnson[1],
Victoria Roemig[1], and Behzad Dariush[2]

[1] Santos Human Inc.
Coralville, IA 52241, USA
[2] Honda Research Institute USA
Mountain View CA 94043
{tim.marler,steve.beck,victoria.roemig}@santoshumaninc.com,
{uv,ross}@mazira.com, bdariush@gmail.com

Abstract. Real-time optimization-based posture prediction has fostered the development of zone differentiation, whereby performance-measure values resulting from a predicted posture are evaluated and displayed for large volumes of target points surrounding an avatar. To date, this tool was limited with respect to computational speed and practical applications. This paper presents a series of improvements and new features, including new algorithms for sphere filling and collision avoidance, significant increases to computational speed, incorporation of whole-body posture prediction, new methods for visualizing results, and multi-dimensional zone differentiation, which is the ability to automatically calculate multiple zones for various sets of problem parameters. These new tools collectively advance human systems integration. They are successfully applied to three example problems and demonstrate the ability to direct product design virtually, based on human performance.

Keywords: Digital human modeling and simulation, zone differentiation, reach analysis, posture prediction.

1   Introduction

Often, the concepts of human systems integration (HSI) or human-centered design relate primarily to fit, access, and range-of motion, but not necessarily broader aspects of human performance. Yet, in order to design products for ease of use and safety, even when focusing on static analysis, one must consider performance. This is true whether one works with experimental protocols or with virtual simulation and analysis. As digital human models (DHMs) become more mature and more prevalent in the virtual design process, the amount and form of the analysis data they present becomes more critical. Distilling a variety of results from many different cases (i.e. millions of potential reach targets) into palatable data that can be used for practical design changes continues to be a challenge. Furthermore, although basic DHMs can be used for geometric package analysis, predictive and analytical capabilities are critical for improving designs as effectively as possible and thus for increasing safety and ease of use. In this vein, optimization-based posture prediction provides a means of not only

V.G. Duffy (Ed.): DHM 2014, LNCS 8529, pp. 136–147, 2014.

studying the interaction of virtual humans with their environment, but also studying their performance as well. Advances with this technology have been substantial over the past decade, but only recently have extensive real-world use cases for digital human models been published.

In response to this state of the art, Santos Human Inc. has developed the next generation *zone differentiation*, which allows one to conduct concurrent virtual design and analysis, and has used this new tool for improving the designs of seats in amusement park rides, hand breaks in automobiles, and seats in heavy equipment. In all cases, one is able to consider biomechanical performance measures like joint displacement or discomfort, when studying products for potential design changes. This in turn provides a novel approach to performance-based design.

Zone differentiation is based on optimization-based posture prediction implemented within the Santos DHM, whereby optimization is used to determine joint angles that optimize a specified combination of performance measures, subject to constraints that represent the task being simulated. This approach is computationally fast, so it is possible to predict and evaluate postures for large numbers of scenarios in a relatively small period of time. Zone differentiation entails automatically running posture prediction with millions of target points, and recording the consequent performance-measure values for each posture. The values are then presented as a 3D contour plot.

To date, this tools use with complex real-world problems and whole-body DHM models has been impractical, because it has not been fast enough, especially with cases that require collision avoidance. A variety of work has been completed with optimization-based posture prediction as summarized by Marler (2005), and zone differentiation is a natural outgrowth from such capabilities. One of the first developments in this regard is provided by Yang et al (2006), in the context of a 21-degree-of-freedon (DOF), one-arm, upper body system. Similar methods and results are presented by Yang et al (2008), albeit with a more extensive description of the discomfort model from Marler et al (2005). Yang et al (2008) extend this work with applications to discomfort analysis within an automobile cab, and with the ability to view preliminary results before the complete zone is calculated. Again, the tool is used for upper-body analysis. The same work surfaces in Yang et al (2009) and Yang and Abdel-Malek (2009), although the latter focuses on analytical determination of reach envelopes.

This paper presents new capabilities for whole-body zone differentiation, including refinements that increase computational speed. First, multi-dimensional zone differentiation allows one to compute and compare multiple zone differentiation volumes calculated with different constraints. Secondly, iso-contour surfacing allows the user to specify desired thresholds for visualizing the performance measures used to calculate zone volumes, thus reducing the final size of the volume. It is then possible to shrink wrap the resulting volume and export and/or manipulate the consequent geometry. Finally, a series of computational enhancements have been implemented to increase the speed of zone differentiation, including parallel processing, with the potential for cloud-based use.

2 Background

This section provides an overview of the underlying human model and the formulation for posture prediction. The work presented in this paper uses the Santos human model (Abdel-Malek et al, 2004) as a platform for further development. The underlying skeletal structure for Santo is modeled as a series of links with each pair of links connected by one or more revolute joints (Figure 1). There is one joint angle for each DOF, and the relationship between the joint angles and the position of points on the series of links (or on the actual avatar) is defined using the Denavit-Hartenberg (DH)-notation (Denavit and Hartenberg, 1955). This structure is becoming a common foundation for additional work in the field of predictive human modeling and has been successfully used with other research efforts (Ma et al, 2009; Howard et al, 2010).

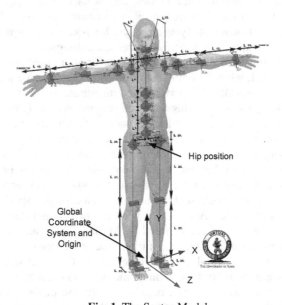

Fig. 1. The Santos Model

Given the structure in Figure 1, postures are predicted using an optimization-based approach first detailed by Marler (2005). Joint angles serve as the design variables, which are incorporated in various objective functions and constraints, the fundamental formulation for which given as follows:

Find: $\mathbf{q} \in R^{DOF}$

To minimize: $f(\mathbf{q})$

Subject to:

$$\text{Distance} = \left\| \mathbf{x}(\mathbf{q})^{\text{end-effector}} - \mathbf{x}^{\text{target point}} \right\| \le \varepsilon$$

$$q_i^L \le q_i \le q_i^U \; ; \; i = 1, 2, \ldots, DOF$$

q is a vector of joint angles, x is the position of an end-effector or point on the avatar, ε is a small positive number that approximates zero, and DOF is the total number of degrees of freedom. With this study, a single model with 113 DOFs is used for the human torso, arms, legs, neck, hands, eyes, and global position and orientation. Including the global DOFs as additional design variables allows one to predict the position and orientation of the body as well.

$f(q)$ can be one of many performance measures (Marler *et al*, 2005; Marler *et al*, 2005b; Marler, 2005; Marler *et al*, 2009). For these studies, joint displacement and discomfort are used. In general, the objective function, potentially composed of of many performance measures, models what drives human behavior.

The primary constraint, called the *distance constraint*, requires the end-effector(s) to contact a specified target point(s). q_i^U represents the upper limit, and q_i^L represents the lower limit. These limits are derived from anthropometric data. In addition to these basic constraints, many other constraints can be used as boundary conditions in order to represent the virtual environment. In particular, in order to model collision avoidance, spheres are used to represent all geometry and all avatars, and *collision constraints* are added such that no one sphere overlaps another. Additional constraints can be created by the user on the fly, in order to simulate infinitely many tasks.

Typically, posture is predicted for a single scenario (a single set of constraints). A single objective function is used, although multiple performance measures may be aggregated to form what is technically a multi-objective optimization problem. However, regardless of the objective function being used, any performance measure can be evaluated at a consequent posture. In fact, zone differentiation involves predicting postures for potentially millions of target points surrounding the avatar, recording the consequent set of performance-measure values for each target, and then displaying the performance values corresponding to each target point within a volume around an avatar. This volume is called the *zone volume*.

3   Method

3.1   Multi-dimensional Zone Differentiation

Although zone differentiation has been a powerful tool for ergonomic analysis, there is been a need to automatically evaluate zone volumes for different conditions. For instance, one may need to evaluate a discomfort zone for different wrist orientations or different loading condition. This is called *multi-dimensional zone differentiation*. This functionality provides one with ways to batch more than one zone differentiation computation based on certain user configurable parameters. With respect to initial use cases, this tool provides a way to batch and compute several different volumes based on changing rotation of a 3D world entity, such as a lever of hand break (Figure 2).

The user specifies the range of rotation around the X, Y, and Z axes. Then, once the user specifies the geometry of interest, the tool automatically detects the axis on which the user may intend to rotate the geometry. The user may then choose the number of volumes for each axis. The total number of zones computed is based $L*M*N$ where L, M, and N indicate the number of volumes chosen per axis. The user may then submit the problem for solution, and the submission window allows the user to preview the orientation of the geometry of interest.

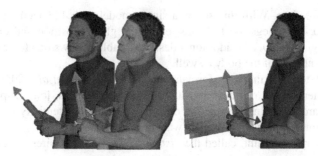

Fig. 1. Computing multiple zone volumes with changes in entity orientation

Multi-dimensional zone differentiation is a compute-intensive process and relies on partial-zone evaluation, parallelization, and batch computation techniques to deliver results in a reasonable amount of time, all of which are discussed in the following sections.

3.2   Computational Speed

Although posture prediction typically requires less than one second to run, running multiple zone volumes with millions of target points can be computationally demanding. Therefore, the following steps have been taken to increase the speed. First, we provide the feature of *sub-zone volume* calculations. This allows the end-user to take a more focused approach and define reduced zone volumes that do not necessarily include the complete volume around the avatar, some areas of which may not be important for the problem at hand.

A single instance of posture prediction can require more time when collision avoidance (Johnson *et al*, 2010) is involved. This is because, in order to incorporate collision avoidance, all avatars and geometry are represented by sphere-based surrogate geometry, and many additional constraints are included in the optimization problem to ensure one sphere does not overlap another. Thus, the second step in increasing the efficiency of zone differentiation entails a modified approach to selecting sphere constraints. Since we know that at most, an avatar will only intersect the spheres in the zone volume, all other spheres are discarded before zone differentiation (and posture prediction) begins. Note that previous work presents a multi-run approach to collision avoidance, which significantly reduces the number of spheres used in collision avoidance (Johnson *et al*, 2009). This method is "smart" in determining which spheres need to be used in avoidance constraints, but it still has to determine which spheres are colliding with the computed posture, and then update the constraint set. Although this approach is faster than considering all spheres in the environment, it is not fast enough for zone differentiation.

Next, one of the most significant improvements in computational time entails eliminating consideration of avatar/object collision spheres that are already in collision when the zone diff volume calculations begin.

In addition to reducing the number of sphere constraints, we implement a *reduced target set*, whereby target points (for posture prediction) that happen to fall within existing geometry are automatically disregarded. It would be impossible to reach such points.

Zone differentiation provides an ideal opportunity for parallelization. Target points inside the zone volume are evaluated independently thereby eliminating data dependency chains. The parallelization of zone volumes is achieved by splitting the volume into smaller fixed size volumes, which are then computed separately and in parallel on all available CPUs. Interestingly, paralleling zone volumes only provides a significant benefit for larger volumes. The amount of effort required to split, compute, and combine smaller volumes outweighs the effort required to compute a small volume using non-parallelized zone differentiation. This break-point volume is approximately 8x8x8.

Since zone differentiation is computationally intensive it makes little sense to block a user's access to the 3D program while the volume is computed. Thus, zone differentiation batch processing provides a way to run zone differentiation out-of-process, whereby a separate program accepts computation requests and executes them one after another.

How fast zone runs is now is determined by how many processors a machine has. The performance boost will be approximately 0.8 * (number of cores).

3.3   Sphere Filling

An integral component of collision avoidance, and thus the effectiveness of posture prediction, is the process by which the avatar and environment are represented with sphere-based surrogate geometry. New developments with the underlying approach to filling objects with spheres have led to substantial improvements in zone differentiation. Sphere filling is more accurate, flexible, and orders of magnitude faster. Specific improvements are summarized as follows.

Now, the avatars are actually filled with spheres based on their morphology, whereas previously, the body-based spheres were fixed. Sphere representation of an avatar can now be completed by separating the avatar geometry into two regions defined by the hands and then the rest of the avatar. This provides the end-user with the ability to obtain highly accurate representations of the avatar hands and fingers for collision avoidance, without significantly increasing the number of spheres used to represent the rest of the avatar body.

In addition, the avatar spheres can be re-oriented on the fly, depending on the posture. Sphere representations of avatars can be dramatically different based on posture. For instance, sphere filling based on a seated posture eliminates overestimation in the hip region, rather than using standing posture and then moving the avatar joints into a seated posture.

With respect to the use of spheres to represent general imported geometry, the underlying inflate algorithms has been improved. First, the algorithm can now lump together various geometry components and consider the results as one piece for filling purposes. This increases the speed with which complex composite objects can be represented. There is a preprocess step to group triangles (fundamental elements for creating geometry) to the grid points (points where spheres are placed) they intersect. Then, grid points that are inside an object are determined differently. Instead of evaluating the orientation of nearby triangles as it fills at every grid point, it now assumes all grid points on the outside of a bounding box are outside the object, and conducts a breadth first search marking grid points as outside until a grid point intersects geometry. Since the algorithm knows which points are inside and outside, it only fills (places spheres at) inside points. With the geometry grouped to grid points, the algorithm only calculates distance to the nearby triangles instead of to all of them.

The culling portion of the algorithm, which subsequently determines which spheres to retain/use, has been redesigned. The old method used a greedy approach, picking the spheres that covered the most grid points and then recalculating the coverage of the other spheres. The new method makes a list of the largest spheres providing coverage to each grid point. It then starts filling by using the smallest spheres first, but only retaining spheres that are the largest spheres for covering a specific point.

Computation time for sphere filling used to dedicate 70% of the time to distance calculation and then 30% to culling. Now time is allocated as 10% for preprocessing, 88% for distance calculation, and 2% for culling (the new culling method is much faster). Overall, sphere filling is more than twice as fast.

3.4   Zone Differentiation Compute Instance (ZDCI)

In addition to developing new zone-differentiation capabilities, an overarching management system has been implemented. This program is responsible for accepting compute requests, batching, monitoring progress, enabling cancel requests, and presenting computation progress. This program is automatically instantiated when it is needed. ZDCI accepts connections over HTTP using a REST-full interface. All needed parameters to run a zone computation are delivered using JSON. The Santos software submits tasks by connecting to ZDCI over HTTP and pushing a request using the POST method with the associated JSON payload.

This tool allows one to run zone differentiation independently from other Santos-related processes. It also provides the opportunity of scaling zone differentiation to external, more powerful, dedicated compute clusters. Since ZDCI communicates over HTTP, any external software package can submit computation requests over the Internet, thereby allowing for cloud computing.

3.5   Iso-contour Surfacing

The color gradients used to present zone differentiation results are called *iso-contour surfaces*, and a suite of capabilities have been developed for manipulating these surfaces. Iso-contour surfacing provides the ability to generate surface geometry from zone differentiation data via a marching-cubes algorithm and an end-user definable zone differentiation data threshold value. The threshold value can be interactively modified to indicate what is of interest (and what is not). Values below the threshold value are considered "of interest" and are visible, while values above the threshold value are made invisible, as shown in Figure 3. Once the desired threshold value is identified, invoking the iso-contouring algorithm creates 3-dimensional surface geometry that encompasses the zone differentiation data. Removal of the orthographic cutting planes, which can help the end-user gain insight into the volumetric data, shows the complete, resulting surface, which can be exported for use with third party systems.

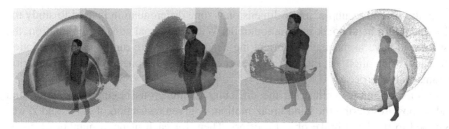

Fig. 2. Modification of threshholds with iso-contour surfaces

4   Results

In this section, three basic case studies are presented to further demonstrate the types of problems to which the new zone differentiation capabilities can be applied. The first example depicts Santos in an amusement park ride. As shown in Figure 4, collision avoidance is used to predict Santos's posture while reaching over a restraint, as if to help another passenger for safety reasons.

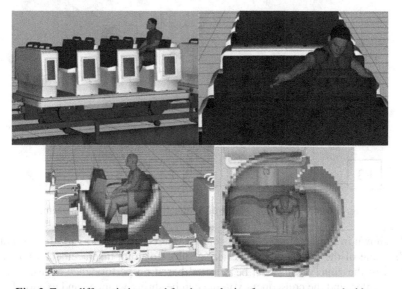

Fig. 3. Zone differentiation used for the analysis of an amusement park ride

Zone differentiation is then used to illustrate the joint-displacement values for all points around Santos. Ranging from green to red, the color scheme demonstrate Santos's difficulty, with red being the most difficult. A fixed volume around the ride was initialized before the test was run. The test shows the difficulty of reaching around the top of the front seat and the ease of touching the seat next to Santos. With respect to design considerations, in order to make sure a parent could reach his/her child in front of them, for instance, the seat would have to be redesigned.

As the second example, multi-dimensional zone differentiation is used to study the placement of a hand break in an automobile. With traditional zone differentiation, the user would have to manually re-orient the hand-brake and re-run zone differentiation for each orientation of interest. However, multi-dimensional zone differentiation automates this process.

Results in Figure 5 illustrate the difficulty of numerous beginning, middle, and ending postures during the hand break motion. A given restriction of X, Y, and Z was assigned to the hand brake object a priori. Then, for each plane, a number of zones were calculated. This example includes four zones. As shown from beginning to end of the avatar's hand brake motion, the green color begins to fade to red, where the red color corresponds to a less comfortable posture. The current location for the hand brake's motion is easily seen as acceptable, since all four postures are located in a green zone. The results do indicate, however, that there could be some benefit to moving the hand break forward slightly.

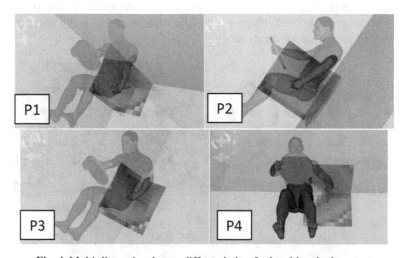

Fig. 4. Multi-dimensional zone differentiation for hand-break placement

As shown in Figure 6, iso-contours can be altered in order to vary the presentation of the scale of the underlying numerical results (for joint displacement values). Any portion of the zone volume can be selected based on performance-measure scale or contour color, and the consequent volume can be shrink wrapped and exported for use in third party design packages.

A third use case demonstrates the use of whole-body zone differentiation for concurrent seat design (Figure 7), whereby multiple ergonomic constraints (hand reach for joysticks, foot reach for pedals, visual target point, etc.) are considered concurrently.

The design criteria were as follows. The location of a point midway between the operator's hips when seated is provided. The range of motion of the seat is 7.2 cm forward of default location and 7.2 cm upward of default location. The joysticks are designed to be used while the elbows rested on the arm supports. The arm supports are not attached to the seat and are not adjustable. The left hand joystick rotates 15-degrees forward and aft. The brake is fully deployed at 17-degrees.

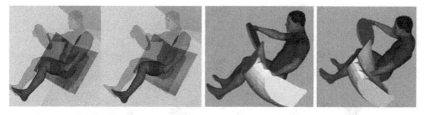

Fig. 5. Variation in iso-contour coloring scale, and shrink wrapped contours

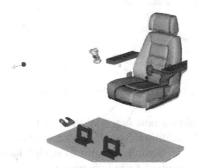

Fig. 6. Seat design example

Posture is predicted by minimizing discomfort while requiring both feet to remain on the pedals and both hands to remain on the joysticks. Zone differentiation is used to determine the discomfort value for the predicted postures when the seat (and avatar) i.e. moved throughout the seat range of motion (ROM). Figure 8 displays the zone volume for the initial seat ROM, and then for a new ROM extended down and to the left. In the first case, the avatar actually has difficulty seeing the target and touching the pedals. When the ROM is extended, more comfortable postures become feasible, and the avatar is essentially able to relax.

5   Discussion

This paper presents new capabilities for optimization-based zone differentiation that yield a tool for human-centric, performance-based design. Improvements to collision avoidance, computational speed, and visualization allow zone differentiation to be used in a wider and more practical set of scenarios. This in turn allows one to automatically consider human performance when evaluating a virtual design. Most novel among the proposed capabilities is multi-dimensional zone differentiation, which allows one to consider variations in problem constraints when evaluating performance.

By leveraging real time posture prediction, this work provides one of the first DHM tools for automatic human systems integration. Especially with the final example, Santos actually determines beneficial design changes automatically while considering how a human interacts with the product. The inherent use of performance measures in the optimization-based posture-prediction construct is a key factor as to why this can be done.

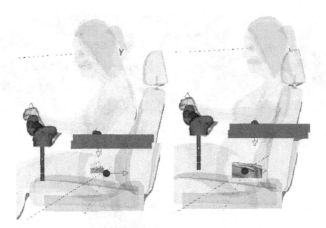

Fig. 7. Whole body seat-based zone differentiation

The presented work offers a new practical tool, and the implications of this work are significant. Ultimately, additional product parameters can be considered and automatically altered within an overarching optimal design loop. Furthermore, one can evaluate the differences in implied design changes when different performance measures are used. How does a seat designed to minimize discomfort differ from a seat designed to minimize joint displacement? Finally, these kinds of capabilities will not only be available within the Santos software, but given the provisions for ZDCI, they could be accessed by co-located users, thus fostering collaboration and concurrent design on a large scale.

References

1. Abdel-Malek, K., Yang, J., Kim, J., Marler, R.T., Beck, S., Nebel, K.: Santos: A Virtual Human Environment for Human Factors Assessment, In: 24th Army Science Conference, Orlando, FL, Assistant Secretary of the Army (Research, Development and Acquisition), Department of the Army, Washington, DC (November 2004)
2. Denavit, J., Hartenberg, R.S.: A Kinematic Notation for Lower-pair Mechanisms Based on Matrices. Journal of Applied Mechanics 77, 215–221 (1955)
3. Howard, B., Yang, J., Gragg, J.: Toward a New Digital Pregnant Woman Model and Kinematic Posture Prediction. In: 3rd International Conference on Applied Human Factors and Ergonomics, Miami, FL (July 2010)
4. Johnson, R., Fruehan, C., Schikore, M., Marler, T., Abdel-Malek, K.: New Developments with Collision Avoidance for Posture Prediction. In: 3rd International Conference on Applied Human Factors and Ergonomics, Miami, FL (July 2010)
5. Johnson, R., Smith, B.L., Penmatsa, R., Marler, T., Abdel-Malek, K.: Real-Time Obstacle Avoidance for Posture Prediction. In: SAE Digital Human Modeling Conference, Goteborg, Sweden. Society of Automotive Engineers, Warrendale (June 2009)
6. Liu, Q., Marler, T., Yang, J., Kim, J., Harrison, C.: Posture Prediction with External Loads – A Pilot Study. In: April, D.M. (ed.) SAE 2009 World Congress, Detroit, MI. Society of Automotive Engineers, Warrendale (April 2009)

7. Ma, L., Zhang, W., Chablat, D., Bennis, F., Guillaume, F.: Multi-objective Optimization Method for Posture Prediction and Analysis with Consideration of Fatigue Effect and Its Application Case. Computers and Industrial Engineering 57, 1235–1245 (2009)
8. Marler, R.T.: A Study of Multi-objective Optimization Methods for Engineering Applications, Ph.D. Dissertation, University of Iowa, Iowa City, IA (2005)
9. Marler, T., Arora, J., Beck, S., Lu, J., Mathai, A., Patrick, A., Swan, C.: Computational Approaches in DHM. In: Duffy, V.G. (ed.) Handbook of Digital Human Modeling for Human Factors and Ergonomics. Taylor and Francis Press, London (2008)
10. Marler, R.T., Arora, J.S., Yang, J., Kim, H.: –J., and Abdel-Malek, K., Use of Multi-objective Optimization for Digital Human Posture Prediction. Engineering Optimization 41(10), 295–943 (2009)
11. Marler, T., Knake, L., Johnson, R.: Optimization-Based Posture Prediction for Analysis of Box-Lifting Tasks. In: 3rd International Conference on Digital Human Modeling, Orlando, FL (July 2011)
12. Marler, R.T., Rahmatalla, S., Shanahan, M., Abdel-Malek, K.: A New Discomfort Function for Optimization-Based Posture Prediction. In: SAE Human Modeling for Design and Engineering Conference, Iowa City, IA. Society of Automotive Engineers, Warrendale (June 2005)
13. Marler, R.T., Yang, J., Arora, J.S., Abdel-Malek, K.: Study of Bi-Criterion Upper Body Posture Prediction using Pareto Optimal Sets. In: IASTED International Conference on Modeling, Simulation, and Optimization, Oranjestad, Aruba. International Association of Science and Technology for Development, Canada (August 2005b)
14. Yang, J., Abdel-Malek, K.: Human Reach Envelope and Zone Differentiation for Ergonomic Design. Human Factors and Ergonomics in Manufacturing 19(1), 15–34 (2009)
15. Xiang, Y., Chung, H.-J., Kim, J.H., Bhatt, R., Marler, T., Rahmatalla, S., Yang, J., Arora, J.S., Abdel-Malek, K.: Predictive Dynamics: An Optimization-Based Novel Approach for Human Motion Simulation. Structural and Multidisciplinary Optimization 41(3), 465–479 (2009)
16. Yang, J., Verma, U., Penmatsa, R., Marler, T., Beck, S., Rahmatalla, S., Abdel-Malek, K., Harrison, C.: Development of a Zone Differentiation Tool for Visualization of Posture Comfort. In: 2008 SAE World Congress, Detroit, MI (April 2008)
17. Yang, J., Sinokrot, T., Abdel-Malek, K., Beck, S., Nebel, K.: Workspace Zone Differentiation and Visualization for Virtual Humans. Ergonomics 51(3), 395–413 (2008)
18. Yang, J., Sinokrot, T., Abdel-Malek, K., Nebel, K.: Optimization-Based Workspace Zone Differentiation and Visualization for Santos. In: 2006 SAE World Congress, Detroit, MI (April 2006)
19. Yang, J., Verma, U., Marler, T., Beck, S., Rahmatalla, S., Harrison, C.: Workspace Zone Differentiation Tool for Visualization of Seated Postural Comfort. International Journal of Industrial Ergonomics 39, 267–276 (2009)

Context-Aware Posture Analysis in a Workstation-Oriented Office Environment

Konlakorn Wongpatikaseree[1], Hideaki Kanai[2], and Yasuo Tan[1]

[1] School of Information Science
[2] Research Center for Innovative Lifestyle Design
Japan Advanced Institute of Science and Technology, Ishikawa, Japan 923-1211
{w-konlak,hideaki,ytan}@jaist.ac.jp

Abstract. Among current research trends, correction of the sitting posture is attracting growing attention. Most office workers suffer several health problems during their work. The two greatest causes of health problems in the office environment are simple things. The first is poor sitting posture. Sitting with poor posture in front of a computer for hours causes cumulative damage. The second is an inappropriate workstation environment. The workstation environment is related to good sitting posture. For example, if the desk is too low, the user has to lean forward to look at the display. To address this problem, we propose a sitting posture recognition system that can recognize both human posture and the context of the workstation environment. The proposed system has three components. First, skeleton tracking is used to create a sideways view of the human skeleton. The skeleton model in this research is used to measure the joint angles of the human body. Second, we detect information on objects using a proposed workstation environment tracking system. Three types of features are used to filter the objects from the depth image. Finally, we compare the overall information with a standard sitting posture in a model-matching component. Experimental studies showed that the system can provide the necessary information for analyzing the human posture. A physician or user can apply this information to achieve correct sitting posture or prevent health problems in the office using the provided results.

Keywords: Sitting posture recognition, skeleton model, workstation environment tracking.

1 Introduction

Office syndrome is a serious problem that is common in office workers, who spend about 6 h/day working at a desk. A study by the American Cancer Society [1] found that sitting in front of a computer for long periods of time can lead to poor health outcomes. For example, men who sit for more than 6 h/day have a 20% higher death rate than those who sit less than 3 h/day. Moreover, an improper sitting posture can also cause several conditions such as inflammation of the muscles, back pain, or shoulder pain. Thus, recognition of the user's ergonomics

V.G. Duffy (Ed.): DHM 2014, LNCS 8529, pp. 148–159, 2014.
© Springer International Publishing Switzerland 2014

while sitting plays an important role in correcting the sitting posture to improve the user's health.

Among current research trends, the analysis of human posture in a workstation-oriented office environment is attracting growing attention. Kikugawa et al. [2] proposed a system for interrupting poor posture when a user is performing a video display terminal task. In their approach, the distance between the user and the display is used to identify poor posture, and then the user is notified by means of a blur effect on the PC's display. Mu et al. [3] presented a sitting posture surveillance system based on image processing technology. In their approach, the face's location and size were used to detect the sitting posture. Although several research works have proposed sitting posture recognition systems, the limitations of existing research leave room for improvement; for instance, when only the upper body is considered, a system cannot recognize poor sitting posture that involves crossing the legs.

To address this problem, the primary goal of this research is to provide a human sitting posture profile and context awareness at the workstation to analyze human posture. To achieve our goal, three components are established in this research. First, we propose a skeleton tracking method. Nine joints on the human body are detected to identify the ergonomics of sitting. Second, workstation environment tracking is developed for recognizing the objects in the workstation space. Information about the desk height, chair height, and distance between the user and the display is considered in terms of the human sitting posture. Finally, all of the observed information is evaluated according to the standard for the ergonomics of sitting. The benchmark for analyzing the ergonomics of sitting is based on that of the U.S. Occupational Safety & Health Administration (OSHA) [4]. The system developed in this study can provide the user's sitting profile to enhance understanding of good and poor sitting posture so that the user can correct poor sitting posture using the provided information.

2   Related Works

A wide range of methods for recognizing human posture has been introduced. However, two main sensing approaches are commonly used for posture classification. The first is a sensor-based approach, and the second is a vision-based approach.

In the sensor-based approach, various types of sensors have been used to capture human motions. The most commonly used sensor in posture classification is the force sensor, which is generally attached to an object to which mechanical force is applied, such as a chair, sofa, or bed. Huang [5] proposed a sitting posture detection and recognition method using the force sensor. Seven force sensors were attached to a chair to recognize four types of sitting posture. Sitting posture classification systems with force sensors have also been studied [6, 7]. Other types of sensors are also used in posture classification. Wongpatikaseree et al. [8] proposed a posture classification system using ultrasonic sensors. Three types of human posture (standing, sitting, lying down) were observed. In their research, ultrasonic sensors were attached to the human body, and the height data for each sensor were extracted to classify the human posture.

The concept of the vision-based approach is to use an image processing technique to extract the human posture from an image. This approach uses primarily a visual sensing device, such as a high-resolution camera or a Kinect camera, to collect image or video files. Liao et al. [9] proposed a vision-based walking posture analysis system. In their approach, four features were extracted from the images: the body line, neck line, center of gravity, and gait width. Along the same lines, Kaenchan et al. [10] also presented a technique for analyzing the walking posture using Kinect cameras. Three Kinect cameras were used to capture the walking posture, and the resulting multiple skeletons were combined into one final skeleton for analyzing the walking posture. In addition, a sitting posture surveillance system was also presented in [3]. The details of the sitting posture, such as the face's location and size, were extracted from the images to identify poor sitting posture.

3   System Architecture

In this research, we propose a sitting posture recognition system for recognizing and analyzing the human sitting posture. The system architecture is designed as shown in Fig. 1. To obtain data, the Kinect camera [11] is used as the main device for recording the depth image. The depth image is sent to two components: the skeleton tracking and workstation environment tracking components. The main task of the skeleton tracking component is to create the human skeleton model in the sitting posture and then analyze the relationship between body parts by measuring the angles of body joints. The workstation environment tracking component tracks the objects around the workstation using three proposed features. Next, the results from the first two components are sent to the model-matching component, which analyzes the ergonomics of sitting on the basis of the benchmark, which is provided by OSHA. Consequently, the results are plotted in graphs, and then a physician or user can determine the cause of the poor sitting posture using the provided results.

4   Skeleton Tracking

Tracking the human skeleton is not a new technique in posture recognition. Several studies attempted to recognize the human posture using a skeleton model. However, in this research, we developed a skeleton model to classify the human sitting posture in a different way. The entire body as seen from a side perspective is used to create the skeleton model. In the skeleton tracking component, we set up the Kinect camera, which gives a 640×480 image at 30 frames per second (fps) with a depth resolution of a few centimeters, next to the user to record the depth image in sideways. Each control point in the image is defined by a position (x, y, z) expressed in skeleton space. Figure 2 illustrates the axes of the coordinates (x, y, z) of the Kinect camera.

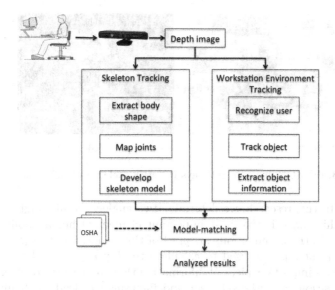

Fig. 1. System architecture

To realize the skeleton model in this research, the main body and shape are extracted from the depth image. Then, this shape information is used to label each joint on the human body. Because we use only one Kinect camera placed to the right of the user, the Kinect camera will label only the joints on the right side of the body. The major joints of a human skeleton are modeled as nine control points (head, center of shoulders, right shoulder, right elbow, right wrist, spine, center of hip, right hip, and right knee), as shown in Fig. 3.

Although we can recognize the sitting posture using the proposed skeleton model, we cannot guarantee that the recognized posture is correct or incorrect. Thus, the skeleton tracking component not only creates the skeleton model, but also measures the angles between joints. These angles can indicate the correct sitting posture. For example, the hip angle should be 90 ° but should not be more

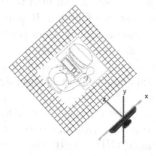

Fig. 2. Axes of coordinates of Kinect camera

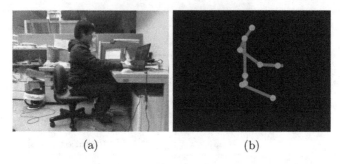

(a)   (b)

Fig. 3. (a) RGB image in sideways (b) stick skeleton model in sideways

than $120°$. In this research, we determine two angles: the hip angle and elbow angle. The hip angle is the most important element of human body posture. The position in three dimensions (x, y, z) of three control points (spine, center of hip, and right hip) are used to calculate the hip angle. Further, the elbow angle is also an important piece of information that we have to consider because improper positioning of the shoulder and forearms can lead to shoulder pain. The positions of the right shoulder, right elbow, and right wrist are detected for measuring the elbow angle. In addition, height differences between two body parts are also investigated to check the correct sitting posture. For instance, the height of the knee joint should be the same as that of the hip joint, whereas the forearms should be straight and parallel to the floor. Examples of the results of skeleton tracking will be described in more detail in Sect. 7.

5 Workstation Environment Tracking

Because the skeleton model alone cannot identify the correct sitting posture accurately, other information might help the user or physician to determine the cause of poor sitting posture. Workstation environment information can be used to analyze the cause of poor sitting posture. For example, the seat height should be adjusted to support the knee and prevent swelling of the leg; in addition, if the position of the armrest is too low, it can lead to shoulder pain because the user has to lean to the side to rest one forearm. Regarding context-awareness at the workstation, it has been proposed that users practice ergonomic principles while working at computers [12]. However, only a few research works propose a practical system that uses context-awareness in ergonomics research. In this research, the context will be analyzed to help the user achieve a good workstation environment.

To extract the information on the workstation environment, the system recognizes the user and then measures the distance between the user and the Kinect camera, called the user distance (UD). Next, the system will define the focus area based on the UD, as shown in Fig. 4. Green indicates the objects, which are located UD $\pm$ 400 mm from the camera. Blue represents the user, and Red denotes the objects, which are placed in the other ranges.

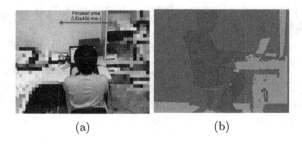

(a)   (b)

Fig. 4. (a) Focused area, (b) focused area in depth image

In this section, we attempt to extract three pieces of information from the workstation environment: the desk height, chair height, and distance between the user and the display. Three features are used to filter these three objects in the workstation environment, as illustrated in Table 1. The pixel matching technique is adopted for filtering the desired objects. First, the desk feature size (25 × 10) is used to recognize the desk in the depth image in Fig. 4(b). The pixels that are consistent with the desk feature size are represented in green; otherwise, the pixels are red, as shown in Fig. 5(a). Second, the extent of the color is adopted in the chair feature for detecting the chair object. The first three lines in the chair feature should be blue, and overall this feature should be about 80% to 90% blue. Figure 5(b) illustrates an example of chair recognition, where the chair object is represented in blue. Finally, to recognize the monitor, the system uses the UD information to filter the objects that are located at the same distance as the user. Then, the monitor feature is used to recognize the monitor, as shown in Fig. 5(c), where green indicates the monitor, and the user is identified in blue.

Table 1. Features for extracting objects

Objects	Feature size	Condition
Desk	25×10 pixels	Green (100%)
Chair	25×25 pixels	Blue (80%-90%) Note: First three lines of feature should be blue
Monitor	7×15 pixels	Green (≥20%) Note: First and last pixel of feature should be green

6   Model-Matching

The model-matching component analyzes the results from the first two components. The benchmark for analyzing the ergonomics of sitting is based on that of OSHA [4]. OSHA provides a basic design for sitting posture and the workstation environment. Several points need to be considered when setting up a computer workstation. In this research, evaluation checklists are established for analyzing

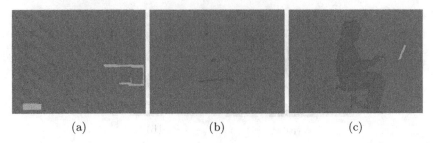

(a)   (b)   (c)

Fig. 5. (a) Desk recognition result, (b) chair recognition result, (c) monitor recognition result

Table 2. Checklist for sitting posture

Working postures (Consider these points when evaluating sitting posture)	
Human body	**Condition**
Wrist and forearms	Roughly parallel to the floor
Elbow	$90 - 120°$
Hip	$90 - 120°$
Thigh	Roughly parallel to the floor

the human sitting posture and the workstation environment, as illustrated in Tables 2 and 3.

To analyze the results, a rule-based technique is adopted for matching the information obtained from the first two components. Using the results of the matching process, the system can explain why the user has poor sitting posture by plotting the results in graphs, as described in more detail in the next section. The physician can use this information to diagnose the cause of conditions such as back pain, shoulder pain, or eyestrain.

7   Experimental Results

7.1   Experimental Setup

To analyze the human sitting posture, the sitting posture recognition system, which has the three main components described above, was implemented in C# using the Microsoft Kinect SDK library. In this experiment, the Kinect camera was set to operate at 30 fps and was located to the right of the user. In the experiment, we asked only that the examinee perform computer tasks for 1 hour, without further instruction. The examinee was free to use any sitting posture during the experiment.

7.2   Results

Figure 6 demonstrates the recognition results of the system after 1 hour. First, Figure 6(a) and 6(b) illustrate the elbow and hip angles, respectively. The blue

Table 3. Checklist for workstation environment

Workstation Environment (Consider these points when evaluating workstation objects	
Object	Condition
Desk	Height should generally be between 50-72 cm.
Chair	Height should be approximately at knee level.
Monitor	User should view the monitor from a distance of at least 50 cm.

line indicates the angle in degrees, whereas the red lines indicate the range of suitable angles, which is defined in Table 2. Second, Figure 6(c) presents the distance between the user and the display, where the blue line represents the distance in centimeters, and the red lines indicate the normal range of distances, which is defined in Table 3. Finally, Figure 6(d) and 6(e) show the difference in height between two body parts. This value is used to check whether the forearm and thigh are parallel to the floor (which is indicated by a value of 0).

From the results, we found that the relationships among parts of the human body affect the ergonomics of sitting. Three sitting postures were identified in the experiment, as shown in Fig. 7.

1. **Leaning forward**
   Normally, this sitting posture can happen easily when the user is typing on the keyboard and is highly attentive to the work. The user tends to sit close to the display by leaning the body forward, as shown in Fig. 7(a). On the basis of the graphs, the system can recognize this posture using the relationships among four data points (elbow angle, hip angle, distance between user and display, and height difference between elbow and wrist). A good example of detection of this sitting posture appears between 10 and 20 min. The angles of the elbow and hip are below the threshold angle, and the distance between the user and the display is small. Further, the forearm will be forced to tilt because the body is too close to the computer, so the height difference between the elbow and the wrist increases. Consequently, this posture will cause the user to suffer from neck pain, shoulder pain, or eyestrain because the main body is not in a straight line, and the upper body is bent toward the front edge of the chair.

2. **Leaning backward**
   The observation suggests that sitting while leaning backward normally occurs after the user has focused on the work for a long time. The user tends to relax his back against the backrest by leaning backward. Thus, the lower back is not supported by the backrest. In the experiment, the system recognized this posture between 35 and 43 min. The distance between the user and the display was increased because the user leaned backward against the backrest. At the same time, the angle of the elbow is greater than usual because the user has to stretch his arm to type on the keyboard, as illustrated in Fig. 7(b). In this posture, the user might experience tension in the upper

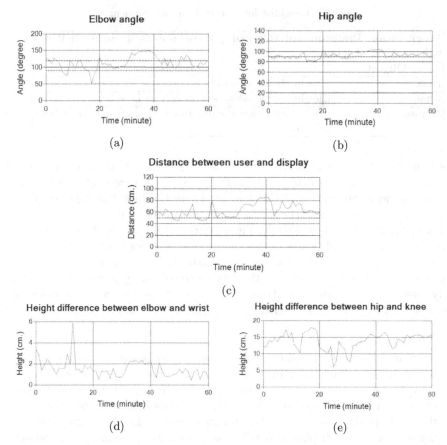

Fig. 6. (a) Elbow angle, (b) hip angle, (c) distance between user and display, (d) height difference between elbow and wrist, (e) height difference between hip and knee

or lower back or the shoulder because the lower back is not supported by the backrest, and the keyboard is too far from the main body.

3. **Correct posture**

The correct posture is a comfortable working posture in which the joints are naturally aligned. In this posture, the user sits with a neutral pelvis; the forearms are straight, in-line, and roughly parallel to the floor, and the elbows remain close to the body and are bent at an angle of $90 - 120°$. Further, the user is upright or leans back slightly. The results indicate that from about 55 to 60 min, the user tended to sit properly. All of the data were consistent with the benchmark, except for the height difference between the hip and knee. Unusual results also appeared in this period of time, which are described in more detail in the next section.

In addition to the results from the skeleton tracking component, we need to consider the workstation environment because good sitting posture is not

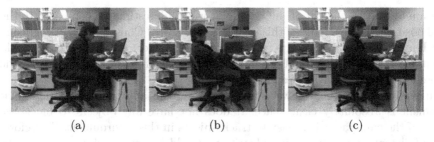

(a)   (b)   (c)

Fig. 7. Three sitting postures: (a) leaning forward, (b) leaning backward, (c) Correct posture

possible without a good workstation environment. Moreover, because we cannot design a good workstation environment that fits every person, it is necessary to establish an appropriate environment for the individual. Thus, we observed three pieces of information: the desk height, chair height, and position of the display. Because most of the workstation environment objects are not moved often, the system will recognized the objects and average the results over 1 hour. Table 4 shows the real positions of the objects and the average results of these three pieces of information in 1 hour.

Table 4. Results of workstation environment tracking

Data	Real position	Recognized position
Desk height	70 cm	77.776 cm
Chair height	50 cm	56.63 cm
Distance between user and display	60 cm	62 cm

7.3 Discussion

As described in Sect. 2, most studies have attempted to recognize the sitting posture using only the human upper body information. Sometimes, however, the use of this information alone cannot guarantee that the user has a proper sitting posture. For instance, using only the distance between the user and the display, the system cannot identify a good sitting posture because a suitable distance does not mean that the user is sitting correctly. The user might be sitting within the distance range but leaning forward or backward. This research aims to solve this problem by capturing the human posture using the entire body in sideways view. The system can perceive the relationship between body parts for identifying good sitting posture.

Although our proposed system can provide the necessary information to the user or physician to analyze the sitting posture, there are several limitations in this research. The first is the recognition accuracy. When the Kinect camera is placed to one side, the skeleton cannot be tracked accurately. The results for the height difference between the hip and knee in Fig. 6(e) are an excellent example.

We found that the height of the knee joint was underestimated compared to the real position. The evidence of this is shown in Fig. 3(b) Consequently, recognizing the human posture in sideways view with a single Kinect camera might not yield accurate results. Using multiple cameras from different angles might provide more accurate recognition results.

In addition, the area between the Kinect camera and the workstation environment is absolutely clear space. It does not have any objects to block the view of the camera, so it is easy to track objects in this environment. Therefore, an intelligent image processing algorithm should be improved or developed to remove objects in real offices that block the view of the Kinect camera.

8   Conclusion and Future Work

In this paper, we proposed a sitting posture recognition system that detected both the entire human body in sideways view and provided context-awareness in the workstation area. This differs from other research that used only the upper body to recognize human sitting posture. Our proposed system can provide the necessary information for identifying good sitting posture. A skeleton model in sideways was created to measure the angles of joints on the human body. Nevertheless, the skeleton model alone cannot determine good sitting posture, and other information should be considered. In this research, three objects (the desk, chair, and monitor) were detected using three proposed features. This information plays an important role in setting up a good workstation environment. In addition, all of the observed results will be evaluated using the standard for the ergonomics of sitting provided by OSHA. With the results of this research, the user or physician can perceive the true cause of poor sitting posture and also prevent health problems such as back pain, shoulder pain, or eyestrain by correcting the sitting posture using the provided information.

Although our proposed system can provide the necessary information for analyzing the human posture, it requires more intelligent techniques for improving the recognition accuracy. For example, a multiple camera technique can be adopted in this research to improve the ability to recognize the features of images in sideways view. Moreover, other objects in the workstation environment, such as the keyboard, mouse, or footrest, need to be tracked.

References

[1] American Cancer Society, http://www.cancer.org (accessed January 16, 2014)
[2] Mariko, K., Hideaki, K.: A system for breaking poor posture in performing vdt tasks using pseudo-negative effects associated with user actions. In: Proceedings of The Sixth International Conference on Collaboration Technologies, vol. 2012, pp. 86–89 (August 2012)
[3] Mu, L., Li, K., Wu, C.: A sitting posture surveillance system based on image processing technology. In: 2010 2nd International Conference on Computer Engineering and Technology (ICCET), vol. 1, pp. V1-692–V1-695 (2010)

[4] Occupational Safety and Health Administration,
    https://www.osha.gov/SLTC/etools/computerworkstations/index.html
    (accessed January 16, 2014)
[5] Huang, Y.R., Ouyang, X.F.: Sitting posture detection and recognition using force
    sensor. In: 2012 5th International Conference on Biomedical Engineering and In-
    formatics (BMEI), pp. 1117–1121 (2012)
[6] Tessendorf, B., Arnrich, B., Schumm, J., Setz, C., Troster, G.: Unsupervised mon-
    itoring of sitting behavior. In: Annual International Conference of the IEEE En-
    gineering in Medicine and Biology Society, EMBC 2009, pp. 6197–6200 (2009)
[7] Kamiya, K., Kudo, M., Nonaka, H., Toyama, J.: Sitting posture analysis by pres-
    sure sensors. In: 19th International Conference on Pattern Recognition, ICPR
    2008, pp. 1–4 (2008)
[8] Wongpatikaseree, K., Lim, A.O., Tan, Y., Kanai, H.: Range-based algorithm
    for posture classification and fall-down detection in smart homecare system. In:
    2012 IEEE 1st Global Conference on Consumer Electronics (GCCE), pp. 243–247
    (2012)
[9] Liao, T.Y., Miaou, S.G., Li, Y.R.: A vision-based walking posture analysis sys-
    tem without markers. In: 2010 2nd International Conference on Signal Processing
    Systems (ICSPS), vol. 3, pp. V3-254–V3-258 (2010)
[10] Kaenchan, S., Mongkolnam, P., Watanapa, B., Sathienpong, S.: Automatic mul-
    tiple kinect cameras setting for simple walking posture analysis. In: 2013 Inter-
    national on Computer Science and Engineering Conference (ICSEC), pp. 245–249
    (2013)
[11] Microsoft, Xbox 360 + Kinect, http://www.xbox.com/en-US/kinect (accessed
    February 02, 2014)
[12] Logaraj, M., Priya, V.M., Seetharaman, N.: Hedge,S.K.: Practice of ergonomic
    principles and computer vision syndrome (cvs) among undergraduates students in
    chennai. National Journal of Medical Research, 111–116 (2013)

Comfort Evaluation of Cockpit
Based on Dynamic Pilot Posture

Hongjun Xue[1], Xiaoyan Zhang[1], Yingchun Chen[2], and Lin Zhou[2]

[1] School of Aeronautics, Northwestern Polytechnical University, Shanxi Xi'an 710072, China
[2] Commercial Aircraft corporation of China, Ltd. Shanghai 201210, China
xuehj@nwpu.edu.cn, zxyliuyan@sina.com

Abstract. Comfortable dynamic pilot posture is the principle for steer design and layout of cockpit design, and is used to study on how to improve the manipulation efficiency. This paper has built a comfort evaluation method considering the consecutive of pilot manipulation based on the static pilot posture, which using the comfort of the dynamic pilot posture to evaluate the comfort of cockpit. The dynamic posture data has be captured by the Measurand@ motion capture system in the cockpit. Then the comfortable evaluation is executed for the pilot postures by fuzzy evaluation method. Form the results, the comfortable evaluation conclusions of cockpit design can be deduced. The better comfortable the pilots have the better design the cockpit is. The result has been validated through the evaluation by JACK software. The conclusion is: the two has the same opinion on the key manipulation equipments, but the new method can analyze the consecutive change of pilot comfort and can discover the interference between pilot and cockpit equipments during the whole manipulation. The evaluation results can instruct the optimization of the cockpit design and improve the control efficiency and flight safety.

Keywords: human-machine interface, comfort evaluation, dynamic pilot posture, cockpit.

1 Introduction

Dynamic pilot posture is a continuous operation process of manipulation system. The comfortable dynamic pilot posture is the basis for flight deck and manipulation equipment design and then improves operation efficiency. The cockpit design and evaluation at present is still limited in the use of static pilot posture [1,2,3,4]. For the equipment evaluation, engineers usually put pilot model that poses a posture as he does the operation, then analysis under this posture if the equipment in the accessible zone, or if the pilot could see the equipment. But the static posture evaluation method can not evaluate the rationality layout of the flight deck and so is the manipulation equipment's position and control run. To evaluate the manipulation system generally and solve the operation efficiency the dynamic evaluation method based on dynamic pilot posture should be built[5]. The dynamic operation process can reflect the cognition performance and motion capability of pilot. Dynamic evaluation method is more sophisticated and general for ergonomic evaluation which evaluates the essence of flight deck ergonomics and ensures the operation efficiency.

V.G. Duffy (Ed.): DHM 2014, LNCS 8529, pp. 160–166, 2014.

2   Comfortable Evaluation Method of Cockpit Based on Dynamic Pilot Posture

Dynamic pilot posture is a continuous process of manipulation system which can be represented as the joint coordinates changes with motion time. The dynamic pilot posture takes advantage on ergonomics evaluation. This method can evaluate controllability of the whole process, and can also detect the intervention problem, reflect the operation efficiency.

Operation comfort is evaluated by joint angles' comfort. The evaluation method Considers both the overall comfort of action process and each key frames' comfort. Fuzzy evaluation method is used to evaluate the dynamic pilot process which is represented by joint angles changing with time. To evaluate the cockpit comfort, the whole pilot process is divided by frame, which is represented by the present joint angle, the angles' comfort is the posture's comfort at this moment. The normalized result of all frames' comfort is the comfort evaluation result.

3   Dynamic Manipulation Data Capture

There are three factors that limit the capture system' choose. First is the cockpit environment. The cockpit is full with electromagnetic environment and also has problem of narrow and small room, and unevenness of luminance; second, the capture system shall not influence the pilot's operating; and the final limit factor is capture system itself which is still combined with the cockpit environment. For example, the optic system demands luminance and room, but the electromagnetic system is limited by the electromagnetic environment of cockpit. The fiber optical motion capture system Measurand@ was chosen to complete the job. The Sampling frequency is 83.3HZ, position resolution is 1-3mm, angular resolution is 0.5°, and the system can capture 18 joints and 40 degrees of freedom.

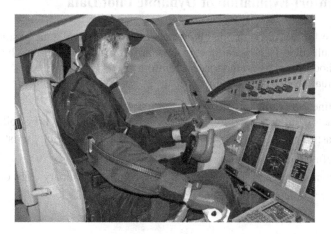

Fig. 1. The scene of pilot dynamic posture capturing

There are 5 pilots completing the experiment on the cockpit simulator. Every pilot do the same action 10 times. The data is recorded by the fiber optical motion capture system.

The original data has been filtered according to the video and data consistency. The data is shown in figure 2. Data is indexed by time including position and angle.

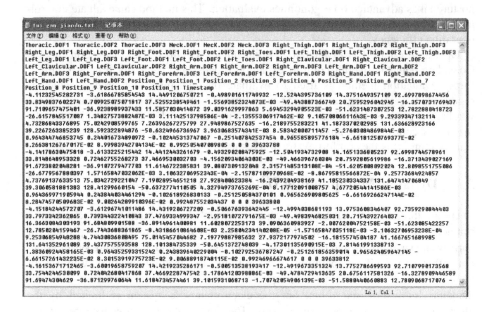

Fig. 2. The captured data sample

4   Comfort Evaluation of Dynamic Pilot Data

The whole pilot process is divided by frame, every frame is a static posture. The normalized result of all frames' comfort is the comfort evaluation result. The fuzzy evaluation method is used to evaluation the comfort.

The evaluation steps are as follows:

1) Define the evaluation factors

The factors influence the final result is defined as factors set. For pilot, the set is simplified as: $U = \{u_1, u_2, \cdots, u_m\} = \{$shoulder joint , elbow joint , wrist joint$\}$

2) Define the comment set

The comment set is $V = \{v_1, v_2, \cdots, v_n\} = \{$comfort , ordinary , discomfort$\}$. For the pilot, every comment corresponds range is shown in table 1.

Table 1. Joint angle range

joint	degree of freedom	angle range (°)		
		comfort	ordinary	discomfort
shoulder joint	flexion/extension	-15~75	-60~-15 75~170	other
	abduction / adduction	0~30	-18~0 30~80	other
elbow joint	flexion/extension	16~100	0~16 100~140	other
wrist joint	flexion/extension	-45~25	-70~-45 25~80	other

3)Define membership

Quantified every factor u_i $(i = 1, 2, \cdots, m)$, and determine the membership R/u_i of u_i to v_i, then the judge matrix is:

$$R = \begin{bmatrix} R/u_1 \\ R/u_2 \\ \cdots \\ R/u_m \end{bmatrix} = \begin{bmatrix} r_{11} & r_{12} & \cdots & r_{1n} \\ r_{21} & r_{22} & \cdots & r_{2n} \\ \cdots & \cdots & \cdots & \cdots \\ r_{m1} & r_{m2} & \cdots & r_{mn} \end{bmatrix}_{m \times n} \quad (1)$$

4) Define weight vector A

$A = \{a_1, a_2, \cdots a_m\}$. Where, $0 < a < 1$ and $\sum_{i=1}^{m} a_i = 1$.

The A is acquired by the analytic hierarchy process. The final weight vector which has passed the consistency test is shown in table 2.

Table 2. Weight vector A

factors	U1	U2	U3	U4	weight value
U1	1	1/3	14/15	7/9	0.157
U2	3	1	14/5	7/3	0.472
U3	15/14	5/14	1	5/6	0.169
U4	9/7	3/7	6/5	1	0.202

5) Evaluation result

Evaluation result $B = A \times R = (b_1, b_2, \cdots, b_n)$

6) Normalized the result

The final result $\bar{B} = (\bar{b}_1, \bar{b}_2, \cdots, \bar{b}_n)$, where $\bar{b}_i$ is membership of evaluation object to V_i .

The final result of pilot operating stick is shown in Table 3.

The comfort evaluation result of joy stick is 78.27 which is not a good score for manipulation system. According to analysis the whole operate process, it suggests that there is not plenty operate room for pilot to finish the action, and all the joints covered here can not extended comfortably, especially wrist joints, during the whole process, the flexion/extension freedom of joint angles are always between 25°and 80°which is the ordinary comfort interval, and the freedom of extension is too big for pilot. For 50 percent pilot the manipulation room of the cockpit is inadequate, according to the analysis and evaluation result above.

Table 3. The final evaluation result

joint angle	com-fort	ordi-nary	discom-fort	evaluation result	final result	norma-lized result
shoulder joint flexion/extension	312	0	0	(1,0,0)	(0.45687,0.54313, 0)	78.27
shoulder joint ab-duction / adduction	158	154	0	(0.51,0.49, 0)		
flexion/extension	108	204	0	(0.35,0.65, 0)		
wrist joint flex-ion/extension	0	312	0	(0,1,0)		

Note: (comfort =(80~100); ordinary = (60~79); discomfort =(0~59))

5   Validation of the Method

The evaluation result by dynamic pilot posture is validated by the result through commercial evaluation software JACK. The researchers have built the same Chinese pilot model in JACK, which has been used to evaluate the comfort of the cockpit. The evaluation result of JACK is shown in figure 3 that represents the comfort of different joints. The joint angles in the box are the joints concerned here. Different color represents different comfort. Yellow means discomfort, green means comfort on the contrary. From figure 3 the wrist is always discomfort, and the discomfort score is about 4.5 which is ordinary discomfort in JACK. The other three joints are all in comfort interval. The result is just the same as the result by the dynamic postures' key frame. The research thinks the correct evaluation process and result means correct final result. So the dynamic posture evaluation method can be thought correct.

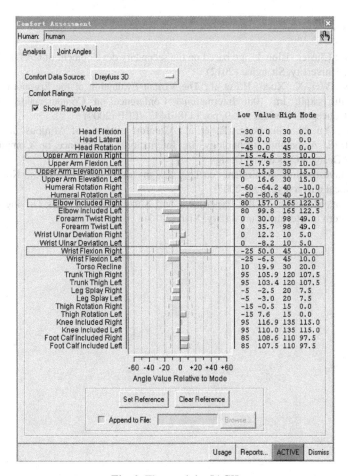

Fig. 3. The result by JACK

6   Conclusion

The whole pilot process is divided by frame, every frame is a static posture. The evaluation is just for the key frame, and the compared result suggests that the dynamic posture evaluation method is effective and correct. The new method can analyze the consecutive change of pilot comfort and can discover the interference between pilot and cockpit equipments during the whole manipulation. The evaluation results can instruct the optimization of the cockpit design and improve the control efficiency and flight safety.

Acknowledgement. The paper is granted under National Basic Research Program of China (No.2010CB734101).

References

1. Fayong, Z.: Cluster vision design based on the secondary development of CATIA. Shanghai Jiao Tong University, Shanghai (2012)
2. Lijing, W., Wei, X., Xueli, H., et al.: The Virtual Evaluation of the Ergonomics Layout in AircraftCockpit. In: 10th International Conference on Computer-aided Industrial Design&Conceptual Design, vol. 9, pp. 1438–1442. IEEE (2009)
3. Fuwu, Y., Yu, N., Shaopeng, T., et al.: Comfort analysis of Minibus driver based on RAMSIS. Automobile technology. In: International Conference on Computer-aided Industrial Design&Conceptual Design
4. Jufeng.: Investigation of airplane cockpit design based on ergonomics. Northwestern polytechnical university, Xian (2007)
5. T. Yanqing.: Research on the Experiment and Simulation of Pilot's Driving Postures. NorthWestern polytechnical university, Xian (2013)

Based on Upper Extremity Comfort ROM of Ergonomic Methods for Household Products Design

Fan Yang[1], Qianxiang Zhou[1,*], Aiping Yang[2],
Huimin Hu[3], Xin Zhang[3], and Zhongqi Liu[1]

[1] School of Biological Science and Medical Engineering, Beihang University,
Beijing 100029, China,
{buaa_yangfan,zqxg,liuzhongqi}@buaa.edu.cn
[2] School of Electronics and Mechanics, Beijing Union University, Beijing 100020, China
289442397@qq.com
[3] Ergonomics laboratory, China National Institute of Standardization, Beijing 100088, China
{huhm,zhangx}@cnis.gov.cn

Abstract. The structure of product demands a higher level of user performance and involves risk that may possibly negatively impact the user's safety and health. For this reason, the evaluation or design of new products requires extensive knowledge of human interaction, including the operation and comfort of motion. This paper presents a technique for assessment of the upper extremity comfortable ROM. The method is based on new experimental data from perceived discomfort of subjects, and uses digital human modeling (DHM) systems to verify the perceived discomfort rank. 55 participants participated in this experiment. They were required to extract and insert pegs from different panels. We get the comfort ROM of subjects according to subjective comfortable ratings and use digital DHM systems to verify the perceived discomfort rank. In this paper, comfortable motion range of the 50th percentile was shown only. Using DHM systems, we can supply upper limb comfortable motion range of different percentile Chinese people for household products ergonomics design.

Keywords: Comfort ROM, DHM, Product design, Ergonomics.

1   Introduction

In order to design household products, we generally need to consider the interaction between the various parts of the body and the product. Activity of joints of the human body is one of the most important factors [1]. We should consider the position of control components (e.g. panel and shelf) of products whether to fit the range of motion (ROM) of the human body. If within the range of motion, we also need to consider whether the joint angle of activity can make people feel uncomfortable.

Unfit and repetitive postures can increase the risk of musculoskeletal disorders. Therefore, the use of effective quantification of the magnitude for physical exposure

---

* Corresponding author.

V.G. Duffy (Ed.): DHM 2014, LNCS 8529, pp. 167–173, 2014.
© Springer International Publishing Switzerland 2014

to poor working postures is important and necessary, if the potential for injury as a result of postures is to be reduced [2]. Since development of the Posturegram, a technique for numerically defining a posture proposed by Priel (1974) [3], various postural classification methods have been developed to identify and quantify postural stress during work. More observation methods have been appliedto the postural classification schemes, such as OWAS (Karhuet al., 1977) [4], RULA (McAtamney and Corlett, 1993) [5], and PATH (Buchholz et al., 1996) [6].

Although the above methods have proved useful for assessment of postural stresses, and contributed to preventing work-related musculoskeletal disorders, they have some disadvantages. First, many of the observational classification schemes are not based on experimental data. In addition, the evaluation criteria was not based on experimental results, but rather relied on the rankings provided by ergonomists and occupational physiotherapists using the biomechanical and muscle function criteria.

A lot of scholars began to made explorations in comfortable ROM by large sample of the experimental data. Genaidy and Karwowski [7] examined the effects of postural dadeviations on perceived joint discomfort ratings assessed under similar working conditions. On the basis of these preliminary findings, Genaidy [8] and Dohyung Kee [9] further developed a ranking system for the stress of non-neutral postures around the joints of the upper extremity. This was based on the ratings of perceived discomfort.

This paper presents a new technique for assessment of the upper extremity comfortable ROM. The method is based on new experimental data from perceived discomfort of subjects, and uses digital human modeling (DHM) systems to verify the perceived discomfort rank.

The DHM is used in ergonomic analyses such as motion capture and simulation, performance measurement, reach-capability check, and visibility check. For example, in the product design, human factors such as positioning, comfort, visibility, reaching, grasping, ingress, and egress can all be evaluated [10].

The important role of the DHM in the design process is in the prototype phase; expensive physical mockups are replaced by virtual prototypes, which can quickly simulate the use of different types of manikins with different percentiles, 5th, 25th, 50th, 95th, etc., male and female. We can change the manikin's data (e.g., stature, weight, leg length, etc.) and build it from similar body dimensions of a real human being.

Meanwhile, digital human models simulating are becoming an effective tool for ergonomics analysis and design. Don B. Chaffin [11, 12] carried out human motion simulation for workplace design. Porter et al. (1998) [13] and Parkinson et al. (2006) [14] studied evaluation and design of driving comfort by DHM systems.

Based on the theory of human-computer interaction, the study of human-products compatibility was carried out. The main goal of the present study was to show human upper limb motion comfortable range and use DHM method for recommended range size of household products' structure.

2   Methods

2.1   Participants

55 participants (28 females, 27 males) participated in this experiment. The age range was between 21 and 70 years old (42±17.1). Participants are all physically active, without any pain or limitation in cubitus, the upper arm, wrist muscle or osteoarticular. Six of them were left handed. Twelve of 55 subjects participated in DHM research.

2.2   Different Heights and Distances Fetching Tasks

Instrument. The functional range of motion (FROM) pegboard (Fig. 1) of BTE-EvalTech assessment system (BTE, Hanove, Germany), operating at a sample frequency of 100Hz.

Experimental Protocol. The subjects were required to extract pegs from panel 2, and insert pegs to panel 3. Test was set up six with distances (based on arm length, AL) and 7 heights (based on shoulder height, SH), as shown in table 1. Participants repeated operation for 1 min, and then gave subjective comfortable ratings (9 scale). Subjects' operation process in different heights was shown in Fig 2.

Table 1. Six distances and seven heights

	1	2	3	4	5	6	7
Distance	1/4 AL	2/4 AL	3/4 AL	4/4 AL	5/4 AL	6/4 AL	/
Height	SH+45cm	SH+30cm	SH+15cm	SH	SH-15cm	SH-30cm	SH-45cm

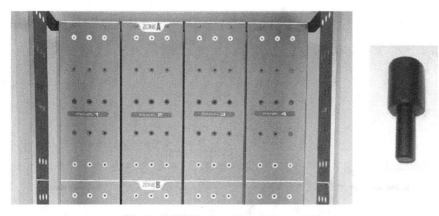

Fig. 1. FROM Pegboard Attributes and Peg

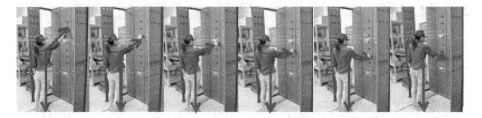

Fig. 2. Subjects' operation process in different heights

2.3 Fetching Tasks of Different Upper Limb Joint Angle

Instrument. Motion capture system (Vicon Motion Systems Ltd. UK) recorded users' actions data. Static Strength Prediction tool of Jack 6.0 (Siemens PLM Software, Germany) [15] analyzed satisfaction of operation action (Fig. 3).

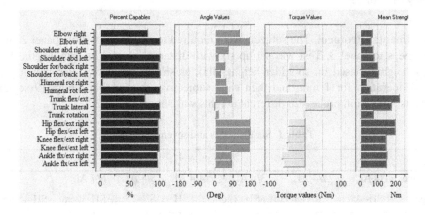

Fig. 3. Static Strength Prediction tool of JACK 6.0

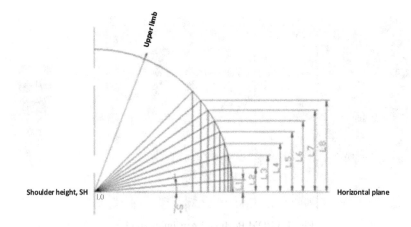

Fig. 4. Test heights

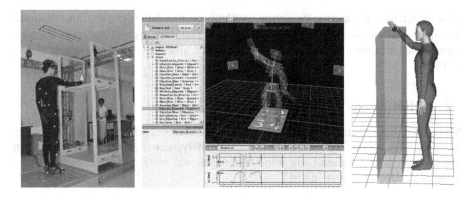

Fig. 5. Experimental schematic diagram

Experimental Protocol. The subjects were required to pick and place bottle (1-2kg) three times in different heights. The test heights was based on the angle of the upper arm in the horizontal plane, 5° intervals increasing (Fig.4). Experimental schematic diagram is shown in Fig.5.

3   Results

3.1   Upper Limb Comfortable Motion Range

By statistical analysis of subjective score after 1 min fetching tasks, the 9 subjective ratings were divided into three grades, from 1-3 (easy), 4-6 (moderate) to 7-9 (hard).

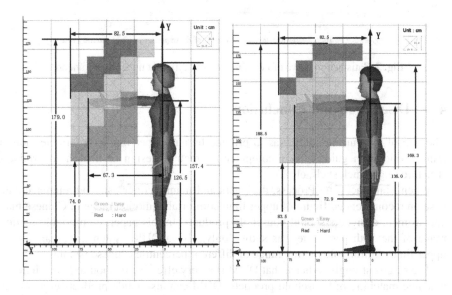

Fig. 6. Upper limb comfortable motion range of P_{50} female and male

Base on Chinese population P_{50} stature (Anthropometric data from the China National Institute of Standardization, 2009) and experimental data, we got the recommended figure of upper limb comfortable motion range of Chinese man and women, as shown in Fig.6.

3.2   DHM Results

The results showed that the participants felt more comfort, when they pick and place bottle in ≤L3 height. By Jack 6.0 ergonomics analysis, when the height is equal or greater than L3, the main body joints and segmental motion satisfaction showed a trend of decline, as shown in Fig.7.

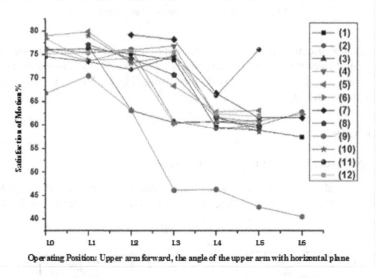

Fig. 7. Satisfaction curve of Fetching tasks of different upper limb joint angle

4   Discussion and Conclusion

The aim of the current study was to provide human upper limb comfortable motion range, which can guide human-computer interaction design of household products structure (e.g. panel, shelf, etc.).

When Manufacturing Process, designers and manufacturer can find reference data base on recommended figure of upper limb comfortable motion range of Chinese man and women, designers should household products. In this paper, comfortable motion range of the 50th percentile was shown only. Using DHM systems, we can supply upper limb comfortable motion range of different percentile Chinese people.

The results strongly indicate that DHM is a very effective method to assess human-machine matching of household products. DHM can also guide products ergonomics design for the recommended and limit value of top shelf height.

Acknowledgments. This work is supported by the Technology Foundation of National Science (A0920132003), the Natural Science Foundation of China (31170895), the opening foundation of the Science and Technology on Human Factors Engineering Laboratory, Chinese Astronaut Research and Training Center (HF2013-K-06), and the basic scientific research project of China National Institute of Standardization (522013Y-3055).

References

1. Sanders, M.S., Mc Cormick, E.: Human Factors in Engineering and Design, pp. 424–512. McGraw-Hill, New York (1993)
2. Andrews, D.M., Norman, R.W., Wells, R.P., Neumann, P.: Comparison of self-report and observer methods for repetitive posture and load assessment. Occup. Ergon. 1(3), 211–222 (1998)
3. Priel, V.Z.: A numerical definition of posture. Hum. Factors 16, 576–584 (1974)
4. Karhu, O., Kansi, P., Kuorinka, I.: Correcting working postures in industry: A practical method for analysis. Appl. Ergon. 8(4), 199–201 (1977)
5. McAtamney, L., Corlett, E.N.: RULA: a survey method for the investigation of work-related upper limb disorders. Appl. Ergon. 24(2), 91–99 (1993)
6. Buchholz, B., Paquet, V., Punnett, L., Lee, D., Moir, S.: PATH: a work sampling-based approach to ergonomics job analysis for construction and other non-repetitive work. Appl. Ergon. 27(3), 177–187 (1996)
7. Genaldy, A.M., Karwowski, W.: The effects of neutral posture deviations on perceived joint discomfort ratings in sitting and standing postures. Ergonomics 36(7), 785–792 (1993)
8. Genaidy, A., Barkawi, H., Christensen, D.: Ranking of static non-neutral postures around the joints of the upper extremity and the spine. Ergonomics 38(9), 1851–1858 (1995)
9. Kee, D., Karwowski, W.: LUBA: An assessment technique for postural loading on the upper body based on joint motion discomfort and maximum holding time. Applied Ergonomics 32(4), 357–366 (2001)
10. Karwowski, W., Soares, M.M., Neville, A.: Stanton: Human Factors and Ergonomics in Consumer Product Design: Methods and Techniques, pp. 325–326. Taylor & Francis Group, Boca Raton (2011)
11. Chaffin, D.B.: Simulation of Human Reach Motions for Ergonomics Analyses. In: Proceedings of SAE Digital Human Modeling for Design and Engineering Conference, Germany, pp. 18–22 (2002)
12. Chaffin, D.B.: Human motion simulation for vehicle and workplace design. Human Factors and Ergonomics in Manufacturing & Service Industries 17(5), 475–484 (2007)
13. Porter, J.M., Gyi, D.E.: Exploring the optimum posture for driving comfort. International Journal of Vehicle Design 19(3), 255–266 (1998)
14. Parkinson, M., Reed, M.: Optimizing vehicle occupant packaging. SAE Transactions: Journal of Passenger Cars–Mechanical Systems 115 (2006)
15. Siemens. Siemens, P.L.M.: software: Jack and process simulate software (2010), http://www.plm.automation.siemens.com/en_us/products/tecnomatix/assembly_planning/jack/index.shtml

Measurement and Analysis of Anthropometric Parameters of Young Male Vehicle Drivers

Qianxiang Zhou[1], Zhongqi Liu[1,*], Fang Xie[2], Sijuan Zheng[2], and Shihua Zhou[3]

[1] Key Laboratory for Biomechanics and Mechanobiology of the Ministry of Education,
School of Biological Science and Medical Engineering,
Beihang University, Beijing 100191, China
[2] General Technology Department, China North Vehicle Research Institute Beijing,
100072, China
[3] Astronaut Center of China, Beijing 100094, China
liuzhongqi@buaa.edu.cn

Abstract. In this study, anthropometric data of 1243 vehicle drivers were sampled and the their age was from 17 to 34 years and averaged 21.85±2.82years. 76 anthropometric static parameters and 11 functional parameters were studied. The 76 static parameters were measured with the Non-contact 3d human boy scanners of VITUS SMART XXL systems while the 11 functional parameters were measured manually with Martin measuring scale. The correlation and fitting formulas of body height, sitting height and other parameters were measured and obtained. We also contrasted measured data with data form GJB 1835-1993. The present analysis showed that the correlation between sizes of body length and sitting height was significant. Sizes of body length and enclosing size and width direction were all increased compared to those in the 1980s. The present results were consistent with other researchers' current research results. The measured data could be an important basis for the data of young male anthropometric parameters and edition of relative standard and design of specific equipment.

Keywords: Anthropometric parameters, Anthropometry, Correlation analysis, Ergonomics.

1 Introduction

Anthropometric measurement method is used to study human body physical features, and acquire the relevant data. Accurate anthropometric data is the basis of engineering system equipment design, space layout, man-machine interface and task design, and also the foundation of human database and all kinds of human body mode.[1][2]. The content of anthropometric measurements includes morphological, physiological measurement and motion measurement. It is a measurement and analysis of anthropometric measurement to the basic human body scale (including contour diameter), surface area, volume and weight measurement, et al, while the measurement mainly focused on static body size.

---

* Corresponding author.

V.G. Duffy (Ed.): DHM 2014, LNCS 8529, pp. 174–181, 2014.

At present, the anthropometric data of Chinese adult mainly comes from GB10000-1988, GB/T 13547-1992 and GJB 1835-1993[3-5]. The data of GB10000-1988 was published in 1988 and it is a nationwide and a large sample measurement. Anthropometric parameters of GJB 1835-1993 measured in 1983 came from armored force. Because of the timeliness characteristics of anthropometric data, the data mentioned above cann't satisfied with the engineering design. According to the investigation and analysis of labor science and social medicine, there is difference in both body figure and growth of different occupation.

According to the investigation and analysis of labor science and social medicine, there is difference in both body figure and growth of different occupation. Especially for some group people, due to long-term professional activities or preference, some body parts have changed the shape because of some special exercise and their body shape is different to the average of people. Therefore, when make a design for a particular career, if conditions permit, it is best to sample from this type of group people to have a anthropometric measurement. For example, in order to make improvement to aircraft cockpit size and layout, and the pilot's life protection and saving equipment, China conducted a series of human body size measurements of air force male pilots which will be a basis of product design[6-9].

Driving is one of the most common work, the requirements to anthropometric data is especially urgent for armored vehicles in the design of man-machine interface. Therefore, this study conducted the measurement and analysis to the youth anthropometric size in a large sample. The results can provide important basis for data accumulation and update of human body, revision of the relevant standards.

2   Method

2.1   Anthropometric Parameters

According to the GB/T 5703-1999, GB10000-1988, GJB 1835-1993 and requirements of armored vehicles and equipment design, the static anthropometric size measurement and functional size of human body were determined in this study which include 76 static anthropometric parameters and 11 functional size parameters(Table 1).

2.2   Anthropometric Method

The overall 76 static anthropometric parameters were measured with VITUS SMART XXL systems which is a non-contact human body 3 d scanner. The system can make a quick and high precise measurement [10][11]. All participants wore uniform measurement cap and put hair within the measuring cap. They wore tight and light color brief with no lace, no obvious fold, and the trousers didn't exceed the umbilical point. If the participants' wears didn't conform to the requirements, they should change one-time measurement trousers that provided by measurement team. They couldn't wear a watch, jewelry and glasses. They were in the environment which its temperature was 20~25°C, noise was 40~50db, atmospheric pressure was the same as the ground. The functional anthropometric parameters were measured with Martin scale.

Table 1. Measured items of anthropometric parameters

	Parameters category	Number	Parameters name
Static parameters	Head parts	7	total head height, auricular height, maximum head breadth, ear to ear breadth, head circum ference, sagittal arc, head length.
	Standing posture	30	stature, eye height, bitragion height, gnathion height, crotch height, shoulder height, upperarm length, forearm length, et al.
	Sitting posture	18	sitting height, eye height sitting, acromion height sitting, elbow height,sitting, Popliteal fossa height sitting, knee height sitting, et al.
	Hand and foot parts	21	hand length, hand breadth at metacarpale, foot length, foot breadth, finger III length, finger IV length, et al.
Functional parameters	Standing posture	5	functional arms span, arms span, middle fingertip height over head, functional upward reach with both arms, akimodo.
	Sitting posture	6	maximum arm reach from back sitting, maximum arm lift length sitting, forearm-hand length, functional forearm-hand length, maximum lower extremity reach sitting, functional maximum arm lift length sitting.

2.3   Participant

The participants were 1243 armored soliders whose age was from 17~34(averaged: 21.85 ± 2.82). The number of effective sample was 1222 and their data was analyzed.

2.4   Data Processing

All measured anthropometric data was analyzed with spss15.0 software. The descriptive statistics was made which include mean value, variance, and percentiles. Also cluster and fitting to the parameters were made.

3   Results and Analysis

3.1   Correlation Analysis

According to the measuring direction and part, anthropometric parameters were divided into six categories: the vertical axis size, which is the height direction size; the transverse axis dimension, that is, the width size; the longitudinal axis dimension, also the thickness direction; the enclosing size; the head and face size; hand and feet size.

It is generally believed that there is certain association between body shape size and stature and weight. Therefore, the correlation analysis was made between body

Table 2. Correlation of stature and sitting height and vertical dimension(R^2)

Parameters	Stature	Sitting height
Knee height sitting	0.894	0.664
Eye height sitting	0.842	0.940
Popliteal fossa height sitting,	0.845	0.569
Maximum arm reach from back sitting	0.791	0.642
Shoulder to elbow length, sitting	0.793	0.627
Forearm-hand length	0.823	0.345
Shoulder height,sitting	0.728	0.824
Cervical height,sitting	0.504	0.556
Maximum arm lift length sitting	0.630	0.515
Functional maximum arm lift length sitting	0.600	0.503
Functional upward reach with both arms	0.694	0.469
Middle fingertip height, over head	0.693	0.468
Functional forearm-hand length	0.487	0.299
Maximum lower extremity reach sitting	0.600	0.324
Lower extremity length	0.981	0.381
Thigh length	0.764	0.559
Leg length	0.766	0.526
Length of upper extremity	0.877	0.685
Upperarm length	0.758	0.572
Forearm length	0.656	0.493
Eye height	0.992	0.865
Gnathion height	0.983	0.851
Bitragion height	0.992	0.861
Crotch height	0.874	0.608
Shoulder height	0.973	0.825
Lower leg-foot length	0.710	0.496
Spinal height	0.981	0.831
Malleolus height	0.293	0.274

shape size and stature, weight, and sitting height. The results showed that there was high correlation between the height direction size and stature and sitting height. The correlation coefficient **with stature** was generally larger than with sitting height($p<0.01$) (Table 2).

The body size of width was positively correlated with height and sitting height ($p<0.05$). The correlation coefficient was in the range of $0.310 \sim 0.674$ which is lower than it was between body size in height direction and stature and height sitting. The body size in thickness direction was positively correlated with height and sitting height($p<0.05$).t he correlation coefficient between body depth sitting and stature was 0.821. The correlation coefficient between back from knee and stare was 0.711. The correlation coefficient of the rest items was between0.101 $\sim$ 0.598. The body size of enclosing was positively correlated with height and sitting height ($p<0.05$). The correlation coefficient was in the range of $0.174 \sim 0.619$. The head and face size was positively correlated with height and sitting height ($p<0.05$). The correlation coefficient was in the range of $0.110\sim0.601$. Among hand and feet size, hand girth, foot length, and foot width was positively correlated with height and sitting height. The correlation coefficient was in the range of $0.134\sim0.301$. The size of the rest parameters was not significant correlative with height and sitting height.

3.2   Fitting Analysis

Linear fitting was made between the parameters that the correlation coefficient was larger than 0.7 and height and sitting height. The fitting result was compared to the part of the relative study[10]. The comparison results were shown in table 3 and table 4.

Table 3. Analysis linear correlation between main human dimensions and height(H)

Number	Parameters	Linear relationship with H	Document fitting
1	Knee height sitting	0.332H - 43.646	
2	Eye height sitting	0.410H + 110.937	
3	Popliteal fossa height sitting,	0.272H – 48.032	
4	Maximum arm reach from back sitting	0.450H + 69.30	
5	Shoulder to elbow length, sitting	0.207H – 5.525	
6	Forearm-hand length	0.259H + 11.072	
7	Shoulder height,sitting	0.306H + 82.610	
8	Lower extremity length	0.517H + 10.075	
9	Thigh length	0.308H – 29.351	0.232H
10	Leg length	0.256H – 53.659	0.247H
11	Length of upper extremity	0.434H + 5.612	
12	Upperarm length	0.188H + 2.531	0.172H
13	Forearm length	0.148H – 17.563	0.109H
14	Eye height	0.936H – 10.434	
15	Gnathion height	0.888H – 46.435	
16	Bitragion height	0.945H – 39.173	
17	Crotch height	0.501H – 116.562	
18	Shoulder height	0.831H – 38.761	
19	Lower leg-foot length	0.272H – 38.354	
20	Spinal height	0.517H – 7.925	
21	Body depth,sitting	0.297H – 28.609	
22	Back from knee	0.367H – 17.826	

Table 4. Linear correlations between main human dimensions and sitting height(H1)

Number	Parameters	Linear relationship with H1
1	Eye height sitting	0.410H + 110.937
2	Shoulder height,sitting	0.306H + 82.610
12	Upperarm length	0.188H + 2.531
14	Eye height	0.936H – 10.434
15	Gnathion height	0.888H – 46.435
16	Bitragion height	0.945H – 39.173
18	Shoulder height	0.831H – 38.761
20	Spinal height	0.517H – 7.925

3.3   Contrast with GJB1835-1993

The anthropometric data could be compared to the corresponding parts of GJB1935-1993. The comparison results was shown in table 5.

Table 5. Comparson between measured data and from GJB1835-1993(P50)(mm)

Number	Parameters	GJB1835-1993	This study
1	Stature	1680	1699.2
2	Sitting height	903	927.9
3	Knee height sitting	496	504.6
4	Eye height sitting	801	808.7
5	Shoulder to elbow length, sitting	345	346.6
6	Maximum arm reach from back sitting	814	834.0
7	Forearm-hand length	448	452.4
8	Lower extremity length	851	888.4
9	Thigh length	497	494.7
10	Leg length	369	382.6
11	Upperarm length	302	321.3
12	Gnathion height	1453	1461.7
13	Bitragion height	1551	1568.4
14	Crotch height	780	734.0
15	Shoulder height	1369	1374.2
16	Lower leg-foot length	418	421.5
17	Maximum lower extremity reach sitting	972	1001.0
18	Functional forearm-hand length	344	332.0
19	Spinal height	942	870.4
20	Akimodo	879	894.0
21	Akimbo span	411	402.0
22	Hip breadth, sitting	320	344.3
23	Cervical height, sitting	653	644.6
24	Body depth, sitting	469	475.3
25	Dorsoventral distance	179	198.1
26	Elbow height, sitting	258	270.8
27	Elbow to elbow breadth, sitting	411	401.4
28	Back from knee	561	604.8
29	Thigh depth	140	144.4
30	Chest circumference	877	921.4
31	Shoulder breadth	373	396.1
32	Chest breadth	275	314.0
33	Eye height	1569	1579.9
34	Total head height	226	238.2
35	Maximum head breadth	154	163.9
36	Ear to ear breadth	192	191.4
37	Head length	188	194.2
38	Auricular height	127	133.6
39	Hand length	186	186.1
40	Hand breadth	88	90.1
41	Foot length	253	257.0
42	Foot breadth	103	105.0
43	Forearm length	241	234.7

It could be seen form table 5 that stature, height sitting, body depth sitting, etc all have increased in vary degree compared to the corresponding part of 1980s, while thigh length, functional forearm-hand length, elbow to elbow breadth of sitting, etc all have decreased. The differences was due to the increased nutrition intake which caused the corresponding changes of the body size and it was a normal phenomenon.

4   Discussion

It could be seen from the correlation analysis that the anthropometric data of the height direction was closely correlated with the data of stature and sitting height. Affected by some other factors, anthropometric data of body width size, the size of body thickness, the enclosing size, the head and face size, hand and feet size was not closely correlated with stature and sitting height.

Parameters which were highly correlated with stature and sitting height were extracted to make linear fitting and a series of fitting equation were obtained. The calculated trend of the fitting equation was consistent with the current experience formula [11]. When the direct measuring data could not be obtained, anthropometric size could be calculated by fitting equation.

Compared with GJB1835-1993, P50 of stature of this study was 1699mm which increased 19mm and the stature showed an increased trend. It said in researcher's study that the stature of male pilots measured from 1974 to 1977 was 1693mm and it was 1711mm measured in 2000[12]. It increased 18mm and the increasing trend was consistent. The weight of P50 of this study was 61.9kg while it was 60.8kg in GJB1835-1993. it increased 1.1kg and showed an increasing trend which was consistent with the other document[12].

Compared with GJB1835-1993, the size of human vertical axis in this study, such as Lower extremity length, eye height, shoulder height, Lower leg-foot length, sitting height, sitting eye height, and sitting knee height ect all increased in vary degree. It reflected not only the overall increase trend of human stature, but also reflected the change trend of proportions. Among the enclosing size, Chest circumference increased by 44.4mm, and the other parameters were not measured in GJB 1835-1993. The body's width size also increased in a vary degree.

Among the functional parameters of this study, 4 items were measured in GJB1835-1993 and only maximum lower extremity reach of sitting changed more. The reason was that the maximum lower extremity reach sitting of this study have increased obviously.

5   Conclusion

A large sample of Chinese young male was made to anthropometry in this study. The analysis showed that the human body size in vertical axis direction was significantly correlated with stature and sitting height. Some formulas were fitted in this study and The result agreed with the relevant studies.

Anthropometric data of this measurement in body length, enclosing size, and width size increased obviously compared with the corresponding data of 1980s which agreed with the air force pilot of the changing trend of anthropometric data.

Thirty seven items static anthropometric parameters and seven items functional anthropometric parameters that have not been measured in GJB1835-1993 were included in this measurement which provided a supplement to the basic data of the same group people.

The anthropometric data of this study was a important reference for accumulation and update of Chinese young males' basic data, reversion of relevant standards, and design of specific equipment.

Acknowledgement. This work is supported by the Technology Foundation of National Science(A0920132003), the Natural Science Foundation of China (31170895) and the opening foundation of the Science and Technology on Human Factors Engineering Laboratory, Chinese Astronaut Research and Training Center(HF2013-K-06).

References

1. Jin, H.Z., Zhou, K., Wang, G.J.: Research on 3D Human Models of Players. Computer Simulation 24(10), 95–98 (2007) (in Chinese)
2. Zhang, Z.X., Zhuang, D.M.: Development of Anthropometric Database. Aircraft Design (4), 38–42 (2006) (in Chinese)
3. GB1000-1988.: Human Dimensions of Chinese Adults (1988) (in Chinese)
4. GB/T13547-1992.: Human Dimensions in Workspaces (1992) (in Chinese)
5. GJB1835-1998.: Man-Machine-Environment System for Armored Vehicles Requirements of Overall Design (1998) (in Chinese)
6. Guo, X.C., Liu, B.S., Xiao, H., et al.: The Linear Dimensions of Human Body Measurements of Chinese Male Pilots in Standing Posture. Space Medicine & Medical Engineering 16(1), 48–54 (2003) (in Chinese)
7. Liu, B.S., Guo, X.C., Ma, X.S.: Data Analysis of Anthropometry for Chinese Male Pilots. Chinese Ergonomics 8(4), 4–7 (2002) (in Chinese)
8. Guo, X.C., Liu, B.S., Xiao, H., et al.: The Head-Face Dimensions of Chinese Male Pilot Population, Space medicine and medicinal engineering. Chinese Ergonomics 9(2), 1–3 (2003) (in Chinese)
9. Wang, M.Y., Liu, B.S.: The Characteristics of Body Composition of the Chinese Fighter and Bomber Pilots. Chinese Journal of Aerospace Medicine 12(4), 201–205 (2001) (in Chinese)
10. Tong, S.Z.: Manual for the man-machine engineering design and application, pp. 98–99. Standard Press of China, Beijing (2007) (in Chinese)
11. Xia, L.: 3 Dimensional Body Measurement Technology in Apparel Industry. Shanghai Textile Science & Technology 34(6), 76–77 (2006) (in Chinese)
12. Liu, B.S., Guo, X.C., Ma, X.S.: Character of Anthropometry Usefulness for Chinese Male Pilot. Chinese Ergonomics 8(4), 1–3 (2002) (in Chinese)

Ergonomics and Human Modelling in Work and Everyday Life Environments

Future Applied Conventional Technology Engineering New Academic Fields from Manufacturing Country JAPAN

Tomoko Ota[1], Atsushi Endo[2], and Hiroyuki Hamada[2,*]

[1] Chuo Business Group, Osaka, Japan
promot1@gold.ocn.ne.jp
[2] Kyoto Institute of Technology, Kyoto, Japan
shootingstarofhope30@gmail.com, hhamada@kit.ac.jp

Abstract. There are various traditional crafts in Japan. They have a long history, and their techniques and cultures have been inherited by many craftspeople. There are various wisdoms in many traditional crafts. In order to create new things, these wisdoms have to be studied by the science technology. Therefore, "Future Applied Conventional Technology Engineering" is defined as becoming the implicit knowledge of traditional manufacturing into formal knowledge by using science technology, and opening up new future for manufacturing by applying them to current manufacturing.

Keywords: Future Applied Conventional Technology Engineering, Traditional Crafts, Manufacturing Country, Implicit Knowledge, Formal Knowledge.

1   Introduction

Future Applied Conventional Technology Engineering was defined as becoming the implicit knowledge of traditional manufacturing into formal knowledge by using science technology, and opening up new future for manufacturing by applying them to current manufacturing. Traditional crafts products have been used by people for many years. There were various wisdoms in many traditional crafts products. It is significant that the various wisdoms are modeled after, understood and applied. On the other hand, the traditional crafts products have been loved and used by many people not as art objects but as articles for daily use. It may be said that people love the products because they are fitted in the daily life. These products are called "Highly cultural products". Characteristics of them are not highly-functional or low-price. It is a product family which is loved and recommended the use of them to other people. Feeling of highly cultural is needed to evolve the manufacturing in the future Japan. Therefore, an analysis on the feeling of highly cultural in the traditional crafts products is of the same importance as understanding of manufacturing. It is characterized as the pillar of the Future Applied Conventional Technology Engineering. This aca-

---

* Corresponding author.

V.G. Duffy (Ed.): DHM 2014, LNCS 8529, pp. 185–196, 2014.

demic field is examined from the viewpoints of manufacturing and products. It is looked like an integrated science including not only engineering but also social science. It was named after engineering for the idea from manufacturing.

Fig.1 showed a study method of the Future Applied Conventional Technology Engineering. There are 3 parts of research method in the Future Applied Conventional Technology Engineering. They are technique, hang and taking the measure. Techniques of traditional craftspeople are understood such as research on hang of speedy work. Especially the craftspeople can not explain the hangs because they learn them, and do not recognize them as special wisdom. The hangs become clear by comparing with another person's manufacturing. Therefore a process checking the hangs to the craftspeople is needed after analysis on various results. Taking the measure is the feeling of decision about product finish. It is the judgment in the final process of manufacturing for maintaining the feeling of highly cultural on the products.

An eye movement analysis on craftspeople was important at the stage of taking the measure for our study. An analysis on the feeling and brain activity was also needed. However craftspeople judge the product finish according to their feeling at the stage of taking the measure. In other words, this is a feeling of good response. In these ways, various scientific studies are needed to understand the manufacturing of the traditional industry.

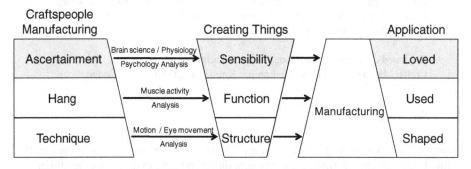

Fig. 1. Study method of the Future Applied Conventional Technology Engineering.

Prof. Hamada and his Laboratory, Kyoto Institute of Technology have studied various traditional crafts in Kyoto. There are many traditional crafts in Kyoto now, because Kyoto had been the capital city for about 1000 years in Japan and these crafts have been inherited by many craftspeople.

Following titles are a part of presentations on the past various conferences.

- A Study of the Effect of the Shape, the Color, and the Texture of Ikebana on a Brain Activity [1]
- A Study on Preference of Shuso Japanese Paper -Comparison of Japan, China and France- [2]
- MOTION ANALYSIS OF WEAVING "KANA-AMI" TECHNIQUE WITH DIFFERENT YEARS OF EXPERIENCE [3]

- SKILL LEVEL DIFFERENCES OF URUSHI CRAFTSPEOPLE IN URUSHI PRODUTS [4]
- STUDY ON THE DEGRADATION MECHANISM OF THE URUSHI PRODUCTS [5]
- Subjective Evaluation of Kyo-Yuzen-dyed Fabrics with Different Material in Putting-past (Nori-oki) Process [6]
- Highly Cultured Brush Manufactured by Traditional Brush Mixing Technique "KEMOMI" [7]
- Influence at Years of Experience on Operation Concerning Kyoto Style Earthen Wall [8]
- Biomechanical Analysis of "kyo-Gashi" Techniques and Skills for Japanese Sweets Experts [9]
- Subjective Evaluation for Beauty of Texture on Metal Surface with Chasing Operation [10]

3 case studies are introduced in the second chapter.

2   Case Study

2.1   Case Study 1: Motion Analysis of Body Movement between the Expert and the Non-expert Clay Plasterers

Background. In Japan, there are many industries based on traditional methods. Plastering a wall with clay, "Tsuchi-Kabe" in kyoto, is one of the traditional industries in Japan. The number of experts in the "Tsuchi-Kabe" industry has decreased with industrial development. Therefore, in order to the Japanese society for preserve the traditions of "Tsuchi-Kabe", effective guideline to improve the skill of craftspeople in wall plastering needs to be developed.

Purpose. This study compares the upper and lower limbs motion between an expert and a non-expert during the plastering of "Tsuchi-Kabe".

Method. An expert plasterer (age54, height 170cm, weight 66kg) with a 26 years experiences and a non-expert plasterer (age37, height 166cm, weight 53kg) with a 4 years experiences participated in this study. Fig.2 showed the scene of experiment. Both subjects wore similar clothing consisting of tops and short pants. Fig.3 showed the 3-dimensional motion analysis system; MAC 3D SYSTEM (Motion Analysis Inc.), which allows optical real-time motion capture. Filming was performed during three trials plastering a wall with clay by expert and non-expert plasterers. Fig.4 showed a measurement on the plastering motion of "Tsuchi-Kabe". A trial was defined as one vertical movement of the right hand from bottom to top while plastering a wall.

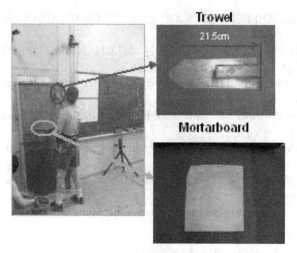

Fig. 2. Plastering "Tsuchi-Kabe" and tools

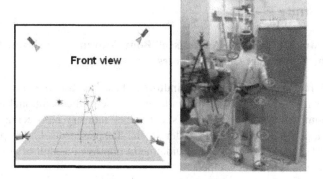

Fig. 3. Cameras and markers setting

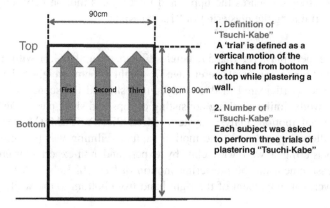

Fig. 4. Measurement of motion during the plastering of "Tsuchi-Kabe"

Results. 1. The upper limb of the expert had less inclination as compared to the non-expert plasterer (Fig.5, 6). 2. Ankle distance was consistent throughout the trails for the expert while the non-expert was not consistent. However, the ankle distance of the expert was longer than that of non-expert (Fig.7). 3. The knee joint angle remained constant after intermediate phase in the expert. However, knee joint angle of non-expert plasterer linearly decreased (Fig.8).

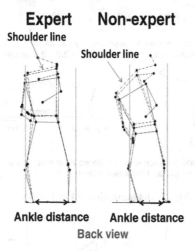

Fig. 5. Typical motion of plastering wall in expert and non-expert

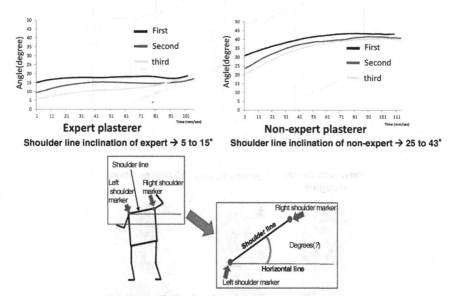

Fig. 6. Inclination of shoulder line

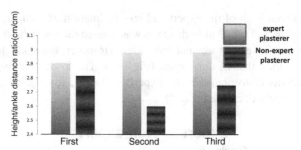

Ankle distance ratio of expert → 2.9 - 3cm/cm
Ankle distance ratio of non-expert → 2.6 – 2.8cm/cm

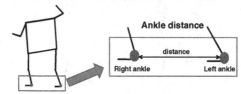

The ankle distance was calculated from distance of
between right and left ankle markers.

Fig. 7. Determination ankle distance

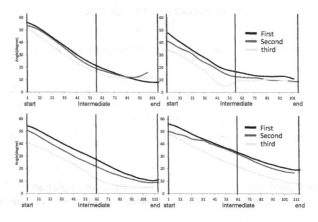

maximum flexion   10 degree flexion   60 degree flexion
0 degree

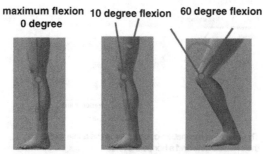

Fig. 8. Definition of the knee joint angle

Summary. Therefore, expert plasterer maintained better stability than the non-expert while plastering "Tsuchi-Kabe". This stability seems to be important for the craftsmen to continue working for longer hours before feeling tired or stressed. The results from this study can be used as an effective guideline for novice plasterers.

2.2   Case Study 2: Effects of Motor Learning on the Edge Shape of Japanese Kitchen Knives

Background. In Japanese traditional food, the Japanese kitchen knife is one of the most important equipment. The effects of motor learning on the Japanese kitchen knife edge had not been reported.

Purpose. The purpose in this study is: 1. To investigate the edge shape of the Japanese kitchen knives in unskilled during 21 days, especially compare with skilled. 2. To investigate the motor learning effects of unskilled human movement in the sharpening Japanese kitchen knives during 21 days.

Method. There were 2 subjects in this study. The information of them was shown in Table 1. Japanese kitchen knife was shown in Fg.9. This knife's blade length was 16.5 cm. Whetstones were used, and its roughness was medium level.

Table 1. Information of subjects

	Skilled A	Skilled B	Unskilled
Age (yrs.)	50	38	18
Career (yrs.)	30	19	none

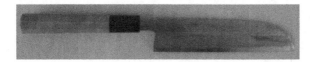

Fig. 9. Japanese kitchen knife

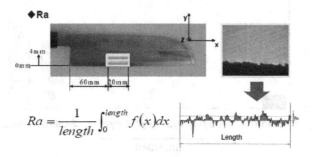

$$Ra = \frac{1}{length} \int_0^{length} f(x)dx$$

Fig. 10. Calculation of Ra

Shape of blade was organized by the optical microscope, its magnification was x200.   Roughness (Ra) was analyzed by the laser displacement meter. Fig.10 showed calculation of Ra. Electromyogram of subject was measured by the electromyography system, and its sampling rate was 1 kHz. Unskilled subject was trained more than 5 times a week. Measurements were conducted 4 times (Day1, Day2, Day7, Day21).

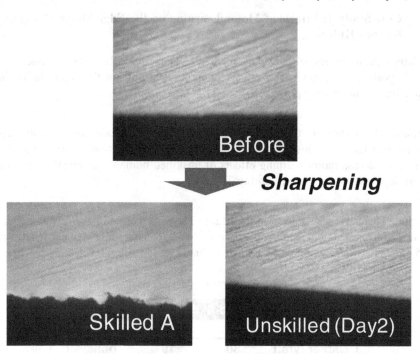

Fig. 11. Edge shape of knife

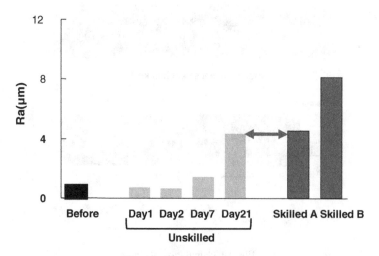

Fig. 12. Change of Ra value

Results. Fig.11 showed the edge shape of knife. There was no roughness in the case of unskilled subject on Day2. Fig.12 showed the change of Ra. Ra value of unskilled subject became similar to the one of skilled A on Day21. The edge shape of unskilled subject was improved little by little.

Fig.13 showed the change of EMG in the case of unskilled subject. EMG of the flexor carpi ulnaris and the deltoid were changed on Day7 and Day21. The knife was more strongly pressed on the whetstone, and it was pulled faster than before.

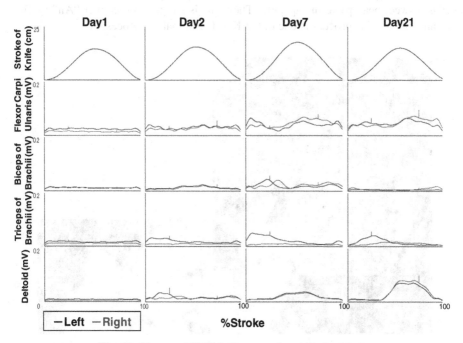

Fig. 13. Change of EMG in the case of unskilled subject

Summary. Training was more improved, the roughness of knife became larger and the EMG of the flexor carpi ulnaris and the deltoid became larger. In this study it was clarified that skill level was increased little by little.

2.3 Case Study 3: Biomechanical Analysis of "Kyo-Gashi" Techniques and Skills for Japanese Sweets Experts

Background. "Wa-Gashi" means the traditional Japanese sweets. "Kyo-Gashi" is one of the Wa-Gashi. It is called that by making in Kyoto. A finger technique is important for Kyo-Gashi, because of making by hands. Especially, subtle finger motion is one of the most important factors. Therefore finger motion skill of the "Kyo-Gashi" expert was analyzed in this study.

Purpose. In order to clarify the making process of Kyo-Gashi sweets, the expert's fingers and hands motion were recorded by the motion analysis system.

Method. Subject was the Kyo-Gashi expert. He was 34years old, and his experience was 14 years. Three dimensional motion capture system was used to analyze the fingers and hands motion on Kyo-Gashi making process. Fig.14 showed measurement scene of this experiment. In this study, an An wrapping process was measured. "An" means a sweet bean paste in Japanese. The "An" is wrapped in another "An" by fingers and hands. This process is one of the Kyo-Gashi making processes.

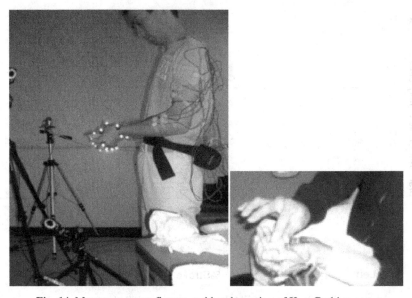

Fig. 14. Measurement on fingers and hands motion of Kyo-Gashi expert

Results. Fig.15 showed An wrapping process of Kyo-Gashi sweets. The An wrapping process was divided into 3 phases.

- 1st phase : first half of an-wrapping (wrapping until two-third from the bottom)
- 2nd phase : last half of an-wrapping (wrapping one-third from the top)
- 3rd phase : final shaping (adjusting the shape)

Fig.16 showed a flexion angle of left second finger in the An wrapping process. In the 3rd phase, left second finger repeated extension and flexion in the range of 50 degrees. Repetitions of extension and flexion were in the 8 to 11 range. Therefore the expert adjusted the number of repetitions to create ultimately similar final products.

Desired weight of sweets was 50 g. Average of weight was 50.5 g. The expert wrapped An with an accuracy of 0.5 g. There was a high repeatability on An wrapping process in the case of the expert.

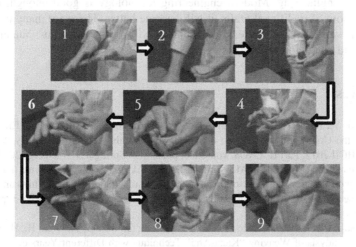

Fig. 15. An wrapping process of Kyo-Gashi sweets

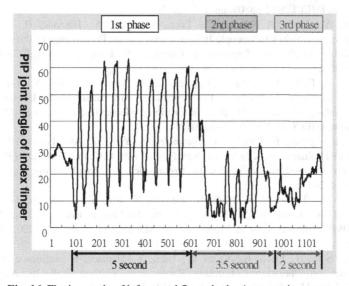

Fig. 16. Flexion angle of left second finger in the An wrapping process

Summary. It was clarified that there was a complex finger motion in the Kyo-Gashi making process. Furthermore expert conducted a sensitive conditioning on An wrapping process.

3   Conclusions

What will Manufacturing Country Japan aim? Japan create a new environment, society, and culture on manufacturing. This is just the Future Applied Conventional

Technology Engineering. Modern engineering technology is good enough, but if it use the wisdom of traditional crafts, it will become better. There are many traditional crafts in the world. In the future, if all countries will use the wisdoms, human beings and the world could go to the next step.

References

1. Ikenobo, Y., Kida, Y., Kuwahara, N., Goto, A., Kimura, A.: A Study of the Effect of the Shape, the Color, and the Texture of Ikebana on a Brain Activity. In: Duffy, V.G. (ed.) DHM/HCII 2013, Part II. LNCS, vol. 8026, pp. 59–65. Springer, Heidelberg (2013)
2. Hongguang HU, Yuka TAKAI, Noritaka SAIKI, Akihiko GOTO, Hiroyuki HAMADA: A Study on Preference of Shuso Japanese Paper -Comparison of Japan, China and France. In: Proceedings of 1st International Symposium on Affective Engineering 2013, pp. 65–69 (2013)
3. K.-i. Tsuji, C., Narita, A., Endo, Y., Takai, A., Goto, G., Sasaki, T., Ohta, H., Hamada, H.: Motion Analysis of Weaving "Kana-Ami" Technique with Different Years of Experience. In: Proceedings of the ASME 2012 International Mechanical Engineering Congress & Exposition, IMECE2012-88809, pp. 1–6 (2012)
4. Shimode, Y., Endo, A., Narita, C., Takai, Y., Goto, A., Hamada, H.: Skill Level Differences of Urushi Craftspeople In Urushi Produts. In: Proceedings of the ASME 2012 International Mechanical Engineering Congress & Exposition, IMECE2012-88288, pp. 1–6 (2012)
5. Shimode, Y., Endo, A., Narita, C., Higashi, S., Murakami, M., Takai, Y., Yasunaga, H., Goto, A., Hamada, H.: Study on the Degradation Mechanism of the Urushi Products. In: Proceedings of the ASME 2012 International Mechanical Engineering Congress & Exposition, IMECE2012 87693, 1–6 (2012)
6. Takashi, F., Atsushi, E., Chieko, N., Tomokazu, S., Yuka, T., Akihiko, G., Hiroyuki, H.: Subjective Evaluation of Kyo-Yuzen-dyed Fabrics with Different Material in Putting-past (Nori-oki) Process. In: Advances in Ergonomics in Manufacturing, pp. 168–177. CRC Press (2013)
7. Shinichiro, K., Toshiyuki, K., Maki, N., Kenichi, N., Hiroshi, T., Akihiko, G., Hiroyuki, H.: Highly Cultured Brush Manufactured by Traditional Brush Mixing Technique "KEMOMI". In: Advances in Ergonomics in Manufacturing, pp. 211–220. CRC Press (2013)
8. Goto, A., Sato, H., Endo, A., Narita, C., Takai, Y., Hamada, H.: Influence at Years of Experience on Operation Concerning Kyoto Style Earthen Wall. In: Advances in Ergonomics in Manufacturing, pp. 153–159. CRC Press (2013)
9. Goto, A., Takai, Y., Hamada, H.: Biomechanical Analysis of "kyo-Gashi" Techniques and Skills for Japanese Sweets Experts. In: Advances in Ergonomics in Manufacturing, pp. 195–204. CRC Press (2013)
10. Nishina, M., Sasaki, G., Takai, Y., Goto, A., Hamada, H.: Subjective Evaluation for Beauty of Texture on Metal Surface with Chasing Operation. In: Advances in Ergonomics in Manufacturing, pp. 187–194. CRC Press (2013)

Comparison of Different Tea Whisk Influence on Bubble Form in Processes of "The Way of Tea"

Tomoko Ota[1,*], Wang Zelong[2], Soutatsu Kanazawa[3],
Yuka Takai[4], Akihiko Goto[4], and Hiroyuki Hamada[2]

[1] Chuo Business Group, Osaka, Japan
promot1@gold.ocn.ne.jp
[2] Kyoto Institute of Technology, Kyoto, Japan
simon.zelongwang@gmail.com, hhamada@kit.ac.jp
[3] Urasenke Konnichian, Kyoto, Japan
kanazawa.kuromon.1352.gentatsu@docomo.ne.jp
[4] Osaka Sangyo University, Kyoto, Japan
{takai,gotoh}@ise.osaka-sandai.ac.jp

Abstract. In this paper, three kinds of Japanese tea whisks' influence on bubble form in "the way of tea" process were investigated. The bubble form and distribution state by each whisk after 100%, 80%, 50% and 30% of tea making finishing time were recorded and analyzed through numerical processing. In order to verify the quality of tea whisk, three kinds of tea whisks' performance were evaluated and compared during the whole tea making process. Consequently, it can be concluded that "Yabunochi" was the most efficient tea whisk for making a perfect Japanese tea.

Keywords: The way of tea, Tea whisk, bubble form, Japanese tea.

1 Introduction

The long Japanese ancient culture accumulated a number of traditional artistic activities including "The Way of Tea" ("Chado"), flower arrangement, "Kendo" and so on. Japanese tea ceremony is developed based on "daily after-meal". "The Way of Tea", also called the "Japanese tea ceremony", is a special ceremonial art preparation and presentation of "matcha"(a kind of green tea powder) to entertain the guests, through the tea ceremony people will achieve temperament, improve the cultural quality and aesthetic view. The essence of "The Way of Tea" is meant to demonstrate reverence and respect between host and guest, both of them can truly experience the artistic conception and taste the most primitive taste of green tea during tea-tasting activity and service process with the tallest state of the etiquette.

"The Way of Tea" is consisted of many specific and strict procedures, whose basic skill just only handed over by oral instructions by expert. Furthermore, the spirit of modern Japanese tea ceremony extends to the exterior and interior decoration of tea house. Appreciating the painting and calligraphy decorated in tea house, enjoying the

V.G. Duffy (Ed.): DHM 2014, LNCS 8529, pp. 197–203, 2014.

gardening design and tea pottery are also the important parts in "The Way of Tea". Among them, using Japanese Tea-whisks stir the tea powder to mixing uniformity and make sure the infusion of the tea leaves combined with the water is the highest technique and important process, which directly affected the taste of tea.

As a an important tool for "The Way of Tea", there appeared some genre of tea whisks with distinguishing shape features and many representative "The Way of Tea" arts masters during the long course of its development. Different genre of tea whisks exhibit has great influence on the development of Japanese tea ceremony. However, the different shapes of tea whisks have different mixing effects and impacts in the whole process of tea making. Basically, tea's mixing uniformity is characteristic by bubble size and distribution attached on the tea surface.

A good tea whisks can mix the green tea power into the hot water with a period of proper time as shown in Fig.1. In order to brewed up a nice cup of tea, masters not only should study and practice for a long time to be an expert and make a high level tea using a user-friendly tea whisk. However, until now the scientific evaluation for the quality of tea whisk is limited. Therefore, it is valuable to conduct some scientific comparison mainstream tea whisks to promote this country cultural treasure and inherit to the next generation effectively.

In this research, 3 types of tea whisks with different shape were investigated as the subject, they were called "Yabunouchi", "Kankyuan", "Ensyu". During "the way of tea" performance, the difference of formed bubbles distribution on the tea surface and temperature variation with different 3 types were inspected and recorded. The characteristic of bubble distribution and the performance of tea whisks were discussed. The bubble form and distribution state after 100%, 80%, 50% and 30% of tea making finishing time described by recording photos were transferred by numerical processing.

As well known, forming process is very critical for the way of tea as a successful tea would depend on the bubble size, distribution and so on. Base on the record of investigation during tea ceremony process, each process's point of degree of mixing and bubble distribution were focused, relationship between timeliness and different tea whisks were extracted and analyzed according to each process.

It is deserved to find that master's action quicker but accurate with the tea whisks of "Yabunouchi". "Yabunouchi" tea whisk made master focus quickly but shift to whisk together green tea powder and water hesitation, which provided a Japanese tea with right temperature and clean tasting for the guests rather than two other tea whisks. It is notify that all type of tea whisk made up the bubble distribution area widely with high foaming degree after 30% of tea ceremony finishing time. Especially, using "Yabunouchi" tea whisk to make sure that it is easier to make the bubble well-distributed on finished tea surface with less heat loss in less time at last, which showed a strong evidence of a good taste for expert's tea.

In a word, this study was focus on the different tea whisks influence on each tea making process of production. Through numerical processing and analyzing, bubble distribution differences and the characteristic of heat loss on the way.

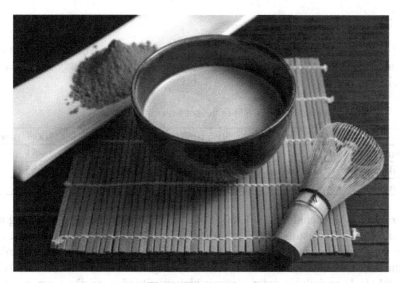

Fig. 1. The way of tea

2   Experiment

2.1   Participants

A Japanese tea master from Kyoto was employed as the participant. The participant has more than 30 years experience in "the way of tea", who can keep the motion of scooping water and ensure the added water weight in the bowl nearly the same for each tea making process.

2.2   Subjects

Three types of Japanese tea whisks were selected for proceeding the experiment called as "Yabunochi", "Kankyuan", "Ensyu", which were the three most popular tea whisks in Japan as shown in Fig.2.

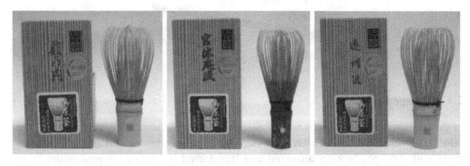

"Yabunochi"   **"Kankyuan"**   **"Ensyu"**

Fig. 2. Three types of Japanese tea whisks

2.3   Experimental Process

1.5g of matcha tea power and approximate 56 g of hot water were dumped into the bowl, and the moisture content of tea was controlled at approximately 97% steadily. The weight of hot water was illustrated in Tab.1.

Table 1. The weight of the hot water in each trial (g)

	30% time	50% time	80% time	100% time
Yabunochi	59.4	58.2	57.6	51.3
Kankyuan	55.6	56.2	55.8	55.6
Ensyu	55.2	55.9	56.1	52.7

Four time stages including 100%, 80%, 50% and 30% of tea making finishing time were focused and investigated for the tea made by three kinds of tea whisks. And bubble form and distribution state after 100%, 80%, 50% and 30% of tea making procedure were also recorded and illustrated by single-lens reflex camera (D40x Nikon CO. Ltd). Especially, in order to obtain high-quality photographs a camera device was employed to support and fix the camera as shown in Fig.3.

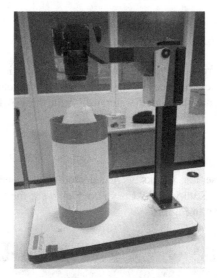

Fig. 3. Camera device

2.4   Image Processing

In this research, all the photos were transformed into the same size as the size of the bowl (Diameter: 12.6cm) firstly. Afterwards, circle region located at the center of bowl with 480 pixels were analyzed and transferred by numerical processing from Fig.4(a) to Fig.4(b). It should be mentioned that only bubble forms larger than

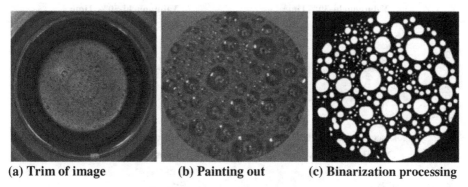

| (a) Trim of image | (b) Painting out | (c) Binarization processing |

Fig. 4. Procedure of image processing

0.03mm2 area was marked. Furthermore, marked bubbles were transformed by the binarization processing method into a white and black two colors as shown in Fig.4(c). The outlines of bubble form and bubbles' distribution state were also sketched on the processed image. Finally, the areas of the bubbles were calculated and converted to the area unit.

3   Results and Discussions

Bubbles' size and the distribution made by three tea whisks in four time stages including 100%, 80%, 50% and 30% of tea making process were presented in Fig.6. The horizontal axis shows the area of the bubble by the logarithm scale and the vertical axis shows the bubble size frequency.

According to Fig.5, it can be found that "Yabunochi" tea whisk is able to produce larger area of bubble at the beginning of tea making procedure as shown in the case of 30% time. However, comparing with "Yabunochi" performance, the medium sized bubbles were appeared intensively for the same 30% time case for "Kankyuan" and "Ensyu" as shown in Fig.6 and Fig.7. The areas of bubble produced by three kinds of tea whisks were showed similar distribution in the case of 50%. And it is easy to find that the bubbles existed in the 50% case was decreased significantly compared with 30% case. Except for "Yabunouchi" performance, the areas of bubble made by "Kankyuan" and "Ensyu" just showed a slight decreasing trend in the case of 50%. It is deserved to find that the majority of bubbles existed in the tea which produced by all three kinds of tea whisks are below 1mm2 when time stage increased to 80%. There were more points concentrated at the higher position in 80% case of "Yabunouchi". It was considered that the tea whisk of "Yabunochi" was presented the wider distribution of small bubbles. Additionally, the sizes of the bubbles after mixing by three tea whisks were concentrated in the 0.05mm2. And bubbles made by "Kankyuan" and "Ensyu" were almost concentrated in the range of 0.2~1mm2.On the contrast, the bubbles showed smaller size after mixing by applying "Yabunochi" tea whisk.

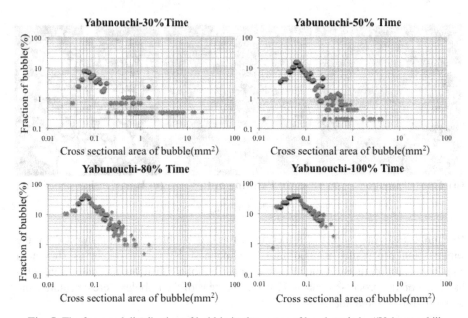

Fig. 5. The form and distribution of bubble in the center of bowl made by "Yabunouchi"

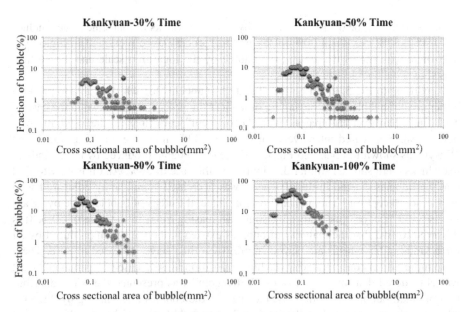

Fig. 6. The form and distribution of bubble in the center of bowl made by "Kankyuan"

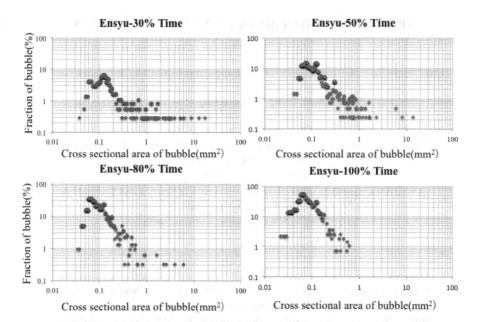

Fig. 7. The form and distribution of bubble in the center of bowl made by "Ensyu"

4   Conclusions

In a word, the tea whisk of "Yabunochi" can produce the most widespread bubbles quickly at the beginning of tea making. Afterwards, big bubble size and area existed in previous time stage was changed into smaller one gradually and effectively until the final tea finishing. In other words, it can be concluded that tea powder and hot water can be efficiently mixed together by applying the tea whisk of "Yabunochi".

References

1. Tujimoto, N., Ichihashi, Y., Iue, M., Ota, T., Hamasaki, K., Nakai, A., Goto, A.: Comparison of bubble forming in a bowl of thin tea between expert and non-expert. In: Proceeding of 11th Japan International SAMPE Symposium & Exhibition (2009)
2. Goto, A., Endo, A., Narita, C., Takai, Y.: Shimode and, Y., Hamada, H.: Comparison of painting technique of Urushi products between expert and non-expert. In: Advances in Ergonomics in Manufacturing, pp. 160–167 (2012)
3. Aiba, E., Kanazawa, S., Ota, T., Kuroda, K., Takai, Y., Goto, A., Hamada, H.: Developing a System to Assess the Skills of Japanese Way of Tea by Analyzing the Forming Sound: A Case Study. In: Human Factors and Ergonomics Society International meeting (2013)

Bedroom Temperature and Sleeping Quality

Hui-Chun Chen[1], Ching-Chung Chen[2], Fang-Ling Lin[3], and Chih-Lin Chang[3]

[1] Business Administration, Hsing Wu University of Science and Technology,
New Taipei City, Taiwan
078011@mail.hwu.edu.tw
[2] Information Management, Hsing Wu University of Science and Technology,
New Taipei City, Taiwan
095165@mail.hwu.edu.tw
[3] School of General Education, Hsiuping University of Science and Technology,
Taichung City, Taiwan
{fingling,salamen}@mail.hust.edu.tw

Abstract. Poor sleeping quality will affect the concentration, reaction and memory ability, and decrease the cognitive abilities such as memory, learning, the ability of expressing complex language, and the capability to make decision firmly. There are some possible causes such as concern about wakefulness, temporary, anxiety or depression, sleep apnea, other illnesses, illuminant, noises and other stimulants etc. Experts agree the temperature of sleeping area and how comfortable people feels in it affect how well and how long they snooze. Many researchers suggest body temperature has connection with the amount of deep sleep an individual gets during the night. However, most of the studies discussed temperature and sleeping quality are conducted in American or European area, however, the situation at tropical area (such as Taiwan) has not been discussed. Therefore, this study set up an experiment performed by Actigraphy to explore the relationships between sleeping quality and bedroom temperature in Taiwan.

Keywords: sleeping quality, bedroom temperature, sleeping disorder.

1 Introduciton

More than 30% of American adults suffer with insomnia-related problems [1]. Asian Sleep Research Society (ASRS) performed a research observed more than 8,000 adults in Taiwan, Hong Kong, Singapore, Malaysia, and Japan in 2003 [2]. The results revealed that more than half of the participants could not sleep well. There were more than 80 percent of the adults who are older than 45 years old believed that they have sleeping problem [1]. Soldatos, Allaert, Ohta, and Dikeos performed a single-day survey in 10 industrialized countries and reported that one in four individuals was suffering from sleeping problem [3]. Poor sleep means a person does not being able to get off to sleep, waking up too early, waking for long periods in the night, and not feeling refreshed after a night's sleep [1]. Poor sleeping quality will affect the concentration, reaction and memory ability, and further induces the decreases of cognitive

V.G. Duffy (Ed.): DHM 2014, LNCS 8529, pp. 204–211, 2014.
© Springer International Publishing Switzerland 2014

abilities such as memory, learning, reasoning and computing, the ability of expressing complex language, and the capability to make decision firmly. Lack of good sleeping quality also increases the risks of reducing productivities at work especially those need highly visual attentions and the operations which are tedious, detail divided, monotonic, repeated, or controlled by machines. When a person lacks of sleep for a long time, he/she might suffer with Hypersomnia and have difficulty to keep awake during most of the time, furthermore, they might also suffer with personality and affective disorders, psychosocial impairment and poor job performance.

Lerner (1982) proposed that the symptoms of poor sleeping quality include bad sleep efficiency, long wake up time, as well as rapid eye movement (REM) and reducing deep sleep [4]. Cohen et al. pointed out once a person has one of the symptoms, sleep time less than six hours, sleep latency (the time between getting to bed and fall asleep) longer than thirty minutes, or wake up more than 3 times per night, the person suffers from poor sleeping quality [5]. In the past, the parameters of the sleep effectiveness on sleeping quality, sleeping incubation, time and period of waking up during sleep were collected by using PITTSBURG SLEEP QUALITY INDEX (PSQI) [6]. The questionnaires are currently useful to collect mass data in a short period of time. The evaluation criteria of this questionnaire include subjective sleeping quality, sleeping incubation, sleeping hours, sleeping efficiency, sleeping trouble, capabilities during day time, and hypnotics use [7].

The methods to evaluate sleep quality can be separated into three categories; (1) subjective self-evaluation, (2) objective equipment measurement, and (3) sleep observation. PSQI mentioned above is one of the subjective evaluation which conducts by asking questions such as the subjective thoughts of sleeping quality, drug or drink using habits, the time before fall asleep, and etc. Polysomnography (PSG) and Actigraphy are used to collect objective information by recording tester sleeping quality, sleeping incubation, the wake up time and etc. PSG is a comprehensive recording of the biophysiological changes that occur during sleep and monitors many body functions including brain (EEG), eye movements (EOG), muscle activity or skeletal muscle activation (EMG) and heart rhythm (ECG) during sleep. Actigraphy is a methodology for recording and analyzing small activity (movement) during sleep and a useful methodology for investigating group differences, and sleep-pattern variations over time. By using PSG, the testees must stay in a specific laboratory and carry a lot of inductance electrode and signal wires which seriously damage testees' sleep quality. Contrary to PSG, the patient remains movable while using actigraphy. Most of the experiment will conduct at testees' home to enhance their comfort and collect the measured data more generally applicable. The subjects will sleep with the device that provided by the testers, and then return the device to retrieve data from it. By analyzing the data collected, the testers could evaluate the testee's quality of sleep. Sleep observation is conducted by testers who watch and record testees' conditions during their sleep in person or by cameras. The results can only provide as the references for total sleeping time, activities while sleeping and some sleep diseases. Therefore, sleep observation is considered as the less efficient way to evaluate the sleep quality.

Poor sleep may develop for no apparent reason. However, there are some possible causes such as concern about wakefulness, temporary, anxiety or depression, sleep apnea, other illnesses, illuminant, noises and other stimulants etc. Many researchers tried to find out the reasons causing sleeping problem. Rodriguez-Munoz et al. shown that the gender makes differences on sleeping quality; the male has better sleeping quality than female [8]. Friedman et al. (2007) reported the personal income also one of the reasons influencing sleeping quality; the lower the income the worse the sleep quality [8]. Singh, Clements, & Fiatarone believed that the person who exercises regularly has better sleep quality [10]. Shilo, Sabbah, & Hadari demonstrated that a person who has irritant stuff such as coffee has poor sleep quality [11]. Kearnes (1989) believed that smokers have poor sleeping quality due to the nicotine [12]. Becker & Jamieson (1992) reported that the aging also is one of the reasons causing poor sleeping quality [13]. Besides all the causes mentioned above, experts also agree the temperature of sleeping area and how comfortable people feels in it affect how well and how long they snooze. Many researchers suggest that temperature between 60 and 67 degrees Fahrenheit (15.56 and 19.44 degree Celsius) is optimal for sleeping, with temperatures above 75 degrees Fahrenheit (23.89 degree Celsius) and below 54 degrees Fahrenheit (12.22 degree Celsius) disruptive to sleep [1]. The reason of this propose might due to sleep is typically initiated during the time when body temperature really starts to decline [14]. That is, body temperature has connection with the amount of deep sleep an individual gets during the night. The cooler body temperatures, the more deep sleep a person can get. However, the researchers did not reach the same agreement on the ideal temperature for sleep. Because sleep can be interrupted by temperature or climate conditions but the situations might vary from person to person. Most of the studies discussed temperature and sleeping quality are conducted in American or European area, however, the situation at tropical area (such as Taiwan) should be totally different. The average temperature in southeastern and southern Asia is normally higher than 20 °C and even reaches 40 °C during the summer. To maintain the room temperature as low as researchers suggestion (lower than 20 °C), air-conditions must be turn on all the time which causes green-house effect and definitely is not good for the environment. On the other hand, the people live in tropical area may use to the warm weather. And large temperature differences between indoor and outdoor may induce sickness. During the summer time, Taiwanese government requests air-condition must be set higher than 26 °C in all the public areas such as department stores, retail stores and government offices. For all these reasons, the authors wondered that the bed room temperature lower than 20 °C might be too cold for Taiwanese people. Therefore, compare to the prior studies, this study performed few experiments to discuss the best sleep temperature for Taiwanese people by using actigraphy.

2   Methods

This study discusses the relationships between sleeping quality and bedroom temperature in Taiwan. The experiments are performed by Actigraphy. Portable actigraphy screening devices SOMNOwatch (figure 1) produced by SOMNO Medics was used to record the data of sleep latency, sleep efficiency, sleep time, wake time and time in bed of study participants. There were 2 male and 2 female volunteers in Taichung participated in this experiment. They all work and live in Taichung, Taiwan. The average age of the participants is 32.5 years old. One of the female is a housewife. The other female works for her husband. One of the male owns a small factory. The other one works at a technology corporation. All the participants wore the SOMNO-watches all day long during the experiment. Study participants were guided to avoid from consumption of alcohol, tea, coffee, nicotine, and sleep altering medications on the day prior to the study night. They also asked to continue their daily routines. The experiments were performed at the participants' own house to reduce the interference from the unfamiliar environment. According to the prior studies, the best bed room temperature for sleeping should be between 15.56 °C and 19.44 °C, and better lower than 23.89 °C. Therefore, the bed room temperature were set at 18 °C, 22 °C, and 26 °C separately in this study. The reasons to use 18 °C is because it is between 15.56°C and 19.44 °C. Using 26 °C is because it's higher than 23.89 °C. Most studies suggested that a slightly cool room promotes good night sleep, so this study also chose 22 °C which is a little bit cooler than 23.89 °C. The room temperature was chosen randomly by testees. Each experiment under same room temperature were set for two days. The bed room temperature was set two hours before the participants went to bed to keep the room temperature under the same level and obtain steady data. The experiment was conducted during the last week of January 2014 right before Chinese New Year. During this period, the average temperature in the areas that participants lived is around 21 °C during the day time (sunrise to sundown). The participants' entire sleep pattern were recorded under different bedroom temperatures.

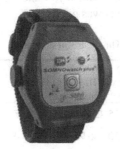

Fig. 1. SOMNOwatch™ plus (copied from http://www.somnomedics.eu/)

3   Results

Sleep is composed of two basic states: rapid eye movement (REM) sleep and non-rapid eye movement (NREM) sleep. The period of NREM sleep consists of stages 1 through 4. A completed sleep cycle is make up of a movement from stages 1-4 before REM sleep is attained, then the cycle starts over again. Each sleep cycle is approximately 90 minutes long. Stages 1 and 2 are called the light stages of sleep; and stages 3 and 4 are called deep stages of sleep. The sleep efficiency is computed by dividing the amount of time a person stay in bed asleep (deducts all the awake time and sleep Latency) by the total time in bed. When the sleep efficiency is higher than 85%, the person should be considered having normal sleep quality. When sleep efficiency is above 90%, the person should be seen as having really good sleep quality [5]. Table 1 shown the means of 4 participants' data under different bed room temperature.

From the results we found out that the time in bed (total sleep hours) for men and women conformed to the suggestion that sleep time should be over 5 hours proposed by Buysse et al. [5]. And the higher the bed room temperature, the shorter the sleep latency. The sleep latency was shortest while the room temperature is set at 26 °C and it was longest while the temperature is set at 18 °C. According to Buysse et al., the sleep latency should less than 30 minutes [5]. Male participants took too long to fall asleep (sleep latency was 44.25 minutes) under the environment that room temperature is 18 °C. This indicated that 18 °C could be bad to sleep quality. Responding to Cohen et al., (1983), if there were more than 3 times waking up, the sleep quality should be considered bad [4]. In this study, male participants wake up more than 3 times while the bed room temperature was setting at 22 and 26 °C. As for male participants' sleep efficiency were under 85% for all room temperature settings which means they did not have good sleep quality.

On the other hand, all female slept more than 5 hours as well and their sleep latency was getting shorter with the higher bed room temperature. The sleep latency for all female were less than 30 minutes and is shortest while the temperature was set at 22 °C. All female participants' wake up time was less than 3 times and their sleep efficiency was higher than 85% under 3 different temperature settings. Female participants slept longer than male in this study which is same as the report from the prior study [15]. According to the sleep latency, wake up time and sleep efficiency, the sleep quality of female participants was good.

Table 1. The means of dependent variables

Gender	Bed Room Temperature (°C)	Sleep Latency (Mins)	Awake Time (Mins)	Wake up Time (Times)	Deep Sleep Time	Time in Bed (Mins)	Sleep Efficiency (%)
Male	18	44.25	29.75	2.75	83.50	361.50	79.72%
	22	15.50	66.75	4	148.00	407.00	76.18%
	26	11.50	59.7	3.25	114.00	391.25	82.79%
Female	18	13.50	9.75	1.25	191.25	457.75	94.84%
	22	7.00	15.00	2	189.25	427.75	94.79%
	26	8.75	11.75	0.75	229.50	478.00	95.15%

AVONA analysis is applied to understand the differences of sleeping quality between various room temperatures and gender. The results are arranged in Table 2. The influences of the room temperatures to all the dependent variables are not significant. However, the gender affects sleep latency, wake up time, awake time, deep sleep time, time in bed, and sleep efficiency significantly ($p < 0.05$). Male needed longer time to fall asleep (sleep latency is longer), and female not only had longer time in bed but also longer deep sleep time, less wake up time and better sleep efficiency.

In Figure 2 and 3, the comparisons of sleep quality variables between male and female are arranged. In total, the sleep quality of female participants is significantly better than it of male participants. This results was interestingly different from Rodriguez-Munoz et al. who suggested that female might more easily suffer from poor sleep quality [7]. From the results of LSD multiple test, this study found out that the sleep latency (28.88 minutes) with the bed room temperature set at 18 °C was much higher than it (11.25 minutes) with temperature set at 22 °C and (10.13 minutes) with temperature set at 26 °C (p=0.037<0.05). While the room temperature set at 22 °C and 26 °C, the sleep latency did not show significantly differences.

Table 2. The results of ANOVA Analysis

		Gender	Bed Room Temperature	Gender ×Temperature
Sleep Latency (Mins)	F	5.51	4.15	2.05
	P value	0.03 *	0.03*	0.16
Wake up Time (Times)	F	16.00	1.78	0.33
	P value	0.00 *	0.20	0.72
Awake Time (Mins)	F	19.18	1.95	1.21
	P value	0.00 *	0.17	0.32
Deep Sleep Time (Mins)	F	15.89	0.98	1.14
	P value	0.00*	0.39	0.34
Time in Bed (Mins)	F	6.50	0.53	0.86
	P value	0.02 *	0.60	0.44
Sleep Efficiency (%)	F	58.51	1.00	0.81
	P value	0.00 *	0.39	0.46

*p<0.05

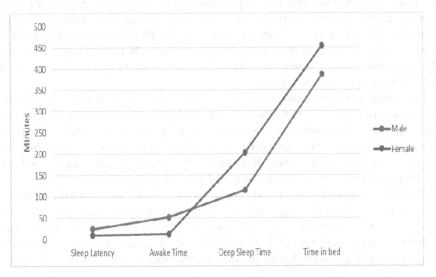

Fig. 2. The comparison of sleeping quality between male and female (A)

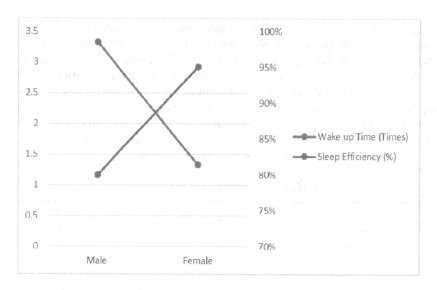

Fig. 3. The comparison of sleeping quality between male and female (B)

4   Conculsion

This study adopted SOMNOwatch, a portable actigraphy screening devices, to evaluate the influences of gender and room temperature upon sleepers' sleeping quality. Different from adopting PSQI, SOMNOwatch is able to record and analyze small activity (movement) during sleep and sleep-pattern variations over time conveniently. The results demonstrated that the temperature only affect sleep latency significantly. That means that the uncomfortable room temperature could only make people more difficult to fall asleep. In this study, the most comfortable room temperature is 22 °C which is a lot warmer than the temperature suggested by National Sleep Foundation. Maybe the bed room temperature which closer to the daytime temperature outside makes sleepers easier to fall asleep.

This results about the female participants had better sleep quality were totally contrary to the proposition about the female is more likely to have poor sleep. The results might be because the experiment was performed in Taiwan. Most of the male earn for their family and endure heavier work pressure. And, the experiment had conduct during the period just before Chinese New Year. All the business activities boomed during this period and reduced male participants' sleep time.

Most experts agree that if a person is in a cooler [rather than too-warm] room, it is easier to get a good night sleep. But people are more likely to wake up, if the room becomes uncomfortably hot or cold. Recommendation about the temperature setting is to keep the room between 15.56°C and 19.44°C, however, the most comfortable temperature setting should depent on whatever that means to the sleeper. Therefore, the best room teperature to sleep in tropic area should be warmer than it in American and European countries. To obtain more useful informations subjet to this topic, the reseach which is including longer measurement period and more participants should be performed. Besides the room temperature, the humidity inside the bed room could also be considered to one of the factors influencing the sleep quality.

References

1. National Sleep Foundation, http://www.sleepfoundation.org/article/how-sleep-works/the-sleep-environment
2. Asian Sleep Research Society. Asian Sleep Research (2003)
3. Soldatos, C.R., Allaert, F.A., Ohta, T., Dikeos, D.: How do individuals sleep around the world? Results from a single-day survey in ten countries. Sleep Med. 6, 5–13 (2005)
4. Lerner, R.: Sleep loss in the aged: implications for nursing practice. Journal of Gerontological Nursing 8, 323–328 (1982)
5. Cohen, D.C., Eisdorfer, C., Prize, P., Breen, A., Davis, M., Dadsby, A.: Sleep disturbances in the institutionalized aged. Journal of the American Geriatrics Society 31, 79–82 (1993)
6. Buysse, D.J., Reynolds, C.F., Monk, T.H., Berman, S.R., Kupfer, D.J.: The Pittsburgh Sleep Quality Index (PSQI): A new instrument for psychiatric research and practice. Psychiatry Research 28(2), 193–213 (1989)
7. Summers, M.O., Crisostomo, M.I., Stepanski, E.J.: Recent developments in the classification, evaluation and treatment of insomnia. CHEST 130(1), 276–286 (2006)
8. Rodriguez-Munoz, A., Moreno-Jimenez, B., Fernandez-Mendoza, J.J., Olavarrieta-Bernardino, S., de la Cruz-Troca, J.J., Vela-Bueno, A.: Insomnia and quality of sleep among primary care physicians: A gender perspective. Rev. Neurol. 47(3), 119–123 (2008)
9. Friedman, E.M., Love, G.D., Rosenkranz, M.A., Urry, H.L., Davidson, R.J., Singer, B.H., Ryff, C.D.: Socioeconomic status predicts objective and subjective sleep quality in aging women. Psychosom. Med. 69(7), 682–691 (2007)
10. Singh, N.A., Clements, K.M., Fiatarone, M.A.: Sleep, sleep deprivation, and daytime activities: A randomized controlled trial of the effect of exercise on sleep. Sleep 20(2), 95–101 (1997)
11. Shilo, L., Sabbah, H., Hadari, R.: The effects of coffee consumption on sleep and melatonin secretion. Sleep Med. 3(3), 271–273 (2002)
12. Kearnes, S.: Insomnia in the elderly. Nursing Times 85(47), 32–33 (1989)
13. Becker, P.M., Jamieson, A.O.: Common sleep disorders in the elderly: Diagnosis and treatment. Geriatrics 47, 41–52 (1992)
14. Murphy, P.J., Campbell, S.S.: Nighttime drop in body temperature: A physiological trigger for sleep onset? Sleep 20(7), 505–511 (1997)
15. Burazeri, G., Gofine, J., Kark, J.D.: Over 8 Hours of Sleep-Marker of Increased Mortality in Mediterranean Population: Follow-up Population Study. Croatian Medical Journal 44, 193–198 (2003)

Comparison of Characteristics Recognition in the *"Mitate"* of *Urushi* Crafts

Atsushi Endo[1,*], Chieko Narita[1], Koji Kuroda[2], Yuka Takai[3], Akihiko Goto[3],
Yutaro Shimode[4], and Hiroyuki Hamada[5]

[1] Kyoto Institute of Technology, Kyoto, Japan
{shootingstarofhope30,soy155apf}@gmail.com
[2] Dai Nippon Printing Co., Ltd., Tokyo, Japan
kuroda-k2@mail.dnp.co.jp
[3] Osaka Sangyo University, Osaka, Japan
{takai,gotoh}@ise.osaka-sandai.ac.jp
[4] Future-Applied Conventional Technology Center,
Kyoto Institute of Technology,
Kyoto, Japan
shimode-yutaro@xa2.so-net.ne.jp
[5] Kyoto Institute of Technology, Kyoto, Japan
hhamada@kit.ac.jp

Abstract. Urushi crafts is one of the Japanese traditional crafts. Urushi painting and "Maki-e" decoration of these Urushi crafts works were removed by usage for many years. Experts of Urushi crafts have repaired and restored them correctly by gain an insight into their conditions, materials and techniques. They can understand the contained information by watching the works. This observation method is called "Mitate". In this study, it was aimed to examine how to conduct Mitate when Urushi craftspeople look at the works. As a result, it is considered that expert craftspeople could ensure the characteristics recognition by gaining and combining more information from the work than the other subject.

Keywords: Mitate, Text mining, Maki-e, Urushi crafts, Craftspeople, Expert and Non-expert.

1 Introduction

Urushi crafts is one of the Japanese traditional crafts. This is understood from the name of "japan" in English-speaking countries in the past. Urushi painting and "Maki-e" decoration of these Urushi crafts works were removed by usage for many years. Experts of Urushi crafts have repaired and restored them correctly by gain an insight into their conditions, materials and techniques. They can understand the contained information by watching the works. This observation method is called "Mitate". Mitate is performed by the naked eye. In the previous study, the observation actions in Mitate were divided into following 7 actions [1]. Fig.1 showed the images of 7

---

[*] Corresponding author.

V.G. Duffy (Ed.): DHM 2014, LNCS 8529, pp. 212–223, 2014.
© Springer International Publishing Switzerland 2014

observation actions in Mitate. It was important to jiggle the work up and down in Mitate. Expert pointed out many characteristics about the work, had many words for representing them.

- Visual contact
  Subjects observed the work by only naked eye.
- Work inclination
  When subjects observed the work, they inclined it greatly.
- Body inclination
  When subjects observed the work, they inclined their bodies.
- Touch
  When subjects observed the work, they touched the work.
- Move
  When subjects observed the work, they moved the work.
- Head inclination
  When subjects observed the work, they inclined their heads.
- Jiggling work up and down
  When subjects observed the work, they jiggled the work up and down.

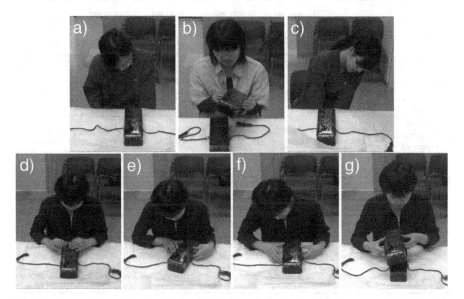

Fig. 1. 7 observation actions in Mitate; a) Visual contact, b) Work inclination, c) Body inclination, d) Touch, e) Move, f) Head inclination, g) Jiggling work up and down

There were various previous studies on characteristics recognition in the past [2]. Study on mechanical recognition [3], and study on characteristics recognition through text-mining approach [4] was made. There also was the study on characteristics recognition based on eye movement analysis [5].

Therefore in this study, it was aimed to examine the characteristics recognition in Mitate when Urushi craftspeople look at the works.

2   Measurements

2.1   Subjects

Table 1 showed the information of subjects. There were 18 subjects in this study. Subject A was expert Maki-e craftspeople. Maki-e is one of the decoration techniques of Urushi crafts. He was 57 years old, and had 39 years of experiences. Subject B and C were non-expert Maki-e craftspeople. Their age was about 30 years old, and their years of experience was about 10 years. Subject D - G were non-expert Maki-e craftspeople. Their age was 20's and 30's, and their years of experience was about 5 years. Subject H - R were the student studying Urushi crafts techniques. Their age was 20's and 10's, and their years of experience was about 1 - 3 years.

Table 1. Information of subjects

Subject	A	B	C	D	E	F
Sex	Male	Female	Female	Male	Female	Female
Age	57	32	31	34	29	28
Years of Urushi crafts experience	39 years	12 years and 2 months	9 years and 6 months	6 years and 6 months	5 years and 2 months	4 years and 2 months
Job	Maki-e craftspeople	Maki-e craftspeople	Maki-e craftspeople	Maki-e craftspeople	Maki-e craftspeople	Maki-e craftspeople

Subject	G	H	I	J	K	L
Sex	Female	Female	Female	Female	Female	Female
Age	23	21	24	21	20	21
Years of Urushi crafts experience	4 years and 2 months	3 years and 2 months	3 years and 2 months	3 years and 2 months	3 years and 2 months	3 years and 2 months
Job	Maki-e craftspeople	Student studying Urushi crafts	Student studying Urushi crafts	Student studying Urushi crafts	Student studying Urushi crafts	Student studying Urushi crafts

Subject	M	N	O	P	Q	R
Sex	Female	Female	Female	Male	Female	Female
Age	23	28	20	20	19	23
Years of Urushi crafts experience	2 years and 6 months	1 years and 2 months	1 years and 2 months	1 years and 2 months	1 years and 2 months	1 years and 2 months
Job	Student studying Urushi crafts	Student studying Urushi crafts	Student studying Urushi crafts	Student studying Urushi crafts	Student studying Urushi crafts	Student studying Urushi crafts

2.2   Mitate Work for This Study

Fig.2 showed a work for this study. Four-handled basin with Maki-e decoration was used in this study. It was made in Edo period (300 - 400 years ago). Urushi was painted in whole area of the work, and its surface was decorated with golden powder by Maki-e technique. The cranes, turtles, pines and bamboos were designed in this work. These were one of the auspicious omens motifs in Japan.

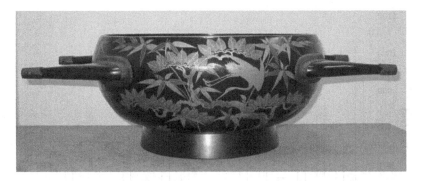

Fig. 2. Four-handled basin with Maki-e decoration [Collection of COSTUME MUSEUM]

2.3   Measurement Condition

Mitate was conducted in a fluorescent lighted room. Four-handled basin with Maki-e decoration was placed on a desk. Points of focus were not specified, and order subject to talk about information from the work point by point. Allow subject to hold and move the work in order to conduct Mitate easily. When subject hold or move the work, require wear of glove in order to protect it. Time limit of Mitate was approximately 30 minutes, because its time was adequate to get the information from the work.

Mitate was recorded by the digital video camera. Time and remark points were analyzed through a movie of Mitate. Remark points were divided into 4 viewpoints. It was "Wooden Base", "Urushi Painting", "Maki-e" and "Other".

Remark sentences were analyzed by text-mining approach. IBM SPSS Text Analytics for Surveys (IBM Japan, Ltd.) was used. "Maki-e", "Urushi Painting", "Golden Powder" and so on were set as a category, relationship on remark sentences were examined.

3   Results

3.1   Time of Mitate

Fig.3 showed a total time of Mitate. Fig.4 showed the average time of Mitate. Expert conduted Mitate for about 1060 seconds. Non-expert with about 10 years experiences conduted Mitate for about 660 seconds. Non-expert with about 5 years experiences conduted Mitate for about 590 seconds. Student with about 3 years experiences conducted Mitate for about 430 seconds. Student with about 1 year experience conducted Mitate for about 230 seconds.

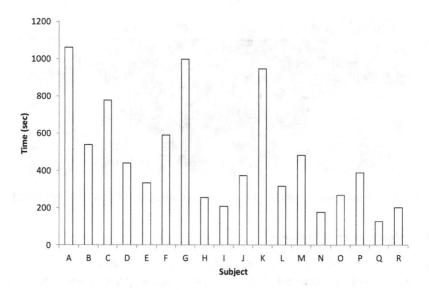

Fig. 3. Total time of Mitate

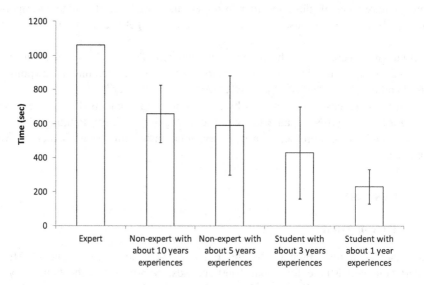

Fig. 4. Average time of Mitate

3.2   Remark Points

Fig.5 showed total number of point in Mitate. Fig.6 showed average number of total points in Mitate. Expert pointed out about 60 points. Non-expert with about 10 years experiences pointed out about 20 points. Non-expert with about 5 years experiences pointed out about 13 points. Student with about 3 years experiences pointed out about 10 points. Student with about 1 year experience pointed out about 5 points.

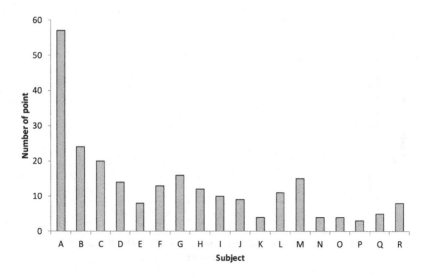

Fig. 5. Total number of point in Mitate

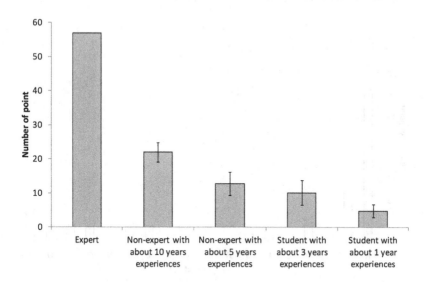

Fig. 6. Average number of total points in Mitate

Fig.7 showed number of point about "Wooden Base". Only expert pointed out 5 points, other subjects did not point out.

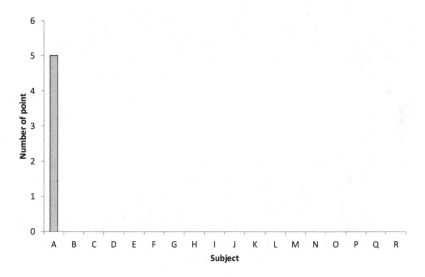

Fig. 7. Number of point about "Wooden Base"

Fig.8 showed number of point about "Urushi Painting". Expert pointed out 21 points, and the other subjects pointed out 0 - 7 points.

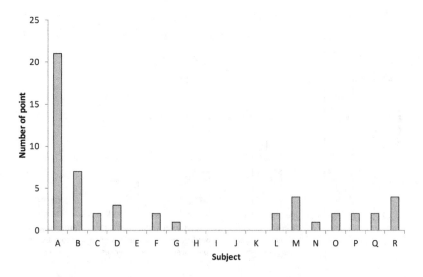

Fig. 8. Number of point about "Urushi Painting"

Fig.9 showed number of point about "Maki-e". Fig.10 showed average number of points. Expert pointed out 27 points. Non-expert with about 10 years experiences pointed out about 17 points. Non-expert with about 5 years experiences pointed out about 11 points. Student with about 3 years experiences pointed out about 9 points. Student with about 1 year experience pointed out about 2 points.

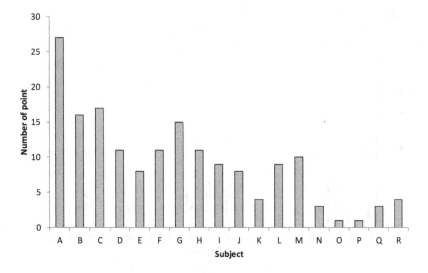

Fig. 9. Number of point about "Maki-e"

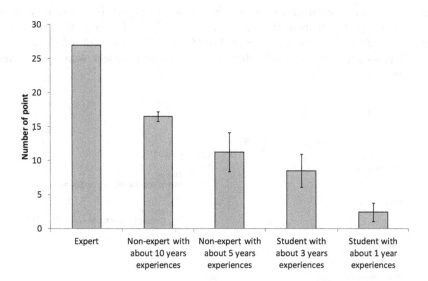

Fig. 10. Average number of points about "Maki-e"

Fig.11 showed number of point about "Other". Expert pointed out 4 points, and the other subjects pointed out 0 - 1 point.

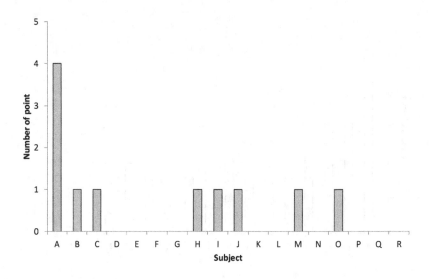

Fig. 11. Number of point about "Other"

3.3   Text-Mining

Fig.12 showed the result of text-mining in the case of expert. Fig.13 showed in the case of non-expert with about 10 years experiences, Fig.14 showed in the case of non-expert with about 5 years experiences, Fig.15 showed in the case of student with about 3 years experiences, Fig.16 showed in the case of student with about 1 year experience.

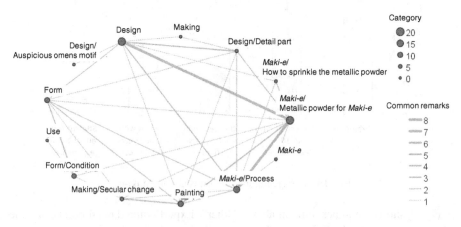

Fig. 12. Result of text-mining in the case of expert (Subject A)

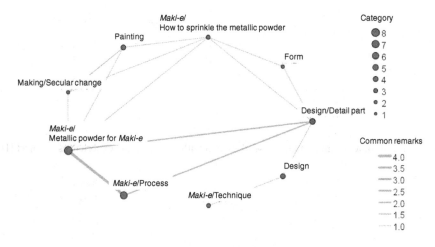

Fig. 13. Result of text-mining in the case of non-expert with about 10 years experiences (Subject C)

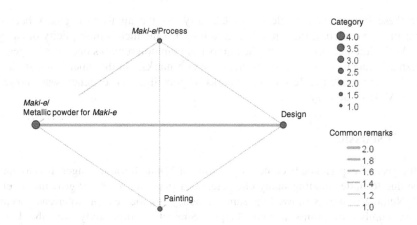

Fig. 14. Result of text-mining in the case of non-expert with about 5 years experiences (Subject D)

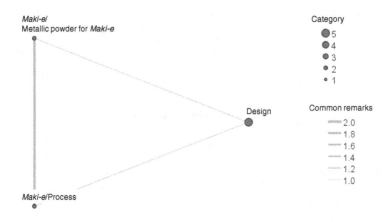

Fig. 15. Result of text-mining in the case of student with about 3 years experiences (Subject H)

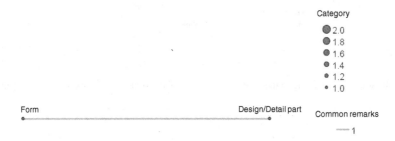

Fig. 16. Result of text-mining in the case of student with about 1 year experience (Subject Q)

In these figures, blue circle means category. As the number of remark becomes larger in each category, the circle becomes bigger. Line means multiplicity of categories. As the line becomes thicker, the number of common remarks becomes bigger.

Expert's remarks were related to many other remarks. On the other hand, student's remarks were related to few other remarks. Especially, this tendency was shown in case of Maki-e category.

4   Discussion

As the year of experience became longer, time of Mitate became longer. It is assumed to be due to understanding many characteristics from the work for growing level of skill. Number of points showed the same tendency. As the year of experience became longer, number of points became bigger. Subject of this study was the Urushi craftspeople, and they specialized in Maki-e decoration. Therefore, number of points in "Maki-e" was bigger than the one of "Wooden Base", "Urushi Painting" and "Other". Especially, number of point in the case of student with 1 year experience was the least in all subjects. They could not point out, because they did not learn the Maki-e decoration techniques in their school.

As the results of text-mining, as the year of experience became longer, the remarks had a relationship with more other remarks. Therefore, as the level of skill was improved more, more information could be understood. Furthermore, it seemed that the characteristics recognition was ensured by combining the information.

5   Conclusion

Urushi craftspeople need to recognize characteristics of the work, because they can understand how to make the work for exact characteristics recognition. Based on the information about the materials and techniques, making process is decided in the case of Urushi crafts. Therefore, this skill is effective for repair, restoration and making an imitation work. In order to improve this skill, Urushi craftspeople need to try to not only get information but also recognize the characteristics by combining information.

Acknowledgment. Four-handled basin with Maki-e decoration is a collection of COSTUME MUSEUM (Located in Shimogyo-ku, Kyoto, JAPAN). We greatly appreciate for their kindness.

References

1. Endo, A., Narita, C., Suzuki, R., Kuroda, K., Takai, Y., Goto, A., Shimode, Y.: Study on "Mitate" of Urushi Craftspeople With Different Years of Experiences. In: Proceedings of 13th Japan International SAMPE Symposium and Exhibition (JISSE 2013), Paper ID 2416, pp.1-5 (2013)
2. Kume, H., Osana,Y., Hagiwara, M.: Neural Network Model of Visual System based on Feature Integration Theory, IEICE Technical Report, 98(674), pp.261-268 (1999)
3. Inouye, T., Kishinami, T., Fumiki, T.: Study of Process Planning based on Feature Dependency of Manufacturing Features (2nd Report) - Improvement for Feature recognition and Creation of Feature Dependency with Manufacturing View. Journal of the Japan Society for Precision Engineering 73(5), 588–592 (2007)
4. Ikemoto, S., Inaba, H., Takai, Y., Goto, A.: Sheet Metal Molding Technique Analysis for Learning System for Car Mechanic. In: Proceedings of 13th Japan International SAMPE Symposium and Exhibition (JISSE 2013), Paper ID 2410, pp.1-6 (2013)
5. T. Sugimoto, Y. Takai, A. Goto.: Comparison of Polishing Process for Metallographic Preparation by Means of Analysis of Eye Movement. In: Proceedings of 13thJapan International SAMPE Symposium and Exhibition (JISSE-13), Paper ID 2415, pp.1–6 (2013)

Evaluation of Kyo-Yuzen-Zome Fabrics
with Different Pastes

Takashi Furukawa[1,*], Yuka Takai[2], Akihiko Goto[2], Noriaki Kuwahara[1],
and Noriyuki Kida[1]

[1] Kyoto Institute of Technology, Kyoto, Japan
t-furukawa@hishiken.co.jp,
{nkuwahar,kida}@kit.ac.jp
[2] Osaka Sangyo University, Osaka, Japan
{takai,gotoh}@ise.osaka-sandai.ac.jp

Abstract. "Yuzen-zome" is a traditional but still popular method of dyeing fabrics in Japan. The products using the Yuzen-zome method and manufactured in Kyoto city are called "Kyo-Yuzen-zome." The dyeing method of Yuzen-zome can be dividing into 10 procedures. A specialized craftsman is in charge of each procedure. During the paste application (Nori-oki) procedure, the expert applies a starch paste or a rubber paste to a fabric. The two pastes create different effect on the dyed fabric. At market, the fabric with a starch paste application is perceived to have a higher value than that with a rubber paste. In this study, the difference of the viscosity between two materials was clarified, and specimens which craftsman dyed were observed. Then how two materials put on fabrics, and the structures of them were measured.

Keywords: Paste, Fabric, Dyeing, Starch, Rubber.

1   Introduction

There are some methods to dye a kimono in Japan such as Yuzen-zome (Yuzen dyeing), Shibori-zome (tie dyeing), Ai-zome (indigo dyeing), and Rou-zome (batik dying). Among these methods, the most widely used dyeing technique is Yuzen-zome. The Yuzen-zome dyed in Kyoto is specifically called "Kyo-Yuzen-zome." Not much literature clarifies the origin of Yuzen-zome; however, the "Genji Hiinagata" published in 1686 indicate the names of Yuzen-zome and Yuzensai, with the descriptions of pattern dying such as Icchin-zome, Chaya-zome, and Edo-zome. Yuzensai Miyazaki is alleged to be a fan painter, Yuzensai Miyazaki, living in Kyoto at that time. Later, Kyo-Yuzen-zome has been supporting the garment industry in Japan together with Kaga-Yuzen and Edo-Yuzen. In the Meiji era, the dyeing technology of the synthetic dye was advanced, and most of the currently used dyes are synthetic dyes. Likewise in the Meiji era, once the technique to dye a fabric using a dyeing stencil was established, a mass production of kimono using Yuzen-zome became possible.

---

* Corresponding author.

V.G. Duffy (Ed.): DHM 2014, LNCS 8529, pp. 224–235, 2014.

The amount of products had been increased and the annual production reached to 16,500,000 bolts in 1971; however, it has been decreased and reached to 840,000 bolts in 2003 along with the lifestyle change [1]. Regarding the market size of Japanese dress industry, it was 627 billion yen in 2003, but was 400 billion yen in 2008, [2], and has been believed to be lower than 300 billion yen in 2013.

Generally, Kyo-Yuzen-zome can be classified into five types: hand-drawn Yuzen, *kata* Yuzen (i.e., dyed with paper patterns), screen printed, machine printed, and inkjet dyeing. Among them, the representative example is the hand-drawn Yuzen which whole production procedure is performed by handwork. This shows the uniqueness that each product has its own character. Each craftsman is in charge of each manufacturing procedure. In the process of producing the hand-drawn Yuzen, the outline of the design was dawn on the fabric with a dayflower extract. Then, using the paper tube, a fine line paste or "itome" is applied to the fabric to mask the line, and insert the dyes within the area with the target color. As this method masks the line of the pattern with a paste, it is also called as Itome-Yuzen.

As the flow chart shows in Figure 1, the dyeing process of hand-drawn Yuzen consists of ten procedures. The first procedure, "preliminary sketch," is to draw a pattern of the design on a white fabric with a dayflower extract. The second procedure called "paste application (i.e., masking)"is a procedure to apply a fine line paste along with the lines of the preliminary sketch to avoid the dyes to bleed other parts when inserting colors on the fabric. Figure 2 shows the scene of a paste application during the paste application procedure. The third procedure, "covering with paste ," is to apply a paste on the pattern to avoid the dyes to penetrate the parts of design in brush dyeing. The fourth procedure, "brush dyeing (or *hiki-zome*)", is a procedure to dye evenly or gradate by a brush, using a combined colors. The fifth procedure, "steaming," is to place the brush dyed fabric in a steamer and steams it at the temperature of about 100℃ for 20 to 50 minutes. By steaming the fabric for 20 to 50 minutes, the ground color (dye) is stabilized on the fabric. The sixth procedure, "sink yuzen, or *mizumoto*,"is to wash the fabric with water to eliminate the excess dyes, medicaments, and pastes from the fabric on which dyes are completely stabilized. The seventh procedure, "inserted yuzen" is a procedure to give colors to the design by using different types of brushes. The eighth procedure, "straightening the fabric or *Yunoshi*" is to steam wrinkles out of the fabric to soften the texture. The ninth procedure, "gold glazing" is to add here gold and silver foils and powders on the dyed fabric to make the product gorgeous. The tenth procedure, "embroidery," is to embroider a part of the design with gold and silver threads and other colory embroidery threads, to add elegance and luxuriousness to the product by giving the design volume.

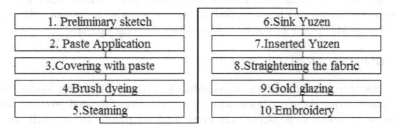

Fig. 1. Flow chart of manufacturing process

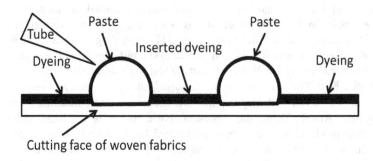

Fig. 2. Model of process about Paste application

2   Paste Application and the Function

2.1   Paste Application

In Japanese dress industry, inventing and deciding the first design to draw on kimono is considered to influence strongly on the end product. Without a high artistic quality or an aesthetic sense for the design, the product will remain unsold regardless of each procedure of making Kyo-Yuzen-zome was completed in a careful manner. The process to draw a design on a silk fabric is a preliminary sketching. The paste application procedure plays a significant role in changing highly artistic product drawn during the preliminary sketching into a manufactured product. Furthermore, recently, in many cases, instead of drawing the preliminary sketch on the silk fabric, a new method is used; a craftsman places a paper template of kimono with designs under the silk fabric and traces the design during the paste application. Therefore, it is very important to complete the putting a paste procedure by tracing the design accurately while taking the artistic quality of the designs drawn during the preliminary sketch or on the paper template.

Materials used for a paste application procedure are a starch paste, a rubber paste, and a flour. The typical materials are a starch paste and a rubber paste, which consists of over 99% of the material used in the process. There is a research on paste application and dyeing technology. In 1984, Kyoto City Senshoku Shikenjou (presently, the Kyoto Municipal Institute of Industrial Technology and Culture) published the "Technology and Techniques of Hand-Drawn Yuzen-Zome" [3], which editor-at-large was the Committee of the Technology and Techniques of the Hand-Drawn Yuzen-Zome. While a starch paste is made from sticky rice, a rubber paste is made by melting a rubber sheet with benzin and gasoline. Currently, more than 90% of hand-drawn Yuzen which were produced in Kyoto uses the rubber paste.

2.2   Objective of Research

On the other hand, in the Japanese dress industry, it is said that dyeing method using a starch paste during the paste application procedure makes the end products have an impression of softness and depth than using a rubber paste. Consequently, the final product value becomes higher when using a starch paste than a rubber paste; in many cases, the product using the starch paste tends to be sold at a higher price than the rubber paste.

In research on the relation between sensitivity evaluation and price setting, if starch paste is used as a result of evaluating the sample dyed using related [4]. Starch paste and rubber paste of the sensitivity evaluation and price setting in the Kyoto yuzen stain which uses different paste using the questionnaire technique, if high-quality increases and rubber paste is used on the other hand, it turns out that clearness increases. Furthermore, it is clear that the factor's which the starch paste is highly set up in a price rather than rubber paste, and has on a price about price setting it is a high-quality feeling. On the other hand, there are the technology and technique of Tegaki-yuzen dyeing which Kyoto Municipal Institute of Industrial Technology and Culture performed in 1984 also as that of Tegaki-yuzen dyeing technology and technique investigating committee editorial supervision in research on the dyeing and finishing technology of paste application or a kimono. However, researches, such as viscosity about the starch paste used for paste application and perviousness with a fiber bundle, are not made.

So, in this research, the structure dyed using starch paste and rubber paste was solved, and it aimed at clarifying relation between structure of paste application, and an impression difference and price setting. Therefore, the viscosity of starch paste and rubber paste was measured and the difference was clarified. Furthermore, by observing the section and the surface of the product produced using starch paste and rubber paste, when starch paste and rubber paste dyed, the influence which it has to a fiber bundle was investigated.

3   Materials

3.1   How to Manufacture Putting Paste

Starch paste steams and kneads rice cake rice flour and rice bran, and it mixes the solution which melted lime, paints red pigment mix it, and it needs it. Finally starch paste is filtered with the cloth of cotton. Since the antiseptic is not contained, it is easy to decompose starch paste. Therefore, it is necessary to put into a container and to save in a refrigerator. When using it again, warming in hot water must be carried out and heat must be applied. Then, rubber paste cuts board rubber finely and pickles it in benzene or gasoline together with Dan Mull liquid. Furthermore, board rubber melts by mixing the ultramarine of paints and soaking for several days, and it becomes rubber paste. The reason of red pigment mixing and mixing ultramarine with rubber paste is for using the mark color of paste at starch paste.

3.2   Viscosity

In the Kimono industrial world, it is said that it is hard to treat starch paste firmly compared with rubber cement. Therefore, the craftsman who can use starch paste is limited to the ability of a craftsman to use rubber cement every paste of all the members.

Then, the viscosity of starch paste and rubber cement was measured. Production of the starch paste and rubber paste which were used for measurement was requested from the craftsman of Paste application, (70 ages, a male, right-handed person) of years-of-experience about 50 year. Indoor temperature is gone into the range of 19~20℃, in order to carry out to viscosity measurement using a viscosity measuring device (ARES G2) . The viscosity of the starch paste at the time of the shear rate 1 (/s) and rubber cement is shown in Fig. 3. As a result, it was shown that starch paste high viscosity about 30 times compared with rubber paste.

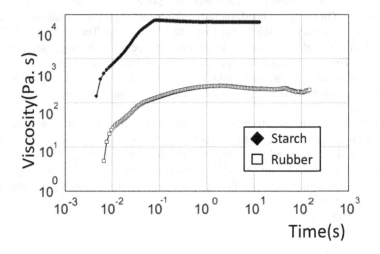

Fig. 3. Viscosity of Starch and Rubber on Shear Rate (1/s)

4   Experiment

4.1   Observation of Cutting Faces

Cloth prepared plain weave of the pure silk fabrics made from Nankyu, Inc. Manufacture was requested from the same craftsman using the same starch paste and rubber paste which were used for measurement of viscosity. The temperature which performed process of paste application was about 18℃. The specimen performed by paste application, dyed the thing of the stage (silk has not dyed) which the ground color is not dyeing, the gradual thing which dyes a ground color and has not removed paste, and the ground color, removed two paste, and prepared the thing of the stage which became the end products. Starch and rubber judged the specimen by silk along with warp, and the observation method observed those sections. It carried out to observation using the done type metallurgical microscope (PME3: made by Olympus, Inc.) of a handstand.

4.2   Observation of Woven Surfaces

In order to carry out surface observation of the part   was given, a total of three things [six] of three sheets and rubber paste use was prepared [the sample to which three craftsmen (more than all the members craftsman history 50 year, a male, a right-handed person) performed the process] for the thing of starch paste use, respectively. The entire sample of six sheets chose the general pattern in the kimono industrial world called "Paddle bucket". "Paddle bucket" is a comparatively linear pattern, and it performed so that it might be parallel at warp and the woof, respectively. The size of the pattern was made into what has all six the same sheets. All were dyed through the manufacture process of the kyo-yuzen shown in Fig. 1. Each time spent on the paste application was about 30 minutes.

Cloth is pure silk fabrics and plain weave. It is a sample of these six sheets IOS D6000. A photograph was taken by make (Canon Co, Ltd). In order to suppress the variation in a light source, the indoor fluorescent light was erased and the window facing north was opened, and it adjusted so that outdoor available light might enter.

5   Results

5.1   Observation of Cutting Faces

The cross-sectional picture carried out every paste with starch paste and rubber paste is shown in the figure 4 ~ 7. Fig. 4 shows the specimen which performs paste application and is not having the ground color dyed. Fig. 5 shows the specimen which mixed dye with starch paste and rubber paste, and performed the same process. Starch paste has blue rubber paste in reddish brown, and this is because the adhe-sion degree of paste and a fiber bundle becomes clearer. Starch paste did not permeate a fiber bundle rather than rubber paste, but adhesion area of rubber paste was larger than Fig. 4 and Fig. 5, and it turned out that it has permeated deeply into a fiber bundle. Fig. 6 shows the specimen before performing dyeing of paste application and a ground color and removing paste continuously. Adhesion area of rubber paste was larger than starch paste, and it turned out that it has permeated deeply into a fiber bundle. Fig. 7 is a sectional view of the same stage as the end products continuously. The part which removed starch paste and rubber paste was enclosed white. Starch paste did not per-meate a fiber bundle deeply, but the dye which dyed the ground color has permeated the back side (back side of a dyeing side) which performed paste application. On the other hand, since rubber paste had permeated to the back side of cloth, it turned out that it has prevented a ground color entering the back side of the marks of paste. Al-though it was said in the kimono industry that starch paste had resist-printing power weaker than rubber paste, and tends to turn around a ground color from the reverse side of cloth, from such cross-sectional observation, rubber paste permeated the fiber bundle deeply and the resist-printing effect kept from being mixed when a ground color is dyed more became clear.

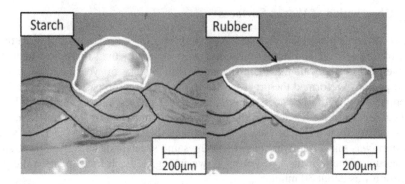

Fig. 4. Cutting faces of fabrics about Starch paste and Rubber paste before dyeing

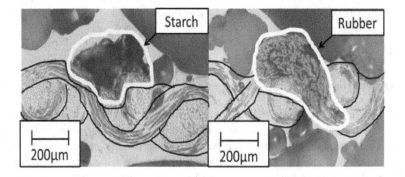

Fig. 5. Cutting faces of fabrics about Starch paste and Rubber paste mixed black dyestuff before dyeing

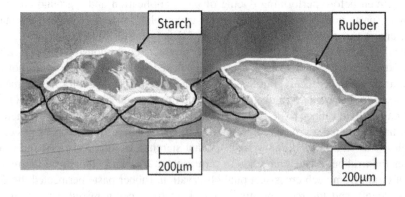

Fig. 6. Cutting faces of fabrics about Starch paste and Rubber paste before washing after dyeing

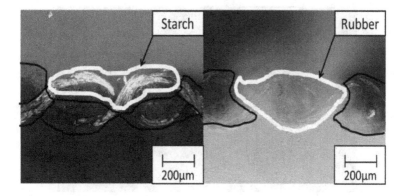

Fig. 7. Cutting faces of fabrics about Starch paste and Rubber paste after washing and steaming

5.2   Observation of Woven Surfaces

The sample used for surface observation is shown in Fig. 8. In the sample dyed with starch paste and rubber paste, the part which surrounded four parts enclosed with circle at a time by circle using selection and picture processing software (Photoshop, Microsoft Corp. make), respectively was cut off. Two cut-off places are perpendicular to warp, and two places which remain are parallel to warp. Four sheets were produced from the sample of one sheet. Therefore, the number of the pictures produced from surface observation is 24. And in order to detect a RGB value from the processed picture, it outputted to the cell of Excel using matrix calculation software (MATLAB).

The average value of the RGB value of the picture which cut off the part of the starch paste 1 and rubber paste 6 are shown in Fig. 9 in the sample measured in Fig. 8. Starch paste had a change of the RGB value from a dyeing side to an achromatic side looser than rubber paste. On the other hand, the change of rubber paset from a dyeing side to an achromatic side was rapid. Furthermore, the average of the RGB value of a total of 24 places enclosed with O to the sample 1 ~ 6 was computed. The sample of six sheets -- turn -- N1 (Starch), N1 (Rubber), N2 (Starch), N2 (Rubber), N3 (Starch), and N3 (Rubber) -- it named, the average value of RGB in every pixel was calculated, and those maximums were detected. Table 1 shows the average value of the maximum of the RGB value of starch paste and rubber paste about the sample of six sheets. As a result of comparing the average of the maximum of starch paste and rubber paste, the difference was seldom seen by the maximum, but the starch paste of standard deviation and a coefficient of variation are larger than rubber paste. It turned out that the maximum of a RGB value varies.

The dyed part (part by which resist printing was carried out with paste) rubber Paste to uniform being dyed firmly and the white of silk remaining firmly compared with starch paste starch paste, According to resist-printing power being weak, a ground color enters into the portion of the remains of a fine line in some places, and the white of silk does not remain completely. From such a thing, it is thought that the variation of rubber paste in an achromatic side is larger than starch paste.

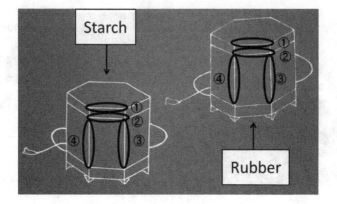

Fig. 8. Specimen for observation of woven surfaces

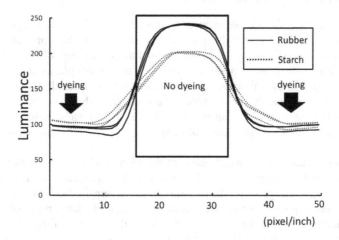

Fig. 9. Average of RGB value

Table 1. Comparison of each average

	Starch paste			Rubber paste			material
	Mean	SD	CV	Mean	SD	CV	F-value
N1	234.2	14.4	6.1%	239.7	7.7	3.2%	3.5 ***
N2	234.6	16.8	7.1%	234.0	9.3	4.0%	3.2 ***
N3	246.1	12.7	5.2%	248.7	5.2	2.1%	5.9 ***

*** p<0.05

6   Discussion

6.1   Cutting Face and Surface

Two materials to a fiber bundle that rubber paste is   "clear" in "superior quality" at sensitivity evaluation, and starch paste has set up price setting highly compared with rubber paste in this research how In order to investigate whether it pasted up and has affected the fiber bundle, cross-sectional observation and surface observation were performed. As shown in the figure 4 ~ 7, starch paste has not permeated a fiber bundle compared with rubber paste. On the other hand, rubber paste has permeated the fiber bundle firmly. Although it is generally said in the kimono industrial world that the starch paste must take care and it must dye it from the reverse side of cloth by that around which dye turns (it spreads) when resist-printing power is weak and carries out Brush dyeing rather than rubber paste, it can be said that it is in agreement with understanding from this and cross-sectional observation. Furthermore, since the resist-printing effect is high compared with starch paste and rubber paste in which giving impression evaluation that starch paste is high-quality and rubber paste is clear has been reported by research of sensitivity evaluation can dye the boundary of a dyeing side and an achromatic side more vividly, it is in agreement with impression evaluation called a clear feeling. The feature of starch paste has high viscosity, resist-printing power falls compared with rubber paste, and the boundary of a dyeing side and an achromatic side does not dye vividly. Therefore, when starch paste is used from this, it is thought that it is in agreement with the result of sensitivity evaluation that a high-quality feeling can be obtained by the impression evaluation to the product of completion.

Furthermore, the sample which performed paste application by three craftsmen was prepared. The same pattern was dyed one craftsman using starch paste and rubber paste. As shown in Fig. 9, as a result of carrying out surface observation of the part in the end products, starch paste had a loose change of the RGB value compared with rubber paste. In order to investigate this result in detail, out of the sample of six sheets, four places and a total of 24 places were chosen, respectively, and surface observation was performed. As a result of calculating an average and standard deviation of each maximum, and a coefficient of variation, the difference was not seen so much by average value, but the big difference was seen by standard deviation and the coefficient of variation. Rubber paste shows from this that variation is uniformly dyed the RGB value of an achromatic side few compared with starch paste.

That is, when rubber paste is used, it is shown that the boundary of a dyeing side and an achromatic side is uniform, and it is shown that rubber paste has the feature which it can be uniform and can be dyed vividly. On the other hand, starch paste has large variation to the maximum of a RGB value, and the boundary of a dyeing side and an achromatic side does not dye vividly, but it can be said that this result is high-quality and relevance with the result which can set up a price highly is suggested.

6.2   Dyeing Model

The result of having performed cross-sectional observation and surface observation according to material is made into a mimetic diagram, and is shown in Fig. 10.

Cross-sectional observation and surface observation to starch paste does not permeate a fiber bundle compared with rubber paste, and its boundary of a dyeing side and an achromatic side is not clear. On the other hand, the resist-printing effect of rubber paste is high, it is uniform and the marks of paste application remain vividly. It is thought that there will be relevance with the result that starch paste is high-quality and rubber paste is clear, from the feature of starch paste and rubber paste.

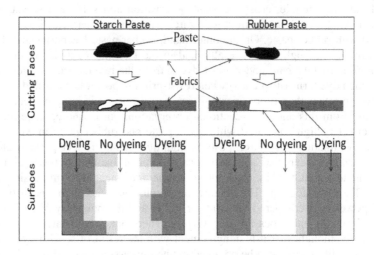

Fig. 10. Relationship between fabrics, pastes and dyeing

7   Conclusion

In this research, it became clear that starch paste has viscosity about 30 times as high as rubber paste. From cross-sectional observation, starch paste was understood that the resist-printing effect is which has little osmosis in a fiber bundle lower than rubber paste. Moreover, as for the starch paste, the boundary of a dyeing side and an achromatic side varies, and it became clear from surface observation that the boundary of rubber paste of a dyeing side and an achromatic side is uniform and that it is clear. Since the number of the samples produced for surface observation is six, I would like to examine whether a sample is increased and the same result is brought by this research from now on. Moreover, although the part perpendicular to warp and parallel was chosen, I would like to also perform observation of a bias part to warp.

Furthermore, comparison with the way a model performs paste application of a fine line type, and the dyeing method in which mass-production called model Yuzen other than Tegaki-yuzen is possible is also required. Moreover, although it is possible in the kimono industrial world to use it if rubber paste has a skillful degree for about one year, in order to master starch paste, it is said that it generally takes for about ten years. Furthermore, although the craftsman who can use starch paste can also use rubber paste, the craftsman only treating rubber paste cannot use starch paste.

That is, since the number of craftsmen which can use starch paste is limited, there is very little production with starch paste than rubber paste, and the starch paste of the ratio which uses starch paste in the number of production in Tegaki-Yuzen is about 10%. Then, although training of the craftsman who can use starch paste is a future subject, I would like to make low the development of rubber paste and the viscosity of starch paste which have a high-quality feeling like starch paste, and to develop the starch paste which is easy to treat also to craftsmen who can treat only rubber paste.

References

1. Kyo-yuzen Kyodoukumiai Rengoukai, Research of production in Kyo-Yuzen and Kyo-Komon (2012)
2. Yano Keizai Kenkyujo, Kimono Sangyo Hakusho (2009)
3. Research Committee of Technique and Skill in Tegaki Yuzen-zome, Technique and Skill in Tegaki Yuzen-zome Kyoto Municipal Institute of Industrial Technology and Culture, pp.67-100 (1984).
4. Furukawa, T.: Relationship between Kansei Evaluation and pricing Decision to Kyo-Yuzen-Zome with Different Pastes, Japan Socuety of Kansei Engineering (2013)

A Task Analytic Process to Define Future Concepts in Aviation

Brian F. Gore[1] and Cynthia Wolter[2]

[1] NASA Ames Research Center, Moffett Field, CA 94035-0001
[2] San Jose State University/NASA Ames Research Center, Moffett Field, CA 94035
{Brian.F.Gore,Cynthia.Wolter}@nasa.gov

Abstract. A necessary step when developing next generation systems is to understand the tasks that operators will perform. One NextGen concept under evaluation termed Single Pilot Operations (SPO) is designed to improve the efficiency of airline operations. This SPO concept includes a Pilot on Board (PoB), a Ground Station Operator (GSO), and automation. A number of procedural changes are likely to result when such changes in roles and responsibilities are undertaken. Automation is expected to relieve the PoB and GSO of some tasks (e.g. radio frequency changes, loading expected arrival information). A major difference in the SPO environment is the shift to communication-cued crosschecks (verbal / automated) rather than movement-cued crosschecks that occur in a shared cockpit. The current article highlights a task analytic process of the roles and responsibilities between a PoB, an approach-phase GSO, and automation.

Keywords: Task analysis, concept evaluation, single pilot operations.

1 Introduction

The task analysis is a methodology covering a range of techniques to describe, and in some cases evaluate, the human-machine and human-human interaction in systems. It is often described as the study of what an operator (or team) is required to do in terms of actions or cognitive processes to achieve a specific system state. Typically, it is characterized by a hierarchical decomposition of how a goal-directed task is accomplished, including a detailed description of activities, task and element durations, task frequency, task allocation, task complexity, environmental conditions, necessary clothing and equipment, and any other unique factors involved in, or required for, one or more people to perform a given task (1). The current task analysis will focus on the process whereby the tasks to safely fly the aircraft with automation are analyzed, documented and outlined (1).

One type of task analysis, the Cognitive Task Analysis (CTA) identifies all of the critical cognitive tasks that the operator is required to perform with the automation (2,3). CTA is a family of methods and tools for gaining access to the mental processes that organize and give meaning to observable behavior. CTA methods describe the cognitive processes that underlie the performance of tasks and the cognitive skills

V.G. Duffy (Ed.): DHM 2014, LNCS 8529, pp. 236–246, 2014.
© Springer International Publishing Switzerland 2014

needed to respond adeptly to complex situations. Knowledge is elicited through in-depth interviews and observations about cognitive events, structures, or models. Often the people who provide this information are subject matter experts (SMEs) – people who have demonstrated high levels of skill and knowledge in the domain of interest (4). The CTA is a complement to traditional task analysis as it adds the capability for designing for the unanticipated by describing the constraints on behavior rather than solely describing the behavior. These approaches feed into a concept-verification phase, where the research concept is verified by a human-system engineer, and preparations are made to implement the results from the task analyses into a model form (5).

The task analysis is an important step when a new concept of operation (CONOP) is being developed as they enable a certain degree of transparency into the required actions to safely operate in a given operational environment. The task analysis both feeds forward and feeds back to HITL simulations. One aviation-related environment currently undergoing such an operational change is the NextGen CONOP associated with Single Pilot Operations (SPOs). The current day flight deck operational environment consists of a two-person Captain/First Officer crew. Current NextGen guidance is to optimize the efficiency of operations where feasible while maintaining the safety that exists in current operations. A CONOP to reduce the commercial cockpit from the current two-pilot crew, to a single pilot termed Single Pilot Operations (SPO) has been suggested as an option to optimize the efficiency of the flight deck and airline operations. The SPO concept has been under study by researchers in the Flight Deck Display Research Laboratory (FDDRL) at the National Aeronautics and Space Administration's (NASA) Ames and Langley Research Centers (6). Transitioning from a two-pilot crew to a single pilot crew will undoubtedly require changes in operational procedures, crew coordination, use of automation, and in how the roles and responsibilities of the flight deck and ATC are conceptualized in order to maintain the high levels of safety expected of the US National Airspace System.

The NextGen SPO environment would modify current day operations by reducing the crew complement onboard from two pilots to one pilot. The ground dispatch operator's tasks would also need to be modified to account for some of the responsibilities that would no longer be in the cockpit, operations like cross checks. One SPO concept maintains that three entities would share in the safe transport of the aircraft; a Pilot on Board (PoB), a Ground Station Operator (GSO), and automation. In this environment, both the PoB and the GSO would be fully trained pilots capable of flying the aircraft alone if incapacitation of one pilot should occur. Possible roles and responsibilities of a PoB, an approach-phase GSO, and automation are explored following a brief explanation of the current day roles and responsibilities.

1.1   Current Day Operations

The traditional roles of the cockpit crew are defined as Captain and First Officer roles. The Captain is the main pilot of the aircraft and the one who remains ultimately responsible for the aircraft, its passengers, and the crew. The Captain sits in the left seat of the cockpit. The first officer is the second pilot of an aircraft. The first officer sits in the right-hand seat in the cockpit. One pilot is designated the "pilot flying" (PF) and the other the "pilot not flying" (PNF), or "pilot monitoring" (PM), alternating during each flight as necessary. Even when the first officer is the flying pilot, the captain is in command and has legal authority for the aircraft. The amount of time either pilot is in control of the aircraft is near equal in normal operations, as the PF designation is passed back-and-forth for each leg (departure or destination) of a flight. In typical day-to-day operations, the essential job tasks are distributed fairly equally but final decisions always remains with the Captain (pilot-in-command). Some have defined the shared roles in the cockpit as being Aviate, Navigate, Communicate, and Systems Management in a task management hierarchy (7).

1.2   Single Pilot Operations (SPOs)

In SPOs, it is entirely possible that three entities will be required to guide the safe transport of the aircraft. These three entities include a PoB, a GSO, and automation. In the proposed SPO environment, both the PoB and the GSO would be fully trained pilots capable of flying the aircraft alone in the event that incapacitation of either human pilot should occur. Pilot Flying and Pilot Not Flying designations would vary between the PoB and the GSO, with possible multiple mid-flight reassignments. Most settings and radio communications would remain solely PNF responsibilities. Current Captain-specific tasks would remain the same and would always fall to the PoB. Both human operators would continually monitor instruments and radio communications, as well as perform crosschecks when notified of a change via voice or automation, and verify that the environment is consistent with their internal schema.

The PoB and the GSO means that the crew is operating essentially as a "separated cockpit". Due to a "separated cockpit", automation will be playing a large role in notifying the PoB and GSO of any changes (radio frequency, altitude, heading, speed, altimeters, CDU inputs/executions, entering/exiting holds, approach mode, speed brake, landing gear, touchdown zone elevation) so that either could verify without undue radio congestion. Advancements in automation may also relieve the human operators of some tasks such as loading expected arrival information, getting ATIS, and setting altimeters. A major notable difference between the current day and the SPO environment is the shift to 'communication-cued' crosschecks (verbal or automated) rather than 'movement-cued' crosschecks that occur in a shared cockpit. Automation will need to account for these overt and covert characteristics associated with a human "good crew member". Automation that mimics the characteristics of a "good crew member" can lead to increased efficiencies; which in turn lead to increased spare capacity to deal with unforeseen events.

1.3   Research Objectives

The objective of this research was to validate and refine sets of tasks associated with likely SPO environments. These tasks are the actions that are required of the crew and are linked together in a string of both sequential and parallel nodes. These nodes represent networks that can then be used to analyze different scenarios and task assignments for their impact on workload, taskload, task bottlenecks, efficiency, and safety. Possessing such task analyses allows researchers to explore the degree to which the location of pilots (remote or co-located) impact the ability of the crew to work as an effective, separated, two-person crew as compared to a co-located two-person crew.

In an empirical study that was used to populate the task analysis, pairs of pilots were asked to complete simulated flight segments in each of two conditions: co-located, and remote (6). The pilots were purposely presented with a critical situation that required problem-solving; one in which the crew encountered severe weather during their flight and needed to divert to an alternate airport. Scenarios added complexity to the diversion task, such as the amount of fuel onboard to support planned or unplanned diversions and system failures such as antiskid that required the crew to recalculate landing weights and distances.

The co-located condition required that pilots work together in a two-person flight simulator, a scenario that corresponded to current-day conditions. The remote condition required that the right and left seats of the cockpit be placed in different rooms, a scenario that represented a SPO concept. The crew in the SPO condition was allowed to communicate freely, however they could not see each other, observe each others' body language or point to information like weather cells on the navigation display. The interaction of the crew would be impacted by this change to SPO and part of the current analysis was to identify how the tasks would change as a function of such SPO operations.

Review of the above-described study was used to generate a preliminary high-level task analysis of both current day and SPO environments and for specific scenario development. Finer level of detail and validation came from subsequent interviews and collaboration with subject matter experts (SMEs).

1.4   Method

Task decompositions were created in the current research that included both a task analysis and a semi-structured CTA of four scenarios (described below) of a planned approach into Denver starting at 37000' ASL with the crew operating under: (1) current day rules, (2) SPO-rules. Each rule set was run in either (3) nominal approach to land, or (4) an off nominal condition requiring the dynamic re-planning to an alternate airport. The task network analyses are represented with time-sequence profiles, task decomposition spreadsheets, 4D profiles, and task network representations.

1.5   Task Representation

Due to the complexity of the operational domains, four representations at varying levels of fidelity (from high level to lower levels) were created to convey the details associated with each approach to land rule set. This breakdown was necessary given the complexity of the tasks and because the tasks shifted from a well-established concept to a new CONOP as is the case with SPO. These representations of the tasks include a time-sequence profile, task decomposition spreadsheets, 4D profiles, and task network model representation.

Time-sequence profile (high level): A high-level time/sequence based profile of both nominal and divert approaches to Denver was developed. This is termed time-sequence based because the analysis is represented along a timeline as the aircraft approaches the landing point and was not broken out by specific operator roles; only the tasks that were required to safely land an aircraft were identified. This process allowed us to identify task groups (not operator-specific) associated with the arrival and approaches. The task groups that were identified and classified were then broken down into a finer level of detail (Figure 1).

- Task decomposition spreadsheet (low level): The task decomposition spreadsheet was created to describe each task and operator roles in a more detailed, organized, in-depth manner to illustrate the task flow and the operator responsibilities. This complex representation of the task network allowed for a more evolved under-standing of both the malleable and rigid associations between tasks (Figure 2).
- 4D profile (mid level): The high level-task groups were decomposed into individual, operator-specific tasks, and organized based on position of the aircraft and its phase of flight. This profile enabled side-by-side comparisons of current day and SPO environments as well as in-flight significant event conditions (Figure 3).
- Task Network Representation (low level): A linear, pictorial representation in Powerpoint was used to visualize the task network and to identify trouble spots where there is an increased task load due to the proposed SPO environment. By creating validated task groups, we can more fluidly re-organize task orders for analysis based on a given scenario (Figure 4).

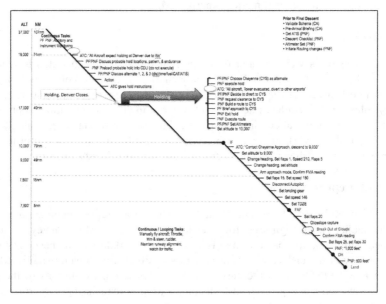

Fig. 1. Time-sequence profile

		(1b) Denver Approach-SPO DEN ILS RWY 16L 800' Cloud Ceiling Category D				
Altitude	Airport Distance	Pilot NOT Flying Ground Station Operator (Cruise)	Pilot NOT Flying Ground Station Operator (Approach)	Pilot Flying Pilot-on-Board (CA)	Automation	ATC
Prior to Scenario Start:		Continuous Tasks: Build a common schema - occurs mainly during cross checks.	Continuous Tasks: Build a common schema - occurs mainly during cross checks.	Continuous Tasks: Build a common schema - occurs mainly during cross checks.		Continuous tasks: Maintain separation
Prior to Final Descent		Continuous tasks: Auditory and Instrument Monitor (continue to TOD)	Continuous tasks: Auditory and Instrument Monitor (continue to TD)	Continuous tasks: Auditory and Instrument Monitor (continue to TD)		Continuous tasks: Maintain separation
					Send flight information to GSO (Approach)	
		Handoff to GSO (Approach) Say current altitude (37,000 ft) and probable arrival (LANDR ILS 16L). Say "United 573, your GSO for approach is Pat."	Connects.	Listen.		
			Say "Good afternoon United 573. Brief me on your flight thus far."			
		Crosscheck.	Listen. Take notes.	Flight briefing. (Any changes since filing flight plan. Weather, turbulence...)		
		Verbally confirm agreement on briefing.	Listen.	Listen.		
		Disconnects.				
			Monitor PF Pre-Arrival Briefing. Crosscheck.	Pre-Arrival briefing. (Taxi Chart, taxi route, gate, flaps, target landing speed, descent speed, brake settings, time of year, geographic position)		

Fig. 2. Task decomposition spreadsheet

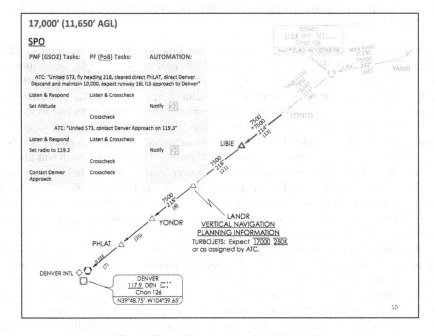

Fig. 3. 4D profile representation of the tasks

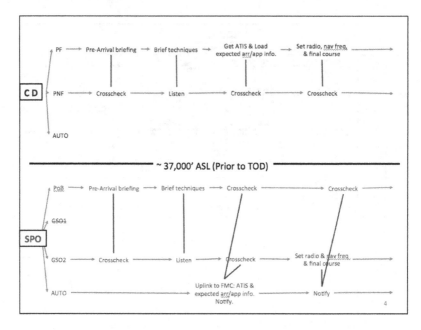

Fig. 4. Task network representation of the task analysis

1.6   Concept Verification Process and the Impact of SPO on Operator Roles and Responsibilities

The task analyses were performed to determine the task differences between the current day and the proposed SPO descent and approach to land phases of flight, in addition to the changes in procedures when the crew is given divert commands from ATC regarding specific significant events (e.g. weather radar failure). Specific variables of interest included the role of communication, role of automation, role of crosschecks and its impact on crew coordination The analysis process began with a pre-existing time / sequence-based profile of a descent into SFO as this task decomposed the approach profile and is a comprehensive NextGen approach to land task analysis.   The SFO approach was altered to represent the tasks required to descend into Denver, enter and exit a hold pattern, decide to divert to Cheyenne, and to safely land the aircraft. This preliminary high-level representation of a significant event scenario was populated through direct observation of the SPO I study (1), SME evaluations and interviews, and published reports of anticipated NextGen tasks and operator errors (8,9,10,11).

After final scenarios were chosen and populated with high-level tasks, they were refined and decomposed through the SPO concept reports and a series of SME interviews. Four spreadsheets of very detailed and ordered tasks representing each scenario were drafted and reviewed by SMEs (one current CA, and one former air traffic controller). The spreadsheets are organized by altitude, airport distance, operator tasks (PNF & PF) with CA assignment, automation tasks, and ATC communications. Using the SME input, the task decomposition spreadsheet was modified to be more representative of the proposed SPO environment (11).

As per SME recommendation, 4D profiles were then created using the updated information from the spreadsheets (11). This representation specifies each task performed by the operators in the current day, and in the SPO environments. The tasks were overlaid onto the ownship's route, indicating the current phase of flight by including location, altitude, and nautical miles to destination. This profile assisted side-by-side comparisons of the differences between current day and SPO crew workload, highlighting high task-load phases of flight that could benefit from an increase in automated assistance. Using this information, tasks were restructured in the 4D profile representation, and both the time-sequence based profile and the task decomposition spreadsheet representations were edited to align with the changes.

All three representations went through a series of edits to create both an accurate representation of a current day environment, and a task distribution capable of representing a future SPO concept. A final SME interview was conducted to confirm the tasks and their orders illustrated in the representations and provide some further editing suggestions. All three representations created up to that point were refined further via the SME input, and the task networks began to be uploaded into Micro Saint Sharp (11).

After the initial SPO concept was evaluated with the HITL simulations, the flight deck crew was then questioned on the technologies and processes that could be included in the SPO CONOP with the goal of guiding future research developments. Initial observations involved both the separated GSO/PoB and the co-located Captain/First Officer verbal and non-verbal communications through the headset and video monitors provided in the experimenter's control room. These observations also included participating in the crew debrief sessions and the GSO and PoB tools training sessions. This served to validate the task analyses already in progress and to provide context and direction for future analyses that more closely align with FDDRL studies.

1.7   Candidate Roles and Responsibilities Considerations

The preliminary evaluation separated the crewmembers to evaluate the kinds of interactions that could be expected when the crew was separated from each other, but needed to coordinate. As a function of being separated, the crewmembers engaged in extra communication tasks in order to insure that both crew members were operating according to a consistent mental map of the approach and the candidate divert options. These additional communication tasks highlight a potential area of concern implementing SPO-like conditions; if the crew needs to take immediate action, they may be faced with fewer cognitive or attentional or even coordinated resources to safely land the aircraft as they are occupied getting to a consistent mental map. Alternatively, during the time period when the crew coordinates their activities, their attentional resources will be occupied to a greater extent than if they were already coordinated. This suggests that additional tasks cannot be added to the crew when in this situation, and it is only through a thorough analysis of the tasks that such bottlenecks can be identified. It is also important to highlight that the SPO study was an experimental simulation focused on examining a limited amount of the social interactions that exist between and among the crew. In the first SPO experiment, the crew was only separated and small changes were implemented in the roles for the crew to perform (the separated crew performed all of the tasks as if they were collocated on the flight deck with the PoB). It has been suggested however that one GSO may be responsible for multiple aircraft during nominal operations. The responsibility for multiple aircraft will change to the GSO being responsible for a single aircraft if the aircraft in question requires additional support or faces some other off-nominal kind of operation.

Transitioning between actively controlling multiple aircraft to actively controlling a single aircraft will be a challenge for the GSO as well as the GSO dedicating him/herself to the additional aircraft. Additional research is needed to further evaluate these conditions and the scenarios that were explored in a second SPO experiment in 2013.

1.8   Future Research

The SPO task analysis and scenarios defined thus far represent two flight conditions and one potential way of assigning tasks between entities. Future effort will take the knowledge gained from the existing task structure and roles and responsibilities to refine the existing task analysis to additional divert locations to parallel ongoing HITL simulations being completed by the Flight Deck Display Research Laboratory (FDDRL). Understanding and correctly populating the operational environment with the required tasks is a vital step to successfully develop and field CONOPs like the SPO. The task analysis highlights the required actions to safely fly the aircraft in various operational conditions. The operational conditions drive the tasks required which, in turn can be manipulated to explore operational feasibility (can a task set be accomplished safely under different scenarios). These tasks can feed into new HITL simulations to verify that the concept works in the anticipated manner. Furthermore, the tasks can be used to design the HITL simulation by identifying points in the simulation that a given experimental manipulation may exceed the operational capacity of the operator.

It is expected that future research will modify the existing scenarios to include the GSO controlling multiple aircraft versus dedicated assistance requests, scenarios comparing different levels of automation (e.g. notification of pilot initiated changes, initiation of changes uplinked from ATC or automated, setting changes), scenarios with significant events other than/in addition to weather (e.g., cargo door open), and evaluate the impact on the number of tasks required of the current GSO, the new GSO and the interaction that needs to occur with the PoB. In the current SPO iterations, flight roles and responsibilities were primarily attended to by the PoB (CA) during cruise through the top of descent. The responsibilities of a typical current day FO are assumed by the GSO at that point and continue to touchdown (i.e., ATC communications, radio frequency settings, heading settings, one altimeter setting, altitude settings, flap settings). In future iterations, other role assignments may show a lessening of task load for both human operators. Analysis of the benefits if the roles of automation are expanded is also planned based on projected automation advancements becoming available in the future. In addition, the GSO and PoB may need to be flexible within their roles and responsibilities and assign tasks differently for each flight based on flight conditions, emergency situations, and experience level. Task type as a function of the operator role under both current day and future SPO operations during additional divert conditions are also possible areas of research for the SPO environment. It is expected that thorough task decompositions of the various scenarios will provide insight into the impact of required and time critical flight crew and ATC tasks under SPO technologies and procedures. Methods that feed the understanding of the task environment such as human-in-the-loop simulations will lead to more comprehensive understanding of the effects of such a conceptual change on the task performance and efficiency of operations of a complex environment such as those as exemplified by SPO.

Acknowledgements. The composition of this work was supported by the Concepts and Technology Development Project of NASA's Airspace Systems Program (NASA POC Dr. Walter Johnson). The authors would like to thank the SMEs Cpt Robert Kotesky, and Vernol Battiste for their invaluable assistance identifying the likely SPO tasks, the entire SPO research staff from the FFDRL, and all reviewers for their insightful comments.

References

1. Kirwan, B., Ainsworth, L.K.: A Guide To Task Analysis. Taylor & Francis, London (1992)
2. Diaper, D.: Task Analysis for Human-Computer Interaction. Ellis Horwood Limited, England (1989)
3. Zachary, W., Ryder, J., Hicinbothom, J.: Cognitive Task Analysis & Modeling of Decision Making In Complex Environments. In: Salas, E., Cannon-Bowers, J. (eds.) Making Decisions Under Stress. American Psychological Association, Washington, DC (1998)
4. Klein, G.: Cognitive Task Analysis Of Teams. In: Schraagen, Chipman, Shalin (eds.) Cognitive Task Analysis, pp. 417–430. Lawrence Erlbaum Mahwah, NJ (2000)
5. Gore, B.F.: Chapter 32: Human Performance: Evaluating The Cognitive Aspects. In: Duffy, V. (ed.) Handbook of Digital Human Modeling, pp. 32-1-32-18. CRC Press/Taylor & Francis, Boca Raton (2008)
6. Johnson, W., Lachter, J., Feary, M., Comerford, D., Battiste, V., Mogford, R.: Task Allocation For Single Pilot Operations: A Role For The Ground. In: HCI Aero 2012 – International Conference on Human-Computer International Aerospace, Belgium, Brussels, pp. 12–14 (September 2012)
7. Schutte, P.C., Trujillo, A.C.: Flight Crew Task Management In Non-Normal Situations. In: Proceedings of the 40th Annual Meeting of the Human Factors and Ergonomics Society, pp. 244–248. HFES, Santa Monica (1996)

8. Gore, B. F., Hooey, B. L., Mahlstedt, E. A., & Foyle, D. C. Evaluating NextGen Closely Spaced Parallel Operations concepts with validated human performance models. Scenario Development and Results (NASA TM-2013-216503). NASA Ames Research Center, Moffett Field (2013)

9. Gore, B.F., Hooey, B.L., Haan, N.J., Socash, C., Mahlstedt, E.A., Foyle, D.C.: A validated set of MIDAS v5 task network model scenarios to evaluate NextGen Closely Spaced Parallel Operations concepts (HCSL 13-03). NASA Ames Research Center, Moffett Field (2013)

10. Gore, B.F., Hooey, B.L., Haan, N., Bakowski, D.L., Mahlsted, E.: A methodical approach for developing valid human performance models of flight deck operations. Paper presented at the 14th Annual HCI International, Orlando, FL, July 9–July 14 (2011)

11. Wolter, C.A., Gore, B.F.: ASP/CTD/SPO Task Summary Report: Single Pilot Operations (SPO) ConOps-related gaps and research issues identified by analysis of SPO Pilot and Controller tasks, technologies and procedures. HCSL Technical Report (HCSL-13-07) Human Centered Systems Laboratory (HCSL). NASA Ames Research Center, Moffett Field (2013)

Application of E-learning System Reality in Kyoto-style Earthen Wall Training

Akihiko Goto[1], Hirofumi Yoshida[1], Yuka Takai[1], Wang Zelong[2,*], and Hiroyuki Sato[2]

[1] Osaka Sangyo University
Department of Information Systems Engineering, Japan
gotoh@ise.osaka-sandai.ac.jp
[2] Kyoto Institute of Technology
Advanced Fibro-Science, Japan
simon.zelongwang@gmail.com

Abstract. In this paper, application of e-learning system in Kyoto-style earthen wall training was introduced and investigated. Simultaneously, a new design of e-learning (on-line) "Kyokabe" coating teaching system was put forward and established focusing on the analysis of motion, electromyography and eye movement. Consequently it was verified to provide a platform to publish the latest quantitative researches and coasting technical skills for assisting beginners to understand the key points in process technique from expert.

Keywords: E-learning system, Kyoto-style earthen wall, clay wall, training, painting.

1   Introduction

In ancient times, timber and clay were played very important roles in the building materials of Japanese house. The timber was applied to reinforce frame structure and the filler wall was adopted with the clay. It could date back to as early as the Nara period, 1300 years ago or even earlier.

The culture of clay way has been deeply entrenched within Japanese people's heart. With the development of building technology, high-strength reinforced concrete frame structure has been extensive application in modern Japanese architecture, which replaces the most of Japanese traditional clay wall. However, clay wall was made of natural materials. The features of moisture conditioning properties and absorption properties of indoor pollutants were one the most excellent performances that cannot be replaced.

Out of respect for traditional culture and considering the advantage of natural material, more and more Japanese people are willing to choose the clay wall to decorate their interior and exterior wall nowadays. Among them, a kind of clay wall called "Kyokabe" was produced in Kyoto, which is famous for thin but strong and able

---

* Corresponding author.

V.G. Duffy (Ed.): DHM 2014, LNCS 8529, pp. 247–253, 2014.

to send out a fragrant smell. "Kyokabe" production is a very complex process and divided into three coating layers. A skilled craftsman has to spend a substantial amount of time and effort to make an excellent "Kyokabe" with a strong wall and beautiful patterns. Additionally, it is very difficult to teach key points for coating technique to beginners by oral transmission and action demonstration. "Kyokabe" beginners have to take about ten years, or twenty years of deliberate practice to become an expert. In the past, beginners were accepted coating training after junior high school. Due to the higher requirements on basic education modern society, most young people starts to coating training after graduating from high school or college, who will become a full-fledged craftsman of "Kyokabe" after 30 years of age. Therefore, it is urgent time to pay attention to reduce time of training cycle and keep healthy development of this traditional industry.

Kyoto Sakan Vocational-technical College is one of the most elite "Kyokabe" training school in the Japan, which always has been seeking a useful and available way to transform these experts' tacit knowledge to explicit knowledge in order to shorten cultivating time and improve the efficiency of training. For this purpose, Kyoto Sakan Vocational-technical College's researchers successfully applied ergonomics techniques and human factors engineering to find key points of "Kyokabe" coating. In past research, motion analysis technology, Electromyography technology (EMG), eye movement technology were carried out to analyze possible differentiation between expert and non-expert. It is unrealistic and high cost to measure the characteristics of each student's operation with test equipment. This requires researchers to use results of related studies to design a standardized training plan.

In this study, a new design of e-learning (on-line) "Kyokabe" coating teaching system was put forward and established. It can provide a platform to publish the latest quantitative researches and coasting technical skills and assist beginners to understand the key points from expert. In the system, the application method of trowel (an main tool for coating) was illustrated in detail by a short and clear video at firstly, which came from the thoughts and experience conclusion from expert. Next, the elements of each engineering process was introduced and summarized, and basic principles and attention points were emphasized as the same time. After that, the most important part was shown that what kind of essentials caused difference for technology during the whole production process between expert and non-expert according to the latest research of human engineering. Finally, each process was comprehensively reviewed and summarized. In this way, by using this e-learning system, the implicit technique from expert craftsman was well taught to beginners, and they can understand and accept it well too.

The target of this research was found a best way to develop "Kyokabe" teaching through set up an e-learning system based on the research achievements of ergonomics. In order to help "Kyokabe" coating beginners are able to become a qualified craftsman in a shorter time.

2   The Present Situation and the Development of Kyoto-style Earthen Wall Training

2.1   The Problems in the Kyoto-style Earthen Wall Training Industry

Kyoto-style earthen is a most outstanding representative of Japanese clay wall as called "Kyokabe", which is especially famous for thin but strong and able to send out a fragrant smell. "Kyokabe" production is a very complicated process, which is divided into three coating layers as lower level, middle level and upper level. The lower level must have sufficient strength to coun-terbalance the whole thin wall, and the upper level is used to decorate wall. The middle level are combined the lower level and upper level, which are required to ensure strength and have a smooth surface so that facilitate to decorate the upper level.   Fig.1 was illustrated a craftsman was making the "Kyokabe."

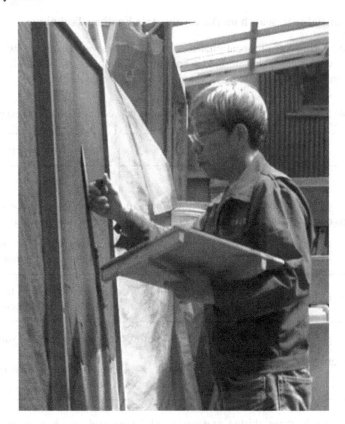

Fig. 1. Kyoto-style earthen wall process

Generally, beginners can obtain system training of the production method and the design essentials of each layer. However, the best learner still takes more than ten years practice to become an excellent craftsman in order to master some imperceptible and indispensable behavioral essentials, which is a tacit knowledge and highly dependent on intuition and experience.

On one hand, Japan is a highly developed country, the urban construction has been completed nearly half a century. Some craftsmen began to make the clay wall as a sideline, who was originally engaged in earthen wall. On the other hand, more capital was spent on national education as economic development proceeds. The college degree and bachelor's degree were used as benchmarks of the finance system of compulsory education to the extent that most young people starts to coating training after graduating from high school or college, who will become a full-fledged craftsman of "Kyokabe" after 30 years of age. It is difficult for them to start work and have their own families at the right time.

The Kyoto-style earthen wall training colleges have to face the pressure on the source of students these two reasons. Therefore, how to shorten the training time is the primary focus of   the Kyoto-style earthen wall training industry.

2.2   Quantifiable Research on the Kyoto-style Earthen Technique

In this study, Kyoto Sakan Vocational-technical College was concerned, which is the first earthen wall college that applied ergonomics techniques and human factors engineering led into find key points of "Kyokabe" coating successfully.

Table 1. Process technique difference summary between expert and non-expert

	Expert	Non-expert
Movement	Straight shoulder Keep upper limb and knees in the span width of both legs Trowel's movement located in the range of shoulder width	Sloping shoulder Left shoulder placed outside of both legs' span width Trowel moved from inside shoulder width to outside
Muscle activity	Applied nessisary minimum limit of muscle activity	Larger power than the nessisary limit was employed
Eye movement	Slight is oftern gazed before moved trowel	Slight is often shifted in forward/backward and upper/bottom directions of moved trowel

In past research, three skilled craftsmens of Kyoto-style earthen, experience between 38 years and 43 years, were employed as experts.   And eleven students from 3 month to 6 years were selected as non-experts. Motion analysis technology, Electromyography technology (EMG) and eye movement technology were carried out to analyze possible differentiation between expert and non-expert. The process technique difference was compared and showed in Table 1.

2.3   The Development Direction of the Kyoto-style Earthen Wall Training

At this stage, it is a very effective way to help students to realize their insufficiencies of key techniques by applying ergonomics technology. However, the spread and development of this method is also hindered to some extent by expensive cost of equipment and low accuracy of prototype part.

It is unrealistic and high cost to measure the characteristics of every student's operation with test equipment. This requires researchers to use results of related studies to design a standardized training plan.

Therefore, how to develop an efficient, low-cost way to popularize research achievement into teaching process based on transform these experts' tacit knowledge to explicit knowledge is a future development of the Kyoto-style earthen wall training.

3   The Realization of E-learning System in Kyoto-style Earthen Wall Training

3.1   The Establishment of E-learning System

As shown in Fig.2, the E-learning system is consisted of two parts to meet the needs of different periods in study process, and each display fifteen minutes.

In the first trial, the griping and moving methods of trowel and the processing flow chart was explained in detail. The key point of each step was emphasized to give a first impression to beginners intuitively. Then, the performance's difference between expert and non-expert were presented by the three dimensional motion animation from various angles in order to strengthen their learning effect and promote the students understand and solidify learning point.

In the second trial, the main detailed points of painting technique have been elucidated through comparing the muscular activity and eye movement's difference between expert and non-expert. Learners can get a good knowledge of earthen wall technique and skill basically after former two trial studies.

3.2   The Usage Method of E-learning System

Basically, e-learning materials can be utilized and read by users' computer, smart phone and the other mobile terminal devices in order to meet social need of using diversity. However, if some parts of e-learning materials only limited in computer utilization we cannot access and read the related content by other devices option. Most importantly, no matter where they are, the learners are able to utilize e-learing system anytime if they bringing the mobile terminal devices.

3.3   The Characteristic of E-learning System

Systematization. Until the current stage, the learners mainly study the painting technique of earthen wall from craftsmen depend on observation and imitation. However, learners have to observe this painting process from the reverse side and profile because the craftsmen paint the wall facing the subject location. Furthermore, some minor muscle activity and eye observation method also are inconspicuous and significant technology.

E-learning course is consisted of two parts, and each display fifteen minutes

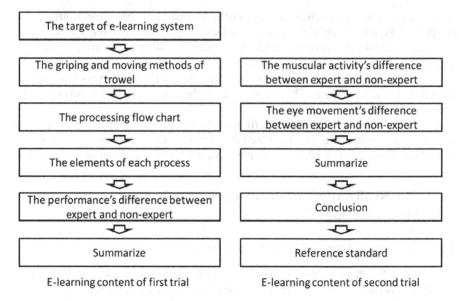

Fig. 2. E-learning system framework content

As shown in Fig.3, the instruction of the trowel, basic performed movement, the technique of muscular activity and eye's gazing track were passed forward to learners step by step. The most professional craftsmen were also employed to explain the key point of each step and share their technical essentials and experience with learners.

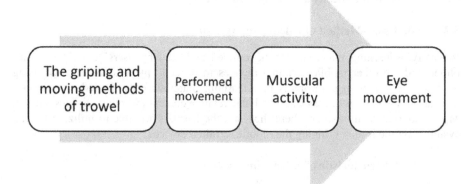

Fig. 3. E-learning material teaching flowchart

Flexibility. The E-learning system was divided into two parts. The first part have six chapters, and the second part have five chapters. Learning content can be freely chosen to view by learners based on the actual learning schedule. E-learning allow people to break through time and space to communicate study insight and obtain guidance from professional masters anytime and anywhere.

4   Conclusions

As well known, traditional skill and technique inherit realization was often investigated by "watching" approach. However, in fact, the opportunity of watching expert's real process technique is very limited due to decreased related job amount in current social period. Therefore, it is urgent and valuable to establish the effective e-learning system for all learners.

In this paper, application of e-learning system reality in Kyoto-style earthen wall training was introduced and explained. It is deserved to find that learners are able to utilize e-learning system anywhere anytime to watch expert process technique repeatedly for mastering and getting a good knowledge of specialized technique and skill finally.

In a word, established e-learning system can support beginner's learning effectively and also contribute to forwarding the latest study progress popularly.

References

1. Sato, K., Sato, H.: Tsuchikabe-Sakan no Shigoto to Gijyutsu, 1st edn., p. 191. Gakugei-shuppansha (2001)
2. Sato, H.: A study on the physical properties, function, and construction method of Kyoto Style Earthen Wall, p. 2, pp. 32–41. Kyoto tsukishuppan (2008)
3. Okamura, S., Goto, A., Kume, M., Sato, H., Hamada, H., Arai, M., Yoshida, T.: Effect on years of experience for coating operation on earthen wall. Japan Ergonomics Society Kansai Branch pp.107-110 (2009)
4. Shirahase, K., Takai, Y., Goto, A., Sato, H.: Process Analysis and Eye Motion Analysis on Midle Coat Process of Kyoto Style Earthen Wall. Japan Ergonomics Society Kansai Branch pp. 127-130 (2012)
5. Shinoda, Y., Yoshida, K., Matsumoto, S., Kawaguchi, K.: Learning activities and thinking characteristics of learners in the teaching materials of e-learning model. In: 2011 PC Conference, pp.278-279 (2011)

The Influence of Shift Workers Sleeping Quality upon Job Performance

Yu-Ching Huang[1], Fang-Ling Lin[2], Hui-Chun Chen[3],
Ching-Chung Chen[4], and Chih-Lin Chang[2,*]

[1] International Business Management, Hsiuping University of Science and Technology,
Taichung City, Taiwan
{fishkt@salamen}@mail.hust.edu.tw
[2] School of General Education, Hsiuping University of Science and Technology,
Taichung City, Taiwan
{fingling,salamen}@mail.hust.edu.tw
[3] Business Administration, Hsing Wu University of Science and Technology,
New Taipei City, Taiwan
078011@mail.hwu.edu.tw
[4] Information Management, Hsing Wu University of Science and Technology,
New Taipei City, Taiwan
095165@mail.hwu.edu.tw

Abstract. In the past few decades shift workers are highly needed to meet the demands of globalization and the 24-hour society worldwide. There are about 20% of labors doing shift jobs in America and European. In Taiwan, there are almost 35.5% of labors work shift jobs. Shift and night shift workers usually sleep 15-20% less than the regular workers, and, the sleeping quality during the day time is not as good as during the night. This study discusses the relationships between sleeping quality and job performance of shift workers on various shifting working hours by reviewing the previous literatures and researches. On the other hand, the study further compares the two methods of measuring sleeping quality and discusses the advantages and weakness of different testing methods. The results could provide more useful references to researchers who are interesting in the issues of sleeping quality and shift works while choosing instrument of testing sleeping quality.

Keywords: sleeping quality, shift workers, sleeping disorder.

1 Introduction

Cohen et al.[4] pointed out that poor sleep quality refers to less than six hours of sleep duration and sleep latency (if the duration is over thirty minutes or if a person wakes up more than three times during his sleep; the occurrence of either represents poor sleep quality). Sufficient sleep allows the body to repair itself, regulate physiological needs, and store energy; it is also helpful to coping with work stress, illness or work

---

[*] Corresponding author.

V.G. Duffy (Ed.): DHM 2014, LNCS 8529, pp. 254–262, 2014.
© Springer International Publishing Switzerland 2014

requirements. When poor sleep quality occurs, the body's immunity decreases or the person feels drained, causing an impact job safety, cognition, and judgment. At the workplace, it can also cause absenteeism, decreased productivity, increase of incidence rate in occupational hazards and accidents as well as the decline of job satisfaction [21].

1.1 Sleep Quality

Numerous factors affect poor sleep quality; demographics show women's sleep quality are more vulnerable than men [31]. People with lower socioeconomic status or household income experience worse sleep quality[12] [30]. In terms of personal factors, those who exercise regularly have better sleep quality [33] [24]; those who take stimulating drinks (such as coffee) has worse sleep quality[32]; long-term smokers experience insomnia due to the excitement of the central nerve caused by the stimulation of nicotine[20]. Moreover, nightcap or taking sleeping pills can shorten the time to fall asleep, but will increase the number of awakenings at night, resulting in more abnormal psychological and physiological symptoms[26].

At the workplace, many related factors have an impact on sleep quality, including workshift[26], prolonged labor[21] hazardous physical and chemicals elements in the working environment[37], and the nature of the work itself[29][19]. For the sleep quality of workshift workers, the total hours of sleep during daytime, sleep cycles, and length of REM after a night shift are all significantly shorter than nighttime sleep [15].

1.2 Sleep Quality of Shift Workers

Shift workers refer to workers in the condition when the work is completed by several people at different times in order to increase productivity and utilization rate of the machines and equipment[3]. National Institute of Occupational Safety and Health defines shift work from the perspective of working time and refers to work that is not between 7am and 6 pm.

The most direct impact of shift work is on sleep issues. Humans have so-called circadian Rhythm, which can, based on the change of time, organize time sequence that is most suitable to organism survive, adapting to the different needs of each period and carrying out different physiological actions. However, shift work patterns is a direct violation of the human biological clock, working during the day and sleeping at night, causing the phenomenon of day and night rhythm desynchronization[36].

Sleep quality of shift workers include sleep duration and quality. In terms of sleep duration, shift workers slept an average of 15-20 % less than non-shift workers [1][23]. Night shift workers sleep approximately 5.1 to 5.9 hours; their sleep duration is usually less than 6 hours[17]. Related research also pointed out that the average sleep duration for shift workers is 5.5 hours per day; 32% of shift workers have insomnia and excessive daytime sleepiness, while only 18% of workers who have typical working hours experience these concerns [7]. In addition, in terms of sleep quality, deep -sleep is an important period to repair the fatigue of the body. Night shift workers demonstrate shorter duration of deep-sleep. An observation of the sleep patterns through brain waves discovered a main decrease of rapid eye movement and second phase in non-rapid eye movement, leaving less impact on the third and fourth phases. In terms of sleep latency, day shift workers have shorter sleep latency while night shift workers have longer ones, making it more difficult for shift workers to fall sleep and affecting sleep quality[17].

Japanese scholars conducted sleep studies on middle-aged male employees and pointed out irregular shift workers face higher mortality rate due to ischemic heart attack, hypertension, overweight, as well as drinking and smoking habits[13]. In related studies about the impact of different workshift system on sleep quality, the research on sleep quality of overnight shift, night shift, and day shift workers discovered that overnight shift workers have the worst sleep quality[34]. In addition, Ohayon, Lemoine, Arnaud-Briant & Dreyfus[28] study indicates that the sleep quality of the overnight shift workers is worse than that of the night shift workers and fixed daytime staff. Overnight shift workers have the shortest sleep duration while accident rate for workshift workers is two times higher than that of the fixed daytime staff and night shift workers; the sick leave rate in the first 12 months is 62.8 %, higher than 38.5% of the fixed daytime staff. It can thus be proven that when shift workers take on overnight shifts, their unhealthy sleep quality leads to drowsiness at work, work accidents, and sick leave.

In summary, shift workers are physiological affected by the disorder of day and night rhythm and experience worse sleep quality compared to daytime workers. The impact incudes longer time needed to fall sleep (sleep latency) and shorter sleep duration. In terms of the influence on different shifts, overnight shift (00:00 to 08:00) experience most severe impact, followed by night shift (16:00 to 24:00).

1.3   The Impact of Sleep Quality on Work Efficiency

Although the nature of work for each shift worker varies, workshift possess a considerable degree of impact on the interruption of life quality, including physical, psychological, as well as family and social adaptation. In terms of physical and mental health, numerous physical and psychological risk factors increase for shift workers [22]. When sleep disorder occurs, shift workers tend to leave their jobs due to lack of adequate sleep[2]. Lack of sleep leads to employees' decreased alertness and increased sleepiness at work, escalating accidents rates and causing harm to the safety of the individual employee, enterprises, and society[10].

Shift workers demonstrate higher fatigue index and have greater chance of sick leave and accidents compared to daytime workers[18][16]. U.S. research report pointed out that the chances of shift workers dozing off while driving to work or experiencing accidents due to sleepiness is twice as high compared to normal daytime staff. Severe incidents may cause traffic accidents, occupational injuries, and major occupational accidents[14].

When a worker has poor sleep quality, the brain's ability to focus, reaction rate, and memory are all affected. Work quality and efficiency will thus decline, especially for those with heavy vision workload, precise division of work, monotony operation, long duration of same activity, and machine controlled work pace. Related studies show that in fixed work shift systems, shift schedule and number of working days have significant influence on production volume and yield rate; job performance of the day shift has higher production volume and yield rate than night shifts and overnight shifts[25]. Folkard, Monk & Alexander[11] use five factors to evaluate staff job performance, including error rate, sleep and degree of accumulated fatigue, degree of interruption of the biological clock, absence rate, and accident rate. Results show that night shift workers have the highest error rate, are most difficult to fall sleep, have insufficient sleep, are irritable, tend to be absent from work, and demonstrate the highest chance in accidents; therefore, night shift workers have the worst job performance.

In summary, job performance of shift workers will be influenced by their shift schedules; the impact includes efficiency, quality of work, and occupational accidents. Followed by night shifts, overnight shift faces the greatest impact.

1.4   Assessment Method of Sleep Quality

The assessment of sleep quality can be determined from subjective and objective standards. Subjective assessment allows study subjects to express their subjective feelings through methods such as subjective evaluation chart, survey, interview, and sleep journal. Objective assessment, on the other hand, uses equipment or a third party to convey the sleep condition of the study subject. The following illustrates survey procedures for sleep quality from the perspectives of subjective and objective assessment methods [5][8][6].

Subjective Sleep Assessment Method. Questionnaire is a self-assessment survey evaluating sleep quality and issues in the past month. In terms of subjective assessment methods, the most common assessment scale is the questionnaire for sleep quality compiled by scholars such as Buysee from the University of Pittsburgh in 1988[35]. Pittsburgh Sleep Quality Index survey include a total of 19 questions; a global score for the overall sleep quality and scores for seven different sleep-related components can be derived through calculation. The seven components include: subjective sleep quality, sleep latency, sleep duration, sleep efficiency, sleep disturbances, use of sleeping medication, and daytime dysfunction. The components of the scale and assessment content are organized in Table 1.

Table 1. Seven components of the Pittsburgh Sleep Quality Index survey

Component	Assessment
Subjective sleep quality	An individual's subjective overall evaluation of the sleep
Sleep latency	Time needed to fall asleep would be best if it is under thirty minutes
Total number of sleep hours	The recommended individual sleep duration is five hours and above
Sleep efficiency	Total number of sleep hours /duration of lying in bed, should be above 85%
Sleep disturbances	The continuity of the impact on the sleep caused by the disturbances
Use of sleeping medication	Yes or no, frequency of use
daytime dysfunction	Including bad mood, irritability, and lack of concentration

Objective Sleep Assessment

1. Multi-channel physiological recorder. This is thus far the most detailed and accurate testing method. Standard clinical multi-item sleep records include continuous EEG of the parietal lobe and occipital lobe, EOG, and chin EMG. These items are used to record the structure and stages of sleep, such as (1.) EEG, (2.) EOG, (3.) EMG, (4.) ECG, (5.) nose and mouth breathing flow, (6.) abdominal and chest breathing exercises, (7.) blood oxygen, (8.) the number of times snoring. Generally, various examinations at a night sleep laboratory need to last for seven to eight hours[5].

2. Sleep observation. Sleep observation is conducted by medical personnel or laboratory personnel observing the sleeping condition of the research subjects. The advantage is that the instrument will not interfere with the subjects' original sleep behavior, yet it requires tremendous manpower and time to conduct the observation and record; photographic recording can also be used to reduce the burden in human resources.

3. Activity recorder. Activity recorder (actigraphy) is an instrument shaped like a watch, and is also worn on the feet or wrists like a watch. It can be set to record the activity of the wrist at fixed intervals of time (2 seconds or 60 seconds). Due to the "sleep-wakefulness" cycle and "rest –activity" cycle, the devise must worn 24 hours a day except taking a shower; the data stored up in the activity recorder can range from several days to several weeks and even months.

Summarizing the above subjective and objective assessment methods, a comparison of the two assessment methods is conducted (as in Table 2). While collecting data, subjective assessment tools can collect a large number of samples quickly and with a low cost; this is the advantage of surveys and is the method preferred by researchers. On the contrary, objective assessment tool, multi-channel physiological recorder, and sleep observation must be conducted under particular conditions and it requires significant expense for the needed equipment and manpower. The results, moreover, can only include the observation of total sleep duration, sleep activity, and certain sleep disorders; it cannot provide full-time recording data like the activity recorder. In addition, objective assessment tools need to be evaluated by an instrument or observer, which is time-consuming and is suitable for small-scale samples.

Sleep quality assessment tools each has its own advantages and disadvantages. Considering that the quality of sleep is related to "time", observation of its changes over a period of time is needed through objective data collection techniques in order to clearly present the research result. Therefore, the use of activity recorder is suggested in the study of sleep quality assessment methods. Through instrumental measurement, full-time observation of a work shift worker's personal condition and schedule can be recorded; activity situation can be recorded anywhere and anytime in order to obtain accurate and complete information on sleep quality.

Table 2. Comparison of subjective and objective sleep quality assessment method

Data collection method	Subjective assessment tool (PSQI)	Objective assessment tool		
		Multi-channel physiological recorder	Sleep observation	Activity recorder
Number of samples	Big scale	Small scale	Small scale	Small scale
Assessor	Self-assessment	Equipment	Observer	Equipment
Assessment period	Recall	Sleep duration	Sleep duration	Full-time record
Data collection	Fast and convenient	Time-consuming and inconvenient	Time-consuming and inconvenient	Time-consuming and convenient
Cost of collection	Low	High	Medium	Medium

Past studies related to sleep quality requested shift workers to conduct self-assessment of sleep quality with the Pittsburgh Sleep Quality Index; although large amount of research samples can be obtained in a short time, those are still subjective information. Sleep quality is the observation result over a period of time; objective assessment method would be appropriate (activity recorder) to work along with the shift workers' personal condition and schedule, recording their activity condition anywhere and anytime. Hence, the research can be conducted with greater objectiveness and can record the research subjects' schedule at work or at home. Compared to the Pittsburgh Sleep Quality Index commonly used by past scholars, sleep quality related information can be collected with higher accuracy. Meanwhile, a comparison of the activity recorder data and the Pittsburgh Sleep Quality Index items (Table 3) shows that component related self-assessment items that can be found in the Pittsburgh Sleep Quality Index can all be obtained in the activity recorder, without shift workers conducting self-assessment on the sleep quality in the past.

Table 3. Data comparison between the activity recorder and the PSQI

Activity Recorder	Pittsburgh Sleep Quality Index
Number of Sleep hours	Total number of sleep hours
Sleep efficiency	Sleep efficiency
Sleep latency	Sleep latency
The number of dozing	Daytime dysfunction
Awake duration and the number of times	Sleep disorders
Activity levels while awake	Daytime dysfunction

2   Result and Suggestion

According to the discusses of shift workers sleep quality and related job performance in this study, shift workers are affected by the physiological disorder of the day and night rhythm, their sleep latency period becomes longer, sleep duration is shorter, resulting in poor efficiency in job performance and increase of quality defect rate and work-related accidents. Among the various work shifts that are affected, overnight shift faces most serious impact, followed by night shift. In response to the issues arising from these shift workers, this study suggests companies to make adjustments about the shift workers and the performance standards of night shifts. First, regarding the shift workers themselves, companies should consider the health and family condition of the employees while making the night shift personnel arrangements, minimizing the factors that affect sleep. Secondly, regarding the job performance of night shifts, priority should be given to ensuring work quality and avoiding increase of defect rate and accident caused by the struggle to achieve the same efficiency rate as the daytime staff.

In terms of the measurement method for sleep quality, questionnaires are survey tools used by many domestic scholars in the research of sleep quality[22][19][16], researching the subjective perception of a period of sleep time; the information collected in this cross-sectional research method only reflects "a frozen section of a substance" or an "one-time snapshot" of the research context[9]. This data collection method cannot provide meaningful information across a time period, and certainly cannot verify the before and after change between incidents; it can only be used for relationship analysis in the basic behavior logic.

This study compared objective and subjective sleep quality assessment method and analyzed different objective measurement tools. Pittsburgh survey utilizes self-assessment method to collect massive sleep quality samples at a low cost in a short period of time in order to achieve statistical power to verify the quality of sleep. However, sleep quality is the result of observation through a period of time and requires long term record of the research sample's schedule at work or family; it would be appropriate to adopt objective measurements (activity recorder) to record daily activities anywhere and anytime.

Finally, in practical research, activity recorders are not research tools that can be easily obtained and implemented by general researchers. First, the acquisition cost of each tool is approximately NT$100,000, which is not affordable for general researchers. Second, it is even more difficult to find research subjects who can work with long hours of recording. However, benefitting from the emergence of wearable technology access to measurement tools is no long a problem that cannot be solved. Currently there are sleep quality measurement products in the market, for example Jawbone UP is NT$5,000 each and Fitbit one is NT$4,000; the sleep quality data they provide meets the analysis needs of the researchers. At the same time, these products are easy to wear and can handle long hours of record, increasing the willingness of the subjects to participate in the research.

References

1. Akerstedt, T., Froberg, J.E.: Interindividual differences in circadian patterns of catecholamine excretion, body temperature, performance, and subjective arousal. Biological Psychology 4(4), 277–292 (1976)
2. Akerstedt, T.: Shift work and disturbed sleep/wakefulness. Occupational Medicine London 53(2), 89–94 (2003)
3. Benjamin, G.A.: Shift workers: Improve the quality of life for employees who aren't on the 9-to-5 routine. Personnel Journal 63(6), 72–76 (1984)

4. Cohen, D.J., Eisdorfer, C., Prize, P., Breen, A., Davis, M., Dadsby, A.: Sleep disturbances in the institutionalized aged. Journal of the American Geriatrics Society 31(2), 79–82 (1983)
5. Cornelia, W., Andreas, M., Brandmaier, von Oertzen, T., Müller, V., Gert, G., Wagner, M.R: A new approach for assessing sleep duration and postures from ambulatory accelerometry. PLOS ONE 7(10), e48089 (2012), doi:0.1371/journal. pone. 0048089
6. Deng, J.R.: Discussion of Regular Exercise and Sleep Quality of the Seniors. Journal of Physical Education, National Taiwan Normal University 5, 185–192 (2003)
7. Drake, C.L., Roehrs, T., Richardson, G., Walsh, J.K., Roth, T.: Shift work sleep disorder: Prevalence and consequences beyond that of symptomatic day worker. Sleep 27(8), 1453–1462 (2004)
8. Edwrs, G.B., Schuring, L.M.: Pilot study: validating staff nurses' observations of sleep and wake states among critically ill patients, using polysomnography. American Journal of Critical Care 2, 125–131 (1993)
9. Finkel, S.E.: Causal analysis with panel data. Sage Publications, Thousand Oaks (1995)
10. Folkardt, S., Tucker, P.: Shiftwork, safety and productivity. Occupational Medicine 53, 95–101 (2003)
11. Folkard, S., Monk, T.H., Alexander, A.I.: Maintaining safety and high performance on shiftwork. Applied Ergonomic 27, 17–23 (1996)
12. Friedman, E.M., Love, G.D., Rosenkranz, M.A., Urry, H.L., Davidson, R.J., Singer, B.H., Ryff, C.D.: Socioeconomic status predicts objective and subjective sleep quality in aging women. Psychosom. Med. 69(7), 682–691 (2007)
13. Fujino, Y., Iso, H., Tamakoshi, A., Inaba, Y., Koizumi, A., Kubo, T., Yoshimura, T.: Japanese Collaborative Cohort Study Group. A prospective cohort study of shift work and risk of ischemic heart disease in Japanese male workers. Am. Journal of Epidemio. 164(2), 128–135 (2006)
14. Gold, D.R., Rogacz, S.L.: Rotating shift work sleep, and accident related to sleepiness in hospital nurse. American Journal of Public Health 82(7), 1011–1014 (1992)
15. Hossain, J.L., Reinish, L.W., Kayumov, L., Bhuiya, P., Shapiro, C.M.: Underlying sleep pathology cause chronic high fatigue in shift-workers. Journal of Sleep Research 12, 223–230 (2003)
16. Hsu, S.Y., Guo, H.R., Su, S.B.: A Study of the Sleep Quality of TFT-LCD Photoelectric Industry Shift Workers. Chinese Journal of Occupational Medicine 13(3), 157–167 (2006)
17. Hsu, T.L.: The Influence of Shift Work on Physiological Conditions, News-letter of Labor Safety and Health. Institute of Occupational Safety and Health 40, 24–30 (2000)
18. Janssen, N., Kant, I.J., Swaen, G.M., Janssen, P.P., Schroer, C.A.: Fatigue as a predictor of sickness absence: results from the Maastricht cohort study on fatigue at work. Occupational Environmental Medicine 60(suppl. 1), i71–i76 (2003)
19. Ji, Y.Z., Wu, C.L., Lee, Y.S.: A Study on Related Factors that Impact Sleep Quality. Health Promotion & Health Education Journal 30, 35–61 (2010)
20. Kearnes, S.: Insomnia in the elderly. Nursing Times 85(47), 32–33 (1989)
21. Kivistö, M., Härmä, M., Sallinen, M., Kalimo, R.: Work-related factors, sleep debt and insomnia in IT professionals. Occupational Medicine 58, 138–140 (2008)
22. Lien, J.W., Liu, B.S.: The Impact of Age and Daily Rhythm Pattern on the Sleeping of Worshift Healthcare Personnel. Journal of Ergonomic Study 3(1), 57–63 (2011)
23. Lin, G.Y.: Sleep and Labor Safety and Hygiene. Newsletter on Occupational Head Safety 85, 4–5 (2007)

24. Lin, Z.C., Fu, H.S.: The Impact of Regular Exercise on the Sleep Condition of Shift Workers. Quarterly of National Sport of Physical Education of the Republic of China, Vol 19(2), 1–9 (2005)
25. Liou, T.S., Wang, M.J.: Rotating-shift system vs. fixed-shift system. Industrial Ergonomics 7, 63–70 (1991)
26. Mendelson, W.B.: Sleep after forty. American Family Physician 29(1), 135–139 (1984)
27. Nakata, A., Ikeda, T., Takahashi, M., Haratani, T., Hojou, M., Fujioka, Y., Swanson, N.G., Araki, S.: Impact of psychosocial job stress on non-fatal occupational injuries in small and medium-sized manufacturing enterprise. American Journal of Industrial Medicine 49, 658–669 (2006)
28. Ohayon, M.M., Lemoine, P., Arnaud-Briant, V., Dreyfus, M.: Prevalence and consequences of sleep disorders in a shift worker population. Journal of Psychosomatic Research 53(1), 577–583 (2002)
29. Ota, A., Masue, T., Yasuda, N., Tsutsumi, A., Mino, Y., Ohara, H.: Association between psychosocial job characteristics and insomnia: an investigation using two relevant job stress models—the demand-control-support (DCS) model and the effort-reward imbalance (ERI) model. Sleep Medicine 6, 353–358 (2005)
30. Pallesen, S., Nordhus, I.H., Nielsen, G.H., Havik, O.E., Kvale, G., Johnsen, B.H., Skjøtskift, S.: Prevalence of insomnia in the adult Norwegian population. Sleep 24, 771–779 (2001)
31. Rodriguez-Munoz, A., Moreno-Jimenez, B., Fernandez-Mendoza, J.J., Olavarrieta-Bernardino, S., de la Cruz-Troca, J.J., Vela-Bueno, A.: Insomnia and quality of sleep among primary care physicians: A gender perspective. Rev. Neurol. 47(3), 119–123 (2008)
32. Shilo, L., Sabbah, H., Hadari, R.: The effects of coffee consumption on sleep and melatonin secretion. Sleep Med. 3(3), 271–273 (2002)
33. Singh, N.A., Clements, K.M., Fiatarone, M.A.: Sleep, sleep deprivation, and daytime activities: A randomized controlled trial of the effect of exercise on sleep. Sleep 20(2), 95–101 (1997)
34. Sudo, N., Ohtsuka, R.: Sleep pattern and sleep disorders among female workers in a computer factory of Japan. Human Ergology Society 28(1-2), 39–47 (1999)
35. Summers, M.O., Crisostomo, M.I., Stepanski, E.J.: Recent developments in the classification, evaluation and treatment of insomnia. CHEST 130(1), 276–286 (2006)
36. Van Mark, A., Spallek, M., Kessel, R., Brinkmann, E.: Shift work and pathological conditions. Journal of Occupational Medicine and Toxicology 1, 25 (2006)
37. Vouriot, A., Hannhart, B., Gauchard, G.C., Barot, A., Ledin, T., Mur, J.M., Perrin, P.P.: Long-term exposure to solvents impairs vigilance and postural control in serigraphy workers. Int. Arch. Occup. Environ. Health 78(6), 510–515 (2005)

The Classification Tendency and Common Denomination of the Points Paid Attention in Ikebana Instruction

Yuki Ikenobo[1,*], Noriaki Kuwahara[1], Noriyuki Kida[2],
Yuka Takai[3], and Akihiko Goto[3]

[1] Department of Advanced Fibro Science, Graduate School of Science and Technology,
Kyoto Institute of Technology, Kyoto, Japan
hanahana@ikenobo.jp, nkuwahar@kit.ac.jp
[2] Department of Applied Biology, Graduate School of Science and Technology,
Kyoto Institute of Technology, Kyoto, Japan
kida@kit.ac.jp
[3] Department of Information Systems Engineering, Faculty of Design Technology,
Osaka Sangyo University, Osaka, Japan
{takai,gotoh}@ise.osaka-sandai.ac.jp

Abstract. "Ikebana" is one of the representative aspects of Japanese Culture. However Ikebana arranging skill has been passed down as an oral tradition from master to disciple, rather than in a systematic educational system. This research examines the words used by a teacher with regard to ikebana arrangements created by a beginner and an experienced arranger, examines what parts of the arrangements are focused on and evaluated, and looks at the points ikebana teacher pay attention to in correcting arrangements. It is possible that clarifying the criteria for evaluation and correction of arrangements will contribute to establishing a logical and scientific method of teaching ikebana in the future.

With respect to the arrangement created by a beginner, there were many comments about the "tai" portion rather than evaluation of the overall form of the arrangement. So "tai" is supposed to be a difficult part of Ikebana arrangement for beginner. Regarding the arrangement created by the experienced arranger, it is possible that overall balance of the arrangement made the viewer have a positive impression of the whole work. However, a few positive comments were also made about the overall arrangement created by the beginner. Although the beginner's arrangement was not as accomplished as the work by an experienced arranger, it appears that viewers don't always look negatively at an arrangement created by a beginner. Next concerning correction of the arrangement, Comments for correction of Ikebana arrangement occurred both for beginner and for experienced arranger, though experienced arrangers followed the standard method. These results indicate that comments made during the correction of an arrangement can be categorized into two types: "comments made because of discrepancy with the one standard arranging method," and "comments made because of disagreement with the aesthetics of the viewer." The former type of comment occurs only for the arrangement made by a beginner,

---

* Corresponding author.

V.G. Duffy (Ed.): DHM 2014, LNCS 8529, pp. 263–272, 2014.
© Springer International Publishing Switzerland 2014

as opposed to many positive comments for the arrangement made by an experienced arranger. The latter type of comment seems to be made for arrangements both by an experienced arranger and a beginner.

Keywords: Correction, arrangements, comments, aesthetic, evaluation, standard method.

1   Introduction

In Ikebana, teachers evaluate ikebana arrangements made by disciples and correct them along certain criteria, in order the output be accomplished. This is called "Tenaoshi (Correction)". Teachers correct ikebana arrangements made by disciples, however, there are many different ways of correcting, and thus, there is still no common way of guidance.

In addition, although there are primary curriculums[1], already established for "Rikka" and "Shoka", the typical formats of Ikenobo Ikebana, criteria vary by the degree of the experience of the teachers, which is sometimes hard for students to understand.

This research examines the words used by a teacher with regard to ikebana arrangements created by a beginner and an experienced arranger, and investigates what parts of the arrangements are focused on and are evaluated. By drawing out teachers' knowledge and comments about Ikebana, and putting them in order, it would be possible to categorize the points focused by teachers when they correct, and to clarify a common point and a tendency from the guidance. For example, by comparing the words and comments made by teachers when assessing ikebana arrangement, the difference between the experienced and the beginner would appear clearly. By doing so, it would be possible to integrate the criteria, which had traditionally been evaluated by teachers' experience and aesthetics.

In addition, it enables teachers to instruct based on systematic knowledge, which would also be helpful for less experienced teachers. For students and disciples as well, they will be enabled to acquire knowledge and skills even faster by such scientific guides.

2   Method

2.1   Outline

In this investigation, six experienced teachers evaluated each piece of Shoka arrangement created by an experienced arranger and a beginner (Fig 3, Fig 4). Teachers were asked to evaluate each piece of work by oral words, and then describe what was wrong and what should be improved. By doing so, it enabled us to extract typical and core phrases used to evaluate, and to categorize them in order.

2.2   Teachers

The six teachers in this investigation were the ones who are experienced in ikebana for more than ten years, and also experienced in teaching for more than five years. The details are shown as below:

Table 1. List of participants (Interviewees)

	Age	Years of Ikebana Experience	Years of Teaching
Teacher A	35	20 years	7 years
Teacher B	58	40 years	13 years
Teacher C	50	32 years	12 years
Teacher D	66	40 years	11 years
Teacher E	70	50 years	30 years
Teacher F	69	47 years	31 years

2.3   Arrangers and Place Taken

The arrangers in this experiment were the ones who were well experienced and less experienced. Their profiles are as follows:

Table 2. List of participants (Ikebana arrangers)

	Age	Years of Ikebana Experience
The Experienced	42	21 years
The Beginner	27	4 years

In this research, "experienced arranger" was defined as an arranger who has more than ten years of ikebana experience, since it requires roughly ten years to be certificated as a teacher of ikebana[2], and "beginner" was defined as an arranger who had less than five years of ikebana experience.

The experiment was taken in a meeting room where the frontage width was five meters and the depth was ten meters long, and was surrounded by white walls with a window faced south.

The arrangers were asked to arrange ikebana on a table right beside the wall, and were asked to work back to back with each other, in order not to mutually influence their works.

When two arrangers accomplished their works and departed from the room, teachers entered the room evaluating both works and corrected them by oral. The arranged works were exhibited one at a time so that each work had been evaluated and corrected independently by the teachers. This serial procedure was repeated for each teacher, thus, six times.

2.4   Format and Materials Used

The arrangers were asked to arrange ikebana in "Shoka" style, using four to six branches of cornus albas and two to three flowers of small chrysanthemums. Shoka has its own rules to be obeyed, and because cornus albas, the main material in this task, are relatively elastic, this task was practical to see the difference of the well experienced and the beginner.

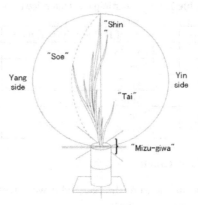

Fig. 1. Form of "Shoka"

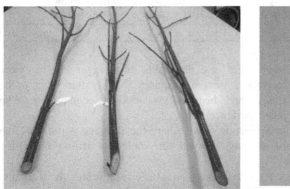 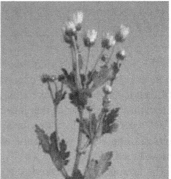

Fig. 2. Materials for Ikebana arrangement in this experimentation

2.5   Collecting Date

Data of evaluations and corrections spoken by the teachers were collected in the same place as the experiment was conducted. We, first, asked the teachers to assess the overall evaluation of each work independently, and asked to give reasons why some particular points should be corrected and how. We also asked them questions when needed. There was no regulation in time length when each teacher made comments, but came out approximately five to ten minutes.

This evaluation process was recorded by a video camera, and every comment was archived in words afterward.

Although a various range of comments were made depending on the age and the linguistic environment of the teachers (as shown in Table 3), there are similarities in each comment, and therefore, we categorized such comments and integrated them in simple words. Table 4 shows typical comments made by the teachers. As shown in the table, most comments were mainly concerned in the overall impression and the partial points.

Table 3. Chart of representative comments for experienced arranger by the teachers

	Experienced Arranger
Overall Impression	• I assume that the work was arranged by someone who is highly skilled. • This is not a work made by someone ordinary. • It is very free and easy. • The Shin has strength and is excellent. • Tai seems confused. • It is hard to arrange in such a beautiful way. ...and more.

Table 4. Chart of typical comments by the teachers

	Experienced Arranger	Beginner
Overall Impression	• Skillful. • Free and easy. • Well arranged. • Skillful in making and is based on the Shoka format. • Assembled in clear and straightforward way. • A skill of arranging it natural.	• Lacking sense of "free and easy". • The balance and the height are in format. • Need to put materials in order.
Corrections	• Tai and Soe should be more balanced. • There should be more coarseness and fineness in small branches.	• There should be more variations in expression. • Small branches in Soe should be cut off. • Tai should be in order and should make variations.

2.6   Categories of Comments and Structuring the Categories

In order the data to be liable, all recorded comments were double checked by the teachers themselves. The average number of comments made in each work, including evaluation and correction, was 16. Those comments can be categorized as follows, and these are the main categories to assess arrangements based on Shoka format:

1. Overall evaluation and correction.
2. Evaluation and correction about "Shin".
3. Evaluation and correction about "Soe".
4. Evaluation and correction about "Tai".
5. Evaluation and correction about "Mizugiwa".

These main categories can also be broken down into some sub-categories, such as follows:

1. Overall evaluation
2. Shin – synthetic evaluation
i. An arrangement of Shin
3. Soe – synthetic evaluation
i. An arrangement of Soe
4. Tai – synthetic evaluation
i. Flowers and buds
ii. Leaves
iii. Tai-saki
5. Mizugiwa – synthetic evaluation

Nejime in Tai, in this case, belongs to Mizugiwa, the core of Shoka format, and is the important part of balancing overall impression. Tai-saki means the edge of Tai. Depending on teachers, they sometimes comment based on botany such as flowers, leaves, and buds, whereas others express them by using technical phrases of ikebana such as Nejime and Tai-saki. Though those comments sometimes correspond, their nuances may vary in a wide range, and are not always the same. In this research, we tried to specify the points the teachers were focusing on as precise as possible, and categorized them in order. Also, an "arrangement" in this study means supplementary works processed to the main materials such as Shin and Soe, in order to strengthen the materials and add tastes and elegance in it. Arrangement should be done only when needed.

In addition, the comments about corrections made after the overall evaluation can be categorized as follows:

1. Shin
i. Balance and space
ii. Position and direction
iii. Quantity and Length
2. Soe
i. Balance and space
ii. Position and direction
iii. Quantity and Length
3. Tai
i. Balance and space
ii. Position and direction
iii. Quantity and Length
4. Mizugiwa
i. Balance and space
ii. Position and direction
iii. Quantity and Length
5. Work as a whole
i. Synthetic evaluation
ii. Balance and space

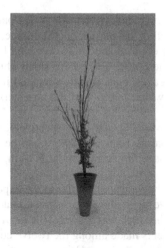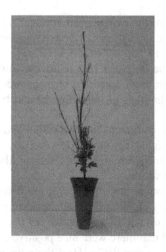

Fig. 3. The works for experiment (Left: by expert, Right: by beginner)

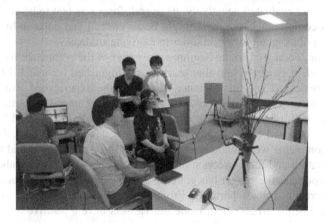

Fig. 4. The scene of the expert interviews in the actual Ikebana arrangements

Afterward, we categorized pros and cons made by the teachers about each of the total arrangement. And then, we calculated frequencies of the comments made in each category.

It should be noticed that corrections are made in some parts where they should be amended, and thus, there are no positive comments there. Based on this premise, we calculated frequencies of the comments made in each category.

3   Result

In overall evaluation, positive comments for the experienced arranger's work appeared 49% and were overwhelming. Other than that, Tai was the only part where 30% of the comments appeared, whereas other parts had been referred only 1-7%. This implies that there was more weight on evaluating overall form of the work. In addition, for the experienced arranger, many comments were made in Tai part, which implies that the experienced have managed well in Tai part among Shin, Soe, and Tai. Especially in Tai, the experienced were positively evaluated in flowers and buds part, whereas the beginner had relatively low values in it. Tai, where small chrysanthemums were used, consisted of many weeds, leaves, buds and flowers, and it required higher techniques to treat flowers and buds, which might lead the arrangers to such difference.

Positive comments made for Shin and Soe were 7% and 1% respectively, and were both not highly appeared. However, by comparing Shin and Soe, it can be said that the experienced arranger had successfully managed to arrange more in Shin, the main part of the whole.

On the other hand, comments made for the beginner, as similar to the experienced, were mostly about the overall work, too. However, it should be noticed that negative comments do not always appear just because the work was made by the beginner. It is rather said that there were nice positive comments made among the twelve comments, which means that $9/12=3/4$ of the comments were positive. However, partially looking, we can find many negative comments in Shin, Soe, and Tai. Although parts of the arrangement were evaluated negatively, its overall form was tent to be evaluated positive, and this could be because there might be an educational purpose by teachers to find out good points in any work, in order to motivate students.

In correction, compared to the beginner, only half of the comments were made for the experienced. It is easily said that teachers distinguished technical difference between the experienced and the beginner. However, the experienced arranger who is not supposed to be given corrections, were still asked to amend the arrangement. In fact, 24% and 40% of the corrective comments were made in Shin and Tai parts respectively. As opposed to the highly evaluated comments on the overall form, only 16% of the comments were made in correction for the overall form, and this implies that the evaluation and the correction are said to be coherent. On the other hand, although the experienced arranger has gotten positive evaluation in Tai part, there were also some corrections made partially. From here, it can be concluded that although overall balance of the arrangement made the viewers have a positive impression as a whole, it appeared not enough for the teachers' aesthetics in order the work to be accomplished.

On the other hand, about 50% of the corrections were made in Tai portion for the beginner. Since 21% of the comments were also made in Shin, it is said that there is a certain difficulty in arranging Tai and Shin portions. Especially in Tai portion, many corrections had been commented both for the experienced and the beginner, and thus it is said to be the most difficult and most seen part in ikebana arrangement. Although Shin is essentially the main portion in ikebana, more attentions were paid in Tai, which could be due to the nature of the materials used. In this experiment, Shin and Soe were consisted of cornus albas, which had no leaves, whereas Tai consisted of small chrysanthemums with leaves and flowers crowed. This peculiar situation could have lead teachers to pay attention in Tai more. These results indicate that corrections made for the beginner were mostly the comments that were made because of discrepancy with the standard arranging method, whereas the corrections for the experienced were mostly the comments that were made because of disagreement with the aesthetics of the viewers.

Table 5. Chart of comment appeared for overall

No.	Parts	Categories	The experienced			The biginner		
			Positive	Negative	Appearance	Positive	Negative	Appearance
a.	Shin		4	1	0.074626866	2	6	0.126984127
1		Synthetic Evaluation	3	0	0.044776119	2	1	0.047619048
2		Arrangement	1	1	0.029850746	0	5	0.079365079
b.	Soe		1	0	0.014925373	2	5	0.111111111
1		Synthetic Evaluation	0	0	0	2	5	0.111111111
2		Arrangement	1	0	0.014925373	0	0	0
c.	Tai		16	6	0.328358209	1	20	0.333333333
1		Synthetic Evaluation	2	5	0.104477612	1	12	0.206349206
2		Nejime	4	0	0.059701493	0	0	0
3		Flowers and buds	10	0	0.149253731	0	4	0.063492063
4		Leaves	0	0	0	0	1	0.015873016
5		Tai-saki	0	1	0.014925373	0	3	0.047619048
d.	Mizugiwa		3	0	0.044776119	3	0	0.047619048
1		Synthetic Evaluation	3	0	0.044776119	3	0	0.047619048
e.	Meterials		3	0	0.044776119	0	0	0
1		Synthetic Evaluation	3	0	0.044776119	0	0	0
f.	Overall Form		33	0	0.492537313	9	3	0.19047619
1		Synthetic Evaluation	33	0	0.492537313	9	3	0.19047619

Table 6. Chart of comment appeared for correction

No.	Parts	Categories	The experienced		The biginner	
			Number of Comments	Appearance	Number of Comments	Appearance
g.	Shin		6	0.24	10	0.21
1		Balance and Space	3	0.12	1	0.02
2		Position and Direction	2	0.08	5	0.1
3		Quantity and Length	1	0.04	2	0.04
h.	Soe		3	0.12	6	0.12
1		Balance and Space	0	0	1	0.02
2		Position and Direction	2	0.08	1	0.02
3		Quantity and Length	1	0.04	4	0.08
i.	Tai		11	0.44	25	0.53
1		Balance and Space	2	0.08	6	0.12
2		Position and Direction	7	0.28	12	0.255
3		Quantity and Length	2	0.08	7	0.14
j.	Mizugiwa		2	0.08	2	0.04
1		Balance and Space	0	0	0	0
2		Position and Direction	1	0.04	1	0.02
3		Quantity and Length	1	0.04	1	0.02
k.	Overall Form		4	0.16	4	0.08
1		Synthetic Correction	1	0.04	1	0.02
2		Balance and Space	3	0.12	3	0.06

4   Considerations

It could be said that throughout evaluation, teachers were seemed to see abilities of the experienced and the beginner, and assessed each of them fairly and appropriately. The comments made during the correction of the arrangement can be categorized into two types: "comments made because of discrepancy with the standard arranging method" and "comments made because of disagreement with the aesthetics of the viewer". The former type of comments was found only for the arrangement made by the beginner, whereas the latter type of comments appeared in both. These two categories must be thoroughly investigated in the future, with relation to the materials used or levels of the arrangers. Also, the reason why the work was positively evaluated as a whole, even though there were some negative comments in parts, was because there would be an educational consideration for students to motivate themselves.

5   Conclusion

Teachers are seemed not only to evaluate abilities of students throughout assessment, but also to consider them from educational aspects as well, and they give two different types of corrections according to students' abilities.

Since aesthetics and what they perceive from the work vary by teachers, more testees would be required in the future, in order to investigate how it affects the process of corrections done by teachers.

Also, the comments made because of discrepancy with the standard arranging method, which were found only for the beginner, can be examined more carefully, so that it would be helpful when guiding beginners. It is also one of the concerns that I would like to investigate in the future.

References

1. Ikenobo Origin of Ikebana Eds.: Curriculum of Rikka for begginers 1&2. Ikenobo Origin of Ikebana (2011)
2. Ikenobo Origin of Ikebana Eds.: Qualified ranking list for Ikebana. Ikenobo Origin of Ikebana(established in 1978, revised in 2007)
3. Hirohide, S., Sen'ei, I. (eds.): Easy Ways to Understand the Ikenobo Ikebana's Shoka, pp. 12–13. Nihon Kodansha Company Ltd. (1997)
4. Kim, E., Fujii, E.: A fundamental study of physiological and psychological effects of colors of plants. J.JILA 58(5), 141–144 (1995)
5. Hasegawa, S., Shimomura, T.: Comparison of psychological effects on workers between a small interior plant and a large interior plant. Journal of the Japanese Society of Revegetation Technology 36(1), 63–68 (2010)
6. Hasegawa, S., Shimomura, T.: Influences of the plants' shape, size, and distance to the estimator on the impression evaluation of the indoor plant. Landscape Research Japan (Online Journal) 4, 24–32 (2011)

Analysis and Comparison of Ergonomics in Laparoscopic and Open Surgery – A Pilot Study

Kristian Karlovic[1], Stefan Pfeffer[1], Thomas Maier[1], Karl-Dietrich Sievert[2],
Ralf Rothmund[3], Monika A. Rieger[4], and Benjamin Steinhilber[4]

[1] Institute for Engineering Design and Industrial Design, Research and Teaching Department Industrial Design Engineering, University of Stuttgart, Germany
{kristian.karlovic,stefan.pfeffer,
thomas.maier}@iktd.uni-stuttgart.de
[2] University Department of Urology, University Hospital Tuebingen (UKT), Germany
[3] University Department of Gynecology and Obstetrics,
University Hospital Tuebingen (UKT), Germany
[4] Institute of Occupational and Social Medicine and Health Services Research,
University Hospital Tuebingen (UKT), Germany
{karl.sievert,Ralf.Rothmund,Monika.Rieger,
Benjamin.Steinhilber}@med.uni-tuebingen.de

Abstract. This pilot study systematically analyses and compares ergonomics of laparoscopic and open surgery in gynecology and urology. The results will help to identify and describe elements for ergonomic optimization in these professions. Further a supporting technical system to reduce physical demands shall be developed on the basis of assessment. A multiple measurement approach including subjective and objective methods was used with regard to the complex setting in surgery units. Subjective and objective methods indicate musculoskeletal strain for both types of surgery. Several indications for low ergonomics and static work have been found.

Keywords: Ergonomics, healthcare, supporting system, workload.

1 Objective

Physical discomfort and harm due to suboptimal working postures have been shown by surveys among surgeons [1] [2]. With the aim to reduce the physical load on surgeons and surgery staff a research project has been established to investigate the ergonomics of laparoscopic and open surgery. By means of this pilot study, key elements for ergonomic optimization should be described. In a second step, these key elements will be addressed in order to develop a supporting technical system that reduces physical demands (e.g. the reduction of static work). Surgeons and operating procedures of two surgical units (one urological and one gynecological) were investigated.

During this pilot study, the instruments for the systematic analysis of ergonomics, physical demands and musculoskeletal health status among surgeons of the mentioned

V.G. Duffy (Ed.): DHM 2014, LNCS 8529, pp. 273–281, 2014.

professional disciplines were developed. This paper presents the respective data resulting in differences between open and laparoscopic surgery. In addition, ideas are given to the question whether ergonomic improvements and technical supporting systems should be developed separately for these two kinds of surgery or whether universal concepts might be sufficient.

2 Significance

Work intensification among surgeons [3] and an increasing risk of medical error [4] are reported in the literature. The tendency towards work intensification (more operations per day) and consequently an aggregation of physical demands has also been reported by the surgeons participating in this research project. Furthermore they mentioned critically that higher physical demands may lead to less concentration and an increased risk of errors. As a consequence, this might contribute to less quality in health care and increased costs for further medical treatments.

In this context the improvement of ergonomics in surgery seems to be important for maintaining the workforce of surgeons and surgery staff and to support high quality work of surgical units.

3 Methods

Data was collected from 6 surgeons during 20 surgical interventions (10 laparoscopic hysterectomies, 6 laparoscopic prostatectomies, 4 radical prostatectomies) lasting 20 to 180 minutes. A multiple measurement approach consisting of subjective and objective methods was used. Subjective methods included the NASA TLX [5] and the Nordic Questionnaire [6]. The questionnaire NASA TLX determines the workload during a specific work task according to its six dimensions: physical demand, mental demand, temporal demand, performance, effort and frustration. This questionnaire provides an Overall Weighted Workload Score (OWWS) including all of the mentioned dimensions and more detailed the scores of every single dimension. Higher scores indicate higher demands. The Nordic Questionnaire was used to obtain information about musculoskeletal complaints of the last 12 months and the last week.

The objective methods included muscular strain assessed by surface electromyography (sEMG) and life record data. The electrical activity (eA) of the trapezius muscle (descending part) as the root mean square value of the bipolar sEMG was measured continuously throughout surgery. A reference measurement with an anteversion of both straight arms holding an external load of 2 kg in each hand was conducted before surgery and was used for sEMG normalization. The trapezius muscle has been shown to be an import indicator for physical demands in laparoscopic surgery [2]. Life record data was also determined continuously throughout the whole surgery by a 3-perspective videoanalysis (3 cameras) in order to observe the whole body of the surgeon and to get information about movements, postures and the surgeons' procedures. The camera positions were arranged to realize the back, front and side view of the observed surgeon. The settings of the laparoscopic and the open surgery are shown in figure 1 as well as the positions of the cameras.

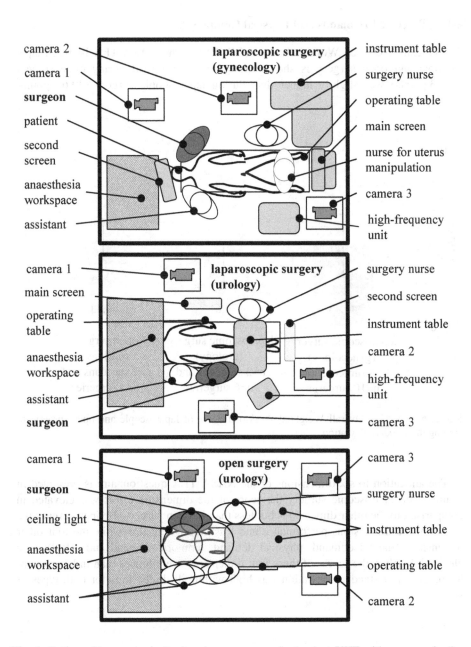

Fig. 1. Setting of laparoscopic (top) and open surgery (bottom) at UKT with cameras for 3-perspective-video-analysis

4   Results

4.1   Perceived Demands and Physical Complaints

The Overall Weighted Workload Score (OWWS) of the NASA TLX between laparoscopic and open surgery is shown in figure 2. Workload during open surgery (49,33 points) was slightly higher than during laparoscopic surgery (39,61 points, 46,43 points).

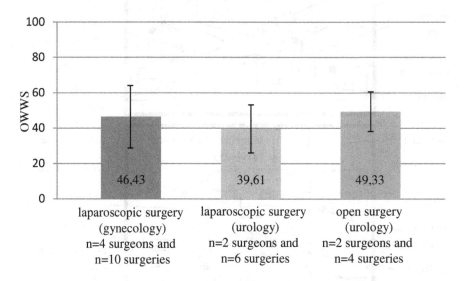

Fig. 2. NASA TLX Overall Weighted Workload Score of laparoscopic and open surgery including the standard deviation

The allocation to six dimensions of the NASA TLX questionnaire is presented in figure 3. In laparoscopic surgery the score of the dimension effort was elevated in comparison to the other dimensions but less than in open surgery. In open surgery the scores of the dimensions performance and frustration were low while the four other dimensions (mental demand, physical demand, temporal demand and effort) were elevated. Further, the scores of these four dimensions were higher than in laparoscopic surgery. The standard deviation was high within all dimensions for both types of surgery.

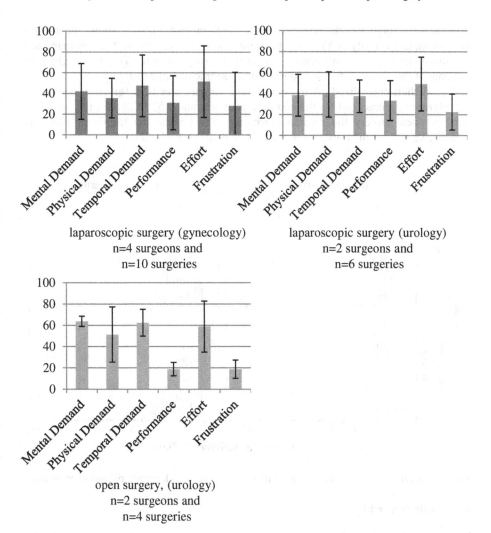

Fig. 3. Examination of NASA TLX dimensions of laparoscopic and open surgery

The results of the Nordic Questionnaire suggested high prevalence of neck or low back pain and therefore confirm the data from literature.

4.2   Muscular Strain (sEMG)

For analysis of muscular strain assessed by electrical activity (eA), only the data derived from the urological unit are used (data from 2 urological surgeons, 3 open surgical interventions, 4 laparoscopic surgical interventions).The measurements performed by the gynecological surgeons were excluded due to differences in monitor height, patient positioning and surgical procedures. In addition, the participating gynecological surgeons were more specialized in laparoscopic surgery and did not perform open surgery in the scope of this research project. Figure 4 shows the normalized electrical activity (eA) of the trapezius muscle, separated to the dominant and the non-dominant arm (only data of the urologic surgical unit). This figure gives an estimate of the physical demands during laparoscopic and open surgery.

The median normalized eA in laparoscopic surgery was 0.54 [given in percent of the reference contraction] for the non-dominant arm and 0.57 % 2kg for the dominant arm. In open surgery the median normalized eA for the non-dominant arm was 0.68 % 2kg and for the trapezius of the dominant arm 0.63 % 2kg.

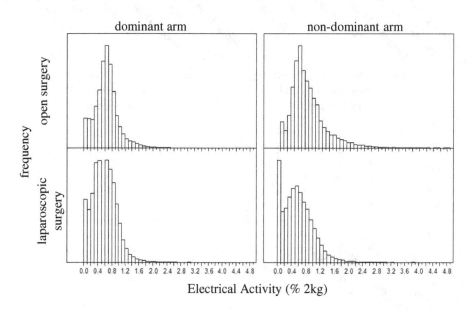

Fig. 4. Frequency distribution of the normalized trapezius eA in laparoscopic and open surgery

4.3   Life Record Data

Life record data showed position changes and body postures of the surgeons in dependence to setting, task and individual factors. Some selected results will be shown in this chapter.

The most obvious difference between open and laparoscopic surgery is the visual reception of the operating field. In laparoscopic surgery the surgeon looks at a screen which shows the videostream of the laparoscope, therefore the surgeon has an indirect view on his surgical task. In contrast, during open surgery the surgeon looks directly at the operating field. This difference induces different body postures especially of the surgeons' head. Figure 5 shows two examples from laparoscopic surgery (left) and two examples from open surgery (right). The angle α for laparoscopic surgery is bigger than the analogous angle β for open surgery (α > β).

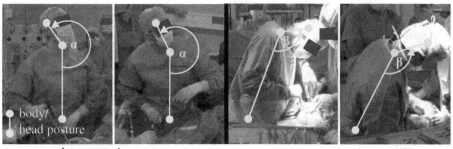

laparoscopic surgery   open surgery

Fig. 5. Head posture in dependence of surgery type

Both types of surgery are characterized by periods of static postures, especially of the arm, lasting for several minutes. Hence, figure 6 shows observed typical and significant head/body and arm postures of the surgeon for laparoscopic (left and middle) and open surgery (right). In laparoscopic surgery, the typical arm posture consists of the bent right arm beside and in front of the body and the bent left arm in front of the body. This posture is persistented for several minutes without moving the arm or upper body. Consequently this is leading to static work and is observed in the preparation period of laparoscopic surgery in particular. In open surgery, the extreme head flexion position (fig. 6, right) is remarkable and is maintained during most of the time of the surgical intervention. The arm posture shown on the right side of figure 6 is common for open surgery.

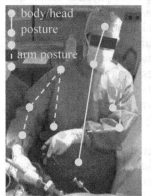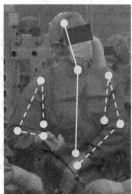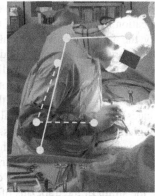

laparoscopic surgery   open surgery

Fig. 6. Significant body and arm postures in laparoscopic (left) and open surgery (right)

However, the surgeon changes his position, body posture and tasks during open surgery as shown in figure 7. On the left side every picture shows one of the three main positions. On the right side these positions are shown from the top.

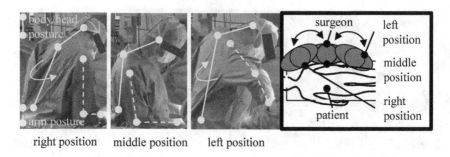

right position   middle position   left position

Fig. 7. Positions of the surgeon at open surgery (urologic clinic)

In summary both types of surgery show non ergonomic body postures. Given the data of this pilot study, open surgery exhibits more changes in positions and postures and is characterized by a large head flexion angle compared to laparoscopic surgery. Laparoscopic surgery seems to consist of more static and akinetic body and arm postures. Thus, the musculoskeletal strain is a result of static postures and tasks.

5 Discussion and Conclusion

A tendency towards higher demands in open surgery as compared to laparoscopic surgery was shown by NASA TLX questionnaire. This is supported by the results of the sEMG analysis of the trapezius muscle showing higher activity in open surgery. The explanation for this is given by the information of the video analysis. In open surgery more frequent changes of body position indicating more physical action was observed as well as extreme head flexion positions which are persisted over time. The allocation to six dimensions of the NASA TLX questionnaire show that for open surgery the four dimensions mental demand, physical demand, temporal demand and effort were elevated and in addition higher than in laparoscopic surgery. In laparoscopic surgery the score of the dimension effort was a bit less than in open surgery but elevated in comparison to the other dimensions. The results from the allocation to six dimensions may indicate that the use of a technical system in laparoscopic surgery reduces the perceived physical demand and consequently relieves the operator although the effort is slightly less.

Already published data of this research project considered sEMG of laparoscopic surgery from gynecological surgeons [2] indicating a substantial proportion of static work and asymmetric physical demands of the trapezius muscle. In this recent analysis, the strain of the trapezius of the dominant arm was significantly higher than of the non-dominant arm.

However, this could not be shown for laparoscopic surgery in urology. Differences in monitor height and patient positioning between both settings may be possible reasons for these findings. Thus, this indicates that not only the type of surgery but also the setting might be the reason for increased physical demands.

Ergonomic improvements should therefore include a pre- and post-evaluation of body postures and perceived demands of the surgeons or surgical staff. Considering the two investigated surgical units, ergonomic improvements should focus on strategies to improve the head and the arm posture of the surgeon. Unphysiological head positions were documented in both types of surgery and may lead to physical complaints [7]. Physical demands in the trapezius muscle may be reduced by a supporting technical system. For laparoscopic surgery the supporting system might be sufficient if the dominant arm is addressed. For open surgery it is obvious that a supporting system should consider both arms. Furthermore, short rest periods (several seconds) to enable muscular recovery and to prevent potential muscle fatigue should be considered. Especially routine surgery, as investigated in this study, might not be compromised by such rest periods.

Although both types of surgery require an ergonomic optimization, a supporting technical system will be developed for laparoscopic surgery. The more static character of this type of surgery makes a transfer into practice more realistic and the fact that the supporting system is focused on the dominant arm reduces the complexity of the required system.

Acknowledgement. The study is a component of the "Industry on Campus" project IOC-103 (Ministerium fuer Wissenschaft, Forschung und Kunst Baden Wuerttemberg, induced by Interuniversitaeres Zentrum fuer medizinische Technologien Stuttgart-Tuebingen) with the title "Interaktionsbasierte manipulatorgestützte Assistenz" in cooperation with FESTO and TRUMPF Medizin Systeme [2].

References

1. Miller, K., et al.: Ergonomics Principles Associated With Laparoscopic Surgeon Injury/Illness. Human Factors 54(6), 1087–1092 (2012)
2. Pfeffer, S., Hofmann, A., Maier, T., Rothmund, R., Sievert, K., Seibt, R., Rieger, M., Steinhilber, B.: Ergonomics of Selected Laparoscopic Procedures – Need for Action? In: Biomedical Engineering/Biomedizinische Technik, Band 58, Heft SI-1 Track J, Usability. Risk Management & Regulatory Affairs (2013)
3. Bohrer, T., Koller, M., Schlitt, H.J., Bauer, H.: Quality of life of german surgeons: results of a survey of 3652 attendees of the annual meetings of the German Surgical Societies. Deutsche Medizinische Wochenschrift 136(42), 2140–2144 (2011)
4. Mc Cormick, F., Kadzielski, J., Landrigan, C., Evans, B., Herndon, J.H., Rubash, H.E.: Surgeon fatigue: A Prospective Analysis of the Incidence, Risk, and Intervals of Predicted Fatigue-Related Impairment in Residents. Archives of Surgery 147(5), 430–435 (2012)
5. Hart, S., Staveland, L.: Development of NASA-TLX (Task Load Index): Results of empirical and theoretical research in Human mental workload. In: Hancock, P., Meshkati, N. (eds.), pp. 139–183. North Holland, Amsterdam
6. Kuorinka, I., et al.: Standardised Nordic questionnaires for the analysis of musculosceletal symptoms. Applied Ergonomics 18(3), 233–237 (1987)
7. Kilbom, A.: Neck. In: Mager Stellman, J. (ed.) Encyclopaedia of Occupational Health and Safety, 4th edn., ch 6.14. International Labor Organization, Geneva (1998)

Effect of Wall Material of a Room on Performance in Long Monotonous Work

Hiroki Nishimura[1], Yuka Takai[2], Akihiko Goto[2], Atsushi Endo[3],
and Noriaki Kuwahara[3]

[1] ARC EDU Co. Ltd., Osaka, Japan
arc-nnlervmenve@arc-edu.com
[2] Osaka Sangyo University, Osaka, Japan
{takai,gotoh}@ise.osaka-sandai.ac.jp
[3] Kyoto Institute of Technology, Kyoto, Japan
shootingstarofhope30@gmail.com, nkuwahar@kit.ac.jp

Abstract. A decline in concentration and physical/mental fatigue induce the occurrence of errors in monotonous work, or a decline in work efficiency. The efficiency of monotonous work is closely related to the environment of a room. Historically, Japan incorporates natural materials, such as clay, grass, bamboo charcoal in the interior construction of rooms. Natural materials used for interiors characteristically have properties which adjust to moisture levels and absorb contaminants in a house. We thus, expect the possibility of utilizing these specific effects to improve work efficiency while performing tedious work. The purpose of this study is to clarify how materials, such as wallpaper, clay wall and bamboo charcoal board, used in the construction of an interior, influence work efficiency and fatigue during long monotonous work. In this study, subjects sorted literature to represent the monotonous work used in the research. The status of work was recorded via video camera and the brain waves of the participants were measured. Fatigue levels, before and after the experiment, were also recorded.

Keywords: long monotonous work, interior environment, clay wall, bamboo charcoal, fatigue.

1 Introduction

It is generally considered that the decline in work efficiency, or the occurrence of error in monotonous work, is caused by a decline in concentration, or physical/mental fatigue [1]. However, studies show that the efficiency of monotonous work is also closely associated with the interior environment of a work room. The humidity and temperature in the room greatly influence the alertness of a worker engaged in monotonous work (for example [2]). Moreover, the smell in a room is also closely related to the alertness level of a worker (ex. [3]).

In Japan, we utilize indoor construction materials made from natural substances, such as clay wall. Some researchers report that clay wall contains properties which adjust to indoor humidity and absorb pollutants in a house (for example [4]). It is also

V.G. Duffy (Ed.): DHM 2014, LNCS 8529, pp. 282–291, 2014.
© Springer International Publishing Switzerland 2014

considered that the smell of grass emitted from a clay wall influences the efficiency of monotonous work.

It is common in Japan to utilize charcoal made from the chamber of bamboo to assist in the elimination of bad odors from a house. Bamboo has an exceptional microstructure, and after carbonization, displays high absorption ability. Bamboo charcoal is also used to purify water, removing organic impurities and odors. Because of its ability to remove substances which have an adverse effect on the environment, such as formaldehyde, the function of bamboo charcoal has been assessed [5]. Moreover, bamboo charcoal emits far extending infrared rays. Reports have revealed that these far extending rays emitted from bamboo charcoal improve blood circulation [6]. The far reaching infrared rays from bamboo also have a deodorizing effect which could influence the outcome of monotonous work.

The purpose of this study is to clarify how materials used for interior construction, such as wallpaper, clay wall and paper board made of bamboo charcoal influence work efficiency and fatigue while performing long monotonous work. Subjects sorted literature to represent the long monotonous work used in this research. The status of the participants work was recorded via video camera and their brain waves were measured. Fatigue levels were also measured pre and post experiment. Water generated during the work was also observed and analyzed. The results were based on the findings from three types of rooms: one room with a paper wall, one with a clay wall, and one with a bamboo charcoal board wall. We compared and analyzed the percentage of efficient work time and the occurrence of error per subject, per room.

2   Method

2.1   Subject

The data of the subject is as shown in Table 1. All nine subjects were male.   And the breakdown by age is as follows: 5 in their 20's, 2 in their 20's, 1 in his 40's and 1 in his 60's.

Table 1. Fig. 1. Table 2. Subjects

Subject	Gender	Age(years)	Height(cm)	Weight(kg)
A	Male	21	172	58
B	Male	23	173	74
C	Male	24	175	80
D	Male	23	172	64
E	Male	31	181	55
F	Male	23	183	75
G	Male	41	174	73
H	Male	63	172	70
I	Male	28	171	84

2.2   Measurement Environment

For our research, three rooms were created with identical layouts in the same facility. However, each room had a different wall material. As shown in Figure 1, the wall material used by room was wallpaper, clay, and bamboo charcoal board. Wallpaper is the most common interior material utilized in Japan.   A clay wall is a traditional Japanese wall made from clay, sand and straw. Since the clay wall is made from only natural materials, it emits a peculiar smell, but contains properties which have a positive effect on moisture levels. Bamboo charcoal is known to emit far reaching infrared rays, and has effective properties which absorb and remove odors, prevent electromagnetic waves, purify water and improve soil. Although bamboo charcoal board has not been widely used as a wall material in Japan, its positive effects have spread in various fields such as clothing and environmental products.   Recently, a charcoal board product has been developed by molding finely powdered bamboo charcoal. The charcoal board is flat so that it can be utilized as material for a wall. We expect that the application of bamboo charcoal will spread in the future.

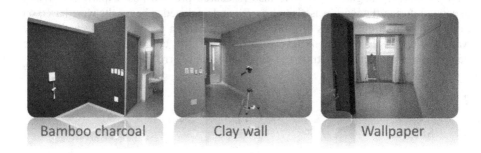

Bamboo charcoal   Clay wall   Wallpaper

Fig. 1. The status of each room used for experiment

2.3   Measurement Method

The subjects were engaged in monotonous work over a long period of time in three different rooms. Measurements were conducted on 3 separate days: March 28, 2012, April 18, 2012, and May 9, 2012. Although the measurements were conducted during a three day period, the time the measurements took place remained consistent. So, the subjects were measured at the same time each day over the course of three days. Subjects were assigned to each room in a random order to obtain unbiased experiment results. We asked the subjects to sort papers which represented the long monotonous work. The material utilized for sorting were application booklets for graduate school. The booklets consisted of text, resumes and envelopes. The booklets were classified into seven sections (1) cover and back cover, (2) resume, (3) mailing labels, (4) a large sized envelope, (5) a small sized envelope, (6) recyclable paper and (7) waste paper.   The subjects sorted 200 booklets in one trial. Desks and chairs were installed in each room with a layout of the room shown in Figure 2. Seven boxes, which contained the classified documents, were placed on each desk.   Prior to the experiment, instruction was given to the subjects pertaining to the booklet. Next, the subjects were told to begin work by sorting through all the booklets until they were finished. A particular method was not given as to how to remove a document from the literature.

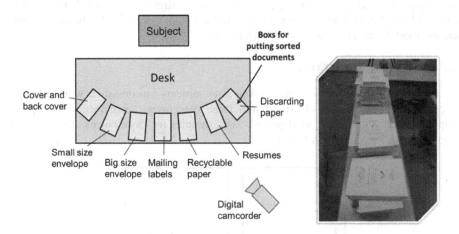

Fig. 2. Experimental Environment

2.4   Video Recording

The movement of the subjects during work was recorded by a digital camcorder. The entire time subjects engaged in work was measured and recorded via video.

2.5   EEG Measurement

Electroencephalogram (EEG) (MindSet NeuroSky) was used to measure the EEG of the subjects during work. The MindSet technology was developed for leisure. It is easy to use and low in cost. Three dry electrodes placed on the ears and chin are able to capture neural activity. By applying the algorithm, it decrypts neural activity. MindSet can detect information regarding the brain band activity of a user, and can also measure the delta, theta, alpha, beta and gamma output levels. The subjects closed their eyes for three minutes before and after work while their EEG output was measured. The EEG used for this study can calculate the the degree of attentiveness and meditation. On the assumption that the EEG of the subjects while resting was 100%, we normalized the EEG during work.

2.6   Fatigue Survey

Fatigue associated with work was surveyed before and after the course of work by using the "Survey for Awareness", published by The Industry Fatigue Committee of Japan Society for Occupational Health. This questionnaire was developed to evaluate the tendency of fatigue from the work performed, and whether the consistency in the factorial validity was confirmed. The questionnaire consists of 25 questions to be classified into five groups and five factors.   The questions include; "Feeling of sleepiness" indicating sleepiness, "sense of instability" indicating mental fatigue, "discomfort" indicating symptoms of autonomic imbalance, "sense of tiredness" indicating physical dissatisfaction and "feeling blurry" indicating complaints of eye strain.   The answers for each question were prepared in advance to include, "Not at all true", "slightly true" "a little true" "quite true" and "applies very well." Then, we assigned a 5 point system, with 5 being the highest and most intense, and summed up each factor.

2.7   Survey of Work Error

Photographs of the documents were taken after subjects finished their work with the documents. Then, it was classified into three categories; "torn pieces of paper", "ripped paper" and "miss-sorted paper". The examples for "torn pieces of paper" and "ripped paper" are shown in Figure 3.

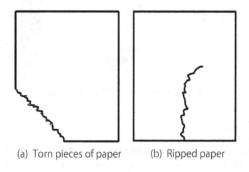

(a) Torn pieces of paper   (b) Ripped paper

Fig. 3. Working Error Examples

3   Results

3.1   EEG Measurement for Fatigue Survey

Although previous findings regarding EEG measurements, fatigue survey and work time have been covered, a summary of the results are listed [7]. The EEG results measured the degree of attentiveness and meditation. We observed the levels of attentiveness in each room.   The results revealed that attentiveness was greatest in the bamboo room. The clay room was the second highest, followed by the wallpaper room. The level of attentiveness declined during work when compared to the "resting" level of all subjects. The attentiveness observed in the bamboo charcoal board room was significantly higher than the clay wall and wallpaper rooms. The meditation degree was highest in the wallpaper room, followed by the clay wall room and lastly, the bamboo charcoal board room.

The meditation degree in the clay wall-room indicated a significantly higher rate than the wallpaper and bamboo charcoal rooms.   And the degree of meditation in the bamboo charcoal room was significantly higher than wallpaper room.

The average time worked in all rooms was 2 hours, 6 minutes and 43 seconds. The average time worked in the bamboo charcoal room was 2 hours and 43 seconds. The wallpaper room was 2 hours, 3 minutes and 24 seconds and the clay wall room averaged 2 hours, 16 minutes and 2 seconds. The least amount of hours worked were observed in the bamboo charcoal board room. The fatigue level tendency was shown to increase in all rooms, especially the wallpaper room. A significant degree of complaints of "local pain or dullness" were expressed in the wall paper room.

3.2   Work Time, Total Number of Sorted Papers, Number of Ripped Papers and Torn Papers

Table 2 shows the aggregated results from hours worked per subject, the number of sorted papers, and the number of torn pieces of paper and ripped paper.   Based on this data, we found a correlation among error occurrence, working time and working efficiency by each subject.

Table 2. Result of Worke Time, Total Number of Sorted Paper, Number of Ripped Papers, and Torn Paper of each Subject

Wall material	Subjects	Work time hh:mm:ss	Total number of sorted paper	Total number of ripped paper	Total number of torn paper
Wall paper	B	1:31:41	467	0	2
	C	2:26:12	339	23	9
	F	1:03:53	603	2	3
	G	3:10:29	1522	197	5
	H	2:17:46	811	5	0
Clay wall	B	2:14:53	437	15	0
	D	1:47:12	501	8	5
	E	1:27:41	382	0	1
	F	1:13:05	828	6	1
	G	3:57:17	1804	2	5
	H	2:32:24	943	50	2
Bamboo charcoal board	A	2:05:49	416	3	0
	B	1:27:11	478	11	0
	C	2:18:43	491	6	1
	D	1:29:48	439	9	0
	F	1:12:37	905	29	1
	G	3:16:28	536	49	0
	I	2:04:15	1268	42	8

3.3   Correlation between Work Time and Error

We normalized the number of errors according to the total number of sorted paper per each subject. In the wallpaper room, the subject who worked a long period of time showed a high tendency to make errors. However, in the bamboo charcoal room and the clay wall room, the tendency to make errors declined. All the samples were in the range of three sigma.

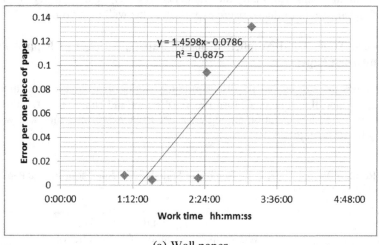

(a) Wall paper

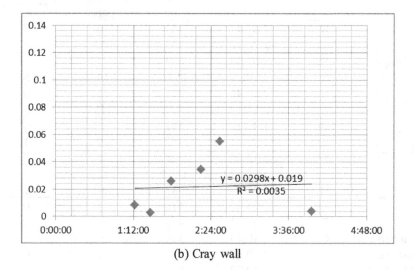

(b) Cray wall

Fig. 4. Correlation between Work Time and Error per One Piece of Paper

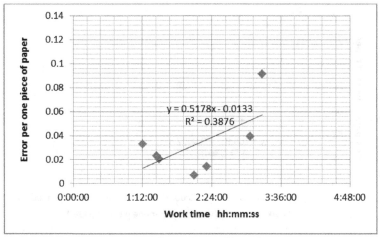

(c) Bamboo charcoal board

Fig. 4. (*Continued.*)

3.4   Correlation between Work Efficiency and Error Per One Piece of Paper

The work efficiency was calculated by dividing the total number of sorted paper, which is the time required for sorting one piece of paper. In either room, the subjects with low working efficiency, which means a long working time, showed a high tendency towards error occurrence. However, all subjects showed only a weak correlation, and a significant difference was not observed. All the samples were in the range of three sigma.

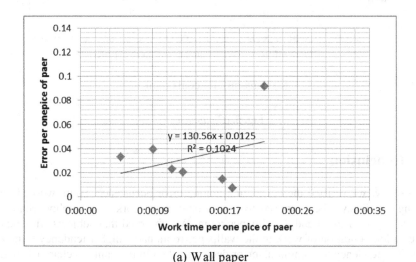

(a) Wall paper

Fig. 5. Correlation between Work Efficiency and Error per each Paper

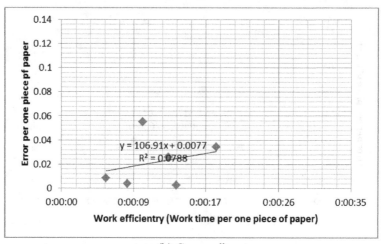

(b) Cray wall

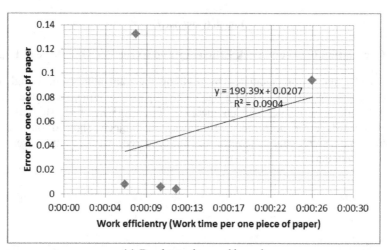

(c) Bamboo charcoal board

Fig. 5. (*Continued.*)

4   Conclusion

In this study, we verified the correlation among error occurrence, hours worked and working efficiency when exposed to long monotonous work in a bamboo charcoal room, a clay wall room and a wallpaper room. We observed that subjects who experienced a long duration of work in the wallpaper room had a higher tendency to make errors. The tendency to commit an error declined when in the bamboo charcoal room, followed by the clay wall room. The correlation between error occurrence and work efficiency was weak in all rooms. And no significant differences per each wall material were observed. Our research suggests a room with bamboo charcoal walls could possibly reduce the amount of error when exposed to long monotonous work. We believe we need to further our study to reveal more findings.

References

1. Kuroda, A., Ishibashi: Analysis of human factor. Japan Industrial Safety & Health Association, pp. 38–39 (2006)
2. Wargocki, P.: The Effects of Outdoor Air Supply Rate in an Office on Perceived Air Quality, Sick Building Syndrome (SBS) Symptoms and Productivity. Indoor Air 2000, 10 (2000)
3. Kimura, M., Mori, T., Suzuki, H., Endo, S., Kawano, K.: EEG Changes in Odor Effects after the Stress of Long Monotonous Work. Journal of International Society of Life Information Science 19(2), 271–278 (2001)
4. Iwasaki, H., Kamiyama, T., Tawata, T.: Cigarette Smoke Adsorption-Emission Characteristics of Mud Wall. Summaries of Technical Papers of Annual Meeting Architectural Institute of Japan 2006, 933–934 (2006)
5. Asada, T., Ishihara, S., Yamane, T., et al.: Science of Bamboo Charcoal: Study on Carbonizing Temperature of Bamboo Charcoal and Removal Capability of Harmful Gases. Journal of Health Science 48(6), 473–479 (2002)
6. Harikae, N., Inadomi, K., Sakai, Y., et al.: Changes of peripheral skin blood flow and skin temperature of healthy humans with using a bamboo charcoal bedding. Bulletin of the School of Nursing Yamaguchi Prefectural University 7, 89–92 (2003)
7. Takai, Y., Goto, A., Takao, K., et al.: A Pilot Study Investigating the Impact of Indoor Wall Construction on Performance during Long Monotonous Work. In: Proceedings of the Human Factors and Ergonomics Society 57Th Annual Meeting 2013, pp. 516–520 (2013)

Comparative Study on the Feature of Kitchen Knife Sharpening Skill between Expert and Non-Expert

Yuka Takai[1,*], Masahiko Yamada[1], Akihiko Goto[1], Wang Zelong[2], and Akira Ii[3]

[1] Osaka Sangyo University, Department of Information Systems Engineering, Japan
gotoh@ise.osaka-sandai.ac.jp
[2] Kyoto Institute of Technology, Advanced Fibro-Science, Japan
simon.zelongwang@gmail.com
[3] Kyoto Culinary Art College, Japan
iakira@taiwa.ac.jp

Abstract. Sharpening is one of basic culinary for a cook. In this study, 10 experts and 10 non-experts from Kyoto culinary art college were employed to investigate the gesture of sharpening. The feature of processing was recorded and summarized by a force plate and two cameras. All participants' main movement elements were counted and summarized. The most representative subjects of expert and non-expert in each type were observed and analyzed by Digital Microscopy. The movement gesture performing with right hand deeply holding the knife was the recommended knife position.

Keywords: Sharpening, Expert, Non-Expert, Gesture.

1   Introduction

Sharpening is one of the basic culinary skills you must get a good knowledge in order to be a successful and serious cook. Generally, the beginners have to receive detailed sharpening related training and experience in the cooking college before be-coming a formal internship in restaurant. There are a lot of experienced cooks teaching sharpening technology in cooking college, who had formed their own super technique during long cooking work. However, nearly all of sharpening skill and knowledge were passed to beginners by oral teaching and action imitation. Therefore it is very difficult for most of beginners to master and duplicate those excellent skills. They have to take considerable time and effort to practice sharpening again and again with the aid of indescribable motion perceiving.

In the ancient period, numbers of old craftsmen sought various ways to head to Kyoto for serving the Emperor so as to improve their skill. There is no exception in cooking occupation. Kyoto cuisine is one of representative Japanese dishes (Fig.1) combined taste and delicate design together. Achieving a high-quality sophistical Kyoto cuisine, cooks pursued to prepare the food material with remarkable cutting techniques basically. Therefore, mastering good knowledge with knife is a critical

---

* Corresponding author.

V.G. Duffy (Ed.): DHM 2014, LNCS 8529, pp. 292–300, 2014.

step for becoming a successful cook and fulfilling a good taste and delicate assigned dish. Furthermore, a good Kitchen knife sharpening skill is particularly important for Kyoto cuisine. Usually, kitchen knife sharpening operation is taught by real practice and oral explanation in cooking colleges during training. However, it is very difficult for the students to catch the key technical point of sharpening motion only based on teachers' demonstration. In other words, scientific understanding for expert's kitchen knife sharpening is urgent and useful in the real teaching application.

By far, some studies were conducted related to mastery knowledge of the kitchen knife employment. Hayashi et al. clarified the different cutting motion for cucumber and carrot by three-dimensional motion capture system. Niikawa et al. investigated sound effects' stimulation on manipulation skill of the slicing of the cucumber at the constant distance. Hoshi et al. showed appropriate learning time for the kitchen knife skill from the primary schoolchildren. However there were little literatures which focused on kitchen knife sharpening skill. Akaike et al. paid attention to perturbation influence on the rhythmical movement of kitchen knife sharpening. In previous work, we have already demonstrated sharpening motion, muscle activity by expert cooks during the sharpening process.

In current research, 10 teachers and 10 students from cooking colleges were employed as expert and non-expert investigated subjects respectively. A single edged Yanagiba knife(Japanese sashimi knife) was selected as exclusive subject. All participators' press force directly beneath the knife during the whole sharpening process was measured by reaction force plate in the z (vertical) directions. All tested motion process of sharpening was recorded by 2 digital video cameras. Experts and non-experts' finger location and gesture for holding and pressing the knife during sharpening were focused. That phenomenon was applied to distinguish expert and non-expert's process each other well and clarify the reflected force trace and force differences. And after sharpening process, cross-section of knife's edge was embedded and observed by optical microscope. As a result, a lot of jagged edges were existed in the kitchen knife sharpened by expert cooks. It can be considered that experts pushed the kitchen knife against a whetstone with a steady rhythm under bigger power and also employed larger whetstone surface.

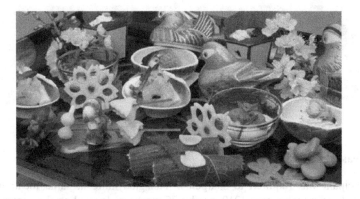

Fig. 1. Kyoto cuisine-representative Japanese dish

The purpose of this study was to clarify the main difference of sharpening gesture between expert and non-expert through numeric measurement and analysis the effect of knife's edge by microscopy. Base on this study, our final goal is to establish self-study tool system to help students to train the sharpening skill.

2   Experiments

2.1   Participants

10 teachers and 10 students from Kyoto culinary art college were employed as expert and non-expert respectively. As shown in Tab.1, average sharpening experience of expert was more than 19 years. There are two experts have more than 30 years sharpening experience. Average experience of non-expert was shorter than 1.3 years.

Table 1. A summary of participants' sharpening experience

Expert	A	B	C	D	E	F	G	H	I	J
Years	36	30	26	25	20	14	13	13	11	5
Non-expert	a	b	c	d	e	f	g	h	i	j
Years	3	2	1	1	1	1	1	1	1	1

2.2   Subject

24-centimeter-long Japanese Yanagiba knives were selected to proceed this experiment as shown in Fig.3, which was normally used to slice the sashimi. (Yagi Chubo-kiki Seishakusyo Inc.) Twenty Yanagiba knives with similar level of blunt were prepared for following sharpening tests.

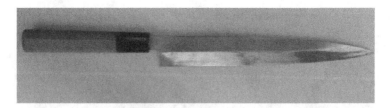

Fig. 2. Japanese Yanagiba knife

2.3   Measurement Setting

Each participant was required to sharpen a Yanagiba knife at same location for 30 seconds. A diamond whetstone (210 mm by 75 mm) was located on the center of force plate (TF-3020-A, Tec Gihan Co., Ltd.). At the same time, reaction force was measured by Force plate and recorded in the x (transverse), y (front-back) and z (vertical) direction as shown in Fig.3. The movements of participants were recorded by two cameras during the overall sharpening process. One was located in front of force plate, and the other one was located on the force plate's side direction which illustrated in Fig.4.

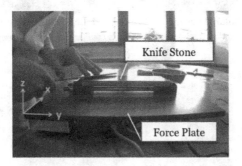

Fig. 3. Testing apparatus

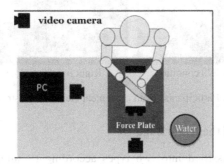

Fig. 4. Testing environment

2.4   Processing Investigation

Participants' main movement elements were counted and summarized by watching the video. The gesture of right hand holding the knife shallowly or deeply was judged according to the little thumb grip on the handle as shown in Fig.5.a. Pressure of right hand's middle finger on the edge of apart from knife blade surface or not was recognized as Fig.5.f. On the left hand, finger numbers and crossed finger pattern pressed on the knife like Fig.5.b & e were also chose the parameter. Additionally, lumbrical muscle's condition and wrist located direction were focused and illustrated in Fig.5.c and Fig.5.d respectively.

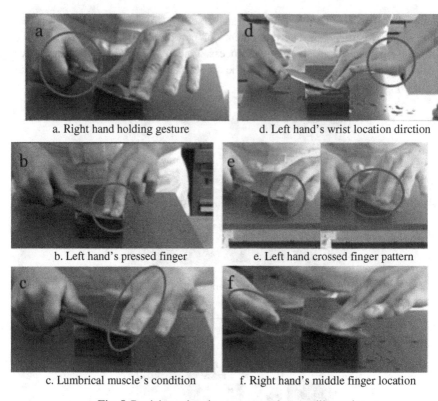

a. Right hand holding gesture   d. Left hand's wrist location dirction

b. Left hand's pressed finger   e. Left hand crossed finger pattern

c. Lumbrical muscle's condition   f. Right hand's middle finger location

Fig. 5. Participants' main movement elements illustration

2.5   Observation of the Knife Edge

The subjects were classified into two types according to summarize participants' sharpening movement elements. The most representative subjects of expert and non-expert in each type were observed and analyzed by Digital Microscopy (VHX-900, KEYENCE). Knife edge from blade top-point to predetermined distance (named as " I ", " II " and "III" region) was observed by reflection microscope which displayed in Fig.6.

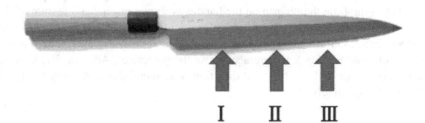

I   II   III

Fig. 6. Observation region along the knife edge

3   Results and Discussions

3.1   Process Analysis Results

Every participant's real movement elements for both hands were obtained and sum-marized according to the characteristic elements illustrated in Fig.7. According to participants' right hand holding knife gesture (shallowly or deeply), tested partici-pants were divided into two categories. One was performed as right hand held knife handle deeply accompanied with its fingers gripped around the handle, called as "Type 1". The other operation category was shallowly holding knife handle by right hand cooperated with little finger wrapping the handle, which was considered as "Type 2".

According to Fig.7's classification flow chart, it is notified to find most of experts performed the movement posture of "Type 1" classification. Additionally, there were half of experts sharpening the knife with the same gesture. Their right hand held knife deeply and index finger also gripped around the handle. The thumb and lumbrical muscle of left hand applied the pressure on knife blade and the wrist always kept straight direction. Experts employed "Type 1" movement posture by adjusting their pressed finger number and gesture to achieve a most suitable sharpening technique during knife sharpening process personally. But only two experts put their right index finger on the knife edge opposite to blade side. In general, most of participants used lumbrical muscle and more than 2 fingers pressed on the blade.

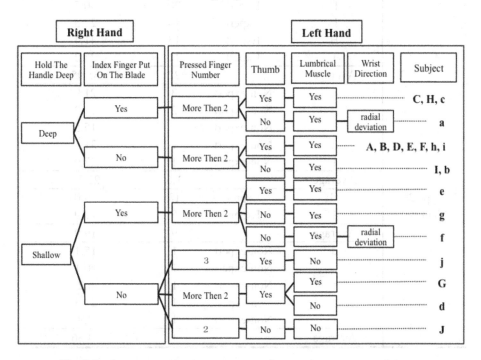

Fig. 7. Real movement element summary and comparison among participants

All the participants' detail information were divided into two types and gathered in Tab.2. Both expert and non-expert's average years of experience in "Type 1" were longer than "Type 2". The expert and non-expert's average years of "Type 1" were 22 years and 1.6 years, which longer than "Type 2" with around 12 years and 0.6 year correspondingly. Among of "Type 1", there were five experts' experience more than 20 years, and two experts' experiences showed more than 30 years. In the contrast, only two experts with 13 and 5 years of experience grouped into "Type 2". Referring to the comparison between "Type 1" and "Type 2", it was deserve to find that the average down force values of expert and non-expert of "Type 1" were almost higher than "Type 2". In an overall view, it can be considered that the gesture of "Type 1" was more suitable for sharpening the knife than "Type 2" as the people can push up the knife easily by holding knife deeply.

Table 2. Participants' testing results comparison related to experience

Type	Participant	Experience	Year	Down Force(N)
Type 1 (Deep)	A	Expert	36	29.0
	B	Expert	30	35.9
	C	Expert	26	41.8
	D	Expert	25	46.5
	E	Expert	20	40.5
	F	Expert	14	27.3
	H	Expert	13	41.4
	I	Expert	11	25.2
	Average		22	35.95
	a	Non-expert	3	21.9
	b	Non-expert	2	17.2
	c	Non-expert	1	15.5
	h	Non-expert	1	31.3
	i	Non-expert	1	27.0
	Average		1.6	22.58
Type 2 (Shallow)	G	Expert	13	19.0
	J	Expert	5	17.9
	Average		9	19.9
	d	Non-expert	1	15.1
	e	Non-expert	1	20.1
	f	Non-expert	1	5.2
	g	Non-expert	1	22.5
	j	Non-expert	1	8.9
	Average		1	14.36

3.2   Knife Blade Edge Observation

As displayed in Fig.8 a & b, three different positions' photos of most representative case for expert and non-expert in "Type 1" classification were taken by digital camera. It was easily to note that the knife's edge by expert in "Type 1" system presented the significant zigzag appearance. Normally, serrated blade is considered to be qualified for heavy task and precision cutting. The photos of non-expert were shown a slight toothed appearance and a straight trend. Relatively, the photos of digital microscopy by expert and non-expert in "Type 2" were illustrated in Fig.8 c & d. Both of them presented a smooth edge trend without toothed structure. The blade edge of expert was show mild slope rather than a straight blade edge for non-expert. It is considered that the gesture of "Type 1" was more beneficial to grind the knife sharp with zigzag shape.

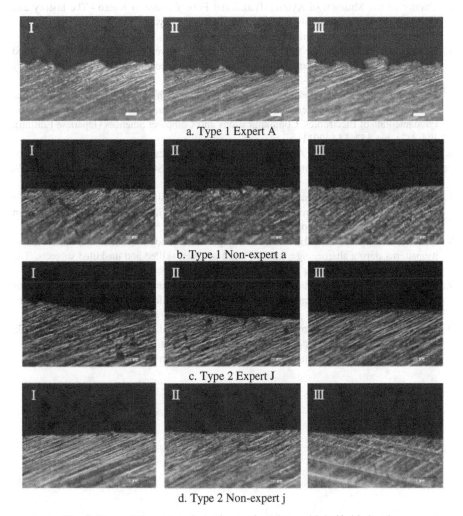

a. Type 1 Expert A

b. Type 1 Non-expert a

c. Type 2 Expert J

d. Type 2 Non-expert j

Fig. 8. Three different locations observation along with knife blade edge

4   Conclusions

In a word, movement gesture performing with right hand deeply holding the knife was a very important procedure during sharpening process as it can sharpen the knife sharp with serrated margin. Furthermore, right fingers grip on the knife handle cooperated with all right hand's fingers grasp the handle together, the left wrist keep straight direction and the thumb, lumbrical muscle of left hand put pressure on the blade are all the key movement elements for sharpening process.

References

1. Kadokami, T.: Kyo-ryouri oagariyasu, 1st edn. Kozaido (2001)
2. Curator of the Museum of Kyoto.: Traditional Food Culture in Kyoto –The history and charm of Kyoto cuisine and vegetables. The Museum of Kyoto (2006)
3. Shibata, S.: Houtyou to toishi. Shibata Shoten (1999)
4. Hayashi, T., Yanagisawa, Y.: Comparison of the movement of knives cutting food between expertsand non-experts by motion analysis techniques. Journal of Cookery Science of Japan 37(3), 299–305 (2004)
5. Niikawa, T., Andachi, S., Nakamura, M., Hagino, C., Onishi, K., Hisaki, K.: The Influence of Pacing Sounds on Mastery of Edge Cutting Technique. The IEICE Transactions on Fundamentals of Electronics, Communications and Computer Sciences (Japanese Edition), J94-A(7), pp. 552–554 (2011)
6. Hoshi, S., Nishikawa, Y.: A Study on Systematic Education to Master the Basics of Cooking. Focusing on Cutting Skills. Studies in Teaching Strategies Ibaraki University 29, 111–120 (2010)
7. Akaike, T., Ohgi, Y., Yasumura, M.: Perturbation Analysis of Coordinative Structure on Knife Grinding Task. In: Proceedings of Symposium on Sports Engineering, Symposium on Human Dynamics 2006, pp. 199–204 (2006)
8. Shirato, M., Miyamoto, N., Hamada, A.: Comparison of body movement and muscle activity patterns during sharpening a kitchen knife between skilled and unskilled subjects. The Journal of Science of Labour 83(4), 139–150 (2007)
9. Miyamoto, N., Shirato, M., Hamada, A.: A kinematic and electromyographic study of skill acquisition for sharpening a Japanese kitchen knife. The Journal of Science of Labour 84(3), 89–98 (2008)
10. Kawasaki, T., Ii, A., Nishimura, Y., Shirato, M., Hamada, A., Nakai, A., Yoshida, T.: Relationship Between the Edge Shape and Sensory Evaluation of Japanese Kitchen Knives Sharpened by Experts. Journal of Cookery Science of Japan 42(2), 123–128 (2009)

Visual Behavior in a Japanese Drum Performance of *Gion* Festival Music

Katsuma Yamada, Masaru Ohgiri, Takashi Furukawa, Hisanori Yuminaga,
Akihiko Goto, Noriyuki Kida, and Hiroyuki Hamada

Kyoto Institute of Technology, Kyoto, Japan
haagen-kattsu@nike.eonet.ne.jp, summersoniclove@yahoo.co.jp,
t-furukawa@hishiken.co.jp, {hhamada,kida}@kit.ac.jp
Kansai Vocational College of Medicine, Osaka, Japan
yuminaga@kansai.ac.jp
Osaka Sangyo University, Osaka, Japan
gotoh@ise.osaka-sandai.ac.jp

Abstract. The purpose of this study was to focus on the gaze shift in a coordinated musical performance and experimentally clarify its role in the matched timing of the players. To summarize the results obtained in the present study, (1) the number of gaze shifts for the expert was less than that for the non-expert; (2) the expert's gaze shifts decreased significantly at the moment of a beat; (3) the expert did not turn his gaze on the drum surface, but turned his gaze between his drum and the opposite person's drum; and (4) the percentages of gaze location on the drum surface of the self and the drum surface of the opposite person were higher in the case of the non-expert.

Keywords: Gaze, percentages of gaze location areas, Expert, Non-expert.

1 Introduction

The "Gion Festival," which is considered to be one of Japan's three greatest festivals, is said to have begun in AD 869 in order to assuage an infectious disease that was prevalent in Kyoto at that time. When Kyoto City was devastated by the Onin War that broke out in the Muromachi period (15 century), the Gion Festival also stopped. However, citizens that later become more prosperous revived the festival. The parade of luxuriously and splendidly decorated floats, Yama-Hoko, is believed to have reached its present form around the same period, and the original style of Ohayashi (Japanese orchestras) called the Gion Festival Music is also said to have originated around this time. Of the 33 Yama-Hoko floats that currently paraded, 12 floats perform the Gion Festival Music, and the Yama-Hoko event of Kyoto Gion Festival was registered as an Intangible Cultural Heritage by UNESCO in 2009 (Figure 1).

The origin of the *Gion* Festival Music is considered to be the *Dengaku* Dance and *Rokusai Nenbutsu* Dance of the Medieval Period, but it is said that *Noh* and *Kyogen* also had a great influence on this dance, and that *Ohayashi*, incorporating a loud and cheerful gong (*Sho*) from the elegant spirit was established. The *Gion* Festival Music

V.G. Duffy (Ed.): DHM 2014, LNCS 8529, pp. 301–310, 2014.
© Springer International Publishing Switzerland 2014

is characterized by the sound of gong, "*konchikichin*," and consists of three types of instruments, including the gong that beats a rhythm, the flute that carries the melody, and the drum that controls the tempo. The *Gion* Festival Music players are known as "*Hayashi-Kata*." Since each instrument is played by multiple *Hayashi-Kata* simultaneously, not only the high performance technique of each player, but also matching of the players' timing is required. In some music pieces of the *Gion* Festival Music, the speed of the music gradually changes, or sometimes nothing is played for several seconds in the middle of a piece, which can be very difficult to perform.

When multiple players perform together, the players need to adjust their timing by communicating with each other. A study on joint musical performances quantified the gap in timing between 2 piano players. Another study measured eye movements in a joint performances. When visual information is collected, an eye movement occurs to visually search the object or target area that contains necessary information and to capture the image of the object with the central retinal fovea. Eye movements in motion can be objectively observed, using a head mounted eye tracker, even if head movements are not restricted. A great deal of research on these shifts in the gaze has been conducted in the fields of music, including singing and playing instruments: It has been demonstrated that the scope of pre-reading a musical score, frequency of gaze fixation, and area of fixation are determined in relation to the phrases, chords, and counterpoint [1-8], and there are also studies that have examined joint violin performances.

However, with regard to performances that are passed down through oral tradition without musical scores and rules for the tempo, such as the *Gion* Festival Music, no research to date has studied the role of gaze shifts while playing from the viewpoint of timing adjustment. Therefore, the purpose of this study was to focus on the gaze shift in a coordinated musical performance and experimentally clarify its role in the matched timing of the players.

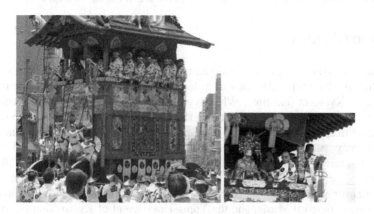

Fig. 1. Gion Festival (Kanko-Hoko)

2   Methods

2.1   Participants

Participants were 2 drum-*kata* (drum players) who belonged to the *Kanko-Hoko* Preservation Society. One of them was a 26-year-old male who had 21 years of experience in the *Gion* Festival Music with 5 years of drum experience, and the other participant was a 52-year-old male who had 42 years of experience in the *Gion* Festival Music with 34 years of drum experience. Although the former participant is a drummer at the *Gion* Festival, his 5 years of experience was the shortest of the drum-*kata* at the Festival. Therefore, he was treated as a non-expert, as opposed to the latter participant who was considered an expert. The participants had normal vision (20/20 vision or better, or corrected eyesight). We obtained the participants' informed consent prior to the experiment.

2.2   Experiment

In order to re-create the actual environment of the festival as far as possible, the experiment was conducted in *Kanko-Hoko* Building of the *Kanko-Hoko* Preservation Society that is used as a practice space by festival musicians. Practice drums were used, and 4 drum-*kata*, 8 flute-*kata*, and 10 gong-*kata* were arranged so that the situation would be identical to actual practice (Figure 2). Similar to a real performance, participants were to play face to face in Drum Position 4 (See Figure 2), so that they would be able to recognize each other's body motion.

A series of music pieces with a relatively slow tempo called "*Debayashi*," which are played on *Sijo-Dori*, the first main street of the *Yama-Hoko* parade in *Gion* Festival, were used in the experiment. The six music pieces, "*Komatsu*," "*Kagura*," "*Karako*,""*Hakusan*," "*Jibayashi*," and "*Waka*" were played continuously in that order, and *Komatsu* was analyzed.

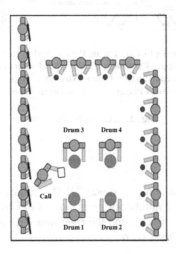

Fig. 2. Experimental environment

2.3   Acquisition and Processing of Gaze Data

Eye Mark Recorder (EMR-8, made by NAC, Tokyo) with a sampling rate of 60 fps recorded the eye movements of the participants. The viewing angle of Eye Mark Recorder was 90 degrees. The participants mounted the Eye Mark camera on their heads. A nine-point calibration was performed prior to the start of the experiment.

The gaze from the beginning till the end of the piece "*Komatsu*" was analyzed. Areas of gaze location were obtained using frame-by-frame analysis. The areas of gaze location were categorized into three major sections, "the self," "opposite person," and "others" (Figure 3). Furthermore, the self was divided into three subcategories: "right upper extremity," "left upper extremity," and "drum surface;" the opposite person was divided into 5 subcategories: "Face," "right upper extremity," "left upper extremity," "trunk," and "drum surface;" and other was grouped into 3 subcategories: "between players," "outside of players," and "between drums." In addition, we visually obtained the time when the stick hit the drum surface, using video footage.

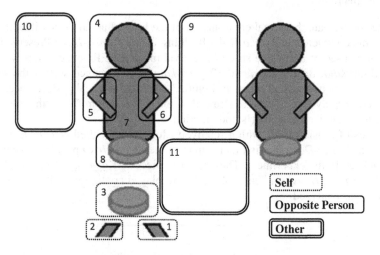

Areas 1 to 3 are Self, Areas 4 to 8 are Facing Person, and Areas 9 to 11 are Other.
Subcategories: 1 Right Upper Extremity, 2 Left Upper Extremity, 3 Drum Surface, 4
Face, 5 Right Upper Extremity, 6 Left Upper Extremity, 7 Trunk, 8 Drum Surface, 9
Between Players, 10 Outside of Players, and 11 Between Drums.

Fig. 3. Areas to be analyzed

3   Results

The performance time of the non-expert was 248.0 seconds, whereas that of the expert was 258.8 seconds. The total number of beats was 64 (45 by the right hand and 19 by the left hand). The number of beats and the right-and-left order of beating were identical for the non-expert and the expert.

3.1   Number of Gaze Shifts

The number of gaze shifts in the areas of gaze location for the non-expert was 301, whereas it was 76 for the expert. The mean time that a gaze remained in a certain area of gaze location was 0.82 second with a standard deviation of 1.02 seconds for the non-expert, whereas the mean time was 3.36 seconds with a standard deviation of 4.55 seconds for the expert.

Figure 4 shows the total number of gaze shifts that occurred every 15 frames (250 ms) during 2 seconds around the beat time. When the numbers before and after the beat were compared, the non-expert shifted his gaze more often after the beat than before, in particular, between 0.75 second and 1.0 second after the beat. On the other hand, the expert shifted his gaze more frequently before the beat, particularly between 1.0 second and 0.5 second before the beat. Additionally, the number of gaze shifts by the expert was considerably low during 0.5 second around the beat time.

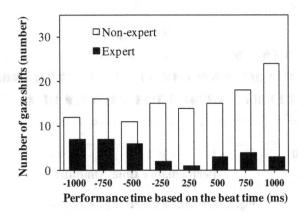

Fig. 4. Numbers of gaze shifts based on the beat time

3.2   Percentage of Gaze Location

Figure 5 shows the areas of gaze location and the beat times during the entire performance in chronological order. The results of calculating the percentages of gaze location by area (Figure 6, Table 1) for the non-expert indicated that the percentages of time in which his gaze was on the self, on the opposite person, and on Other areas were approximately 40%, 45%, and 15% of the total, respectively. During the first minute from the start of performance, gaze on the opposite person and other was observed frequently, and gaze on the self was more often observed after the first minute. When we focused on the subcategories of the areas, he turned his gaze particularly on drum surface of self and opposite person, and the percentage of time in which his gaze was on the drum surface was more than 60% of the total.

In contrast, in the case of the expert, the percentage of time in which his gaze was on the self and the opposite person were 12% and 2%, respectively, and his gaze was on the Other areas over 85% of the time. His gaze was most often on other areas, consistently from the start of the performance, and his gaze shifted to the opposite person only a few times. With regard to the subcategories of areas, his gaze was particularly focused on the drum surface, on the self and on the opposite person, similar to the non-expert; however, the percentage of time in which his gaze was on the drum surface was a little less than 15% of the total. As for the other area, the expert's gaze was between drums, which accounted for over 85% of the total.

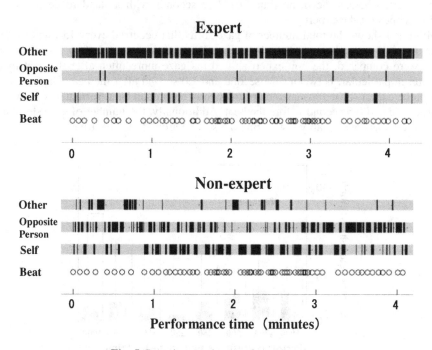

Fig. 5. Beat times and areas of gaze location

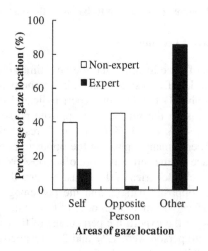

Fig. 6. Comparisons of percentages of gaze location

Table 1. Percentages of gaze location by area (%)

	Non-expert	Expert
Right Upper Extremity	4.2	0.4
Left Upper Extremity	1.6	0.0
Drum Surface	33.9	11.7
Self	**39.7**	**12.0**
Face	2.3	0.0
Right Upper Extremity	6.0	0.0
Left Upper Extremity	4.1	0.0
Trunk	3.5	0.2
Drum Surface	29.6	2.0
Opposite Person	**45.5**	**2.1**
Between Players	8.8	0.0
Outside of Players	6.1	0.0
Between Drums	0.0	85.8
Other	**14.9**	**85.8**

3.3   Time-Series of Gaze Location

Figure 7 shows the percentages of gaze location areas for all 64 beats per frame around the beat time. In comparison to the expert, the non-expert was more likely to turn his gaze on the self between 1.0 seconds and 0.7 seconds before the beat. Then the percentage of his gaze on the opposite person increased once, but the percentage gaze on the self again rose immediately before the beat. His gaze on the self gradually decreased after the beat, while that on the opposite person increased, and these proportions were reversed 0.8 second after the beat.

On the other hand, the expert's gaze was on the self approximately 20% of the 64 beats 1 second before the beat. However, its percentage decreased when approaching the beat time and was reduced to about 10% at the beat time. Moreover, the percentage of his gaze on the self was at the lowest point, 0.3 seconds after the beat. Furthermore, gaze location on the opposite person was not observed after 0.5 seconds before the beat.

Figure 8 compares the percentages of gaze location areas for the right-and-left-hand beats between the expert and the non-expert. When the drum was beaten with the right hand, gaze location on the self was more common than was the case when the drum was beaten with the left hand. This was true for both the expert and the non-expert, and this tendency was particularly notable for the non-expert.

In the case of the non-expert beating the drum with his left hand, his gaze location on the self increased from 1 second before the beat, whereas the percentage of his gaze on the self tended to decrease when beating the drum with his right hand. Additionally, gaze location on the self was not observed between 0.1 second before- and 0.6 second after a left hand beat in the case of the expert.

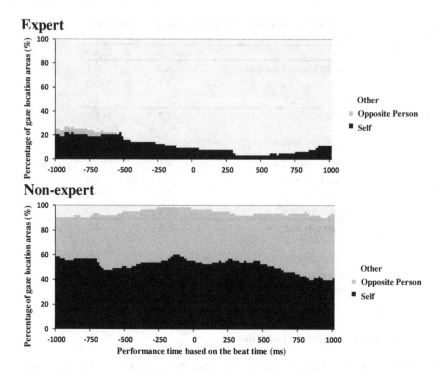

Fig. 7. Time series variation of percentage of gaze location areas

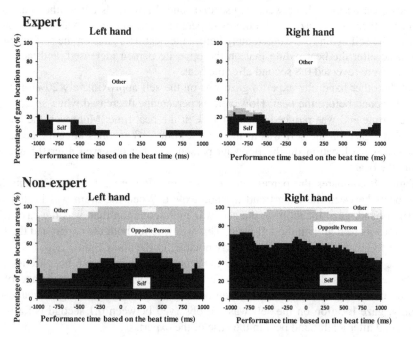

Fig. 8. Percentage of gaze location areas for the right-and-left hand beats

4   Discussion

The performance time of the non-expert was approximately 95% that of the expert, which was about 10 seconds shorter. This is probably because there is no conductor in *Gion* Festival Music, and the tempo of musical pieces is not prescribed, therefore the performance time varies depending on the player. In the actual *Yama-Hoko* parade, as a large number of *Yama-Hoko* floats parade in order, the speed of the advancing procession differs every year, depending on the condition of the floats in front and behind. Thus, it is thought that the tempo of musical pieces is loosely prescribed in order to adjust the length of each piece according to the time required for the parade. Therefore, although there was a difference in the length of time of the performance between the participants, by approximately 10 seconds, it was about a 5% difference and we were determined to analyze it, because it could be compared.

To summarize the results obtained in the present study, (1) the number of gaze shifts for the expert was less than that for the non-expert; (2) the expert's gaze shifts decreased significantly at the moment of a beat; (3) the expert did not turn his gaze on the drum surface, but turned his gaze between his drum and the opposite person's drum; and (4) the percentages of gaze location on the drum surface of the self and the drum surface of the opposite person were higher in the case of the non-expert.

As for the expert, the number of gaze shifts was low, which decreased considerably around the beat time. Moreover, the area of gaze location was on between rums. Therefore, the expert is assumed to have been playing the drum using visual information obtained by peripheral vision. On the other hand, the number of gaze shifts was very high for the non-expert, and the area of gaze location was often on the drum surface of the self; thus, he is assumed to have obtained visual information regarding the beat location mainly by central vision. It seems that the non-expert frequently turned his gaze on the self in order to confirm the position of drum surface so that the stick would hit the surface, as well as to confirm the movement of his raised stick.

In contrast, because the expert had acquired a highly refined performance technique for beating the drum, he did not need to confirm the beat location, or his motions by using his gaze, he was able to perform without looking at the self, or the drum surface. This is the automation of the beating technique, and it seems that when the player has room to turn his/her gaze on things other than the self, he/she can pay attention so as to match timing with other drum-*kata*, flute-*kata*, and gong-*kata*. However, in this experiment, neither the expert nor the non-expert turned his gaze on flute-*kata*, or gong-*kata*. One reasons for this might be that the experiment was conducted immediately after the *Gion* Festival, and there was a long time before next year's Festival. In other words, it was likely to be the time for them to practice basic drum beating techniques and coordination among drum-*kata* above all, rather than with flute-*kata* and gong-*kata*.

Furthermore, the non-expert frequently turned his gaze on the drum surface of the opposite person. In the drum performance of the *Gion* Festival Music, the tempo of a musical pieces is not prescribed, but the drum players need to beat by matching the timing with others. Therefore, it is inferred that the percentage of gaze location on the drum surface of opposite person was high, so as to measure the timing of the other players.

5   Conclusion

To summarize the results obtained in the present study, (1) the number of gaze shifts for the expert was less than that for the non-expert; (2) the expert's gaze shifts decreased significantly at the moment of a beat; (3) the expert did not turn his gaze on the drum surface, but turned his gaze between his drum and the opposite person's drum; and (4) the percentages of gaze location on the drum surface of the self and the drum surface of the opposite person were higher in the case of the non-expert. The present study focused on visual information processing, and examined the characteristics of coordinated performance of drum-*kata*, by comparing an expert and a non-expert, by using data from an Eye Mark Recorder. Thus, it was not possible to investigate the relationship between expertise and performance, such as the gap in the timing of a beat and the strength of a beat. By evaluating the relationship between performance and body motions and sounds, in addition to visual information, it would be possible to further clarify coordination of drum performances that are conducted without using musical scores.

References

1. Kawasaki, T.: Eye movements of sight reading and musical expertise. Mie University Kiyo Kyoiku 33, 49–66 (1982)
2. Banton, L.J.: The role of visual and auditory feedback during the sight-reading of music. Psychology of Music 23(1), 3–16 (1995)
3. Lehmann, A.C., Ericsson, K.A.: Performance without preparation: structure and acquisition of expert sight-reading and accompanying performance. Psychomusicology 15, 1–29 (1996)
4. Lehmann, A.C., McArthur, V.: Sight-reading. The Science and Psychology of Music Performance, 135–150 (2002)
5. Goolsby, T.W.: Profiles of processing: eye movements during sightreading. Music Perception 12, 97–123 (1994)
6. Sloboda, J.A.: The eye-hand span: an approach to the study of sight reading. Psychology of Music 2, 4–10 (1974)
7. Sloboda, J.A.: Visual perception of memory. Quarterly Journal of Experimental Psychology 28, 1–16 (1976)
8. Waters, A.J., Underwood, G., Findlay, J.M.: Studying expertise in music reading: use of a pattern matching paradigm. Perception & Psychophysics 59, 477–488 (1997)

Advances in Healthcare

Understanding and Facilitating the Communication Process among Healthcare Professionals

Janaina Cintra Abib[1,2], André Bueno[1], and Junia Anacleto[1]

[1] Federal University of São Carlos - São Carlos/SP, Brazil
[2] Federal Institute of São Paulo - Araraquara/SP, Brazil
janaina@ifsp.edu.br,
{andre.obueno,junia}@dc.ufscar.br

Abstract. We present a system for e-health considering natural user interactions for mobile through analysis of healthcare professionals' activities. The healthcare professionals have to manager patients´ care and their activities, take notes of all of them and share information. Communication between healthcare professionals is carried out through notations on paper, verbally and sometimes through messages by mobile. These procedures make the communication process inefficient and slow. We studied the relation between healthcare professionals, how they interacting and how they communicate in a hospital to propose a better way of communication, supported by technology. The analysis of activities ensured that the needs of the healthcare professionals were hit and the routine of these professionals was maintained, making this interaction more natural. This experiments show us how the healthcare professionals communicate themselves, to do regular activities related to their work, to exchange experience and to talk about trivial matters. The use of technological accelerated the communication, and the tasks disseminated through big screen TV, allowed that everyone could share the tasks and resolve them quickly by the team.

Keywords: Natural user interface, communication process and information.

1 Introduction

We are presenting a study solution to software development regarding e-Health using concepts of Natural User Interfaces (NUI) for mobile through analysis of healthcare professionals' activities and communication. Healthcare professionals deal with several patients per day and each patient has especial needs, mainly in a chronic mental care hospital, where patients stay for a long period, even their whole life [1, 2]. The healthcare professionals have to manage all patients´ care and their activities, take notes of all information in day-by-day tasks and share all the collected information with the team of professionals, aiming at supporting patients in their normalization process into society. Although professionals working in these conditions, not only share professional activities, but also activities, their personal life and patients feelings, like a big family and the exchange of experiences among them is a mix of moments of personal and professional life.

V.G. Duffy (Ed.): DHM 2014, LNCS 8529, pp. 313–324, 2014.

Communication among healthcare professionals is carried out through notes basically on paper, verbal medical recommendations for patients and sometimes through SMS (mobile phone messages). These not structured procedures usually drive the communication process in an inefficient and slow path, and may also cause inconsistencies and rework in patient´s care.

The communication process in a hospital is essential in the patient's treatment - data from Manhattan Research [19] shows that, in 2012, 85% of U.S. physicians used smartphones to professional propose and patient's interactions - and we have been studying the relation among healthcare professionals, trying to learn how they interact and share information in a certain mental care hospital. This hospital is considered a model for their high degree of expertise and efficiency in patient´s treatments, although their communication is totally paper-based and verbal-based. Using the opportunity to observe this highly qualified group, we are learning how to design Information and Communication Technologies (ICT) solutions to propose a better communication channel for hospital's staff in general, supported by technology. Even though their paper based communication process is really good, it still have some problems, which we want to address and solve with our proposed solution. Their communication is slow and sometimes some healthcare professionals not receive informations, or messages, communicated by paper.

The paper is organized as follow. Related works are presented in section 2. Section 3 presents the context and the hospital of this research. The Collab system and how we validate it are show at section 4. Section 5 presents the conclusions.

2   Related Works

Normally, the use of ICT resources in healthcare turns to use of internet and information systems to improve access, efficiency, effectiveness and quality of clinical processes related to patient treatments, usually for supporting critical situations or as support diagnoses. These systems tend to be patient-centred (electronic health records, to aid professional decision making) or administrator-oriented (better tracking of costs and care systems for decision making) [11]. The papers [12, 16, 17] are focused on aspects of the patient experience, providing better feedback to patients, contributing to the patient's motivation or improvement of a therapeutic process. Similarly, other studies are made to streamline and record information from the hospital to improve workflow and patient record management, in [14].

However, these works are more oriented to the administration and management of the flow of information, including patient information over time. Furthermore, this hospital, to be a hospital for treatment of mental disorders, where patients spend a lot of time, mostly living all their lives in the hospital, the relationship among professionals and patients have the peculiarity of mixing professional and personal life, as a large family. Our research approach follows the path of other studies [11, 12, 15, 18] that have been made in the implementation of ICT solution in hospital´s contexts with many different objectives, such as improving the processes of communication between the hospital staff, providing more accurate diagnostic tools and treatments, support care´s processes, enhance patient adherence to medication, among others. Typically these studies use user-centred design approaches, adapted from the traditional software engineering. In this work we use adopted participatory design approach, involving users throughout the design process to developing interfaces with more natural interactions.

3   Contextualization

In work environments where professionals have to walk in different places/rooms and change their activities' location all the time, it's important to manage the communication among them. In a hospital context, for example, these healthcare professionals are nomadic and provide them some technical resources in order to facilitate the communication in their activities could be helpful.

We intent to study and support the communication process across healthcare professionals to improve messages and task exchange and support their daily activities in their work environment. We aim to improve the current communication process used by them nowadays across the hospital staff. This study was done in a hospital in Brazil without infrastructure for ICT. We prepared the infrastructure and introduced our system to facilitate the communication among healthcare professionals.

3.1   Infrastructure of Clemente Ferreira Hospital

We have a partnership with a Brazilian Hospital called CAIS Clemente Ferreira that is a chronic care hospital witch takes care of neurological and mental disorders patients. This hospital has 3 floors with 6 wings (units) and hosts 800 patients and 600 professionals distributed. Figure 1 shows an aerial view of the hospital.

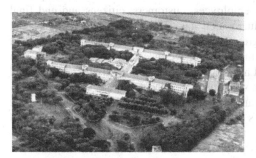
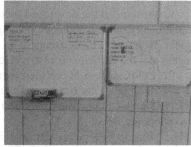

Fig. 1. Clemente Ferreira Hospital   **Fig. 2.** Whiteboard Used at CAIS (Nursery Room)

Previous studies in the same hospital were reported in Calderon [3, 4]. In those studies it was observed that banter between healthcare professionals is essential for interpersonal communication. In almost all cases the exchange of information among professionals starts with an informal greeting. This behavior, typical among Brazilians, must be registered, it is not a universal behavior, and characterizes relations between Brazilians.

Calderon [3. 4] reports that there is a clear need for communication among healthcare professionals in that community, where exist information and communication practices are based on informal socialization conducted in the workplace. It is a big challenge to investigate how to supporting ICT to conduct workflow in this community. Figure 2, shows how healthcare professionals communicate without technologies resources, using a whiteboard to take notes and send messages.

Healthcare professionals working in this community have little or no previous experience with ICT use in their workflow, then, it was also possible for us to investigate the characteristics of ICT that could support the existing flow of information and communication practices among them. One of the patterns of information sharing and monitoring adopted by that community can be explained as a system of sending messages, where tasks are communicated publicly and can be created or performed by members of the work team. Based on this observation, a digital system that replicates that sending messages has been developed to observe the effects of adopting this technology in such environment.

3.2   Developing Collab: Participatory Design Sections

Participatory behavior is a collaborative process that takes isolated people around a common problem and validates their experience as a base to understanding and critical reflection, contextualizing issues and weakness, linking them to political realities and development activities [8]. On Participatory Design (PD), it's also possible to have a direct participation, where the system's stakeholders are included into the development process, while in the indirect participation only a set of stakeholders participate [7].

As the user participation is essential to the development of the proposed environment - [13] says "[...] the most effective way of understanding what works and what doesn't in an interface is to watch people use it and that the user has to participate in design process", the DP must involve employees, customers, citizens and end final users to ensure that the developed product match stakeholders needs and if it's usable. Consequently, all stakeholders must agree with what will be done in order to make it a clear goal to all. In our sections at the hospital, we discussed the communication process and the participants discovered new insights regarding the living situation and the effect of these insights on their own situation. It is expected in PD section, according to [6], where users can be well aware of their everyday political role to trace the society. The resulting artifacts and PD´s characteristics were the main reasons that led us to adopt the DP.

The proposed PD approach on this work aims to involve user participation on the development process through techniques that enable user to actively participate on the definition about what will be developed. We used some techniques, such as: interviews, workshops, prototype, group dynamics, ethnographic studies, social networks and scenarios. The resulting scenarios, interviews and artefacts of PD section are reported in [9]. Figure 3 shows a scenario from meetings among nurses and their team in nursery room.

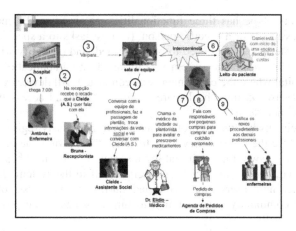

Fig. 3. Scenario for Nursery Room

4   Collab System

Collab is a system to test and improve communication among healthcare professionals using mobile technologies and it is an evolution of the research presented by Calderon [4], where a task management system was deployed among healthcare professionals in this same community aiming to investigate the challenges in using ICT solutions in observing the healthcare professional's behavior in that community. The analysis of the data collect was also performed by Calderon and can be seen in [3].

Collab is a system to test and improve communication among healthcare professionals using mobile technologies and it is an evolution of the research presented by Calderon [4], where a task management system was deployed among healthcare professionals in this same community aiming to investigate the challenges in using ICT solutions in observing the healthcare professional's behavior in that community. The analysis of the data collect was also performed by Calderon and can be seen in [3].

Collab was developed by Oliveira [5] and implemented experimentally in a partner hospital for conducting experiments and collecting data on homophile, communication, activities and work relationships among healthcare professionals.

Collab was projected to use mobile and portable devices because most participants already have a mobile device of their own. In this case, we decided to stick the design focusing on mobile devices as well. For those who didn't have a mobile device, we provided them a seven-inch tablet, that fits in their pocket work aprons and they resemble to the other's mobile devices, trying to make it less disruptive as possible. Another component of the system is a large video displays that shows public messages and tasks. We installed the large video display in the main ward corridor where the research was conducted. We believed that the presence of an information panel where everyone can see messages and notifications of pending tasks also promotes a greater share of awareness among healthcare professionals. With that, everyone can be aware and attentive to the events in their work environment. This system was developed and described in [5].

The Collab prototype has three functionalities: (a) send public messages to all healthcare professionals or a specific person, (b) post tasks to a specific person or to all healthcare professionals that need to be performed, and (c) notify when and whom completed a pending task. The system was installed on an application server within the partner hospital where the experiment was conducted. All devices were connected to the wireless network, thus, healthcare professionals could access the system via browser through their devices.

All the participants healthcare professionals were previously registered in the system. In order to use the system, they have to select their own name on a list of users and   type his/her password in the initial login screen. If some healthcare professional was not registered, he/she can register himself/herself in the system. This new functionality (register new users) was requested during primary tests of the system, because in that community it is common to hire new healthcare professionals and volunteers sporadically.

After logging in, users are directed to a menu containing two large buttons, "Messages" (Figure 4 - A) and "Tasks" (Figure 4 - B), to facilitate users' access to Collab's functionality, beyond the "Exit" button (Figure 4 - C), where users can leave the system and return to the login screen.

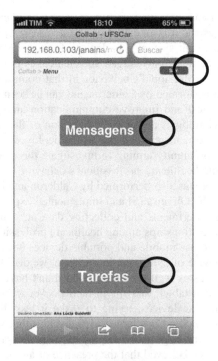

Fig. 4. System´s Options Access

In the message preview screen, users can see all the messages sent previously using the system (Figure 5 - A), besides, s/he can also see the messages that were sent only to him – choosing "For Me" tab (Figure 5 - B). Messages are displayed in descending order, where in the top are shown the most recent posts and all the messages have a header with more information about each of them. In this interface there is also a "New Message" button (Figure 5 -C), which allows users creating and, after that, sending a new message. Users can also go to the task functionality pressing the "Task" button (Figure 5 – D). Finally, to logout of the system, they can press the "Exit" button (Figure 5 – E).

Figure 6 shows the screen responsible for the task functionality in the system, showing to the user the pending and solved tasks (Figure 6 - A and B). Pending tasks are displayed in an increasing time order, i.e., tasks posted previously are shown at the top. Once a healthcare professional solves a task, s/he needs to mark it as completed by pressing the "Done" button (Figure 6 - C). When a task is marked as done, it leaves the to-do list and goes to the list of solved tasks. In the top of the screen, there is the "New Task" button (Figure 6 - D), which allows users creating and posting a new task. To create a new task, the user can select a specific professional to relate the task with, i.e., defining who needs to execute that task, or post the task without marking anyone, what means that any of the healthcare professionals can execute it. Tasks pre-defined to be solved by a specific professional do not appear on the Big Screen TV. This whole task process is similar to the messages that can be sending to a specific person or to all healthcare professionals. In this screen, users can also go to the message functionality pressing the "Message" button (Figure 6 – E) or logout of the system pressing the "Exit" button (Figure 6 - F).

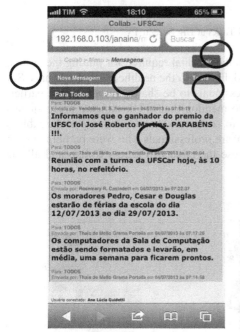
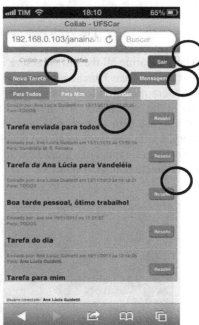

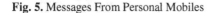

Fig. 5. Messages From Personal Mobiles   **Fig. 6.** Tasks From Personal Mobiles

Another common practice among the healthcare professionals at CAIS is the use of papers and white boards to record tasks and messages (Figure 2). Thinking about that, in our experiment we installed a large video display (TV set) at the main ward corridor where the research was conducted, where all the messages and pending tasks are shown. By doing that, we would like to see if this new method using technology could replace their old method and make it more efficient.

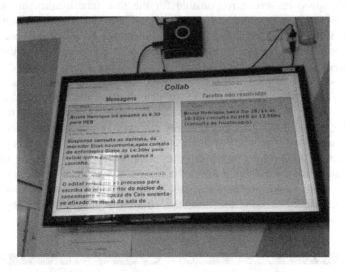

Fig. 7. Messages and Tasks at Big Screen TV

After preparing all the infrastructure in the hospital required for putting the system to start running, the 7-inch tablets were delivered to the healthcare professionals. Six tablets were delivered to healthcare professionals to be shared among all the participating in the experiment. It's important to mention that, the healthcare professionals could also use their own mobile devices to access and use Collab. Upon the tablet's delivery, a talk was given to all the healthcare professionals who were participating in the experiment explaining them how to use the tablets to access Collab and all the system's functionalities (Figure 8).

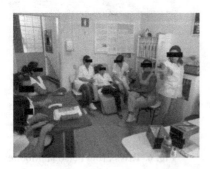 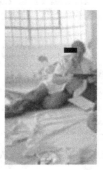

Fig. 8. Learning How to Use Collab

4.1   Collab Experiment and Data Analysis

We track the Collab usage from May, 2013 until October, 2013 to observe the adoption of the system. During this experiment we observed the healthcare professionals and their interaction with Collab. We collected all the data and also we conducted interviews with the healthcare professionals that used Collab (those that work at the nursery room). Analyses of data collected and interviews are reported below.

The experiment was conducted with the participation of 39 healthcare professionals included in the system, but just 26 effectively used Collab during the experiment. As a result we collected: all outgoing messages and tasks - a total of 122 messages and 121 tasks. In interviews with the healthcare professionals they said that they use "Messages" for more informal notes and other ordinary communications. When they post "Tasks" they mean it is an activity that must be done.

Out of the total messages number, 94 messages (77%) were sent to all, i.e., the messages were sent to each participant and were exposed in big screen TV (Figure 8 – Blackboard Used at CAIS   in the Nursery Room) allowing all the hospital staff that circulated in the hallway, used in experiment, could read the messages. Even though they were broadcast messages, i.e., to everyone, 23% of them were directed to a specific person. By using Collab system, our automated tool for sending messages and task´s notifications, we notice that messages and tasks are about extra activities that happen during the workday and these are not formalized as a regular activity.   Many of these messages (75% of total) are related to the patients and only 25% are specific from or to the team.

Analyzing published tasks and type of professional who made the posting in Collab, only 16 healthcare professionals sent a task using Collab. We realized that 25% of 121 tasks were posted by nurses, but there were only 2 nurses in the hospital in our research. The physiotherapist and occupational therapist were responsible for 19% and 21% of posted tasks, respectively (Figure 9).

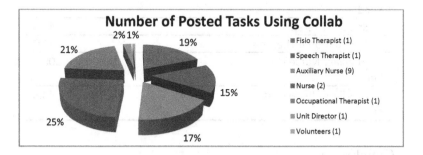

Fig. 9. Professionals X Posted Tasks

Among 75% of messages involving patients, 17% are related to medication and / or medical procedures. Only 7% are messages about feeding patients and 3% involve hygiene procedures. All messages are related to activities outside of the routine of patients, such as "information about a patient who refused the food" or "a patient who needed an extra medication because he is too agitated".   This shows that Collab allows non-routine activities are recorded for later analysis about the extra activities performed by health professionals – this reflects the whiteboard at the nursery room: almost all notes are about non regular activities.

We even notice that occupational therapist does not have activities at nursing station, but she used Collab often for posting tasks and sending messages. Their activities toke place mostly in the hospital corridors, in therapy rooms and patient´s restaurant, but professional believed it was important to share messages and tasks with the entire team.

By comparing the collected data by the system and the analysis of the videos and interviews made by Calderon [3, 4], we can highlight that the professional's communication process in there is something really complex and that has the objective of solving problems. When an emergency or something out of their routine happens, it is essential to inform everyone about the tasks that must be done and ensures/facilitates the work of those healthcare professionals who are going to execute them. Also, through the experiment, we observed that many tasks have been solved by the own professionals who posted them. thus, we concluded that the system was often used as a task schedule (a reminder tool). For example: the speech therapist solved 44% of the tasks that she posted; the occupational therapist did the same, she solved 40% of her own posted tasks. In Table 1, we can observe the percentage of tasks that were posted and executed by the same professional.

Table 1. Posted and Solved Tasks by the Same Professional

Healthcare Profession- al	Percent of Task Posted and Solved
Fisio Therapist	9%
Nurse Number 1	30%
Nurse Number 2	25%
Auxiliary Nurse Num- ber 1	67%
Speech Therapist	44%
Occupational Therapist	40%
Auxiliary Nurse Num- ber 2	100%
Auxiliary Nurse Num- ber 3	33%

5   Conclusion

The communication process in a hospital is essential in the patients treatment, especially procedures and treatments, formalized or not, applicable to patients. The informal communication often helps faster in solving problems and it is the choice of many healthcare professionals.

In the experiments and observations we did, the exchange of messages and the send notification using Collab software, the most activities is not part of daily routine in hospital, and these messages and notification were rapidly communicated to all involved. With the use of an automated tool for sending messages and task´s notifications, these extra activities are recorded and the process of communication can be improved by analyzing the type of task and message. In recent interviews, the health-care professionals, who used the Collab, said they are already so used to new way of sending / receiving messages and notifications of tasks, that they do not use paper neither white board anymore - all communication at nursery room has been made through Collab, which was approved by the staff.

Collab is an experimental study for our first step in developing natural information and communication technology. Collab provided a virtual communication platform which staffs used to deal with unexpected situation beyond daily routine workflow, including solving problem on patient, temporary changing in work, organizing a collaborative task, or strengthen personality relationship, etc.

In this experiment, although certain professional categories seldom used the Collab (this might be due to their work content), some professional categories adopted the Collab system, and some healthcare professionals are using the Collab much more than others. By observing this, we understood that this indicated that each category had different requirements to find a way to strengthen their communication with others. In this case, Collab system allowed them sharing and reporting their working situation, even though their job was is mostly executed independently to the other healthcare professionals. This shown us that Collab just provided the channel to satisfy an undiscovered need among the healthcare professionals and, more than that, the system helped them supplying this needs.

Acknowledgements. We thank all team from LIA/UFSCar by the collected data gathered with observations and interviews in the hospital and the proposed scenarios. We also thank Jônatas Leite de Oliveira by the proposed and developed Collab system.

References

1. Anacleto, J.C., Fels, S., Silvestre, R.: Transforming a Paper Based Process to a Natural User Interfaces Process in a Chronic Care Hospital. In: Proceedings of the 4th International Conference on Software Development for Enhancing Accessibility and Fighting Info-exclusion (DSAI 2012), vol. 14, pp. 173–180 (2012)
2. Anacleto, J., Fels, S.: Adoption and Appropriation: A Design Process from HCI Research at a Brazilian Neurological Hospital. In: Kotzé, P., Marsden, G., Lindgaard, G., Wesson, J., Winckler, M. (eds.) INTERACT 2013, Part II. LNCS, vol. 8118, pp. 356–363. Springer, Heidelberg (2013)
3. Calderon, R., Fels, S., de Oliveira, J.L., Anacleto, J.: Understanding NUI-supported nomadic social places in a Brazilian health care facility. In: Proceedings of the 11th Brazilian Symposium on Human Factors in Computing Systems, Brazil, pp. 76–84 (2012)
4. Calderon, R., Fels, S., Anacleto, J.E., Oliveira, J.L.: Towards supporting informal information and communication practices within a Brazilian healthcare environment. In: CHI 2013 Extended Abstracts on Human Factors in Computing Systems, pp. 517–522. ACM Press, New York (2013)

5. Oliveira, J.L.: Sistema de Recomendação para Promoção de Redes Homófilas Baseadas em Valores Culturais: Observando o impacto das relações hemofílicas na reciprocidade apoiada pela tecnologia. Dissertação (Mestrado). Universidade Federal de São Carlos. São Carlos, Junho p.79 (2012)

6. United Nations. E-Government Survey 2008: From e-Government to Connected Governance. United Nations publication, New York, http://unpan1.un.org/intradoc/groups/public/documents/un/unpan028607.pdf

7. Trimi, S., Sheng, H.: Emerging Trends in M-Government. Communications of the ACM 51(5), 51–58 (2008)

8. Moon, J.: From e-Government? Emerging practices in the use of m-technology by state governments. IBM Center for the Business of Government (2004)

9. Brito, T.C.P., Abib, J.C., Camargo, L.S.A., Anacleto, J.C.: A Participatory Design Approach to use Natural User Interface for e-Health. In: 5th Workshop on Software and Usability Engineering Cross-pollination: Patterns, Usability and User Experience, vol. 1, pp. 35–42 (2011)

10. Fels, S., Anacleto, J., Silvestre, R.G.: Designing a Health-care Worker-Centred System for a Chronic Mental Care Hospital. In: INTERACT 2013 Workshop on Human Work Interaction Design, HWID (2013)

11. Li, J., Wilson, L., Stapleton, S., Cregan, P.: Design of an advanced telemedicine system for emergency care. In: OZCHI 2006 Proceedings of the 18th Australia conference on Computer- Human Interaction: Design: Activities, Artefacts and Environments, 2006, pp. 413–416 (2006)

12. Doyle, J., Kelly, D., Caulfield, B.: Design considerations in therapeutic exergaming. In: Pervasive Computing Technologies for Healthcare (PervasiveHealth) and Workshop, pp. 389–393 (2011)

13. Mcclosky, M.: Turn User Goals into Task Scenarios for Usability Testing. In: Nielsen Norman Group Publication (January 2004)

14. Vegoda, P.: Introduction to hospital information systems. Journal of Clinical Monitoring and Computing 4(2), 105–109 (1987)

15. Schönauer, C., et al.: Chronic pain rehabilitation with a serious game using multimodal input. In: International Conference on Virtual Rehabilitation (ICVR) 2011, pp. 1–8 (2011)

16. Alankus, G., et al.: Towards customizable games for stroke rehabilitation. In: ACM Conference on Human Factors in Computing Systems (SIGCHI 2010), pp. 2113–2122 (2010)

17. Tanaka, K., et al.: A Comparison of Exergaming Interfaces for Use in Rehabilitation Programs and Research. Loading The Journal of the Canadian Game Studies Association 6(9), 69–81 (2012)

18. Geurts, L., et al.: Digital games for physical therapy: fulfilling the need for calibration and adaptation. In: International Conference on Tangible, Embedded, and Embodied Interaction, pp. 117–124 (2011)

19. Camargo, I.: Um infográfico sobre o uso de smartphones e tables na saúde Americana. In: InfoMonday – From Manhattan Research (January 2014)

PEGASO: Towards a Life Companion

Stefano Carrino[1], Maurizio Caon[1], Omar Abou Khaled[1],
Giuseppe Andreoni[2], and Elena Mugellini[1]

[1] University of Applied Sciences and Arts Western Switzerland, Fribourg
{Maurizio.Caon,Stefano.Carrino,Omar.AbouKhaled,
Elena.Mugellini}@hes-so.ch
[2] Politecnico di Milano
Giuseppe.Andreoni@polimi.it

Abstract. In the frame of the PEGASO European project, we aim at promoting healthier lifestyles focusing on the alimentary education and physical activity. This paper presents the concept of health companion as the main tool to inform and push the user towards a healthier lifestyle. This companion is an advanced interface that assists and entertains the user, providing him an adequate knowledge about alimentary and physical education. The companion is based on a knowledge model of the user and its behavior; it is composed of three main facets: is tailored to the user, is based on affective design and is designed to be a life companion.

Keywords: smartphone, health, obesity.

1 Introduction

Lifestyle has been identified as the main preventive methods for several health risks [1]. Among the main emerging problems, overweight ranks probably at first place. Overweight could also easily become obesity, which is now epidemic in many countries so that a general alarm has been issued worldwide [2]. Several researches have demonstrated that health risks are associated with overweight and obesity, e.g., [3-7]. If for adults this could be a result of a joint pathology, in teenagers counter fighting over-weight with proper strategies could be a win-win model for a real prevention of future pathologies.

Obesity is due to several factors as genetic contributors, metabolic conditions (e.g. diabetes and hypertension), psychological and behavioral issues. Concerning the last two factors, an important role is played by an inadequate education [8], in particular about health literacy. We deal with the promotion of healthier lifestyles in an ongoing European project (PEGASO) aiming at developing a complete services' ecosystem that would be able to motivate teenagers to learn and to apply a healthy life-style effortlessly. In particular, one of the most important parts of this system is represented by the digital health companion.

The role of a health companion is to address the challenge to help individuals and their families to achieve self-management in different aspects linked to health [8]. Our companion is an advanced interface that assists and entertains the user, providing him an adequate knowledge about alimentary and physical education.

V.G. Duffy (Ed.): DHM 2014, LNCS 8529, pp. 325–331, 2014.

An important aspect of the proposed companion is the presentation of the information using gamification approach. Gamification is defined as "the use of game design elements in non-game context" [9]. In particular, the PEGASO companion engages and motivates the user towards a healthier life style. The companion proposes games and supports him/her in the social community. It can propose challenges (like soccer matches) or workout group meetings (based on the common interests of the community) to promote the social aspect of exercising. The companion will follow the user in his/her everyday life and will learn his/her preferences and recognize his/her behavior. The companion aims at establishing a special and affective relationship with the user that should last for years, maybe all the rest of his/her life.

In Section 2, we present the PEGASO ICT system, which constitutes the hardware and software base for the realization of the health companion.

In Section 3, we discuss the importance of the affective design in order to strengthen the tight between the companion and the user.

In Section 4, we describe the importance of providing tailored solutions and how the companion can be adapted from a general to a specific, user-dependent model.

In Section 5, we show how the health companion can become a *life* companion and follow the user during all his life.

Finally, Section 6 concludes the paper summarizing the main features of the health companion model and presenting the future steps.

2   The PEGASO ICT System

The multi-dimensional ICT system of the PEGASO ecosystem plays a key role for the human-companion interaction possibilities. Fig. 1 depicts the PEGASO ICT system with some components highlighted. This system includes game mechanisms and social activities to influence users' behaviors in order to fight and prevent overweight and obesity in the younger population by encouraging them to become co-producers of their wellness and take an active role in improving it.

This form of education aims at generating self-awareness about the risks associated to an unhealthy behavior, at sustaining motivation to take care of their health with both short and long terms perspective and at changing behavior towards a healthy lifestyle based on balanced diet and adequate physical activity.

At the base of the PEGASO ICT System, there are the wearable and mobile sensors and devices such as smart garments, scales and smartphone. This layer allows acquiring implicit information about the user behavior and his/her daily habits. While implicit mechanisms will process the information linked to behavior of the user, explicit dialogs will prompt the user for information that is difficult to acquire automatically and also to establish an affective contact with the user (e.g., "what have you eaten today?"). In the first part of the project, the smartphone is designed as the main physical interface with the user. It acquires the signals from the different external or embedded sensors and presents the feedback to the user in a context-aware manner.

As presented in Fig. 1, the interface can be one or multiple applications and different games and social activities. However, not all the information is contained in the smartphone; most of the data will be encrypted and made available on the cloud to the healthcare stakeholders (the user family, the doctors and/or the researchers).

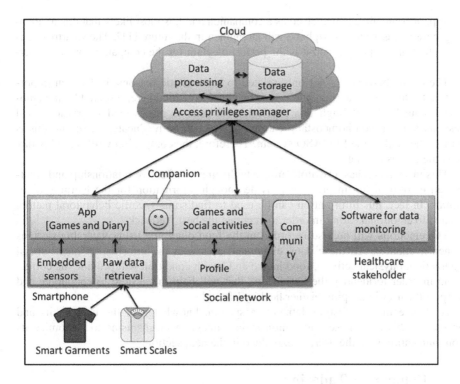

Fig. 1. The PEGASO ICT system

Finally, from an interaction perspective, the health companion constitutes the main interface between the user and the system. This interface is bi-directional: to the user, suggesting activities and games and providing information, and from the user with explicit and implicit interaction.

3 Affective Design

Changing lifestyle is often a challenging task. In order to foster the user engagement and to facilitate the adoption of the proposed activities, it is important to create an emotional link between the user and the health companion. In fact, a modification of the emotional state means switching among different ways of thinking. In particular, positive affects increase intrinsic motivation and has some effects on cognition.

Not only the affective design will encourage the prolonged use of the system but it will improve the learning of the proposed concepts. In fact, affective learning is based on the idea that emotions are intertwined with cognitive capabilities and several researches demonstrate its influence in conditioning the rational behavior and the decision making of the learner [10].

Embedding the companion in the users' smartphone is an appropriate way to make it perceived in a positive way (especially, thanks to a good tailoring). Indeed, the smartphones are already perceived as a companion and it is most likely that this relationship between user and smartphone will strengthen in the future [11]. The smartphone is ubiquitous and is private, and it is the perfect medium for the companion, which is personal.

The eating behavior is not only related to homeostatic reasons. In fact, an important factor that influences people's need and choice of food is represented by the emotional state [12]. Although this psychological state is intertwined in physiological responses, these non-homeostatic eating patterns can be reeducated [13]; and this is part of the goal of the PEGASO system. Therefore, the companion will ask every day how the user is feeling.

This mechanism has a twofold aim: establishing an affective relationship and creating an emotional log in order to provide enough information for the learning algorithms. In fact, this information can be used to find some specific behavioral pattern related to emotional eating in order to generate the best feedback.

The emotions will be also recorded in the food diary and using wearable systems (when available). All these data, elaborated also with the information about social interaction, physical activity, food intake and health condition will provide the correct trend in order to identify the key factors that will help the system to encourage and support the user in keeping his/her healthy life style.

A change in the lifestyle demands a specific knowledge of the user habits and needs, for this reason the companion should integrate mechanisms to customize its communication with the user, as explained in the next section.

4   Companion Tailoring

The proposed companion is based on a dynamic, personalized model. In fact, a crucial characteristic is the possibility to specialize, to tailor the interaction between the user and the system. The companion starts from a general model provided by clinicians and psychologists, then progressively it gets to know the user's preferences and according to the most successful strategies it will keep supporting the user [14]. The tailoring takes into account several aspects:

- The companion learns when and how is best providing a reminder or a message.
- The companion learns to know the user and to become a personal counselor. In fact, the companion is able to make personalized interventions, which provide the users with information that is based on their individual characteristics (e.g., dietary behaviors, motivations, attitudes, and culture). Tailored interventions make the information personally relevant and researches demonstrate that computer-tailored health education is more effective in motivating people to make dietary changes [15] and that it could be also a good practice to promote physical activity [16].

Personalization is based on both user settings and automatic tailoring involving machine learning techniques that specialize and personalize the model. The companion personalization is also aesthetic to reflect the user's personality and style in order to strengthen the emphatic relationship between the user and the companion [17].

The European dimension of our study will allow us to take into account also the different ethnological specificities impacting on adolescents' lifestyle and that should be taken into account in the companion. This will open the possibility to define socio-cultural facets in our tailoring approach. During the PEGASO project, three pilots in different countries will take place (Italy, Spain and United Kingdom). These pilots will allow us to examine the cultural differences that may impact on teenagers' life-style and to adapt the model underlining the companion accordingly.

5   Towards a Life Companion

The companion will know the user's personality and will establish with him/her an affective relationship.

The companion will participate to the whole user's life in order to become a real life companion. Different ages have different requirements and the companion has to be able to continuously adapt to novel needs and propose appropriate activities.

While in the first phase of the project, the smartphone will incarnate the compa-nion, the companion idea is not linked to a unique physical device but it is ubiquitous and will change form over time. The companion will be an interactive teddy bear when the user is a child and will become a smartphone during the adolescence; the companion can follow also an adult to support his/her work as a laptop or will accom-pany him/her during the old age as a smart bracelet (Fig. 2).

Such an evolution will allow designing the human-companion interaction on the user needs and specificities over time.

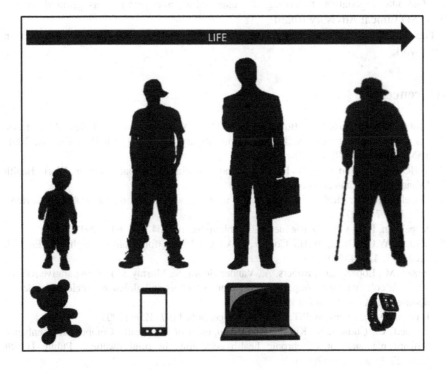

Fig. 2. The life companion vision

6   Conclusion

In this paper, we have presented the concept of life companion in the framework of the PEGASO European project. PEGASO focuses on the development of a complete services ecosystem that would be able to motivate teenagers to learn and to apply a healthy life-style. A crucial component of this ecosystem is the health companion that is introduced in this paper.

Tailored user's model, affective design and over-time adaptive algorithms are the main aspects if the proposed concept. Tailoring allows the companion to shift from a generic model to a personalized, user-specific instance. The affective design aims at establishing an emotional link with the user. The over-time adaptive algorithms enable the companion to become a life companion that can follow the user during all his/her life.

As next step, we plan to develop a mobile application in which to instantiate the life companion having the teenagers as target.

In a later stage, three pilots in different countries will take place (Italy, Spain and United Kingdom). These pilots will allow us to examine the cultural differences that may impact on teenagers' lifestyle and to adapt the model underpinning the companion accordingly.

Acknowledgements. The PEGASO project is co-funded by the European Commission under the 7th Framework Programme. The project is compliant with European and National legislation regarding the user safety and privacy, as granted by the PEGASO Ethical Advisory Board.

The authors of the paper wish to thank all the project partners for their contribution to the work.

References

1. Mokdad, A.H., Ford, E.S., Bowman, B.A., Dietz, W.H., Vinicor, F., Bales, V.S., Marks, J.S.: Prevalence of Obesity, Diabetes, and Obesity-Related Health Risk Factors, 2001. JAMA 289(1), 76–79 (2003)
2. WHO Consultation, Obesity: Preventing and managing the global epidemic. World Health Organization technical report series (2000)
3. Kopelman, P.G.: Health risks associated with overweight and obesity. Obesity Reviews 8(1), 13–17 (2007)
4. Kopelman, P.G.: Obesity as a medical problem. Nature 404, 635–643 (2000)
5. Willett, W.C., Dietz, W.H., Colditz, G.A.: Guidelines for healthy weight. N. Engl. J. Med. 341, 427–433 (1999)
6. Ezzati, M., Lopez, A.D., Rogers, A., Vander Hoorn, S., Murray, C.J.: Comparative risk assessment collaborating group, Selected major risk actors and global and regional burden of disease. Lancet 360, 1347–1360 (2002)
7. Haslam, D.W., James, W.P.T.: Obesity. Lancet 366, 1197–1209 (2005)
8. Weinert, C., Cudney, S., Kinion, E.: Development of My Health Companion to enhance selfcare management of chronic health conditions in rural dwellers. Public Health Nurs. 27(3), 263–269 (2001)

9. Deterding, S., Dixon, D., Khaled, R., Nacke, L.: From game design elements to gameful-ness: Defining gamification. In: Proceedings of the 15th International Academic MindTrek Conference on Envisioning Future Media Environments - MindTrek 2011, pp. 9–15 (2011)
10. Picard, R.W., Papert, S., Bender, W., Blumberg, B., Breazeal, C., Cavallo, D., Machover, T., Resnick, M., Roy, D., Strohecker, C.: Affective Learning - A Manifesto. BT Technol. J. 22(4), 253–269 (2004)
11. Kennedy, C.M., Powell, J., Payne, T.H., Ainsworth, J., Boyd, A., Buch-an, I.: Active assistance technology for health-related behavior change: An interdisciplinaryreview. Journal of medical Internet research, vol 14(3), e80 (2012)
12. Brug, J., Oenema, A., Campbell, M.: Past, present, and future of computertailored nutrition education. Am. J. Clin. Nutr. 77(suppl. 4), 1028S–1034S (2003)
13. den Akker, H.O., Moualed, L.S., Jones, V.M., Hermens, H.J.: A self-learning personalized feedback agent for motivating physical activity. In: Proc. 4th Int. Symp. Appl. Sci. Biomed. Commun. Technol. - ISABEL 2011, pp. 1–5 (2011)
14. Baylor, A.L.: Promoting motivation with virtual agents and avatars: Role of visual presence and appearance. Philos. Trans. R. Soc. Lond. B. Biol. Sci. 364(1535), 3559–65 (2009)
15. Siewiorek, D.: Generation smartphone. IEEE Spectr. 49(9), 54–58 (2012)
16. Science, C., Kapoor, A., Johns, P., Rowan, K., Carroll, E.A., Czerwinski, M., Roseway, A.: Food and Mood Just-in-Time Support for Emotional Eating. ACII 2013, 252–257 (2013)
17. Gilhooly, C.H., Das, S.K., Golden, J.K., McCrory, M.A., Dallal, G.E., Saltzman, E., Kramer, F.M., Roberts, S.B.: Food cravings and Energy Regulation: The characteristics of craved foods and their relationship with eating behaviors and weight change during 6 months of dietary energy restriction. International Journal of Obesity 31(12), 1849–1859 (2007)

Biomechanical Study of Foot Force Pattern in Hallux Valgus (HV) Patients

Saba Eshraghi and Ibrahim Esat

School of Engineering and Design, Brunel University of London, UK
saba_eshraghi@yahoo.com, Ibrahim.Esat@brunel.ac.uk

Abstract

Background: Hallux valgus is the angulation of the big toe of more than 15 degrees. Many people during their lives are challenged with this condition. The occurrence is 3 times more in women to men. However one of the causes of the condition is congenital but the other important factor is wearing narrow toe box and high heel shoes. There are some devices measuring the foot kinematic or sole pressure for identifying such condition but as there are lots of variations in foot kinematics and pressure the identification of the disease becomes more challenging. Many previous works are published regarding to foot sole pressure pattern but still early recognition of the condition is needed.

Method: To see the existence of force pattern out of gait experiments, Rs-Scan device used to take the kinematic data of the one complete foot contact. 10 trials were conducted of each volunteer with the full right foot contact with the pressure mat. 3 valid trials have been chosen for final analyses. With this method the load/pressure measurement under the 10 anatomical regions of the foot have been recorded and used to recognise people with and without deformity. Furthermore, Motion Capture cameras were used to capture the first and the second metatarsal movements in HV and Non HV volunteers to see whether there is a joint laxity of the metatarsals in HV patients.

Results: It was observed that the load pattern in forefoot in people with HV was significantly different compared to non HV volunteers .So independent sample T-Test done and the statistical difference less than 0.05 observed in Toe1,Metatarsal 1,Metatarsal 2, Metatarsal 3, Metatarsal 4 and Metatarsal 5. So just there was no difference load pattern on the Toe 2-5. Hence, the maximum load was on the 2nd and 3rd metatarsal heads in people with HV which is already published by previous authors but the walking speed showed a significant effect on the force variations in both group. The relative movements captured by 7 cameras in Motion Capture laboratory were monitored and it has shown the greater movement of first and second metatarsal heads in patients with HV.

Conclusion: The observed force pattern was changing trial to trial in each individual to have a consistent reading they asked to walk 10 times over the pressure mat. After getting this, it was discovered that there is a relationship between walking speed and maximum load applied to the forefoot. Also there was rising load on the 2nd and 3rd metatarsal heads in HV patients. Hence, the 6

V.G. Duffy (Ed.): DHM 2014, LNCS 8529, pp. 332–339, 2014.
© Springer International Publishing Switzerland 2014

regions on the forefoot including Toe1, Meta1, Meta 2, Meta 3, Meta 4, Meta 5 were statistically different while comparing HV and control group. It should be indicated that HV group also had more lateral movement of the first metatarsal head comparing to control group.

Keywords: Hallux valgus, Foot force pattern.

1   Introduction

Hallux valgus is the lateral deviations of the big toe of more than 15 degrees[1]. The statistics shows that 23% of the people developing this condition during their lives [2]. The measurement of articular surfaces of the foot showed that female bones had a potential for more movement to occur in the direction of adduction [3]. Also recent studies shown that women are more predisposed to HV than men by the ratio of 2 to 1[4].

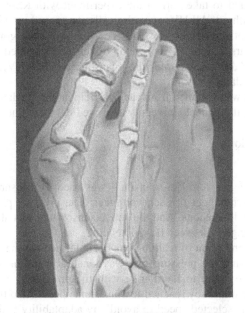

Fig. 1. The foot with the HV deformity [5]

However one of the causes of the deformity is congenital but wearing narrow toe box shoe and high heels have direct effect on the formation of condition.

Changes in the force pattern underneath the foot can change the shape of the first metatarsal bone in individuals.

Inadequate distribution of forces under the sole of the foot can lead to the abnormal movements [6]. Accordingly in people with the normal feet, heel bears about 50% of the body weight while the first and second metatarsals can stand about 25% of body mass and the other metatarsals bear the rest 25% [7]. But people with HV have different pattern of applied force over their feet compared to Non HV individuals.

One study shows the plantar pressure was lower under the 1st and the 2nd toes and higher peak force under 3rd to 5th metatarsal heads but other studies show higher peak force under the 1st to 3rd and lower force under 4th and 5th metatarsal heads in HV patients [8].

One conducted study on plantar pressure and patients with Hallux valgus presents that the highest pressure are on the third, second, first, fourth and fifth [9].

In this study the RS-scan device has been used to analyse the force pattern in individuals with and without HV condition. Moreover, Motion capture laboratory has used to distinguish the laxity of the first metatarsal joint in HV compared to control group.

2   Methodology

2.1   Subjects

20 volunteers recruited to take part in the experiment with RS-scan device, 10 with deformity and 10 without. All HV were clinically diagnosed with HV by an HV specialist or the angle of their right foot was measured with the goniometer so people with the first metatarsal angle of more than 15 degrees counted as HV volunteers. *Foot-scan advanced & hi-end system* (RS-scan International NV, Belgium) has been used to collect force data.

Informed consent was obtained from each participant before data collection and the ethical committee of the Brunel University approved the experimental procedures.

2.2   Data Collection

Foot Scan Device

The plantar measuring system [Rs-scan Inc.] was used to measure the plantar force distributed over the right foot of each volunteer. The pressure plate was 578 mm x 418 mm x 12 mm in dimensions. And the active sensor area was about 488 mm x 325 mm. The pressure range is between 0 – 200 N/cm2.

The start and the end point of walking has been defined for the volunteers, the distance was 6 meters and the pressure mat was located in the middle and before the actual test, they were asked to familiarise with the process by walking some times between the distance until they reached to consistent speed. Also they were requested to walk with the self- selected speed to avoid any adaptability while passing the mat until a full contact of the right foot with the mat achieved.

10 trials have been gained and inconsistency trial to trial in the same individuals observed so their force distribution under their feet was so varies among trials. So speed of walking showed to have the most important effects on the distribution of the force. It is investigated that individuals with steadier way of walking had more repeatable force distribution pattern. To achieve steadier walking pattern volunteers asked to walk with around 4.6 second speed when they are passing the pressure mat. So 10 valid trials collected from each volunteer. To complete each trial they should have had a full contact of the right foot from the heel to the toe off position with the mat.

For the next step they were asked to increase their walking speed by 20% of their normal speed for this stage also 10 valid trials have been achieved.

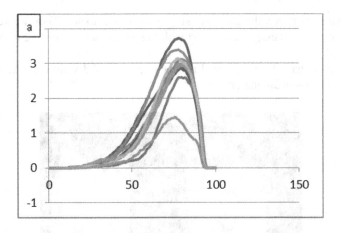

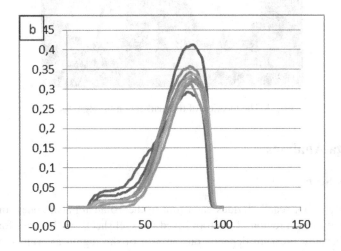

Fig. 2. Force distribution pattern on 2nd metatarsal (a) in the fast speed (b) in the normal speed

Motion Capture Cameras

10 volunteers with and without deformity took part in the experiment. Vicon Blade software has been used to calibrate the 7 cameras and the start and end point of walking has defined. The start and the end points were identified after calibration has done many times to find the best place in which individual could walk and camera had the best view in the space.

Two markers stick to the bare foot of the right foot of each individual.

To avoid any limitation in the natural walking style of each person the markers stick with the blue tag directly to the skin.

First marker located on the first metatarsal head and the second one on the 2nd metatarsal head.

The distance between the start and stop point was 3 meter. They walked 5 times before actual test for being familiarised with the experiment procedure to be constant in their speed.

10 valid trials have been achieved for each person and 3 valid trials have been selected for comparison among groups.

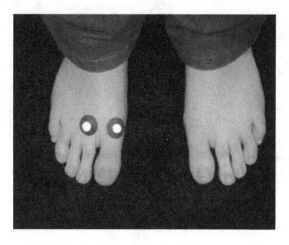

Fig. 3. The location of the markers on the right foot

3   Data Analyses

3.1   Foot Scan

The software, "foot scan", divides each foot to the 10 anatomical zones, the relative forces related to each region of the foot saved in excel sheets. In this case force option is chosen because pressure depends on the size of the region as well as the actual force value, whereas force value is the total force carried by each region which seems to be more meaningful. The force values recorded are normalised against the body weight. For each region the time axis was also normalised.

The maximum force are analysed and metatarsal 2nd and the 3rd bearing the most pressure in both groups but the peak force on these regions were higher in HV group compared to control group.

The amount of force in each region has changed by the changes in the speed of walking. By increasing the speed the force that applied to the foot is about 2 times body weight and more speed means more impact pressure that applies to the sole of the foot [10].

The IBM SPSS Statistics 20 was used to compare the applied forces in both groups to see the existence of significant differences.

Then the force data related to each region of the foot from excel sheets just copy and pasted in the Data View of the software. So in this stage importing the data was completed and the final stage of the analysis was conducted. By going to Analyse toolbar and then Comparing Means Icon and clicking on Independent sample T-Test, the final results appeared in the created table.

The comparison has been done in forefoot which contains Toe1, Toe2-5, Meta1, Meta2, Meta3, Meta4, and Meta5.

The comparison between HV and Non HV groups has conducted to see whether the force pattern is different among groups. The results achieved from the software presents the statistical significance different of less than 0.05 in the First metatarsal in both groups.

The results indicate that there is a significant difference in Levene's Test for equality of variances and also for equality of means which was less than 0.05 in all forefoot regions except toe2-5 in which no significant difference was observed.

So the regions including 1st, 2nd, 3rd, 4th, 5th and Toe1 showed significant difference by less than 0.05 in HV group compared to control group. Just toe2-5 in both groups did not present any significant difference.

3.2   Motion Capture

Each participant's walking movements have been captured by Vicon cameras and the data related to the movement of first and second metatarsal heads were given by 3 coordinates (x, y, and z).

The two markers were glued to the right foot of individuals so in all cases the motion of the right foot had been analysed.

The start time that the software start recording was the same in all participants and in all trials. The X, Y and Z coordinates were saved with the (trc) format on the notepad file then the data just copied and pasted in the excel file to be able to do the analyses. To find out the relative movement of the first and second metatarsal heads regarding to each other the distance between these two regions has been achieved by the Pythagoras formula for each selected trial. And the graphs achieved based on the distance in millimetre (mm). Figure4 shows repetitive fluctuations while walking in HV volunteer.

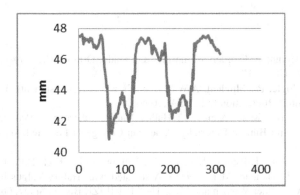

Fig. 4. The distance between markers while walking in HV patient

Other factors that may have impact on the data collection and the results were the way of walking of each volunteers, However they walked 3 times for the preparation for the experiment but still at some stages the error may happen due to the nature of motion but they tried to be steady for the experiments which were repeated 10 times passing between start and the end points.

Furthermore, the way of sticking the markers on the barefoot was an issue because they shouldn't constraint the natural movement of the feet so they glued directly to the skin with blue tag.

For having comparison between HV and control groups the range between maximum distances in each trial minus the minimum distances in the same trial has been obtained and then the average of 3 selected trials was calculated. So for each volunteer one number was calculated for making the comparison between 2 groups.

4   Conclusion

Foot scan data regarding to the force distribution over the 10 anatomical regions of the foot shows to be varied in the same person trial to trial. So consistency is an essential issue that being achieved to get the less variable results in the same person. It is concluded that the speed of walking has an important effect on the variability of the force distribution pattern also the style of walking was another factor to have effect on the force pattern.

Consequently forces on the 2nd and the 3rd metatarsal regions are higher in HV group compared to control group. Moreover, by increasing the speed the magnitude of force rises considerably as many previous published studies neglected the importance of the speed of walking.

Also the relative distance between 1st and 2nd metatarsal heads is significantly higher in HV patients compared to non HV individuals and this an important indicator of lateral laxity of the first metatarsal heads' joint which can be the firm indication of the condition.

References

1. Milner, S.: Common disorders of the foot and ankle, Orthopaedic surgery, pp. 514–517. Elsevier Ltd., UK (2010)
2. Drake, L., Vogle, R., Mitchell, A.W.M.: Gray's anatomy for students. Elsevier Inc. Ian Dick and Antbits Illustration Ltd., USA (2005)
3. Vidal, K.P., Solé, M.T., Antich, J.: Hallux Valgus Inheritance: Pedigree Research in 350 Patients with Bunion Deformity. American College of Foot and Ankle Surgeons 46, 149–154 (2007)
4. Nguyen, U.S.D.T., Hillstorm, H.J., Li, W., Dufouri, A.B., Kiel, D.P., ProcterGray, E., Gagnon, M.M., Hannan, M.T.: Factors Associated with Hallux Valgus in a Population-Based Study of Older Women and Men: The MOBILIZE Boston Study. Osteoarthritis and Cartilage 18, 41–46 (2010)

5. http://www.abbotslangleyclinic.co.uk/
   index.php?pg=foot_pain_explained
6. Donatelli, R.A.: The Biomechanics of the Foot And Ankle, 2nd edn., pp. 3–8. F.A Davis Company, Philadelphia (1996)
7. MCMinn, R., Hutching, R., Logan, B.: A colour atlas of foot and ankle anatomy. Wolfe Medical Publications Ltd., London, London (1982)
8. Wen. J, Ding. Q, Yu. Z, Weidong Sun. W, Wang. Q, Wei. K, Adaptive changes of foot pressure in hallux valgus patients. Gait & Posture (2012)
9. Plank, M.J.: The pattern of forefoot pressure distribution in hallux valgus. The Foot 5, 8–14 (1995)
10. McLester, J., Pierre, P.S.: Applied biomechanics: Concepts and connections. Thomson Wadsworth, Canada (2008)

An Environment for Domestic Supervised Amblyopia Treatment

Giancarlo Facoetti, Angelo Gargantini, and Andrea Vitali

Department of Engineering, University of Bergamo (BG), Dalmine, Italy
{giancarlo.facoetti,angelo.gargantini,andrea.vitali1}@unibg.it
http://3d4amb.unibg.it

Abstract. *Amblyopia* (also called lazy eye) is a condition in which the eye and the brain do not work properly together; this condition causes poor vision in the lazy eye. It involves around 4% of the children. We have devised a system for the diagnosis and treatment of amblyopia by using *3D technology*. To be successful, the proposed treatment must be enjoyable and suitable for domestic use (for instance by watching TV) and carried out with a constant supervision by the doctors. We present a system in which patients and doctors exchange information about the prescribed activities.

Amblyopia (also called lazy eye) is a condition in which the eye and the brain do not work properly together; this condition causes poor vision in the lazy eye. It is a neurological process, as the problem is caused by poor transmission of the visual stimulus through the optic nerve. If amblyopia is not diagnosed and treated in the first years of life, the lazy eye becomes weaker and the normal eye becomes dominant. The traditional way to treat amblyopia is carried out wearing a patch over the normal eye for several hours a day, through a treatment period of several months. This treatment has some drawbacks: it is unpopular, not well accepted by the young patients, and sometimes can disrupt the residual fusion between the eyes.

Our group has been involved in the use of computer technologies for disabilities [3] for several years. The project 3D4AMB exploits the stereoscopic 3D technology, that through glasses with active shutters permits to show different images to the amblyotic eye and the normal eye. We developed some software both for amblyopia diagnosis and treatment that uses this kind of 3D technology. Since the patients are young children, we decided to implement the diagnosis and treatment modules in a form of videogame, in order to make the treatment fun and not boring. The final aim of the project is to give the patients a complete domestic computer based treatment that can be used at home. In fact, a common personal computer mounting a commercial 3D board and a 3D monitor or TV is enough to run the software developed for the 3D4AMB project.

In this work we present a complete environment for domestic and supervised amplyopia treatment. At this stage the environment is under development and validation in collaboration with medical personnel. The treatment begins with the evaluation of the patient in presence of the doctors. Once the amblyopia level

V.G. Duffy (Ed.): DHM 2014, LNCS 8529, pp. 340–350, 2014.

is evaluated and patient case file is created, the treatment stage can be carried out at home. We have developed several software modules in order to emulate the two main types of treatment which are defined as passive and active treatments. The difference between them is based on the interaction of patients during sessions. The passive treatment consists of a video player with some filters applied to the normal eye, such as blurring and luminosity and contrast decreasing. The patient, wearing the 3D glasses, can watch movies and cartoons, and the software will apply the filters to the normal eye in a gradual way and following the parameters set by the doctors in the patient case file. This treatment emulates the classical patching, but it allows partial and dynamic occlusion.

The active module consists in a videogame platform. This choice is based on clinical results which demonstrated the increase of brain skills (in particular visual-spatial skills) on children with visual disorders after some videogame sessions. The games include a modified tetris, a space invaders, and an open source Mario Bros clone to which we have added the stereoscopic 3D vision. In the stereoscopic version, every character of the game can be shown either to the normal eye or to the weak eye (binocular vision). It is also possible to show a character to an eye for a given percentage, and to the other for the remaining value (for example, 70% to the weak eye and 30% to the normal eye). This allows to differently exercise the two eyes (as shown in the image above). As always, how to show the game characters and the left/right eyes percentages has been initially set by the doctors in the patient case file.

During the home treatment, our software records some parameters like the time spent viewing the clips and movies (passive treatment) and playing video-games (active treatment). Periodically the user is tested for stereoacuity at home and this measure is used to judge a possible improvement of the sight. Such data are sent to the doctors through the Internet periodically so they can follow patient progress and intervene if necessary. The doctor can set the treatment parameters in the patient case files according to these results. Moreover our software can autonomously decide to change (under certain bounds) the parameters of the treatment and to suggest some types of activity in order to improve efficiency.

Section 1 introduces amblyopia, the classical treatments and our 3D-based proposal. We present in Section 2 the extension of our environment to a distributed scenario in which patients and doctors exchange data about the treatments by Internet. The architecture of the system is presented in Section 3.

1   Using 3D for Amblyopia Treatment and Diagnosis

Amblyopia, otherwise known as 'lazy eye', is reduced visual acuity that results in poor or indistinct vision in an eye that is otherwise physically normal, or out of proportion to associated structural abnormalities. Typically amblyopia is present in only one eye and is generally associated with a squint or unequal lenses in the prescription spectacles. This low vision is not correctable (or only partially) by glasses or contact lenses.

There exist several causes of amblyopia. Anything that interferes with clear vision in either eye during the critical period (birth to 6 years of age) can result in amblyopia. The most common causes of amblyopia are constant strabismus (constant turn of one eye), anisometropia (different vision/prescriptions in each eye), and/or blockage of an eye due to trauma, lid droop, etc. If one eye sees clearly and the other sees a blur, the good eye and brain will inhibit the eye with the blur. The brain, for some reason, does not fully acknowledge the images seen by the amblyopic or lazy eye. Thus, amblyopia is a neurologically active process. The inhibition process (*suppression*) can result in a permanent decrease of the vision in that eye that can not be corrected with glasses, lenses, or surgery. This condition affects 2-3% of the population, which equates to conservatively around 10 million people under the age of 8 years worldwide. Children who are not successfully treated when still young (generally before the age of 7) will become amblyopic adults. As amblyopic adults, they will have a normal life, except that they are prohibited from some occupations and they are exposed to a higher risk of losing the good eye due to injury or eye disease and became seriously visually impaired.

Amblyopia is currently treated by wearing an adhesive patch over the non-amblyopic eye for several hours per day, over a period of several months. This treatment was introduced in the 18th century and is commonly used also nowadays. This conventional patching or occlusion treatment for amblyopia often gives disappointing results for several reasons: it is unpopular, prolonged, and it can sometimes make the squint worse because it disrupts whatever fusion there is [6]. These issues frequently results in poor or *non-compliance* and since the success of patching depends on compliance, it performs on average very poorly. The treatment by itself works well, but it is often abandoned because it is too much trouble to take. Very often, children are averse to wearing a patch and parents found occlusion difficult to implement [4]. As noted in [11], a treatment whose unacceptability is greater than the motivation of the patients to apply it, will be often abandoned. And if the treatment of patching is not continued, it will eventually fail [10]. For this reason, the orthoptists and ophthalmologists are continuously looking for a more acceptable solution to the problem, i.e. an effective treatment that is also complied with and so really works [9].

There exist several attempts to introduce variations to occlusion which could perform nearly as well as the occlusion without the problem of compliance and the risks of disruption of any existing binocularity. In particular, *partial occlusion* consists in wearing an adhesive filter to attenuate the vision of the good eye [2]. This method is also known as *penalization* and it can be also performed optically by using defocusing lens or pharmaceutically by using atropine which causes blurring of the sound eye. In [1], the authors experimented the occlusion of the lens over the preferred eye with a translucent tape. This technique permitted uninterrupted and prolonged occlusion, with a successful visual outcome. However, this kind of treatment has still some problems of compliance and applicability (e.g. pharmaceutical penalization must be administered by a physician). There are some attempts to use computer systems to implement a sort of virtual penalization, called *rebalancing*. In [5], the authors introduce a vision system based on a head mounted display (HMD) which performs rebalancing of the vision by using a simultaneous enhancing/attenuation image adjustment. The image presented to the normal eye is attenuated while the image presented to the amblyopic eye is enhanced. The main problem of such system is that binocular HMDs have a limited wearability for young children, they either have a very low resolution and a limited weight or a good resolution but a considerable weight, they are costly, and not easily extensible.

The main goal of our research project has been devising a system for vision rebalancing that is accessible. With the term "accessible" we mean: inexpensive (with a low cost), friendly to use, suitable for domestic use, enjoyable, and easily extensible.

All the characteristics listed above should reduce the compliance problem and make the proposed treatment acceptable. In [7] we have presented a system, called 3D4AMB, which is based on 3D vision technologies and which is extended in this paper in a complete environment for domestic supervised amblyopia treatment. The devised system is based on the 3D technologies, although its goal is not to provide the patients with the 3D experience but to allow binocular vision. The classical use of a 3D system is to provide the two eyes with two different images of the same scene with a slightly offset viewing angles which correspond to the different viewpoints of our left and right eye. This vision produces an illusion of real depth of the scene and it is the basis of the *3D virtual reality*. We exploit only the capability of the 3D system to send two different images to the eyes while we do not want to recreate a virtual reality.

The working prototype of the proposed system we have already built, is based on the NVIDIA® 3D Vision™ technology, although other 3D technologies may be supported as well in the future. The NVIDIA 3D Vision technology is one of the most accessible 3D technologies available on the market today, it requires a standard personal computer with a NVIDIA graphic card (also entry level NVIDIA graphic boards work), a monitor 3D Vision ready, which is capable of a refresh rate of 120 Mhz, and a NVIDA 3D glasses. The NVIDIA 3D vision is based on LCD active shutter technology. With this technology, the left and right eye images are presented on alternating frames, but since the monitors used are capable of 120Hz, each eye still sees a full 60Hz signal that is equivalent to the refresh rate on LCD monitors today. This offers a number of advantages with respect to other stereoscopic technologies like polarized or anaglyphs glasses or head-mounted displays, including: **full image quality per eye**, wide viewing angle for 3D, and acceptable cost. The system we have developed for 3D4AMB consists in a normal PC desktop connected to a 3D monitor (3D Vision-Ready Display). The PC must be 3D capable and have all the 3D4AMB software installed on it. The patient wears the NVIDIA active LCD shutter glasses that allow viewing a different image from the left and right eye. The scenario is depicted in Figure 1 and explained below.

Diagnosis. The first use of 3D4AMB software is for the detection and measurement of amblyopia. We have developed some specific diagnosis software

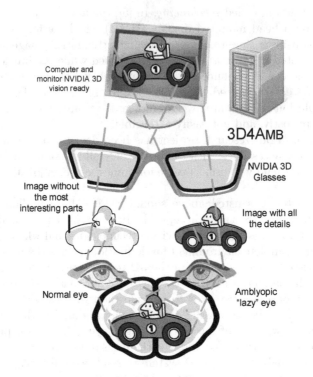

Fig. 1. Video rebalancing: basic principle

that replicates and improves the traditional tests for amblyopia diagnosis and stereoacuity measurement [13]. The tests are presented through the software in a form of videogame and can highlight the presence of amblyopia. Furthermore, the tests give as output the level of weakness of the lazy eye, using a contrast-based measurement of suppression. The contrast balance point can be computed by exploiting the dot stimulus concept. The amblyopic patient watches visual stimulus presented dichoptically (separated images for each eye). Stimuli and noise-stimuli are represented with visible points on the screen, grouped in two sets, named signals and noise. Signals move along horizontal direction and noise moves in random directions. The patient has to guess in what direction the signals are moving. The patient interaction should be minimal, he/she only should say which the right direction is. The difficulty is defined as the number of signals shown to the user when he/she chooses the correct direction. The difficulty is modified through variation of signals number, but the system keeps the number of stimuli constant.

Vision Rebalancing by Video. In [8] we have presented a vision rebalancing system for videos. The basic principle of the system is that the amblyopic or 'lazy' and the normal eye can be shown two different images or videos. This principle can be used in practice for video rebalancing, where the amblyopic eye is shown an enhanced version of a video, while the non-amblyopic or 'good' eye is shown a penalized version of the same video (as shown in Fig. 1). The video to be shown by the patient is duplicated by 3D4AMB in two versions and each version is then modified: one for the right eye (the amblyopic eye in the Figure) is enhanced and one for the left eye (the good eye in the Figure) is penalized. The 3D4AMB software decides how to process the video depending on the type of the desired treatment. In this way, the lazy eye of the child is more stimulated to work, but the non-amblyopic eye is not patched. The patient brain joins (or fuses) the two video versions in one unique vision experience. To make sure that the patient can join the two videos, the two versions must be not too much different. Note that the final video is a bidimensional video because the goal is not to stimulate the stereo vision of the patient (at least initially). We plan to work on the use of real 3D stereo video streaming to combine vision rebalancing with depth perception.

Videogames. We created a rehabilitation environment in a form of video games. To this end, we exploited an open source clone of the well known game Mario Bros, adapting it to our needs. In particular, in the rendering module of the game, we added stereoscopic vision functionalities. In this way, we can select video signal quality independently for the two eyes. (As previously said) The underlying idea is to degrade only the image shown to the normal eye, in order to stimulate the weak eye. To provide the game with an univocal reference scale, we replicated through software the effects of the common occlusion filters. On the user interface it's possible to set the occlusion rate among the following values: 0.0, 0.1, 0.2, 0.3, 0.4, 0.6, 0.8, 1.0, like one would do with the traditional occlusion patches. It's also possible to allocate images on the both two eyes with different percentages. For example, we can send an image with 80% opacity to the weak eye, and the remaining 20% to the normal eye. In this way fusion between the two eyes is stimulated.

We provided the rehabilitation game with two different way to operate: in the first option, we apply the software occlusion filters to the whole image shown to the weak eye. In the second options, we apply filters only to some characters and not to the whole image. For examples, we can occlude partially just the main character, or some enemies, leaving the background untouched. A similar work has been presented also in [14].

2   Use Cases for a Distributed Environment

In this paper we present an extension of the 3D4AMB environment for the diagnosis and treatment of ambliopya in a geographically distributed setting. The basic assumption is that the patient can perform his/her exercises without the need of an actual visit to the hospital or clinic by exploiting our software which is suitable for domestic use. However, she/he is constantly followed by a physician which can supervise (supported by an automatic system) the patient activities, change prescription and recall the patient for a visit if needed.

First of all we have homogenize all the different types of activities presented in the previous section. Every activity has the following attributes:

- **eye** to be penalized, left or right (the normal eye),
- **target** intensity (from 0.1 to 1 with the analogous of the Bangerter foils),
- temporal kind of application, which can be: **instantaneous** (the intensity is applied from the beginning of the exercise at prescribed value), **periodic** (the intensity is applied periodically over the duration of the activity), or **ramp** (the intensity in gradually increased).

We have devised the following scenario, represented in Fig. 2.

1. A patient goes to a physician (an ophthalmologist or an orthoptist).
2. The physician performs the necessary medical tests (possibly by using also the 3D4AMB software) and saves the patient data on a server. The tests give as output the level of weakness of the lazy eye, to be stored in the patient case file. The doctor can add some information such as treatment time lasting and the level of exercise to be performed by the lazy eye. She/he prescribes a series of activities, each with its attributes (type, target intensity, and application kind).
3. The patient periodically starts the (daily) activity at home with his/her computer to which the 3D4AMB software is installed. At the beginning the PC connects with the sever and updates the activities prescriptions, if necessary. Depending on the prescriptions and on the activities already done by the patient, the software suggests to start a certain kind of exercise with suitable parameters (intensity and temporal application). The user is still free to choose what to do, but the PC desktop logs every user choice. At the end (or whenever it is possible) the software client sends information to the server.
4. Periodically the physician logs into the server and checks how the patient is performing. If needed, the doctor can adjust the treatment and recall the patient.

3   Distributed Architecture

The system structure has been designed by following principals guidelines of Health Information Tehcnology (HIT). HIT is the application of information processing involving both computer hardware and software that deals with the storage, retrieval, sharing, and use of health care information, data, and knowledge for communication and decision making [12]. In the last decade, many healthcare software have been developed among which a small set under Free license, such as Health GNU (http://health.gnu.org), FreeMED (http://freemedsoftware.org) and OpenEMR (http://www.open-emr.org). The most important feature of this system is the distributed web design that permits to manage health care information according to the final user (e.g., patient, physician and healthcare personnel) and his/her credentials.

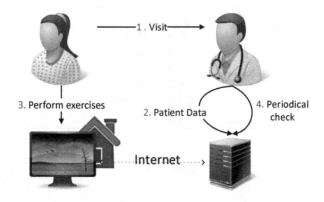

Fig. 2. A typical scenario for domestic supervised treatment

Our system uses the same approach to only manage treatments of visual diseases. The architecture is based on Model-View-Controller pattern for web applications (Fig. 3).

The Model is defined by different modules which permit to manage both patient and treatment data. The information are divided in different modules:

- *Patient Data.* They are composed by both personal information (i.e., first and last name, sex, age) and visual pathologies. In particular, visual pathologies describe the eye condition in terms of visual acuity and improvement level during the rehabilitation. These information are accessible from each actor that uses the distributed platform.

- *Diagnostic Tests.* The doctor associates a set of visual tests in order to make improvements of eye skills. This module contains many parameters, for example the type of diagnostic test, the average duration of each session and medical parameters. The last ones are used from physician to make an evaluation of patient.

- *Rehabilitation Data.* It is a set of parameters which permit to describe the patient's performance during each session of treatment (e.g., duration, level of difficult, number of executed sections).

The modules are managed using database created on server side and it is queried exploiting MySQL DBMS.

The Controller part manages data exchange between database and final user. In particular, the interchange format is defined using XML language which permits to describe information in a consistent way. In order to introduce a standardization of health information, we chosen to use ICD-10 to standardize the description of visual pathologies. For example, instead of typing an arbitrary name for the condition, the doctor will be able to choose from over 14000 mutually exclusive classified

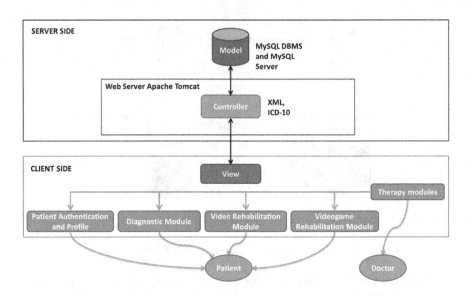

Fig. 3. 3D4AMB system architecture

diseases (http://www.who.int/classifications/icd/en/). In particular, some visual diseases are classified as showed in table 1.

Table 1. Some example of ICD-10 codes about visual disease

ICD-10 Code	Description
H53.009	Amblyopia, unspecified, unspecified eye.
H53.039	Strabismic amblyopia, unspecified eye.
H53.010	Subjective visual disturbances, unspecified.
H53.139	Sudden visual loss, unspecified eye.
H53.2	Diplopia.
H53.30	Disorder of binocular vision, unspecified.
H53.34	Suppression of binocular vision.
H53.33	Simultaneous visual perception without fusion.

The View is defined from both web pages and software for diagnosis and therapy. Furthermore, a data sharing policy has been defined to distinguish information which are only accessible from physicians or generic health personnel. This choice has been made because the patients may wrongly interpret some medical parameters without a medical explanation.

This part defines the client side of 3D4AMB that is formed by applications used from either patient or doctors. A patient can access to his/her health profile through the use of an authentication module released from hospital. The patient profile shows a summary of each treatments which the patient is undergoing. The other patient's modules (i.e., *diagnostic module*, *video rehabilitation module* and *videogame rehabilitation module*) are downlodable applications which permit to execute the prescribed therapy.

A physician can use patient data by exploiting the therapy module. This module is a set of web pages which permit the doctor to manage therapy information for his/her patients. In particular, he/she prescribes activities by modifying some parameters of treatments modules. Furthermore, therapy module allows the doctor an evaluation of therapies. Therefore, doctor delivers the prognosis that will be showed to the patient through the web page of patient profile.

4   Conclusions

We have presented in this paper an environment for providing the treatment for amblyopia in a geographically distributed setting. The proposed system allows a more continuous control by the physicians of the actual progress of the patients, which on the other side, can perform the activities at home without the need of frequent visits to the hospital. We are validating the proposed environment with the collaboration of the local hospital. We are also evaluating the threats to the validity of the current approach. One is that there is no real control over the identity of the patients and (more seriously) about the actual use of the system. For instance, the patient could not wear the glasses or not actually watch the movies as prescribed. We are studying some counter-measures about these problems (for instance by checking periodically during the activities if the user is actually using the system as prescribed).

References

1. Beneish, R.G., Polomeno, R.C., Flanders, M.E., Koenekoop, R.K.: Optimal compliance for amblyopia therapy: Occlusion with a translucent tape on the lens. Can. J. Ophthalmol. 44(5), 523–528 (2009)
2. Charman, W.N.: Optical characteristics of transpaseal as a partial occluder. Am. J. Optom. Physiol. Opt. 60(10), 846–850 (1983)
3. Colombo, G., Facoetti, G., Rizzi, C.: A digital patient for computer-aided prosthesis design. Interface Focus 3(2), 82–84 (2013)
4. Dixon-Woods, M., Awan, M., Gottlob, I.: Why is compliance with occlusion therapy for amblyopia so hard? a qualitative study. Arch. Dis. Child. 91(6), 491–494 (2006)
5. Fateh, S., Speeg, C.: Rebalancing the visual system of people with amblyopia "lazy eye" by using HMD and image enhancement. In: Shumaker, R. (ed.) Virtual and Mixed Reality. LNCS, vol. 5622, pp. 560–565. Springer, Heidelberg (2009), http://dx.doi.org/10.1007/978-3-642-02771-0
6. Fawcett, S.L.: Disruption and reacquisition of binocular vision in childhood and in adulthood. Curr. Opin. Ophthalmol. 16(5), 298–302 (2005)
7. Gargantini, A.: Using 3D vision for the diagnosis and treatment of amblyopia in young children. In: International Conference on Health Informatics HEALTHINF (2011)

8. Gargantini, A., Bana, M., Fabiani, F.: Using 3D for rebalancing the visual system of amblyopic children. In: 2011 International Conference on Virtual Rehabilitation (ICVR), pp. 1–7 (June 2011)
9. Gregson, R.: Why are we so bad at treating amblyopia? Eye 16(4), 461–462 (2002)
10. Newsham, D.: Parental non-concordance with occlusion therapy. British Journal of Ophthalmology 84(9), 957–962 (2000)
11. Searle, A., Norman, P., Harrad, R., Vedhara, K.: Psychosocial and clinical determinants of compliance with occlusion therapy for amblyopic children. Eye 16(2), 150–155 (2002)
12. Thompson, T.G., Brailer, D.J.: The decade of health information technology: Delivering consumercentric and informationrich health care. US Department of Health and Human Services, Washington, DC (2004)
13. Vitali, A., Facoetti, G., Gargantini, A.: An environment for contrast-based treatment of amblyopia using 3D technology. In: International Conference on Virtual Rehabilitation 2013, Philadelphia, PA, U.S.A, August 26-29 (2013)
14. Wei, H., Zhao, Y., Dong, F., Saleh, G., Ye, X., Clapworthy, G.: A cross-platform approach to the treatment of amblyopia. In: 2013 IEEE 13th International Conference on Bioinformatics and Bioengineering (BIBE), pp. 1–4 (November 2013)

Active Prevention by Motivating and Engaging Teenagers in Adopting Healthier Lifestyles:

PEGASO Strategy in Designing Future Healthcare Pillars

Renata Guarneri[1] and Giuseppe Andreoni[2]

[1] Fondazione Politecnico di Milano, P.zza L. Da Vinci, 32 – 20133 Milan, Italy
renata.guarneri@fondazione.polimi.it
[2] Politecnico di Milano, Design Dept. Via Durando 38/A – 20158 Milan, Italy
giuseppe.andreoni@polimi.it

Abstract. Prevention in Healthcare is a mandatory strategy for the next future. Health system sustainability together with lifestyle quality improvement are strictly related to this strategy. PEGASO is a EU funded research project addressing these goals in young people through an integrated approach and system dealing with: human modeling 2.0, wearable technology, and social serious gaming for promoting the adoption of a healthier and happy lifestyle. Such an approach related to social and happiness factors rather than to constraints and limitations is fundamental to ensure long term compliance and efficacy for prevention. User requirements will be addressed by the project including a vision that integrates a lifestyle of healthy habits with an environment that promotes healthy living by encouraging exercise and making healthy food affordable and pleasurable.

Keywords: prevention, social serious gaming, human modeling 2.0, teenagers.

1 Introduction

Health is for everyone a primary, reference, essential and indispensable value. For this reason it is always at the top of the list of both individual and social goals. Nowadays, the term HealthCare is proposing a process that provides a clinical service not exclusively addressed to security and provision of treatment to the individual (which is and remains the main point), but which supports the concept of quality of life for the same individual, his/her family and all the health professionals who interact with him/her every day. In a simple word, we have to move from the concept of "cure" to the concept of "Care", term that embeds the philosophy of quality of care or of "taking care" of the whole person [1]. Thus it is to create a new complex and multifactorial process in which technological factors, organizational, and human dimensions must find a balanced mix for a full success.

At the same time, the growth of expenses for the National Healthcare Systems is no longer sustainable, For this reason new strategies should be identified for future Healthcare. On this issue the European Commission in preparing the Visions for Horizon 2020 evidenced that prevention should become the key strategy for next-generation

V.G. Duffy (Ed.): DHM 2014, LNCS 8529, pp. 351–360, 2014.

healthcare services. Establishment of a European Strategic Action for Healthier Citizens is also recommended, to assist in strategic long-term healthcare research, planning, including preventive measures, and delivery of best practice across Europe [2, 3].

To deliver these services a common and agreed technological platform should be identified as main tool: the rapid development of the ICT, and in particular mobile technologies, together with their increasing diffusion among the EU populations (> 60 millions of person only in EU-5), offers an important opportunity for facing these issues in an innovative manner introducing the possibility of a new technological framework to re-design the healthcare system model.

Always according to the European analysis and vision, one specific target should deal with the huge health problems related to overweight and obesity. Prevention is of obvious importance and there is an urgent need for further research into how physical activity and training, in addition to nutrition, can prevent the steadily increasing average body mass index of Europeans.

These are the three main assumptions behind the development of the PEGASO project and concept. PEGASO (that is the acronym of Personalised Guidance Services for Optimising lifestyle management in teen-agers through awareness, motivation and engagement) is a EU funded research project facing the prevention of obesity and related diseases in younger population though an innovative integrated system, starting from a user-centered perspective so considering the human modeling in three main elements: 1) physical factors, 2) physiological factors, and 3) psychological and social factors. These user requirements will be addressed by the project including a vision that integrates a lifestyle of healthy habits with an environment that promotes healthy living by encouraging exercise and making healthy food affordable. This paper presents the overall methodology and the ongoing results in system design.

2   Methodological Approach

2.1   Identifying the Users and Their Needs

The methodological approach to be followed is strictly related to the specific and sometime critical features of the target users (the younger population) to obtain really motivation and compliance to the PEGASO integrated service system. The starting point is a new user model integrating the three main personal dimensions as explained in Figure 1.

In this view, user-driven and user-centered design is not an option but it is really mandatory. In fact PEGASO will develop a multi-dimensional and cross-disciplinary ICT system that includes game mechanics to influence behaviors in order to fight and prevent overweight and obesity in the younger population by encouraging them to become co-producers of their wellness and take an active role (the said motivation and compliance) in improving it by:

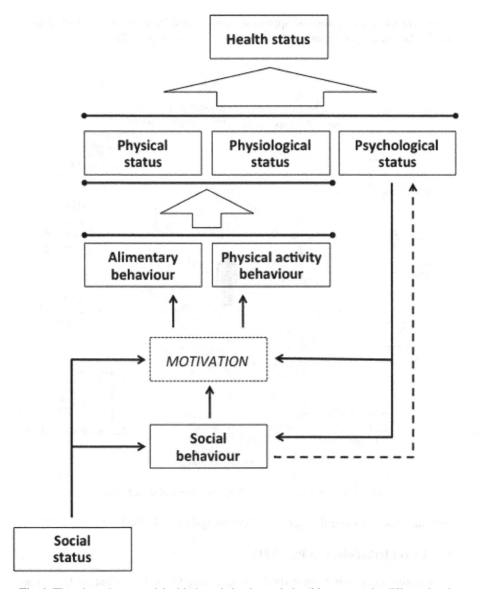

Fig. 1. The adopted user model with the existing interrelationships among the different levels

1. generating self-awareness (acknowledgement of risks associated to unhealthy be-haviors),
2. enhancing and sustaining motivation to take care of their health with a short/medium/long term perspective,
3. changing behavior towards a healthy lifestyle based on healthy diet and adequate physical activity.

However the methodological approach should consider also the complex ecosystem of stakeholders participating the Healthcare process (Figure 2).

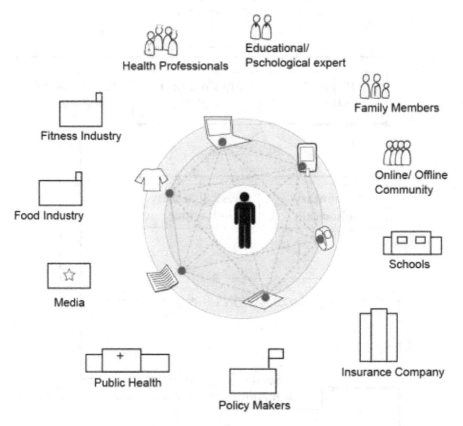

Fig. 2. The user centred PEGASO ecosystem of stakeholders

For this reason, a more detailed and wider analysis was defined.

2.2   UCD Methodology in PEGASO

The proposed analysis is been carried out according to the User Centred Design approach (UCD) [4] by considering our target population (i.e. teenagers) at the centre of the system in a palingenetic process (Figure 3). This approach is useful to motivate and engage users, which is an essential requirement for systems' acceptance and efficacy rather than forcing to accommodate technologies, products, or services. It should be underlined that PEGASO, as tool for prevention, is addressed in general to healthy people. Recruitment of teenagers has been done through schools, focusing on fostering communities of interest (i.e. all students in a class), rather than students with identified risk factors. This step is still on-going to have a very wide and representative sample.

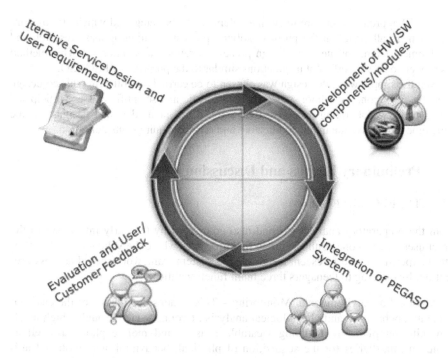

Fig. 3. The UCD approach applied to PEGASO project

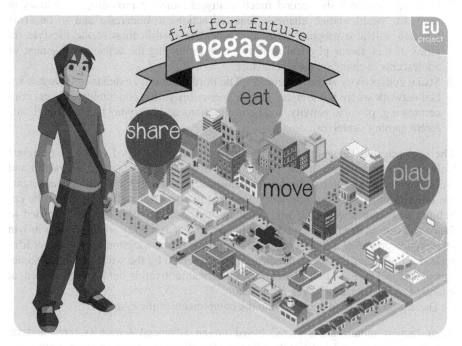

Fig. 4. One of the co-designed home page for the Pegaso System web-site

In UCD approach, there are three main elements to be integrated which are: user involvement in all stages of the problem solving process, multidisciplinary research and development team, and iterative design process to refine the solution set. This method has proven to be very efficient in situations similar to the purposes of PEGASO.

Even the simple web-site design was chosen to be carried out following this co-design principle. 30 secondary school students of humanistic and scientific classes participated in this activity elaborating and cross-evaluating different models and designs. At the same time they drove the initial architecture and service requirements definition.

3   Preliminary Results and Discussion

3.1   The PEGASO Features

From the preparatory analysis [5] and also confirmed by the early interviews to the target user panel in one country among the three sites where the validation and exploitation experiments are foreseen, the PEGASO system framework should address prevention, by offering to teenagers three main functionalities:

1. Individual & Environmental Monitoring – This dimension consists of the environmental, behavioral and physiological analysis of young users, through a high level-monitoring platform including wearable sensors and mobile phone as well as multimedia diaries for the acquisition of physical, behavioral and emotional attitude of adolescent.
2. Feedback System - the second functionality is aimed at providing a feedback in terms of "health status" changes, required actions to undertake and so on. This function will also propose personalized healthy modification of the lifestyle (in terms of diet and/or physical activity), thus promoting the active involvement of adolescents in changing their behaviors.
3. Social connectivity and engagement - The third dimension extends to include a social network where the user can share experiences with a community of peers concerning e.g. physical activity, food consumptions and everyday habits through different gaming strategies.

The user selected keywords to clarify these concepts are listed in the co-designed web-site shown in figure 3: Eat, Move, Play, Share. *Eat* is related to my health and wellbeing status together with *Move* because the regular physical activity represents the prevention strategy but also an indicator of the personal wellbeing and of the capability to obtain rewards for my avatar in the game. So *Play* is strictly related to *Move* and also to engagement and compliance. In teenager *Play* could be the win-win strategy to carry over a long term prevention through the adoption of a healthier lifestyle. Last but least the social dimension is represented by the willingness and sometimes need to *Share*, so to have not only a personal motivation but a group or even, at a larger level, a social motivating dimension.

These goal have been declined into the components of the system:

1. an "active monitoring system" based on an advanced sensor systems and on both exergames and social/networked games allows to discover at an early stage

potential risks of developing obesity and related co-morbidities and encouraging lifestyle changes; technology innovation and fashion trends help this point thanks to the diffusion of wearable technologies embedding monitoring capabilities passing from simple Apps to be mounted into the smartphone to a set of activity trackers and up to sensorized garments;

2. a set of serious games, that are expected to be a key tool to support the education of teen-agers towards healthier lifestyles;
3. the educational level, obtained starting from physical seminars to teachers and parents by means of online educational modules engaging the educational environment (families and schools) reinforce the delivered messages;
4. the global social dimension for integrating all the actors and stakeholders of the healthcare prevention service and system through the information accessibility and sharing; this will support the improvement of stakeholders decisions and provision of specific and personalized services.

About these last global and social dimension of the PEGASO approach, it is important to underline how it is highly important to focus on the interactions points between end users and levels of their influences, in particular where end user is able to give their own decisions, or where the intervention of services and persuasion to healthier lifestyle changes will be acted upon these opportunity areas. This could really exploit motivation and persuasion that in teenagers could be the most difficult targets to be reached also for the "critical age". If we succeed in this persuasion strategy we obtain the passage from youth rebels to future healthcare co-producers, a new engaged and motivated generation. This challenge is high but stimulating.

3.2   The PEGASO Architecture

The user centred PEGASO system can be split into the following three components: a) a first technological frame, including the all the ICT products (multimedia diaries, embedded sensors systems, mobile & web platform) offering a non-intrusive behavior measuring system and, at the same time, the technological endpoint to provide the user with the personal guidance system; thanks to the mobile technology worldwide diffusion we argued also about the smartphones as the ideal possible sustainable solution for achieving a technologic al convergence towards a common platform (apart from OS differences), b) a services frame that try to give a personalized answer to user needs and desires in real time/not real time, for example stakeholders services to provide answers to users' needs, from the health companion to the serious gaming and social experiences; c) an experts layer which provide the teenagers at individual level and relationship, with filtered accurate and needed information to reach their objective.

About the technological frame, we have based our assumptions of the observation that teens are familiar with Internet, social networks, mobile phones and apps, video gaming and, in general, with all the ICT platforms. Smartphones also assures the highest level of technology acceptance. This key issues are assumed as technological starting point to define the PEGASO architecture and to define a successful strategy to empower the teen-agers awareness about healthy lifestyle. The huge amount of personal and social exchanged and/or stored data includes also health records, thus posing severe reliability and security requirements that will be effectively managed through a cloud platform. Finally, PEGASO apps and games from the software layer, as well as wearable sensor and other more traditional systems (balance board for instance) complete the PEGASO technology frame.

Concerning the services frame, we have started from the obvious and undoubted statement that "social" is the key word for service development especially in teenagers: this imply a mass-customized approach in all the main pillars of the proposed intervention (Eat, Move, Play, education). In practice this could be an individual support both for data entry through multimedia apps that simplify and engage the users (for instance through multimedia diary compilation or through the health companion interaction). The social level also helps the diffusion of the approach, of the data and system among all the stakeholders, the PEGASO experts but including the Food Industry, Public and Private health Policy actors, Fitness industries, Media, Schools, and Insurance companies, at different levels.

To the Experts layer belong knowledgeable groups of people from different disciplines - medical/psychological/educational – able to interact with the user and with the system. This integrated pool of experts have to promote motivation and engagement by means of gaming strategies will be integrated with healthier lifestyle. All the information from the users must be "handled" and processed and the corresponding feedback provided. This means building an expert layer that is able to analyze all the data and deliver the resulting answers to the teenagers. A part of this layer will be composed by automatic algorithm (for real-time processing and feedback provision when applicable); a second building block will be the experts' team who will integrate the previous assessment to better stimulate the teenagers' consciousness about obesity and their motivation to adopt a healthy lifestyle. The role of experts in PEGASO project is assumed to be twofold: 1) to personalize information for each individual's physical and psychological models (i.e. personalized care) in order to reach the full acceptance by each teenager and guarantee a correct interpretation; and 2) to follow up of each teenager healthy status. As a consequence, psychologist and educational experts as well as medical experts must be involved in the definition of the system concept e.g. which are the most potential successful tools, and/or what kind of educational model can help influencing the prevention intention of the users.

A specific remark could be dedicated to serious games methodology applied in healthcare. Gaming seems to be a very promising strategy [6-8]. Principles of gamification have been proposed [9], but understanding how to design video games to maximize their health behaviour–enhancing effects is in the earliest stages [10]. Recently, a review of English-language journal articles from 1998 to 2011 using EMBASE and PubMed was conducted [11]. Thirty-four studies concerned with children, video games, physical, and/or nutritional outcomes were included. Results of these studies that showed some benefit (increased physical activity and nutritional knowledge as a result of gaming) demonstrate the possibility of video games to combat childhood obesity, looking beyond the stigma attached to gaming.

4   Conclusions

We as PEGASO consortium believe that we are at a key turning point in the history of the Internet. Convergence of major trends is occurring which is driving changes in people behavior and expectations. These trends include the exponential rise in use of smartphones and tablets, increased Internet access speeds, new business models driven by online commerce and app stores, the impact of social online communication, and software delivery transitioning from prior PC/internet models to cloud-based services accessed with touch-based devices (smartphones and media tablets). With more than five billion mobile users worldwide and a massive global network, for the first time in history mobility is attracting significant attention among the healthcare and life sciences community. This wide ICT platform offers today a unique opportunity to develop innovative healthcare services.

According to the personal, social and institutional needs, including the economical aspects, new services and models needs to be identified for the healthcare in 2020 and beyond. Quality of life and prevention have been identified and key and un-factors to be considered. Starting from this assumptions the PEGASO Project is promoting the adoption of an individual and social healthier lifestyle through motivating and engaging multiuser serious games.

Integrating mobility, gamification and life science has the potential to motivate individuals to adopt healthy lifestyles, through the use of personalization techniques and incentives that will be delivered through the PEGASO system. In fact we believe that for future healthcare services with efficient and long term compliance the key strategies to be exploited i.e. the Persuasion Levels for Disease Prevention are: Develop Awareness, Affective learning, Create Motivation, and Enable Behaviour Change [12].

These are the new prevention pillars we assumed and we will try to apply into the PEGASO approach.

Aknowledgements. This work has been funded by the European Commission: FP7-ICT-2013.5.1 - Grant Agreement n° 610727. The Authors would like to thank all the partners of the PEGASO consortium for their proactive collaboration in the project.

References

1. Andreoni, G., Costa, F., Mazzola, M., Fusca, M., Romero, M., Carniglia, E., Zambarbieri, D., Santambrogio, G.C.: A multi factorial approach and method for assessing ergonomic characteristics in biomedical technologies. In: Duffy, V.G. (ed.) Advances in Human Aspects of Healthcare. Advances in Human Factors and Ergonomics Series, 760 pages. CRC Press (2012) Print ISBN: 978-1-4398-7021-1 eBook ISBN: 978-1-4398-7022-8 (eBook), pp. 3-12 (2012)
2. Visions for Horizon 2020- Copenhagen Research Forum (2012)
3. World Health Organization. Population-based prevention strategies for childhood obesity: Report of a WHO forum and technical meeting, Geneva, pp. 15–17 (December 2009)
4. Sanders, E.B.: From User-Centered To Participatory Design Approaches. Design, pp. 1-7. Taylor & Francis (2002)
5. Arslan, P.: Mobile Health for Social Interaction - Applying Mobile Technologies for a Healthier Lifestyle. PolimiSpringer Brief (in press)
6. Przybylski, A.K., Rigby, C.S., Ryan, R.M.: A motivational model of video game engagement. Rev. Gen. Psychol. 14, 154–166 (2010)

7. Cullen, K., Baranowski, T., Smith, S.: Using goal setting as a strategy for dietary behavior change. J. Am. Diet. Assoc. 101, 562–566 (2001)

8. Latif, H., Watson, K., Nguyen, N., et al.: Effects of goal setting ondietary and physical activity changes in the Boy Scout badge projects. Health Educ. Behav. 38, 521–529 (2011)

9. Bunchball. Gamification 101: An introduction to the use of game dynamics to influence behavior (October 2010), http://www.bunchball.com/ (last accessed December 10, 2012)

10. Baranowski, T., Baranowski, J., Thompson, D., et al.: Behavioral science in video games for children's diet and physical activity change: Keyresearch needs. J. Diabetes Sci. Technol. 5, 229–233 (2011)

11. Guy, S., Ratzki-Leewing, A., Gwadry-Sridhar, F.: Moving Beyond the Stigma: Systematic Review of Video Games and Their Potential to Combat Obesity. International Journal of Hypertension, 2011, Article ID 179124, 13 pages (2011), doi:10.4061/2011/179124

12. Fogg, B.J.: A Behavior Model for Persuasive Design. In: Proceedings of the 4th International Conference on Persuasive Technology Persuasive 2009 (2009), ISBN:9781605583761

Robot Patient for Nursing Self-training in Transferring Patient from Bed to Wheel Chair

Zhifeng Huang[1], Ayanori Nagata[1], Masako Kanai-Pak[2], Jukai Maeda[2],
Yasuko Kitajima[2], Mitsuhiro Nakamura[2], Kyoko Aida[2], Noriaki Kuwahara[3],
Taiki Ogata[1], and Jun Ota[1]

[1] Research into Artifacts, Center for Engineering (RACE),
The University of Tokyo, Chiba, Japan
[2] Faculty of Nursing, Tokyo Ariake University of Medical and Health Sciences,
Tokyo, Japan
[3] Department of Advanced Fibro-Science, Kyoto Institute of Technology, Kyoto, Japan
zhifeng@race.u-tokyo.ac.jp

Abstract. In this paper, we proposed a robot patient for the nursing training in patient transfer. The robot patient was developed to reproduce the performance of the patients who are suffering from mobility problems. We targeted on the reproduction of movement of the patient's limbs (arms and legs) with the consideration of physical and voice interaction between the patient and nurse. The robot patient had 15 joints including 2 active joints installed with motors, 4 passive joints installed with electric brakes and 9 passive joints without any actuators. To realize the physical interaction, potentiometer type angle sensors was utilized to detect the rotation angle of the joints of shoulders, elbows and knees. In addition, follow-up control approach was applied to the shoulder joint. By this way the robot could react accordingly when the trainees moved its limbs. A voice recognition module was applied to enable the robot to interact with the trainee by voice. An experiment was performed by a nursing teacher for examine the robot's performance. The robot patient successfully reproduced the patient's movement with physical and voice interaction, including embracing, keeping embracing, standing up, keeping standing and sitting down.

Keywords: nursing skills training, robot patient, patient transfer.

1   Introduction

In nursing care, there are many tasks involving moving the patient's body, such as bathing, giving assistance in dressing, and transferring patient from bed to wheel-chair[1-3]. For the safety of nurses and patients, it is critically important of the nurses to accurately acquire these skills.

In order to improve the skills for nurses and nursing students in such tasks, the mock patient is generally utilized in simulated training to reproduce the real patient's performance. In traditional nursing education, generally, the mock patients are acted by the stationary manikins [4, 5] or the healthy people [6]. However, such mock

V.G. Duffy (Ed.): DHM 2014, LNCS 8529, pp. 361–368, 2014.
© Springer International Publishing Switzerland 2014

patients cannot precisely reproduce the real patients. For example, the stationary manikins cannot reproduce the movements of human's joints. In addition, the stationary manikins are unable to respond to the trainees' operation, such as motions or voice commands. On the other hands, for the healthy people, it is difficult to simulate the movements of the patient with decline of muscle strength and paralysis. The healthy people often move their body unconsciously during simulating the patients and the movements often help the trainees to complete the tasks. In view of this, to develop a robot patient which could accurately reproduce the patient's limb movements and interact with the trainee would be great help for the nurses and nursing students to improve their nursing skills.

Former studies developed robots for various medical trainings, such as trainings of dentist's clinic [7], medical examination [8-9] and air way management [10]. However, there are few researches of robots for reproduction of patients' body limbs' movement. In addition, the physical interaction between trainees and patients (e.g. embracing) was not taken into consideration.

The aim of this paper is to solve the problem of reproducing patient's body limbs movement with the consideration of interaction between trainees and patients. The challenging points are how to realize the body limbs movement by minimal actuators and the reproduction of physical and voice interaction.

The prototype robot patient for patient transfer training was proposed in this paper. Using the stationary mannequin as the base, we design arms and the knee joints of the robot. Utilizing the electric brakes and servo motors, the patient's limbs movement was reproduced included passively standing up and sitting down, actively embracing nurse's shoulder and keeping standing posture and embracing posture. Angle sensors were installed on the limb joints to detect the movement of the robot's limb for the purpose of physical interaction with the training. In addition, the speech recognition technique was utilized for voice interaction.

The remainder of the paper is structured as follows. Section 2 describes the robot's specification. Section 3 details the hardware configuration of the robot including joints mechanical structure and sensors. Section 4 details the control methods. Section 5 presents the results of an experiment carried out by an experienced nursing teacher to examine the robot patient's performance. Section 6 concludes the paper.

2   Design Specification

2.1   Procedures of Transferring a Patient from Bed to Wheelchair

When nurses perform transferring a patient form bed to wheelchair, firstly, they should adjust the sitting position of patients and then assist the patients to embrace to their shoulders. Since the patient's arm is weak, nurse need to lift the patients' arm to complete the embracing motion. After that, nurses assist the patient to bend down and then assist the patient to stand up, turn to the wheelchair and sit down. Patient's low limbs were weak and very easy to fall down. Therefore, during such process above, nurses need to hold the patient's waits and support most of the weight of the patients, especially during standing and siting process.

2.2   Design Specification of the Robot Patient

Based on the typical performance of patients who are with mobility problems and need the patient transfer nursing care, the specification of the robot patient for patient transfer training was defined.

The robot height was set as 160 cm and the weight was 25 kg. The robot's arms should have enough degree of freedom to reproduce the embracing motion. While trainee was lifting the robot's arms, the shoulder joints should be able to provide force to embrace the trainee. In addition, the embracing motion should be able to keep while standing up and sitting down.

For the lower limbs, the knee joints should be able to passively rotate during standing and sitting process. The knee joints should provide enough force to keeping standing posture even although the joints did not expand totally. The minimum expanding angle was set as 165 degree.

The robot should be able to understand the trainee's comments. When trainees ask the robot patient to sitting down, the knee joints should loosen automatically for passive rotation.

3   Hardware Configuration

3.1   Joint Configuration of the Robot Patient

The joint configuration of the robot was shown in Fig. 1. The robot has 15 joints, including 2 active joints installed with motor (Futaba Co., Ltd), 4 passive joints installed with electric brakes (Miki Pulley Co., Ltd.) and 9 passive joints without any actuator.

To detect the rotation angle, potentiometer type angle sensors (Alps Electric Co., Ltd) were attached on the joints: shoulder joint S-y, elbow joints and the knee joints. The shoulder joint S-x was installed with a servo motor which had an angle sensor inside.

The patient robot was with the height of 160 cm. The robot's weight is 25kg, which is similar to the mean of real Japanese elderly patients.

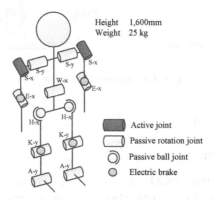

Fig. 1. Joint configuration of the robot patient

3.2   Arms

The robot arm had two degrees in the shoulder joints and one degree in the elbow joints (Fig. 2(a)).

The shoulder joint S-x was installed with a servo motor to reproduce the embracing movement of the patient. The motor was working on 7.4 V and the max output toque is 3.2 Nm. The shoulder joint S-y was a passive joint which was installed a potentiometer type angle sensor.

In the elbow joint, an electric brake was installed. The elbow joints would work in two modes, passive rotation and posture maintaining by controlling the brake to be on or off. The electric brake was working on 24V and its output torque is 2.4 Nm.

3.3   Knee Joints

An electric brake was installed on the knee joint to enable the robot patient to keep standing (Fig. 2(b)). The electric brake was working on 24 V and it output torque is 11 Nm. The torque enabled the robot patient to keep standing even if the knee joints' angle was no totally expended. The minimum open angle of the knee joint in the situation of keeping standing was 165 degree. This design enables the robot patient to simulate the patients' performance that their knee joint is unable to expand to 180 degree totally when keeping standing.

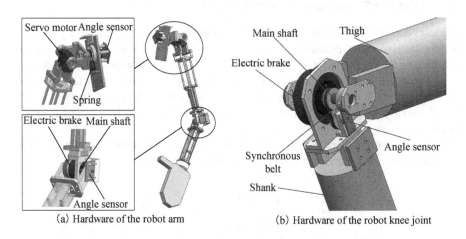

(a) Hardware of the robot arm   (b) Hardware of the robot knee joint

Fig. 2. Hardware of the robot

4   Control Methods

4.1   Voice Interaction

The voice interaction was realized by the voice recognition module (TIGAL KG Co., Ltd). The robot was trained to recognize two words in Japanese: "Hello." and "Please sit down." When the trainee said hello to the robot, the robot would answer "Hello" to the trainee. This interaction happens before the patient transfer begins. This interaction is a required procedure according to the nursing textbook. When the trainee said "Please sit down" to the robot, the robot would answer "I understand." and then release the knee joints to sit down with the help of the trainee. This command is available only when the step of standing assistance was finished.

4.2   Physical Interaction of Body Limbs

Arm. In order to reproduce embracing movement of the patient, the follow-up control approach was applied on the servo motor of shoulder joint S-x. The servo motor's rotation angle based on the rotation angle of shoulder joint S-y.

During lifting the robot patient's arm, the shoulder joints of the robot would slowly rotate to embrace the nurse. Firstly, while the robot's arms were lower than the level of the shoulder, the shoulder joint was unfolding. Second, while the arm was higher than the shoulder level, the shoulder joint would start to fold. Finally, when the embracing finished, the shoulder joints and elbow joints would provide the torques to keep embracing. The torque would maintain until the transfer process finished.

Knee. In the beginning of the patient transfer process, the knee joints' brake was put off to enable the joints to passive rotation with the trainees' assistance. The trainee could adjust the legs' posture freely and then to assist the robot patient to stand up. The knee joints would passively expand during standing up. Once both the expanding angle of the knee joints was bigger than 165 degree, the brake would be put on. The torque of friction of the brake supported the robot patient's weight to keep standing. The robot patient was keeping standing until the turning was finished. Then the trainee would give comment to inform the robot patient to relax the knee joints for sitting down by voice interaction.

5   Experiment

5.1   Procedures

In order to examine the proposed robot patient's performance in patient transfer training, we conducted an experiment with a nursing teacher who is an expert in the nursing field. The teacher performed the steps of standing process and the sitting process to evaluate whether the robot patient would well reproduce the patient's performance, including voice interaction and physical interaction of body limbs.

In addition, the teacher was also asked to perform the same steps to an human mock patient who has up to 30 hours experiences in simulating patient for patient transfer training. The height of the mock patient is 160 cm. The height is the same as the robot.

The head trajectories of the robot were compared with the human mock-patients, since the head trajectories would reflect the movement of the mock patient's whole bodies during standing and sitting processes. We used the camera to record the image sequence of the experiment process. The image processing approach which was developed in our previous work [11] was utilized to extract the trajectories of the head of both robot and human mock patient.

5.2   Results and Discussion

Fig. 3 shows the image sequences when the nursing teacher assisted the robot to embrace stand up and sit down. The robot patient successfully reproduced the patient's movement of body limbs, including active rotation of shoulder joints, passive rotation of elbow joints and the knee joints. In addition, the posture keeping (embracing and standing) was also reproduced.

Fig. 4 shows the trajectories of heads of the robot patient and the human mock patient. The axis of x and y were respectively corresponding to the head's movement in vertical and horizontal direction (Fig. 3). The trajectories of the robot patient were similar to that of the human mock patient during the process of sitting down. The slope of the trajectories was slowly increasing as the decrease of the x.

However, for the standing process, trajectories of the robot patient were different from that of the human mock patient. The difference was caused by the rotation range of the waist of the robot patient which was not enough. The human mock patient bended her back forward during standing while the robot patient bended the back backward.

The nursing teacher's subjective evaluation of the robot patient's performance was also conducted. The teacher was satisfied with physical interaction through the movement of the robot patient's arms. The teacher's comments are follows. The follow-up control of the shoulder joint well reproduced the movement of the weak patient's arms. The keeping embracing was also well reproduced by the patient robot. In addition, the teacher was satisfied with the reproduction of movement of the patient's knee joints, especially the movement when the sitting down process. The teacher commented that the electric brake of the robot patient would well reproduce the situation that the patient's knee joints' force suddenly disappears when the siting down assistance begins. This performance was difficult to reproduce even though by the experienced human mock patient.

From the nursing teacher's view point, this robot patient was suited to the simulated training for the trainees who have the patient transfer experience before hand, such as the senior nursing students or the nurses.

The nursing teachers' advises for improvements were the same as head trajectories analysis results. That is, the robot patient's waist should be improved to enable the robot to reproduce the back bending forward during standing up. This improvement will be considered in our future works.

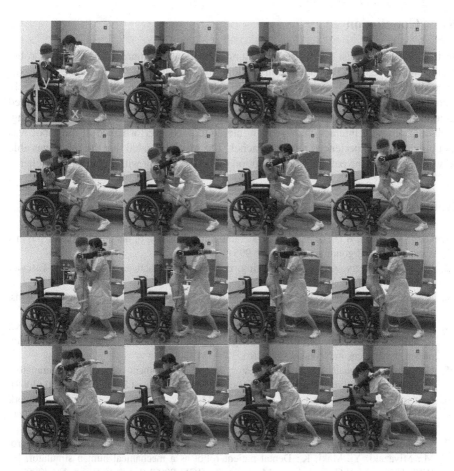

Fig. 3. Image sequences when nursing teacher performed patient transfer using the robot patient: embracing (6s to 10s), standing assistance (11s to 13s), keeping standing (14s to 18s) and sitting assistance (18s to 20s)

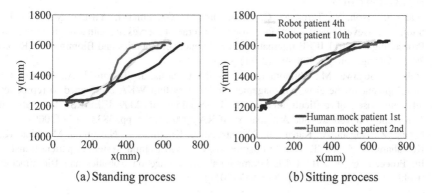

(a) Standing process   (b) Sitting process

Fig. 4. Comparison of head trajectories

6   Conclusion

In this paper, to assist the nurses and nursing student to improve their skill, a robot patient was developed for patient transferring training. The robot was designed to reproduce the patient's limb's motion, including embracing, keeping embracing, passively standing, sitting and keeping standing. Through the potentiometer type sensors installed in joints and speech recognition module, the robot was able to interact with the training, including physical interaction and voice interaction. The performance of the robot was examined by an experienced nursing teacher. The result revealed that the robot was able to well reproduce the patient's limbs motion while interacting with the nursing teacher.

References

1. Garg, A., Owen, B.D., Carlson, B.: An ergonomic evaluation of nursing assistants, job in a nursing home. Ergonomics 35(9), 979–995 (1992)
2. Potter, P.A., Perry, A.G.: Basic Nursing: Essentials for Practice, ch. 25. Mosby Elsevier (2003)
3. Rosdahl, C.B., Kowalski, M.T.: Textbook of Basic Nursing. Lippincott Williams & Wilkins, ch. 48 (2008)
4. Yaeger, K.A., Halamek, L.P., Coyle, M., Murphy, A., Anderson, J., Boyle, K., Braccia, K., Mcauley, J., Desandre, G., Smith, B.: High-fidelity simulation-based training in neonatal nursing. Advances in Neonatal Care 4(6), 326–331 (2004)
5. Cooper, J.B., Taqueti, V.R.: A brief history of the development of mannequin simulators for clinical education and training. Postgraduate Medical Journal 84(997), 563–570 (2008)
6. Johnsson., A.C.E., Kjellberg, A., Lagerström, M.I.: Evaluation of nursing students' work technique after proficiency training in patient transfer methods during undergraduate education. Nurse Education Today 26(4), 322–331 (2006)
7. Takanobu, H., Omata, A., Takahashi, F., Yokota, K., Suzuki, K., Miura, H., Madokoro, M., Miyazaki, Y., Maki, K.: Dental patient robot as a mechanical human simulator. In: IEEE International Conference on Mechatronics (ICM 2007), Kumamoto, pp. 1–6 (2007)
8. Hashimoto, T., Morita, K., Kato, N., Kobayashi, H., Nakane, H.: Depression patient robot for diagnostic training in psychiatric education. In: In Proceedings of 2011 IEEE/ASME International Conference on Advanced Intelligent Mechatronics (AIM 2011), Budapest, pp. 134–139 (2011)
9. Wang, C., Noh, Y., Terunaga, C., Tokumoto, M., Okuyama, I., Yusuke, M., Ishii, H., Shoji, S.: Development of a face robot for cranial nerves examination training. In: Proceedings of 2011 IEEE International Conference on Robotics and Biomimetics (Robio 2011), Guangzhou, pp. 908–913 (2011)
10. Noh, Y., Segawa, M., Shimomura, A., Ishii, H., Solis, J., Takanishi, A., Hatake, K.: Development of the airway management training system WKA-2 designed to reproduce different cases of difficult airway. In: Proceedings of 2009 IEEE/RSJ International Conference on Robotics and Automation (ICRA 2009), Kobe, pp. 3833–3838 (2009)
11. Huang, Z., Nagata, A., Kanai-Pak, M., Maeda, J., Kitajima, Y., Nakamura, M., Aida, K., Kuwahara, N., Ogata, T., Ota, J.: Posture study for self-training system of patient transfer. In: Proceedings of 2011 IEEE International Conference on Robotics and Biomimetics (Robio 2011), Guangzhou, pp. 842–847 (2011)

Evaluating the Healthcare Management System by Usability Testing

Po-Hsin Huang and Ming-Chuan Chiu

Department of Industrial Engineering and Engineering Management,
National Tsing Hua University, Taiwan
No. 101, Section 2, Kuang-Fu Road, Hsinchu, Taiwan 30013, R.O.C
s9834815@m98.nthu.edu.tw

Abstract. To maintain and enhance good health status, many health management products have been developed. However, most of these products are lack of friendliness and usability. This study proposed a new process to evaluate the usability with an aim to improve the user experience. An experiment was conducted that participants played a Kinect sport game based healthcare management system. Results showed that the heart rates of participants were increased while using this product and led to effective exercise. According to the questionnaire results, this study also proposed some suggestions from the participants to improve the healthcare management system usability. The contributions of this study are both on the academic and practical aspects. In the academia, this study created a usability testing process to evaluate and verify a product/system. Practically, the result in this study could enhance the healthcare management system in a more friendly and useful manner.

Keywords: usability testing, user experience, healthcare management system, kinect.

1 Introduction

Healthy means well condition in both mental and physical status. Regular and suitable exercises are very important for people's health. According to the World Health Organization (WHO), "Health is a state of complete physical, mental and social well-being and not merely the absence of disease or infirmity [1]". Hence, proper exercise could avoid or treat health troubles, promote the well mental, and keep healthy of human beings. However, in Taiwan, a lot of workers only had few time for the exercise. This results in worse health status. A healthcare management system is beneficial to keep healthy.

The purpose of a healthcare management system is to assist people to record the variety of physiological data and monitor their health status by themselves. There are already many products in healthcare applications on smart phones or television games. Many Taiwanese used them to maintain health or rehabilitation. However, some of the product interfaces were not designed and evaluated properly which lead

V.G. Duffy (Ed.): DHM 2014, LNCS 8529, pp. 369–376, 2014.

to usability problems. Therefore, products of the healthcare management system are not useful and efficient.

The usability and user experience (UX) plays an important role in the product design and development process. International Organization for Standardization (ISO) defined that usability includes effectiveness, efficiency and satisfaction [2]. UX is the linkage between usability attributes and the corresponding user experience attributes [3]. Furthermore, usability metrics could serve as the instruments to evaluate the UX of product [4].

A new healthcare management system prototype combined with the Kinect motion games were developed by a research team in Taiwan. This study would evaluate that prototype interfaces applying the user experience and usability metrics so as to improve the friendliness and usability of this product.

2   Literature Review

This study evaluated a healthcare management system based on user experience and usability testing. The subsections are introduction of user experience and usability metrics.

2.1   User Experience

User experience (UX) is associated with a variety of meanings, ranging from usability, hedonic and experiential aspects of technology use [5]. UX were mainly programmatic [6], aimed at convincing the Human Computer Interaction (HCI) community to take issues beyond the task-related more seriously. The key is that measures of user experience should concern user performance based on actual usage [7]. Moreover, each of the product, usability and UX would represent a unique but interdependent aspect of usage. Usability metric for user experience is adopted for the subjective assessment of a product application's perceived usability [8].

2.2   Usability Metrics

According to the definition of the International Organization for Standardization (ISO) 9241-11, usability is associated with effectiveness, efficiency and satisfaction as achieved by users [9]. According to the previous research, it was found that usability could address eight main metrics: effectiveness, efficiency, satisfaction, errors, learnability and flexibility [10]. Nielson [11] defined the usability as learnability, efficiency, memorability, errors and satisfaction. Brink, Gergle, and Wood [12] share a similar viewpoint that usability is functionally correct, efficient to use, easy to learn and remember, error tolerant, and subjectively pleasing.

2.3   Summary

Based on the literature review, usability and user experience are two critical factors of a product, service or system, especially for a new health management system. Therefore, this study developed a simple but efficient process to measure the Kinect sport game based healthcare management system performance with usability metrics.

3   Methodology

This study conducted an experiment and designed the usability questionnaire to evaluate the healthcare management system. The research methodology was introduced as the following sections.

3.1   Questionnaire

According to the usability metrics, this study designed the questionnaire to collect and analyze the participant's feedback. The questionnaire was divided into the three parts: regular product usability metrics, create new user account at first time and product interaction customized for kinect product. The product usability metrics has 24 items, the establishment a new user account has 8 items and the product interaction has 15 items.

3.2   Participants

There were 45 participants to execute the tasks in the experimental process. They were including the 29 male and 16 female.

3.3   Design of Experiment

This study conducted an experiment to evaluate the Healthcare Management System. Firstly, the participants' heart rate (HR) would measure before the experiment by blood pressure meter (Fig. 2). Then, the subjects would initialize the healthcare management system by creating new user account. After setting up the new account, the subjects would play sport games in the healthcare management as exercise. Finally, the subjects would measure the HR again and fill in the usability questionnaire after the experiment. The Fig.1 shows the experimental process.

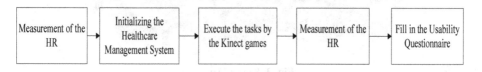

Fig. 1. Experimental Process

3.4 Experiment Equipment

The participants played and evaluated the Kinect sport game based healthcare management system in the experiment. The experimental equipment was blood pressure meter (Fig.2) and system devices (Fig.3 and Fig.4).

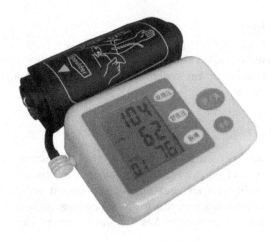

Fig. 2. Blood Pressure Meter

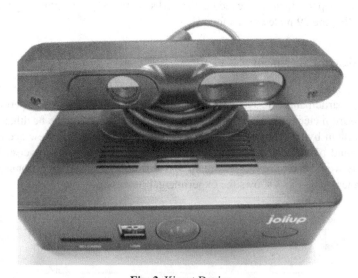

Fig. 3. Kinect Device

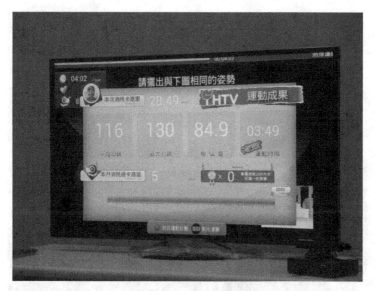

Fig. 4. Monitor Device

4   Results

After the experiment, this study recorded the participant's heart rate before and after the experiment. In addition, this study utilized the Statistical Product and Service Solutions (SPSS) 15.0® to analyze the questionnaire results. The Fig. 5 and Fig. 6 are male and female participants in the experiment.

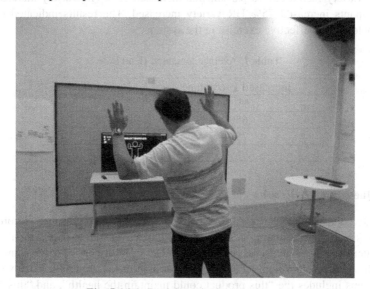

Fig. 5. Male Participant in the experiment

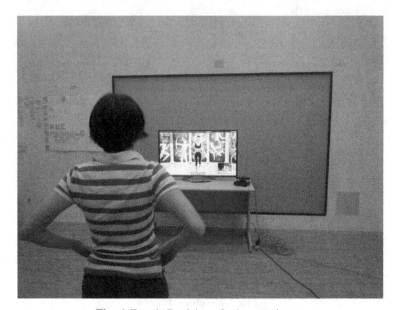

Fig. 6. Female Participant in the experiment

4.1   Heart Rate Variety

Before and after the experiment, this study measured the participant's heart rate (HR) by blood pressure meter. The average increased heart rate is shown in the table 1. There are eight participants had 55% HR variety increased, 11 participants increased 65% HR variety increased, 16 participants increased 75% HR variety increased and 10 participants increased 75% HR variety increased. The results indicated that the users would lead to effective exercise in the system.

Table 1. Average Increased Heart Rate

Increased Percentage	Participants
55 %	8
65%	11
75%	16
85%	10

4.2   Questionnaire Results

This study used statistical t-test to analysis the questionnaire results. According to the results and questionnaire design, the results cover three parts. Firstly, there are two items in the analysis results of the product usability are positive significantly ($p < 0.05$), and the other items scores are bigger than the average. The positive significantly items includes the "this product could maintain the health", and "this product could report correct physiological and physical information". The results showed that this product could assist users in maintaining their health status.

Under created new user account category, one item in the analysis results is positively significant ($p < 0.05$). This item is "ask for unnecessary information in the system". Besides, there are also three items scores are below the average in metrics. They include the "receive operating information efficiently", "create new account in short time" and "not easy to make mistake". The result shows that there are many operating problems in the stage of creating new user account. This indicates that design team should improve the process of new account creation.

Finally, there are three items in the analysis results of the product interaction are positive significant ($p < 0.05$). They are includes the "pay attention in the use the product", "use the product would not tired" and "use the product was uncomfortable". Rest of the items scores in this category are above average. This result shows that the system should focus, stimulate and comfortable in the operating process.

5   Conclusion

By taking advantage of the physiological data and questionnaires of usability in this study, the results would investigate potential healthcare management system usability problems and improve the system regarding efficiency, effectiveness, satisfaction. errors, learnability and flexibility. Furthermore, this study developed a new process to evaluate the product of the healthcare management system. This study improved the healthcare management in terms of the usefulness and efficiency. As a result, this system could assist the people in managing their health and keeping themselves healthy.

This study contributed in both academic and practical perspectives. In academic aspect, this study developed a process to evaluate and verify the Kinect sport game based healthcare management system. Moreover, the subjective and objective data were collected and utilized in the experiment. Practically, this study verified the system that could enhance the system usability and performance which could enhance the healthcare management system in a more friendly and usefully manner.

References

1. World Health Organization,
   http://www.who.int/about/definition/en/print.html
2. International Organization for Standardization Guidance on Usability,
   http://www.usabilitynet.org/tools/r_international.htm
3. Preece, J., Rogers, Y., Sharp, H.: Handbook of Interaction design: Beyond human-computer interaction. Wiley & Sons Publishers Inc., New York (2002)
4. Tullis, T., Albert, W.: Measuring the user experience: collecting, analyzing, and presenting usability metrics. Morgan Kaufmann (2010)
5. Hassenzahl, M., Tractinsky, N.: User experience-a research agenda. Behaviour & Information Technology 25(2), 91–97 (2006)

6. Overbeeke, K., Djadjadiningrat, T., Hummels, C., Wensveen, S.: CHAPTER ONE Beauty in Usability: Forget about Ease of Use! Pleasure with products: Beyond usability 7 (2002)
7. Brooks, P., Hestnes, B.: User measures of quality of experience: why being objective and quantitative is important. Network, IEEE 24(2), 8–13 (2010)
8. Finstad, K.: The usability metric for user experience. Interacting with Computers 22(5), 323–327 (2010)
9. International Organization for Standardization: Ergonomic requirements for office work with visual display terminals (VDT) s-Part II Guidance on Usability (ISO/IEC 9241-11). International Organization for Standardization (1998)
10. Shackel, B., Richardson, S.: Human factors for informatics usability. Cambridge University Press, New York (1991)
11. Nielsen, J.: Usability Engineering. Morgan Kaufmann, San Francisco (1993)
12. Brink, T., Gergle, D., Wood, S.: Designing web sites that work: Usability for the web, 1st edn., vol. 1. Academic Press, San Diego (2002)

Building a Telemedicine Framework to Improve the Interactions between Cancer Patients and Oncology Triage Nurses

Saif Khairat and Venkatesh Rudrapatna

Institute for Health Informatics, University of Minnesota, United States
{saifk,rudra005}@umn.edu

Abstract. As healthcare becomes more complex and data driven, the need and use of telemedicine continues to grow. Cancer patients require substantial amount of assistance and guidance through the chemotherapy process. The traditional telephone interaction between patients and providers shows major limitations such as inaccurate assessments and patient dissatisfaction. For that reason, his paper investigates a novel informatics intervention, which is the utilization of telemedicine to improve patient-provider interaction through videoconferencing technologies. The anticipated outcomes include higher accuracy in triage nursing decisions, higher patient and provider satisfaction rates. The ultimate goal of this research is to provide a study design of a telemedicine framework that aims at improving cancer patient management.

Keywords: Telemedicine, Oncology, Cancer, Patient, Provider, Communication, Management.

1 Introduction

Telemedicine is the use of information technology and telecommunication technologies to provide clinical care and health education to patients and professionals separated by distance [1]. Telemedicine achieved with the telephone is widely used in outpatient management of cancer patients. Adult cancer patients who undergo treatments often experience a multitude of cancer and treatment-related symptoms. It is estimated that during a course of chemotherapy a third of patients will experience mild side effects and another third will suffer from severe side effects [2]. Moreover, many patients experience treatment-related symptoms at home because the majority of chemotherapy and radiation therapies are administered in an ambulatory setting. Thus, the easiest way for patients to communicate with oncology health care providers is by email or telephone [3, 4]. Successfully managing these symptoms via telephone can relieve patient distress and lead to better symptom management, especially for some symptoms that can progress and be life threatening [5]. It has also been found that interventions provided by telephone can also reinforce patient compliance, assess the effectiveness of supportive treatments, provide continuity of care, and increase patient satisfaction [6]. At the Masonic Cancer Center at the University of Minnesota, telephone services are the accepted means of communication for nursing staff to assess,

V.G. Duffy (Ed.): DHM 2014, LNCS 8529, pp. 377–384, 2014.

triage, and manage cancer patients experiencing treatment-related symptoms. The aim of this study is to determine whether video conferencing is a feasible and potentially beneficial technology for use in outpatient management of cancer patients.

The long-term goal of this on-going study is to facilitate the application of new technologies that make outpatient care safer and more effective. Technological advances and the increasing use of computer devices (e.g., smart phones and tablet computers) among the population will drive the need for health care providers and health systems to develop new tools and applications for improving the quality of care and services provided to patients. Video conferencing is a form of telemedicine that uses technology to provide real-time visual and audio patient assessment. Although some studies have assessed the role of video conferencing in non-cancer sub-specialties of medicine [7-9], only a few studies have investigated applications of video conferencing in oncology for the purposes of enabling health professionals to share knowledge. These applications included video conferencing of multidisciplinary meetings, tumor boards, and treatment planning to improve patient care [10]. However, to the best of our knowledge, there are no studies assessing the feasibility and impact of video conferencing on nursing triage of cancer patients. Therefore, this paper plans to further investigate two primary research questions, first, to determine the feasibility of video-conferencing technology in providing oncology nurse triage consultations. The second aim is to assess patient satisfaction and collect triage nursing feedback on the use of video-conferencing technology.

2   Methods

We will conduct a pilot study to evaluate the role of video conferencing in oncology nurse triage care. Patients with newly diagnosed cancer will be eligible for the study only if they have the appropriate internet access and devices needed for video conferencing. We will obtain informed consent from each eligible patient prior to enrollment in the study. Hundred patients will be randomized into 2 groups. Group 1 will consist of 50 patients who will receive the current standard of care (i.e., telephone triage). Group 2 will consist of 50 patients who will receive triage care through two-way video conferencing (i.e., the patient and nurse can see each other in addition to the audio conversation).

We will use Avumedia as the software vendor for this study. The reason for this decision is that Avumedia uses Vidyo technology, a leader in TeleHealth. Figure 1 shows a schematic diagram of the study design for group two.

The patients randomized to the video-conferencing arm will use this technology to communicate with the triage nurse for one month after enrollment on the study. They will revert back to using the standard telephone technique after the defined one month period has ended. In the event the patient is unable to reach the triage nurse using the video-conferencing tool within a stipulated period of time during the study, they will revert back to the telephone service. There is currently no data on patient satisfaction of the nurse triage service at the Masonic Cancer Clinic. The purpose of having the telephone triage arm is to collect baseline and comparative data. This study will not change the scope of practice of the triage nurse, and nurses will continue using the current triage algorithms to make appropriate triage decisions.

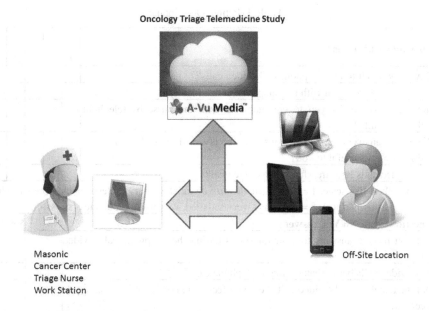

Fig. 1. Telemedicine Oncology Framework for Group 2

The video-conferencing software will be installed at the Triage Nurse workstation in the Masonic Cancer Center. Group 2 patients will be provided with detailed instructions on how to install the software to their home computers, tablets, or smartphones of most manufacturers. Each participant in the study will be able to download the system and a registered user ID will be issued. There will be a training call to explain and test the first use of the system. Participants will have the username ID for the Nurse Triage account. When a participant calls that user ID, an incoming call request will show at the nurse screen, and the nurse will be able to accept the call. Once the call has been accepted and a connection established, both the nurse and patient will see and hear each other through built-in webcams and microphones.

2.1   Patient Satisfaction Survey

Post intervention, study participants and triage nurses will be surveyed to the efficacy of the project. The primary outcomes for the study are satisfaction levels, and the frequency and duration of calls. Therefore, we will assess patient satisfaction through a survey similar to the one outlined below in Table 1. The survey will be presented to patients after the study is completed via electronic and secure online survey tool.

The satisfaction survey is divided into two sections, first, five questions with 5-likert scale answers. The questions target ease of use of telephone and technology, satisfaction with the traditional telephone and telehealth interventions, and the perceived opinion of video calls relative to clinic visits. The second part of the survey includes four yes/no questions that focus on patient's perception and engagement with the telehealth intervention. The goal of the study is further understand patient's perception of telehealth use and whether patients would be interested in further adopting this technology.

Table 1. Patient Questionnaire

Questions with Likert scale	1	2	3	4	5
How easy was it to use telephone calls/video calls?					
How satisfied were you with the telephone calls/video calls?					
How easy was it for you to communicate with the nurse by telephone calls/video calls?					
Were the answers or instructions you received during the telephone calls/video calls useful to you?					
Were video calls less stressful than a clinic visit?					
For the Likert-like scale, 1 = very difficult, very dissatisfied, very useless, much more stressful; 0 = neutral (neither/nor); 5 = very easy, very satisfied, very useful, much less stressful.					

Questions with No/Yes answers	No	Yes
Did you receive answers to your questions during the telephone calls/ video calls?		
Were video calls better than ordinary telephone calls?		
Did the telephone calls/video calls help you feel more confident in the care you received?		
Do you feel that the telephone calls/video calls reduced your need of a visit with your oncology team?		
Comments		

2.2   Triage Nurse Survey

For the nurse questionnaire, we will obtain information about nurses' experiences of and attitudes about the use of video conferencing through a questionnaire similar to the one outlined below in Table2. The triage nurse is responsible to receive calls from cancer patients receiving chemo-therapy, and based on the patient's symptoms the triage nurse makes a decision whether the patient should be seen at the clinic or not. Currently, triage nurses make decisions based on what they hear from the patient however, we argue that triage decisions can be improved when combing patient's complaint with a live video feed that provides the nurse with a visual of the symptoms on the patient's body. In order to identify the efficacy of the telehealth intervention we survey nurses with questions that capture their perceptions of the telehealth intervention.

Similar to patient's surveys, nurses will be asked to fill out the survey post survey. The survey uses 5-point likert scale to assess the ease of use, satisfaction levels, communication, and clinical outcomes from a nursing perspective. There are two yes/no questions that investigate the videoconferencing service is reliable and convenient, and if the nursing staff preferred to use telehealth over telephone.

Table 2. Nurse Questionnaire

Questions with Likert scale	1	2	3	4	5
How easy was it to use video calls?					
How satisfied were you with the video calls?					
How easy was it for you to communicate with the patient by video calls?					
How easy was it for you to assess the patient's status by video calls?					
Questions with No/Yes answers	No		Yes		
Were there any service interruptions during the video-calls					
Were video calls better than ordinary telephone calls?					
Comments					

3   Results

Our preliminary data show that the Masonic Cancer Center triage call-in line received an average of more than 1,000 telephone calls per month from cancer patients during 4 months in 2012 and 2013 (Table 3). Data from three consecutive months were gathered to test the frequency of calls. Data from three consecutive months and one non-consecutive month were sampled to assess the frequency of calls. These data indicate that the triage call-in line is heavily utilized. On average, calls took 1-2 minutes, which is not a markedly long time; On average, calls took 1-2 minutes, which is not a markedly long time per call but cumulatively adds up to an average of 40 hours per month. Currently, on the basis of a patient's response to the triage nurse's question, the nurse will decide the next steps required to resolve the patient's problem. However, it is not known how many patients are referred to the hospital or clinic or how satisfied patients are with the management of their symptoms.

Table 3. Number of Masonic Cancer Clinic Triage Calls

Month, Year	Number of calls	Average talk time (M:S)
February, 2013	1031	2:29
January, 2013	1261	1:35
December, 2012	1097	2:30
July, 2012	1256	1:32

In addition to the surveys above we will be collecting the following additional information through a chart review in EPIC information system.

— Demographic Information including age, gender, distance of residence from Masonic cancer clinic

- Number of calls made by each patient in both study groups during the period of the study
- Duration of the calls
- Emergency room visit or urgent clinic visit within 24 hours of the communication with the nurse while on the study
- Purpose of call - To be characterized as clinical or non-clinical
- Clinical Characteristics including Cancer Type, Stage of Cancer, On treatment, IV and/or Oral Chemotherapy

Post study, data collected will be statistically analyzed through the utilization of tools such as SAS and SPSS. The aim is to find patterns and associations among both study groups, i.e. videoconference and phone. Descriptive analysis will be conducted from each group, and 2 sample t-Tests will be to compare responses from both groups. Moreover, correlation and regression models will be used to identify dependence, identifying any statistical relationship between two survey variables. Anticipated results include statistically significant differences in the aforementioned study outcomes, as well as, an increase in satisfaction levels for Cancer patients and Triage nurses as a result of using telehealth technology. Moreover, data analysis is expected to show improvement in care service through enhancing the ability of Triage nurses to make more accurate decisions with regards to patient symptoms.

4   Discussion

The ultimate goal of this on-going study is to determine whether video conferencing can enable triage nurses to improve the outpatient management of cancer patients. A critical step in the nursing triage process is the initial interaction between the patient and the person answering the telephone call. This two-way communication defines the patient's experience and satisfaction when contacting the cancer clinic. The current telephone system is limited by the inability of the triage nurse to visually assess the patient's clinical condition (e.g., skin rash, jaundice, or pale face). This lack of visual capability often results in the triage nurse having to refer the patient to the nearest health care facility, emergency room, or cancer clinic for further triage. In one study 36.8% of calls led directly to patients being medically assessed [11]. Moreover, referrals not only utilize additional health care resources, but also add to the anguish of the patient and family. Many referrals could be prevented by the use of a live visual feed of the patient. A representative example of this would be a known side effect of a chemotherapy drug, such as capecitabine, causing a hand-foot rash. This side effect can be managed at home, but it is often difficult for the triage nurse to determine the severity of this side effect in the absence of visual data. The potential benefits of visual examination were suggested by a recent study assessing the role Telehealth in people with chronic obstructive pulmonary disorder (COPD). The study found that Telehealth brought "peace of mind" to patients and their families, and the authors hypothesized that this benefit was brought on through two mechanisms: legitimizing contact with health professionals and increased patient confidence in the management of their condition [12].

Currently, triage nurses use the traditional telephone intervention to assess whether a patient should see a care provider specialist, in that case, an appointment is set up and the patient have to travel to the hospital to see their provider. The limitation to this model is that patients need to invest time and money to be seen when in some cases the trip may be unnecessary and consultation could have been done through phone or other communication mediums. Therefore, the aim of this study is to assess the feasibility of telehealth and whether we can reduce the number of unnecessary visits to the clinic by providing the triage nurse with a more accurate communication medium namely, telehealth through video conferencing technologies.

We aim to find that the video-conferencing technology is both feasible and viable as an adjunct or an alternative to telephones in providing oncology nurse triage consultations. We hope that this would improve patient satisfaction and overall experience. The study is intended to be a pilot project. We realize that there may be some limitations to the study including video quality, adaptation of technology, bias towards the younger age group of patient population and variability based on other patient and cancer characteristics.

Successful completion of this study will provide pilot data for a larger study testing the impact and role of video-conferencing on the cost of care, reduction in urgent clinic visits or emergency room visits, and improvements in the quality of care. We envision this technology being incorporated into the workflow in the near future. Additionally, this project will help support our goal of improving Patient-Provider communication and informatics solutions at the point of care in oncology.

References

1. Bashshur, R.L.: On the definition and evaluation of telemedicine. Telemed. J. 1, 19–30 (1995)
2. Larsen, M.E., Rowntree, J., Young, A.M., Pearson, S., Smith, J., Gibson, O.J., Weaver, A., Tarassenko, L.: Chemotherapy side-effect management using mobile phones. In: Conf. Proc. IEEE Eng. 51, 5–5152 (2008)
3. Wilson, R., Hubert, J.: Resurfacing the care in nursing by telephone: lessons from ambulatory oncology. Nursing Outlook 50(4), 160–164 (2002)
4. Reid, J., Porter, S.: Utility, caller, and patient profile of a novel chemotherapy telephone helpline service within a regional cancer centre in Northern Ireland. Cancer Nursing 32, E27–E32 (2011)
5. Behl, D., Hendrickson, A.W., Moynihan, T.: Oncologic emergencies. Critical Care Clinics 26(1), 181–205 (2010)
6. Flannery, M., Phillips, S.M., Lyons, C.A.: Examining telephone calls in ambulatory oncology. J. Oncol. Pract. 5, 57–60 (2009)
7. Taylor, P., Goldsmith, P., Murray, K., Harris, D., Barkley, A.: Evaluating a telemedicine system to assist in the management of dermatology referrals. Br. J. Dermatol. 144(2), 33–328 (2001)
8. Martin-Khan, M., Flicker, L., Wootton, R., Loh, P.K., Edwards, H., Varghese, P., Byrne, G.J., Klein, K., Gray, L.: The diagnostic accuracy of telegeriatrics for the diagnosis of dementia via video conferencing. J. Am. Med. Dir. Assoc. 13(5), 487.e19–487.e24 (2012)

9. Kruse, R.L., Parker Oliver, D., Wittenberg-Lyles, E., Demiris, G.: Conducting the ACTIVE randomized trial in hospice care: keys to success. Clin. Trials. 10(1), 160–169 (2013)
10. Kitamura, C., Zurawel–Balaura, L., Wong, R.K.S.: CurrOncol. 17(3), 17–27 (2010)
11. Reid, J., Porter, S.: Utility, caller, and patient profile of a novel Chemotherapy Telephone Helpline service within a regional cancer centre in Northern Ireland. Cancer Nurs 34(3), E27-32 (2011)
12. Gale, N., Sultan, H.: Telehealth as 'peace of mind': Embodiment, emotions and the home as the primary health space for people with chronic obstructive pulmonary disorder. Health Place 21, 140–147 (2013)

Usability Challenges and Barriers in EHR Training of Primary Care Resident Physicians

Min Soon Kim[1, 2], Martina A. Clarke[2], Jeffery L. Belden[3], and Elaine Hinton[4]

[1] Department of Health Management and Informatics, University of Missouri
[2] University of Missouri Informatics Institute, University of Missouri
[3] Department of Family and Community Medicine, University of Missouri
[4] Center for Education and Development, University of Missouri

Abstract. Current EHRs require a large investment of resources for a user to reach a certain level of proficiency, which is a significant obstacle for new physicians who are not sufficiently trained by their medical schools. Beginning residents in primary care cope with a steep learning curve on EHR use due to EHRs with poor usability, which may lead to medical errors, and decreased quality of patient care. Identifying and addressing early barriers in the learning environment of residents while using an EHR can help improve overall capacity of the new physicians, and save costs for the organization. The goal of this study is to assess current usability challenges and barriers in EHR education and training program at the University of Missouri Health Care (UMHC).

1 Introduction

Primary care physicians (limited to family medicine and internal medicine in this paper) account for a majority of patient visits in a highly interruptive, time-pressured environment [1]. According to the Centers for Disease Control and Prevention, National Center for Health Statistics (CDC NCHS), in 2012, 72% of office-based physicians had use of an electronic health record (EHR) system in their practices [2]. An EHR is defined as a systematic digital record system that gathers a range of patient care data with the potential to enhance quality of health care. Recent research highlights the challenges of EHR implementation [3], which results in lower effectiveness [4], decreased efficiency [5], medical errors [6], and decreased quality of patient care [7]. These issues can be related to "usability", "effectiveness, efficiency and satisfaction" [8]. Although training as a part of the EHR implementation process is critical, a survey shows that nearly 62% of clinicians were not satisfied with many of the best-known EHR systems, with support and training in EHR having the lowest satisfaction [9]. Current EHRs require a large investment of resources for a user to reach a certain level of proficiency (learnability), which is a significant obstacle for new physicians who are not sufficiently trained by their medical schools [10]. In this paper, we define "learnability" as "usability over time," in that how usability improves after repeated use of the system [11].

Many institutions now offer exhaustive EHR trainings for their residents. However, finding sufficient time to train busy physicians, target training to users' needs, and

V.G. Duffy (Ed.): DHM 2014, LNCS 8529, pp. 385–391, 2014.
© Springer International Publishing Switzerland 2014

provide hands-on, on-site support is a challenge [12]. Even though there exists minimal evidence based guidance for effective strategies to train residents on how to use EHRs for patient care [13], Kushniruk et al. examined the association between usability tests and EHR training at an urban medical center, and suggested potentially improving EHR training with usability evaluation [14]. The goal of this study is to assess current usability challenges and barriers in EHR education and training program at the University of Missouri Health Care (UMHC).

2   Method

In order to evaluate the current EHR education and training program, we employed three steps of evaluation strategy: (1) critical discussion with physician champion and EHR training specialists, (2) structural analysis of current EHR education and training program that are offered to resident physicians, and (3) measure of user perceptions on EHR education and training through post training survey from residents.

2.1   Setting

The University of Missouri Health Care (UMHC) is a tertiary care academic medical center located in Columbia, Missouri, with a total of 564 beds. With 626 medical staff at clinics throughout mid-Missouri, UMHC had an estimated 553,300 visits in 2012 [15]. The Department of Family and Community Medicine (FCM) is one of the largest clinical units of UMHC, with more than 70 primary care physicians and manages six clinics, while the Department of Internal Medicine (IM) manages two clinics [16]. In total, both departments admit an average of 30 residents each year into their residential program.

2.2   Electronic Health Record

UMHC's currently uses PowerChart® (Cerner Corporation, Kansas City, MO) and in 2012, HIMSS awarded UMHC with Stage 7 of the Electronic Medical Record (EMR) Adoption Model [17], which translates to complete transition from all-paper to all electronic patient records, use of Continuity of Care Documents (CCD) to share data, and data warehousing is used to analyze clinical data [18]. Less than 2% of hospitals nationwide have reached this advanced stage of EHR implementation [19]. Essentially all data at UMHC is captured in the UMHC database. Evaluating EHR learnability using the fully implemented EHR system within one of the most wired health care setting makes this study ideal to achieve the goal we desire.

3   Results

This section divulges the results from the critical discussion with both the physician champion and EHR training specialists then gives a structural analysis of current EHR education and training program that are offered to resident physicians at the University of Missouri Health Care. There are five EHR training specialists employed as the EHR training team under the Center for Education and Development (CED). The EHR training team develops and administers Web-based training, manages a training database to permit class registration, and provides training to all new staff and clinicians who will be utilizing the EHR at UMHC. There are two parts of EHR training that 1st year primary care residents are required to complete when they start their residency. The first are eighteen inpatient and thirteen outpatient online lecture modules that introduce the basic functionalities of the EHR (e.g., adding diagnosis, document patient summary, entering orders, medication reconciliation) which takes approximately three hours to complete. The second are two sets of instructor-led, in-class, competency training sessions, where the residents get hands-on practice by performing short, scenario-based tasks, designed to use EHR core functionalities in outpatient (4hrs) and inpatient (4hrs) settings, and using the interactive training mode of the EHR. These training sessions take 8 hours for a resident to complete.

According to a recent post-training survey by the CED of 123 residents, they recognized the benefits of EHR training to increase competency when using the EHR, however some potential areas for improvements were identified. First, the length of training time was found to be a massive burden for busy specialist residents. Therefore, residents suggested compact, continuous training and retraining to ensure proficiency. Second, the current EHR training program does not satisfy the needs of specialist physicians but is designed for a general physician audience. Therefore, the training program does not represent unique EHR functionality and features that are frequently used by physicians in specific specialties. As a result, some residency programs plan to include extra 4-12 hours sessions to meet their own specialty needs. Third, there lacks a systematic way to gauge the residents' learning experience as they undergo the training sessions or after the training ends, which may offer critical information that could improve the EHR training program on a continuous basis. Finally, there are very inadequate resources, such as, sufficient experienced staff and time for retraining, available in supporting EHR training, which is a common barrier across health care organizations [20].

4   Discussion

4.1   EHR Usability Issues

EHR adoption across the US is being driven by a significant inflow of capital, with a goal of improved patient care and a reduction in health care costs [21, 22]. Although many studies highlight the potential of a successfully implemented EHR, to enhance quality of medical care [23-32], many negative effects have also been documented, which include: lower effectiveness [4, 33], decreased efficiency [5], decreased team collaboration [34], increased cognitive load [35], medical errors [6], and decreased quality of patient care [7]. This highlights why an effective EHR training is so important.

Primary care physicians account for a majority of patient visits, and because medical advances and socio-demographic changes demand greater primary care performance, the demand for the efficient use of an EHR by primary care physicians may also increase [36, 37]. Residents are medical professionals holding a medical degree who are still in training under supervision by senior residents and attending physicians. Primary care residencies usually enter a three-year program and in each year of training, the residents levels of responsibility increases. Based on their training level and field of concentration, residents participate in diagnostic and treatment procedures.

During the implementation process, the importance of training have been repeatedly stressed in multiple studies on successful EHR implementation [10, 12, 20, 38-46]. For instance, Aaronson et al. [44], surveyed 219 family practice residency programs about the use of EHR systems in the residency program, and found that training changed the residents views on the usability and capabilities of the EHR, such as time management and accuracy of the patient records. Training may have increased the likelihood of residents using EHRs in their practice after their residency. For a user to obtain a certain level of proficiency (learning curve), EHRs now require a large investment of resources for training and beginning physicians who are not sufficiently trained in medical school begin to struggle with competent EHR use [10, 47, 48]. However, according to the "2012 EHR User Satisfaction Survey from 3,088 family physicians," nearly 62% of the respondents were not satisfied with many of the best-known EHR systems, with the area of lowest satisfaction being EHR vendor support and training [9]. Many hospital are now trying to reduce learning curve issues by offering comprehensive EHR trainings for incoming residents, however, finding adequate time to train busy primary care physicians [12, 42, 49, 50], target training to users' needs [42, 50], and provide hands-on, on-site support [12, 38, 41] is another challenge.

4.2   Improving EHR Learnability through EHR Training of Residents

There are limited effective strategies available on EHR training for patient care [13, 51, 52]. Stephens et al. proposed a potential EHR training model, "Reporter–Interpreter–Manager–Educator (RIME)/EHR" for systematic education and assessment of EHR-specific competency [53]. At the Reporter stage, students are expected to have a basic competence to correctly complete a medical history and physical examination [54]. At The Interpreter stage students should be able to analyze and articulate their findings using enhanced clinical reasoning skills. Managers develop patient management skills and are actively involved in developing diagnostic and therapeutic plans based on patient preferences. The Educator stage requires students to be able to the include patient in decision making, search medical literature and integrate evidence based medicine in their practice by sharing this information with the patient and colleagues [55].

Kushniruk et al. examined the association between usability testing and EHR training at an urban medical center in NYC. Five physician users were a part of the study and none had any EHR experience except for the EHR under observation. Physicians participated in a four hour in class training session and then a lab-based usability test was conducted for approximately a month after the training session. The 40 minutes usability test employed think aloud strategy where 2 sets of scenario-based tasks were completed by the participants. The study found areas where physician users struggled to complete their tasks, areas for improvement regarding learnability and usability, and proposed possible improvements to the present training physicians were receiving. Based on the results of this study, usability evaluation may be beneficial in improving EHR training. [14]. Because this study conducted just a single usability test, it is necessary to examine the broader implications of iterative usability evaluations on EHR training.

5   Conclusion

Acknowledging the barriers in the current EHR training and discussions with stakeholders, we suggest mixed method approach usability evaluation methods to evaluate and improve measure varying degrees of physician-user learnability for an extended period to enhance EHR training to improve the learning process.

References

1. Schoen, C., et al.: On The Front Lines Of Care: Primary Care Doctors Office Systems, Experiences, And Views In Seven Countries. Health Affairs 25(6), w555–w571 (2006)
2. Hsiao, C.-J., Hing, E.: Use and characteristics of electronic health record systems among office-based physician practices: United States, 2001–2012. NCHS Data Brief 2012(111), 1–8
3. Scott, J.T., et al.: Kaiser Permanente's experience of implementing an electronic medical record: A qualitative study. BMJ 331(7528), 6–1313 (2005)
4. Koppel, R., et al.: Role of computerized physician order entry systems in facilitating medication errors. JAMA, 2005 293(10), 1197–1203 (2005)
5. Crabtree, B.F., et al.: Delivery of clinical preventive services in family medicine offices. Ann. Fam. Med. 3(5), 430–435 (2005)
6. Ash, J.S., Berg, M., Coiera, E.: Some unintended consequences of information technology in health care: The nature of patient care information system-related errors. J. Am. Med. Inform. Assoc. 11(2), 104–112 (2004)
7. Beuscart-Zéphir, M.C., et al.: The human factors engineering approach to biomedical informatics projects: State of the art, results, benefits and challenges. Yearbook of Medical Informatics, 109–127 (2007)
8. Standard ISO 9241: Ergonomic requirements for office work with visual display terminals (VDTs), part 11: Guidance on usability (1998b)
9. Edsall, R.L., Adler, K.G.: The 2012 EHR User Satisfaction Survey: Responses From 3,088 Family Physicians. Family Practice Management 19(6) (2012)
10. Hammoud, M.M., et al.: Opportunities and challenges in integrating electronic health records into undergraduate medical education: A national survey of clerkship directors. Teach. Learn. Med. 24(3), 219–224 (2012)
11. Elliott, G.J., Jones, E., Barker, P.: A grounded theory approach to modelling learnability of hypermedia authoring tools. Interacting with Computers 14(5), 547–574 (2002)

12. Terry, A.L., et al.: Implementing electronic health records: Key factors in primary care. Can. Fam. Physician. 54(5), 730–736 (2008)
13. Peled, J.U., et al.: Do electronic health records help or hinder medical education? PLoS. Med. 6(5), e1000069 (2009)
14. Kushniruk, A.W., et al.: Exploring the relationship between training and usability: A study of the impact of usability testing on improving training and system deployment. Stud. Health Technol. Inform. 143, 277–283 (2009)
15. 2012 Annual Report. University of Missouri Health Care, Columbia, MO
16. MU 2011 Annual Report. MU Healthcare 2011
    http://www.mydigitalpublication.com/publication/?i=106794
    (cited April 15, 2012)
17. University of Missouri Health Care Achieves Highest Level of Electronic Medical Record Adoption, in University of Missouri Health Care News Releases, Columbia, MO
18. U.S. EMR Adoption Model Trends (2011)
19. Stage 7 Hospitals (2012),
    http://www.himssanalytics.org/emram/stage7Hospitals.aspx (cited October 2012)
20. EHR IMPLEMENTATIONSURVEY: Proactive Consideration and Planning Lead to Successful EHR Implementation. HIMSS, Chicago, IL (2013)
21. Blumenthal, D., Tavenner, M.: The "meaningful use" regulation for electronic health records. New England Journal of Medicine 363(6), 501–504 (2010)
22. Blumenthal, D.: Launching HITECH. New England Journal of Medicine 362(5), 382–385 (2010)
23. Chaudhry, B., et al.: Systematic review: Impact of health information technology on quality, efficiency, and costs of medical care. Ann. Intern. Med. 144(10), 742–752 (2006)
24. Bates, D.W., Gawande, A.A.: Improving safety with information technology. New England Journal of Medicine 348(25), 2526–2534 (2003)
25. Chaudhry, B., et al.: Systematic review: Impact of health information technology on quality, efficiency, and costs of medical care. Annals of Internal Medicine 144(10), 742–752 (2006)
26. Corrigan, J.M., Greiner, A., Erickson, S.M.: Fostering Rapid Advances in Health Care: Learning from System Demonstrations (2002)
27. Donaldson, M.S.: Primary care: America's health in a new era 1996. National Academies Press (1996)
28. Kohn, L.T.: The Institute of Medicine report on medical error: Overview and implications for pharmacy. Am. J. Health Syst. Pharm. 58(1), 63–66 (2001)
29. Maguire, M.: Methods to support human-centred design. International Journal of Human-Computer Studies 55(4), 587–634 (2001)
30. Goldzweig, C.L., et al.: Costs and benefits of health information technology: New trends from the literature. Health Affairs 28(2), w282–w293 (2009)
31. Hillestad, R., et al.: Can electronic medical record systems transform health care? Potential health benefits, savings, and costs. Health Affairs 24(5), 1103–1117 (2005)
32. Holroyd-Leduc, J.M., et al.: The impact of the electronic medical record on structure, process, and outcomes within primary care: A systematic review of the evidence. Journal of the American Medical Informatics Association 18(6), 732–737 (2011)
33. Steele, E.: EHR implementation: who benefits, who pays? Health ManagTechnol 27(7), 43–44 (2006)
34. Han, Y.Y., et al.: Unexpected increased mortality after implementation of a commercially sold computerized physician order entry system. Pediatrics 116(6), 1506–1512 (2005)

35. Tang, P.C., Patel, V.L.: Major issues in user interface design for health professional workstations: summary and recommendations. Int. J. Biomed. Comput. 34(1-4), 139–148 (1994)
36. Grumbach, K., Bodenheimer, T.: A Primary Care Home for Americans. JAMA: The journal of the American Medical Association 288(7), 889–893 (2002)
37. Morrison, I., Smith, R.: Hamster health care. BMJ 321(7276), 1541–1542 (2000)
38. Anderson, L.K., Stafford, C.J.: The "big bang" implementation: Not for the faint of heart. Computers in Nursing 20(1), 14–20 (2002)
39. Ash, J.S., Bates, D.W.: Factors and forces affecting EHR system adoption: Report of a 2004 ACMI discussion. J. Am. Med. Inform. Assoc. 12(1), 8–12 (2005)
40. Brokel, J.M., Harrison, M.I.: Redesigning care processes using an electronic health record: A system's experience. Joint Commission Journal on Quality and Patient Safety 35(2), 82–92 (2009)
41. McAlearney, A.S., et al.: Moving from good to great in ambulatory electronic health record implementation. Journal for Healthcare Quality: Official Publication of the National Association for Healthcare Quality 32(5), 41–50 (2010)
42. Whittaker, A.A., Aufdenkamp, M., Tinley, S.: Barriers and facilitators to electronic documentation in a rural hospital. Journal of Nursing Scholarship 41(3), 293–300 (2009)
43. Yan, H., Gardner, R., Baier, R.: Beyond the focus group: Understanding physicians' barriers to electronic medical records. Jt. Comm. J. Qual. Patient Saf. 38(4), 184–191 (2012)
44. Aaronson, J.W., et al.: Electronic medical records: the family practice resident perspective. Fam. Med. 33(2), 128–132 (2001)
45. Keenan, C.R., Nguyen, H.H., Srinivasan, M.: Electronic medical records and their impact on resident and medical student education. Acad. Psychiatry 30(6), 522–527 (2006)
46. Terry, A.L., et al.: Adoption of electronic medical records in family practice: The providers' perspective. Fam. Med. 41(7), 508–512 (2009)
47. Mintz, M., et al.: Use of electronic medical records by physicians and students in academic internal medicine settings. Acad. Med. 84(12), 1698–1704 (2009)
48. Chumley, H., et al.: First-year medical students document more pain characteristics when using an electronic health record. Fam. Med. 40(7), 462–463 (2008)
49. Carr, D.M.: A team approach to EHR implementation and maintenance. Nurs. Manage, 35(suppl. 5) 15–6, 24 (2004)
50. Lorenzi, N.M., et al.: How to successfully select and implement electronic health records (EHR) in small ambulatory practice settings. Bmc. Medical Informatics and Decision Making 9(1) (2009)
51. Report II: Contemporary Issues in Medicine: Medical Informatics and Population Health. Medical School Objectives Project (1998)
52. Gliatto, P., Masters, P., Karani, R.: Medical student documentation in the medical record: is it a liability? Mt. Sinai. J. Med. 76(4), 357–364 (2009)
53. Stephens, M.B., Gimbel, R.W., Pangaro, L.: Commentary: The RIME/EMR scheme: An educational approach to clinical documentation in electronic medical records. Acad. Med. 86(1), 11–14 (2011)
54. Cate, O., Scheele, F.: Viewpoint: Competency-Based Postgraduate Training: Can We Bridge the Gap between Theory and Clinical Practice? Academic Medicine 82(6), 542–547 (2007)
55. Carter, J.H., American College of Physicians (2003): Electronic health records: A guide for clinicians and administrators, 2nd edn., p. 530. ACP Press. xxi, Philadelphia (2008)

Robotics as a Tool in Fundamental Nursing Education

Yasuko Kitajima[1], Mitsuhiro Nakamura[1], Jukai Maeda[1], Masako Kanai-Pak[1],
Kyoko Aida[1], Zhifeng Huang[2], Ayanori Nagata[2], Taiki Ogata[2], Noriaki Kuwahara[3],
and Jun Ota[2]

[1] Faculty of Nursing, Tokyo Ariake University of Medical and Health Sciences,
2-9-1 Ariake, Koto-ku, Tokyo 135-0063, Japan
{kitajima,m-nakamura,jukai,p-kanai,k-aida}@tau.ac.jp
[2] Research into Artifacts Center for Engineering (RACE), The University of Tokyo,
5-1-5 Kashiwanoha, Kashiwa-shi, Chiba 277-8568, Japan
{zhifeng,nagata,ogata,ota}@race.u-tokyo.ac.jp
[3] Department of Advanced Fibro-Science, Kyoto Institute of Technology,
Matsugasaki, Sakyo-ku, Kyoto 606-8585, Japan
nkuwahar@kit.ac.jp

Abstract. The main purpose of this study was to investigate whether the use of
robotics can contribute to nursing education, using the training for wheelchair
transfers. The most common and extensively used method for practical learning
is role playing. However the nursing student cannot turn into a patient thoroughly. To solve this problem, we proposed the creation of a robot patient for
wheelchair transfer techniques training.

The experiment was performed by a nurse. The nurse attempted to assist the
robot patient by helping it to stand up from the wheelchair, utilizing the basic
techniques and checklist found in the fundamental nursing education textbook.
As a result of this study, we have determined that the utilization of a robot
could contribute to the teaching material for nursing education, and created an
opportunity to reconsider what is accepted as basics or fundamental techniques.

Keywords: Robot patient, Simulated patient, Nursing skill, Nursing Education,
Checklist.

1 Introduction

With the arrival of the advanced medical care and the super-aging of society it is necessary in nursing education to train human resources who can flexibly handle the
changes in the environment which surround society and public health care, and it is
also becoming necessary to work toward the development of nursing as a specialist
profession and train human resources who can meet the needs of people of all health
levels.

Aware of the issue that "the improvement of nursing abilities of college program
graduates is an problem which must be resolved in order for nursing schools to reliably
meet the expectations of society and work for further development", MEXT (Ministry
of Education, Culture, Sports, Science and Technology) compiled nursing ability goals

V.G. Duffy (Ed.): DHM 2014, LNCS 8529, pp. 392–402, 2014.
© Springer International Publishing Switzerland 2014

to be reached at the time of a completion of college program in a 2004 report. One of these goals is "the ability to appropriately execute nursing care techniques" [1].

Practicing of techniques in fundamental nursing education is vital in order for individual students to learn the ability to appropriately execute nursing care techniques. This is because most of the actions performed in nursing techniques involve contact between the nurse and the patient, and nursing techniques which can be safely provided to the patient and which are of a certain standard are required, and they cannot be achieved simply by classroom learning.

Recently, simulators as teaching materials have been introduced which can more elaborately reproduce the conditions of patients such as audio-visual materials and dummies in order to teach nursing techniques. One of these which has been in use for a long time is the practice method wherein students play and experience the roles of both nurse and patient [2]. Of the techniques required in nursing education there are techniques such as simply making up a bed or drawing blood, where the condition of the patient does not largely effect the nursing techniques to be provided, as well as techniques such as wheelchair transfers where there are multiple methods of providing care depending on the condition of the patient or the environment.

In this research we focused on the wheelchair transfer technique, which differs greatly depending on the condition of the patient, to clarify whether robotics can be a useful learning tool in nursing education.

The patients who are the subject of wheelchair transfers in fundamental nursing education textbooks are not fixed because depending on the textbook there is a wide variety of settings and different methods of assistance are adopted based upon the condition of the patients. Also, many textbooks use healthy persons to play the part of the patient, and these patients possess an ADL (activities of daily living) level which allows the nurse who is providing the assistance to transfer them from the bed to the wheelchair alone [3]. When actually transferring a patient into a wheelchair in a hospital, etc., patients have a wide variety of physical conditions, and the textbooks only cover a small fraction of these. Considering these variations, it greatly exceeds the scope of patient settings in other nursing techniques such as drawing blood and bed bathing. The intent of the textbooks is to simply instruct regarding the basic wheelchair transfer technique, and upon learning the basic technique the nurse can apply the assistance method that fits the actual patient's condition. However, there remains the question of whether the ability to apply said assistance in such nursing techniques as wheelchair transfers where the patients' conditions vary widely will be acquired via these teaching methods. The basic technique of the method of wheelchair transfers has not yet been clarified in the first place. When humans take the natural action of moving from a sitting position to a standing position their trunks adopt a forward-bent posture, but in the textbooks for basic nursing techniques there is a tendency toward stating that the method of assisting a person such that their natural movement is not interfered with is the basic f technique or the wheelchair transfer assistance method [4].

Application ability is the concept of taking one thing and applying it to another thing to successfully apply it. As I previously stated, MEXT established "the ability to appropriately execute nursing techniques " [5] as a nursing abilities goal to be reached at the time of completion of a college program, but there is a limit to how much of all nursing techniques students can learn within class time, and students therefore need the ability to apply the nursing techniques which they have learned. I stated that the basic technique of the methods of wheelchair transfers which are the subject of this research has not been clarified, and if that is the case then it should be necessary to test a variety of methods. The learning method which will enable students to acquire application ability is surely one which reproduces as much as possible the condition of patients who cannot cooperate with the person playing the nurse, forcing the students to attempt wheelchair transfers through trial and error.

And this raises the issue of the simulated patient. In current nursing education, practice is generally carried out with the students themselves playing the nurses and patients. It is said that in such cases, the students playing the patients feel bad for the students playing the nurses, especially considering that they themselves are also studying nursing, so they cooperate so that the technique provision will be easier for the student playing the nurse [6]. Therefore, when practicing with other students there is definitely a limit to how well the part of an actual patient can be played. For example, in such cases where the student playing the nurse provided assistance wrongly and this would be likely to result in a fall, the student playing the patient would presumably sense the danger themselves and not entrust everything to the student playing the nurse and collapse.

In order to solve this problem, I attempted to use a robot as a simulated patient in this research. In recent years there are simulators on sale which can elaborately reproduce the ailments of patients. However these are simulators which focus on learning physical assessment and BLS (Basic Life Support), and the simulators themselves are not designed for the purpose of placement in sitting and standing positions. Furthermore, mannequins which simply have the form of a humans, while having movable joints, have no power in their bodies, so they are not suitable for a single caregiver to practice a wheelchair transfer. The robot used in this research replicates a patient who requires assistance in a wheelchair transfer. It can maintain a sitting position, but it cannot stand up under its own power, and it cannot stay standing without the support of a nurse. Furthermore, its standing position is also unstable and it falls easily.

In this research I investigate whether attempting wheelchair transfers with a robot as a simulated patient can be a useful learning tool in nursing education. At the same time, by using a robot which is not a human as a simulated patient, I reconsider the basic actions which have been adopted in traditional basic nursing education and investigate what the key for students to acquire "the ability to appropriately execute nursing care techniques" is.

2   Methods

2.1   Participants

The nurse with more than 10 years of clinical experience was the subjects.

2.2   Procedures

A robot placed into a sitting position in a wheelchair (hereinafter called the "robot patient") was used as a simulated patient. The nurse repeatedly performed the action of assisting the robot patient to stand it up, and then placing it back into a sitting position. The same action was also performed with a healthy person as the simulated patient.

The nurse attempted to stand up and then put back into a sitting position both the robot patient and the healthy person as a simulated patient, following assistance methods which were extracted from wheelchair transfer methods adopted by multiple basic nursing education textbooks (hereinafter called the "checklist") [7]. The checklist was created as an assistance method to transfer patients who are primarily in a sitting square position. There were 21 necessary assistance actions extracted (Table 1), and in basic nursing education this checklist is used to evaluate the state of students' wheelchair assistance technique learning. The target of this experiment was to analyze the actions of standing both a robot patient and a healthy person up from a sitting position in a wheelchair and then returning them to a seated position, so I decided to implement items 5 through 9-b and items 11-a through 11-b from the checklist.

Table 1. Evaluation items for transferring a patient from the bed to wheelchair

No.	Evaluation Items.
1-a	Set wheelchair at the side of the bed with 20 to 30-degree angle.
1-b	Place wheelchair close to the patient.
2	Brake the wheelchair.
3-a	Place nurse's left feet forward and right leg backward when bringing the patient close to the edge of the bed.
3-b	Place nurse's left leg between patient's legs.
4-a	Support patient's hip.
4-b	When bringing the patient close to the edge of the bed, move the patient's center of the gravity to right and left.
5	Bring patient's heels close to the bed.
6	Place patient's both arms around nurse's shoulder.
7	Position of trainee's hands in patient' back.
8-a	Place nurse's left feet forward and right leg backward when patient stands up.
8-b	Place nurse's foot between patient's legs.
9-a	Lowest height of the trainee's waist.
9-b	Bending angle of patients' back before hip away from the bed.
10	Turn patient toward the wheelchair.
11-a	Nurse bends the knees while placing the patient in the wheelchair.
11-b	Angle of patients' back before sit down.
12	Hold patient's forearm from behind the patient and the patient's both the side.
13	Bring the patient's buttocks towards the back of the wheelchair while placing patient's head lower.
14-a	Bring down footrest of the wheelchair.
14-b	Place patient's feet on the footrest.

First of all, the nurse said "Hello" to the robot patient. The robot patient replied "Hello". Next, the nurse was instructed to place and hold both of the robot patient's arms on the nurse's shoulders. After placing the robot's arms on her shoulders, the nurse assisted the robot patient so that it could stand from the wheelchair. After standing the robot patient, the knee joints locked and it was confirmed that it could maintain a standing position with support. Next, the nurse told the robot patient to "please sit", and the robot patient replied "okay" before beginning the sitting action. The nurse unlocked the robot patient's knee joints and assisted it in taking a sitting position as if collapsing to sit it in the wheelchair.

Additionally, the nurse performed the same actions upon a simulated patient played by a healthy person. This simulated patient had 30 hours of experience performing the wheelchair transfer actions as a simulated patient. Furthermore, this simulated patient was 160cm tall, which was almost the same as the robot patient.

In order to analyze the actions with both the robot patient and the healthy person, a camera was used to record the image sequence of experiment. The trajectories of the head of each of the patients when in a sitting position and standing position were extracted and compared.

2.3   Robot Patient

The robot patient was 160cm tall and weighed 25kg. This could be called lighter than the average patient, but this weight was chosen in this research to ensure the safety of the students (Fig.1).

The upper limbs of the robot patient have 3 joints including 2 shoulder joints and elbow joints. The upper limbs can be held on the participant's shoulders and can remain held there. The robot patient cannot hold onto the participant's shoulders by itself, so the participant helps the robot patient to perform the holding action. When the height of the arms is lower than the position of the shoulders, the shoulder joints are not locked. And when the arms are in a higher position than the shoulders, the shoulder joints and elbow joints are locked and the embracing posture is maintained. The posture of this robot patient continues to be maintained during the process of standing from the wheelchair and sitting.

An electric brake is installed in the robot patient's knee joints so that it can maintain a standing position. An angle sensor is also installed to detect the angle of the knee joints. The minimum angle for the knee joints to maintain a standing position is 165 degrees. During the process of the robot patient standing from the wheelchair, the electric brake of the knee joints is turned off so that it moves with the assistance of the participant and can open freely. This is so that the position of the legs can be freely adjusted in the preparations for the participant to stand the robot patient, and also so that assistance in taking a standing position can be given. The electric brake is set to work when the left or right knee joint opens wider than 165 degrees. Furthermore, the torque of the knee joints is set to instantly switch to zero when the electric brake turns off. The reaction time for this to happen is less than 1 second. This reaction speed recreates the way an actual patient's knee joints suddenly buckle when they start to move from a standing to a sitting position [8].

The voice interaction was realized by the voice recognition module. The robot patient is created to recognize the two Japanese phrases "hello" and "please sit". When the participant says "Hello" to the robot patient, the robot patient replies "Hello". And when told "please sit", it replies "okay". The robot patient says "okay" only after it has taken a standing position, and after replying the robot patient releases its knee joints in order to take a sitting position. The torque of friction of the brake would support the robot patient's weight to keep standing. The robot patient maintains a standing position until the participant gives the instruction to "please sit". After recognizing the phrase "please sit" by the participant, the robot patient releases its knee joints and begins to take a sitting position.

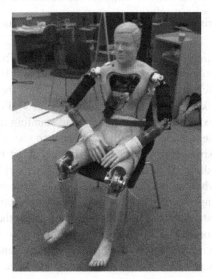

Fig. 1. Robot patient for wheelchair transfer practice

3   Results and Consideration

The nurse who actually participated in the first experiment performed the assistance according to the checklist to assist the robot patient to stand, but was not able to make it stand at all. We will now consider the reasons she was unable to do so. First of all, in checklist 7, "Position of trainee's hands in patient' back", it was predicted from before the trial that the nurse was unable to effectively utilize her power and would have difficulty standing the robot patient. Instead of the robot patient's back, she put her hands under the it's armpits [9] (Fig. 2).

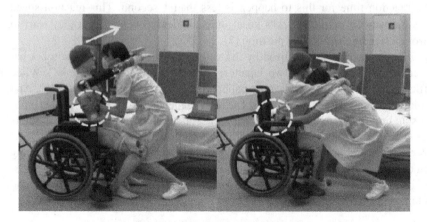

Fig. 2. Comparison of robot and human, position of the nurse's hands

Next, she tried checklist 9-b, "Bending angle of patients' back before hip away from the bed.", but the robot patient's back did not bend and its upper body simply slid down from the wheelchair toward the nurse, and assisting the robot patient to take natural actions to stand like a human was ineffective (Fig. 3). Furthermore, the nurse who participated in the experiment had experience in standing up the healthy human acting as a simulated patient according to the checklist, so she was left with the sense that if she assisted the simulated patient as per the checklist the simulated patient would cooperate in standing. Therefore the nurse didn't exert force from the start upon the robot patient which couldn't move at all under its own power and did not enter the action of making the patient stand, which was presumably the reason she was unable to put it in a standing position. Furthermore, when the standing robot suddenly released its knee joints like an actual patient, there was no chance to attempt checklist 11-a, "Nurse bends the knees while placing the patient in the wheelchair", and 11-b, "Angle of patients' back before sit down.", and there was a risk of letting the robot fall.

The nurse who participated in the experiment was very experienced, so after several attempts she became able to perform the wheelchair transfer upon the robot patient, but the method she used diverged greatly from the checklist (Fig. 4). Looking at Fig. 5, there is a difference between the trajectories of the head when taking a seat from a standing position with both the robot patient and the healthy person as simulated patients. Furthermore, it is clearly shown that there is significant difference in the trajectories of the head when standing from a seated position. In the case of the healthy person as the simulated patient, assisting as if simply performing the natural actions of helping a person to stand from a seated position will achieve a standing position. In the case of the robot patient, unlike the human, the head's trajectories proceeds in an almost strait light toward the return point.

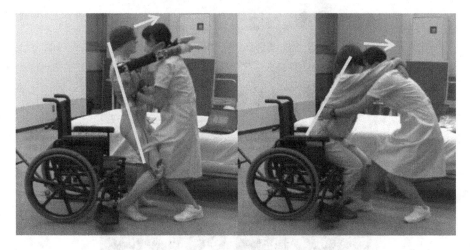

Fig. 3. Comparison of robot and human, bending angle of back

In basic nursing education for assisting patients with physical motions, students are taught to assist in keeping with movements which are naturally inherent to humans [10], and in the checklist to evaluate whether they have acquired said techniques or not as well it is established that actions which are more like helping with a human's natural motions are important actions. However, there are many patients like the robot patient used in this experiment who have some problem which prevents them from performing natural human movements. On the contrary, it could be said that in clinical settings such patients are the majority. In this experiment, we have succeeded in assisting a robot patient in moving from a sitting position to a standing one, as well as from a standing position to a sitting one, without using the assistance methods taught in basic nursing education. The key to the success was the repetition of assistance methods again and again through trial and error until the goal of standing the patient up was achieved. The assistance actions used to achieve the goal were different from those in the checklist, but it led to the result of her mastering the wheelchair transfer assistance method which she thought up by using her own body. If this were a nursing student, it would seem that rather than mimicking the so-called basic movements which are unilaterally taught in basic nursing education, a student using his or her body and head in given circumstances to acquire the technique needed to achieve a goal will come closer to the acquisition of "the ability to appropriately execute nursing care techniques" proposed by MEXT. This was an opportunity to reconsider the idea that has been believed in traditional basic nursing education, namely that application ability follows basic techniques.

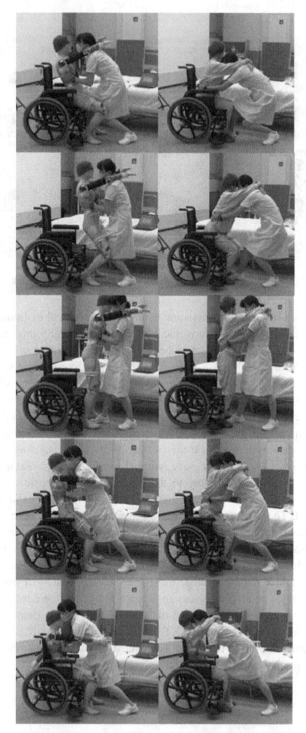

Fig. 4. A sequence of actions of wheelchair transfer methods (Left robot and human right)

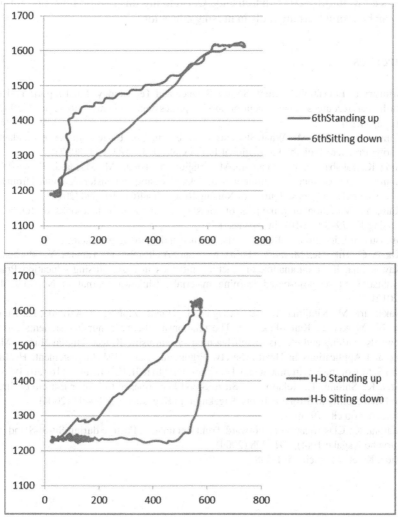

Fig. 5. Comparison of robot and human, the trajectories of the head (Above the robot and under human)

4   Conclusion

Based upon the above, in nursing techniques where the physical condition of the patient has a large influence upon the method of the techniques to be provided, the basic techniques themselves are vague [11], so if students are to acquire application abilities, they must think up and attempt multiple methods repeatedly by themselves upon a simulated patient. For this purpose it is important for the simulated patient to be able to thoroughly reproduce a patient. At the same time, it is also important for there to be no danger of fatigue or injury to the simulated patient during practice. Robot patients can be said to fulfill these requirements. Considering this, we propose that robot patients can be useful learning tools in nursing education.

References

1. Ministry of Education, Culture, Sports, Science and Technology: Final report: Task force for human resources development of nursing professionals in universities, pp. 1–39 (2011) (in Japanese)
2. Tomita, S., Sasaki, M.: What Students Have Learned on Basic Attitude in Fundamental Caring Practice. Tsukuba International Junior College 35, 183–192 (2007)
3. Aida, K., Takabatake, Y., Nakamura, M., Kitajima, Y., Hirata, M., Maeda, J., Kanai-Pak, M.: Comparing the contents of 4 different textbooks: Focusing on transfer techniques from bed to wheelchair. The Japanese Journal of Nursing Research 44(6), 591–598 (2011)
4. Kato, Y.: Variation of principles of transfer sills written in textbooks of fundamental nursing 17, 79–89 (2010) (in Japanese)
5. Ministry of Education, Culture, Sports, Science and Technology.op.cit., 1-39
6. Katata, C., Hiko, K., Murai, Y., Fujita, M., Kato, A., Tambo, K., Tamura, Y., Maruoka, N., Kawashima, K.: Examination of teaching methods in basic nursing education Practical evaluation of scenario-based learning materials. Ishikawa Journal of Nursin 9, 43–51 (2012)
7. Nakamura, M., Kitajima, Y., Ota, J., Ogata, T., Huang, Z., Nagata, A., Aida, K., Kuwahara, N., Maeda, J., Kanai-Pak, M.: The relationship between nursing students' attitudes towards learning and effects of self-learning system using Kinect. Digital Human Modeling and Applications in Health, Safety, Ergonomics, and Risk Management. Healthcare and Safety of the Environment and Transport, DHM/HCII, Part II, 111–116 (2013)
8. Arai, K., Shiomi, T.: Relations of Sit-to-Stand Performance to Lower Extremity Strength and Gait Ability in Stroke Patients. Rigakuryoho Kagaku 19(2), 89–93 (2004)
9. Kato, Y.: op.cit., 79-89
10. Maruta, K.: Classification of Forward Trunk Inclination Posture during Sit-to-Stand. Rigakuryoho Kagaku 19(4), 291–298 (2004)
11. Aida, K., et al.: op.cit., 591-598

Integrated Architecture for Next-Generation m-Health Services (Education, Monitoring and Prevention) in Teenagers

Marco Mazzola[1], Pelin Arslan[1], Gabriela Cândea[2], Ciprian Radu[2],
Massimiliano Azzolini[3], Cristiana Degano[3], and Giuseppe Andreoni[1]

[1] Politecnico di Milano, Design Department, Milan, Italy
{marco.mazzola, giuseppe.andreoni}@polimi.it,
pelinarslan1@gmail.com
[2] ROPARDO S.R.L., Research&Development, Sibiu, Romania
{gabriela.candea,ciprian.radu}@ropardo.ro
[3] Gruppo SIGLA S.r.l., Research&Development, Genova, Italy
{massimiliano.azzolini,cristiana.degano}@grupposigla.it

Abstract. Obesity and other lifestyle-related illness are among the top health-care challenges in Europe. The rapid development of the ICT, and in particular mobile technologies offers an important opportunity for introducing the possibility of a new technological framework. In this paper, the PEGASO system is presented. It will be based on a mobile, social and networked gaming platform, considered as a powerful tool to actively engage the younger population in activities that will stimulate healthier choices in their daily lives. The PEGASO project will implement the User Centred Design approach by considering our target population (i.e. teenagers) at the centre of the system in a palingenetic process. Smartphone is the first and key sensor system. The mobile device also acts as communication gateway towards the other sensors. Basic services, such as those related to location and basic motion sensors to detect physical activity, are provided through sensors embedded within the smartphone.

Keywords: Teenagers Obesity Prevention, Mobile Based Platform, System Architecture.

1   Introduction

Obesity and other lifestyle-related illness are among the top healthcare challenges in Europe. Obesity alone accounts for up to 8% of healthcare costs in the EU[1], as well as wider economy costs associated with lower productivity, lost output and premature death. Childhood overweight and obesity are demonstrated to be strongly related with adult obesity and cardiovascular disease risks, hypertension, metabolic syndrome, fatty liver disease, sleep disturbance and childhood onset type-II diabetes mellitus. [2,3,4]

Obesity in younger age is an alarming predictor for obesity in adulthood, but also entails short term health complications in juvenile age along with greater risk of social

V.G. Duffy (Ed.): DHM 2014, LNCS 8529, pp. 403–414, 2014.
© Springer International Publishing Switzerland 2014

and psychological problems [5]. Knowing how to stay healthy is not enough to motivate individuals to adopt healthy lifestyles, but relevant progress can be achieved through the use of incentives delivered through a combination of processes and mobile technologies [6]. In this landscape, prevention assumes an absolute relevance, and there is an urgent need for further research in how physical activity, training and nutrition can be protective of obesity. With growing rates of childhood overweight and obesity, it becomes increasingly more important to promote healthy eating as poor dietary behaviors are a known risk factor for the development of obesity [7,8].

The main relevant factors tackling childhood obesity prevention result to be related with the Physical Activity, Nutrition and in behavioural education. Addressing the obesity issues requires a comprehensive approach taking into account the individual's physical-physiological characteristics, personality as well as the social and psychological environments influencing decisions and habits in their everyday life. Great relevance should be given to actions developing awareness and enhancing motivation for changing behaviour towards healthy diet (dietary) and physical activity (active lifestyle) [9].

It is demonstrated that Physical Activitiy is protective of obesity. [10-11]. On the contrary, the relation between sedentary time and obesity is not completely defined, but the increased rates of overweight and obesity among children can be attributed to an increase in sedentary pursuits, in relation of the most evidence of higher caloric intake spent in screen time. This fact is relevant because it explains the relation between time spent in, for example, watching television, and the increased amount of food intake as a main cause of overweight.

The rapid development of the ICT, and in particular mobile technologies, together with their diffusion among the EU populations, offers an important opportunity for facing these issues in an innovative manner introducing the possibility of a new technological framework to re-design the healthcare system model. Moreover, establishing healthy behaviors during childhood seems to be easier and more effective than trying to change unhealthy behaviors during adulthood as motivation may be easier to generate while the child is young [12].

The use of technological devices for an active lifestyle monitoring is widely increased in the recent years. As an example, the use of wearable sensors' network has been explored for their application in obesity and activity monitoring [13];

In addition, commercial solutions of monitoring devices are becoming really popular; prove of that is the release of physical activity monitor systems products such as FitBit ultra, sold for 99.95US$ by Fitbit [14], and able to monitor journal activity and sleep patterns. The device includes a 3D accelerometer and an altimeter that permit to track the physical activity. The feedback is provided as estimations of the number of steps, distance, floor climbed, and energy expenditure. As a confirmation of the general interest in this area of technological development, the most influencing brands in ICT, as an example Apple and Samsung, has recently decided to enter this market with smart-watches and specific projects with health purposes.

The behavioural management should be also sensitive to social factors as relations with peers through social network media and personal opportunities focused on increasing awareness and personal involvement in the issues of healthy lifestyles to contrast body mass excess. In this area, the number of projects approaching the education in nutrition and the development of social platform, dedicated apps and serious games is really relevant.

As an example, KickinKitchen.tv [15] from KidsCook Production of Boston, MA, is a web series and online platform based on a musical sitcom for kids ages 8-15 that promotes healthy eating and lifestyles through the creation of a social online environment, including episodes, weekly challenges and special guests contribution.

Another relevant example are the Apps for Healthy Kids challenge [16], promoted by the United States Department of Agriculture, that challenged software developers, game designers, students to develop software tools and apps to encourage children to health nutrition and physical activity. The competition prize was a non cash recognition based on the popularity among visitors and users reached by the developed software.

Video Gaming, concerning serious gaming or exergames, represents another relevant effort in terms of Obesity prevention among children. As an example, Escape From Diab [17] is a serious video game adventure in healthy eating and exercise, released by Archimage in collaboration with experts at the Children's Nutrition Research Center of Houston's Baylor College of Medicine on the project. The video game was designed as an epic adventure, comparable to the experience of commercial quality video and incorporates a broad diversity of behavior change procedures woven in and around engrossing stories.

In this paper, the PEGASO project, an FP7 EU Integrate Project funded by the European Community, and coordinated by Politecnico di Milano is presented through the description of the adopted methodological approach and the System Architecture.

The PEGASO project aims to create a learning platform capable of educating youth through virtual and real-life games and group challenges, in a "social" approach in which they each influence one another. To address these challenges, PEGASO will develop a multi-dimensional and cross-disciplinary ICT system that includes game mechanics to influence behaviours in order to fight and prevent overweight and obesity in the younger population by encouraging them to become co-producers of their wellness and take an active role in improving it by:

- generating self-awareness (acknowledgement of risks associated to unhealthy behaviours),
- enhancing and sustaining motivation to take care of their health with a short/medium/long term perspective,
- changing behaviour towards a healthy lifestyle based on healthy diet and adequate physical activity.

PEGASO will be based on a mobile, social and networked gaming platform, considered as a powerful tool to actively engage the younger population in activities that will stimulate healthier choices in their daily lives.

In consideration of the above, the PEGASO system framework will address prevention, by offering to teenagers – the primary target of PEGASO – three main functionalities:

1. **Individual & Environmental** Monitoring – This dimension consists of the environmental, behavioural and physiological analysis of young users, through a high level-monitoring platform including wearable sensors and mobile phones, as well as multimedia diaries for the acquisition of physical, behavioural and emotional attitude of adolescents.
2. **Feedback System** – The second functionality is aimed at providing a feedback in terms of "health status" changes, required actions to undertake and so on. This function will also propose personalized healthy modification of the lifestyle (in terms of diet and/or physical activity), thus promoting the active involvement of adolescents in changing their behaviours.
3. **Social connectivity and engagement** – The third dimension extends to include a social network where the user can share experiences with a community of peers concerning, e.g. physical activity, food consumptions and everyday habits through different gaming strategies.

2   Methodological Approach

The PEGASO project will implement the User Centred Design approach (UCD)[18] by considering our target population (i.e. teenagers) at the centre of the system in a palingenetic process. This approach is useful to motivate and engage users, which is an essential requirement for systems' acceptance and efficacy rather than forcing to accommodate technologies, products, or services. It should be underlined that PEGASO, as tool for prevention, is addressed also to healthy people.

The main target users in the PEGASO project are teenagers; however there are also several actors (who are also secondary users – Figure 1) and products/systems (the inner circle in Figure 1) involved. The ecosystem of stakeholders and enablers is composed of three main parts that are integrated in the user centred PEGASO system:

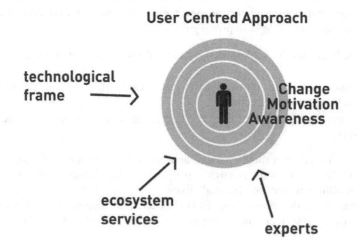

Fig. 1. User Centred Approach adopted in PEGASO

technological frame (multimedia diaries, embedded sensors systems, mobile & web platform), services frame (stakeholders services to provide answers to users' needs and desires in real time/not real time, from the health companion to the serious gaming and social experiences) and experts layer (which are knowledgeable groups of people from different disciplines – medical/psychological/educational – able to interact with the system, who provide them with filtered accurate and needed information to reach their PEGASO objective).

Regarding the ecosystem of the PEGASO project, it is important to consider all personal levels of influence of one's prevention in its environment. Figure 2 below is developed on the basis of the Circles of Influence in Self-Management of Chronic Disease [19] and customized to the target needs of PEGASO, i.e. address prevention management in teenagers.

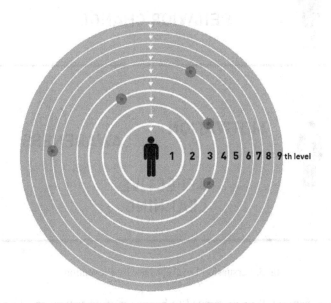

Fig. 2. User's Circles of Influence in Health Management

The circle hierarchy revolving around the end user is not defined in a fixed way; each ring of the concentric circles represents different levels of influence, dispersed around the user: self-management, family involvement, peers influence, experts, school support, community awareness, and environmental measure, industry and policy decisions to the success of the user's prevention management efforts. Therefore for each individual the circles of influence will have different hierarchies, interactions and points (marked in red colour) of decisions for healthy living.

In each circle of influence, the end user has an interaction towards their everyday health. In some circles, the user has the possibility to contribute in decision-making process, in some other they cannot.

Therefore, in the PEGASO project development, it is highly important to focus on the interactions points between end users and levels of their influences, in particular where end user is able to give their own decisions, or where the intervention of services and persuasion to healthier lifestyle changes will be acted upon these opportunity areas. This analysis is important to define for user requirements for the design of the PEGASO persuasion strategies.

Moreover, PEGASO considers the various levels towards persuasion for healthcare[20]. Various types of experts and technologies will feed these levels of persuasion towards healthier decisions. There are four different persuasion strategies: awareness of obesity risks, motivation, affective learning and behaviour change.

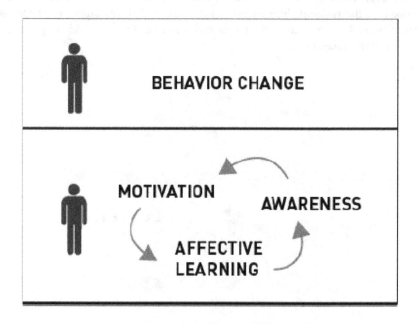

Fig. 3. Persuasion Level for Disease Prevention

- **Develop Awareness:** Teenagers need to be aware of what they are doing; what is right, and what is wrong for their healthy living. Through developing self-awareness and self-reflection, the user can frame the problem or the opportunity area to act upon or intervene.
- **Create Motivation:** It is important to motivate teenagers to change their behaviour and keep this activity in a long-term period. This part is quite challenging, since the motivation depends on many factors as well as emotions, psychological environment and personality of teens.
- Enable **Behaviour Change:** Once teenagers have the awareness and the motivation, it is important to involve experts and use PEGASO system to support the behaviour change process and reinforce existing virtuous behaviours. PEGASO takes a holistic approach involving the teenager's environment and specifically the families, by means of an education process empowered by training that will be provided on location (schools) and on line.

3   System Architecture

Figure 4 represents the architectural scheme of the PEGASO system. The system is designed to be modular, starting from the main device and key functionalities of the application, adding on additional peripherals, more complex services, feedback functions and information.

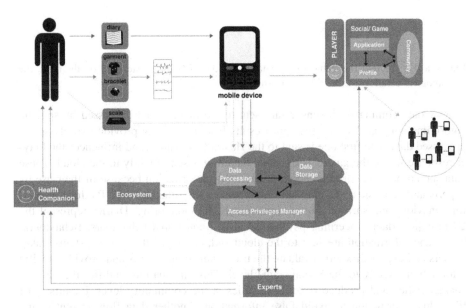

Fig. 4. The PEGASO system Architecture

PEGASO is based on a mobile platform, where the smartphone is the first and key sensor system. The mobile device also acts as communication gateway towards the other sensors. Basic services, such as those related to location (positioning based on GPS and additional algorithms to infer position in the absence of the GPS signal) and basic motion sensors to detect physical activity, are provided through sensors embedded within the smartphone.

Additional sensors that will involve additional hardware, can be added to the system: a bracelet that monitors physical activity; a scale (or balance board) that provides information about weight and body composition; specific sensors to monitor fitness activities.

The behavioural and nutritional data flow (Figure 5a) represents the information that the user provides about its nutritional habits (food intake). These data must be collected through the APP's user interface (UI) directly from the users (e.g. pictures, questionnaires, diaries, vocal annotations etc.).

The physiological data (Figure 5b) can be acquired continuously (this means, accelerometers for the bracelet and, when used, the bio signals from the garment).

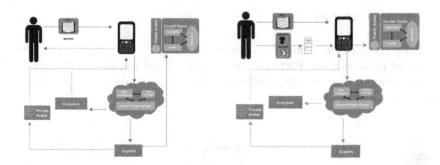

Fig. 5. a) On the left, the Behavioural dataflow of the PEGASO system; b) on the right, the physiological dataflow of the PEGASO system

Raw data coming from sensors are sent to the mobile, and processed by specific algorithms integrated inside the app. Results from processing provide two classes of processed data. The first one is sent to the Health Companion and influences the Player response inside the game. The second dataflow is sent directly to the cloud. These data should be more structured and collect more information because of their use by experts and ecosystem stakeholders. Moreover, a Multimedia Diary Platform is used for behaviour and surrounding environmental data monitoring. Diaries represent the UI to collect data concerning psychological and nutritional behaviours. Behavioural habits and information are sent to the cloud and, consequently, to ecosystems stakeholders and experts. Experts evaluate the user's nutritional habits and provide specific information directly to the Social/Game level. This information modifies the Player's characteristics and produce benefits/penalties at the community level. Experts must filter this information to avoid false information. Another data flow is sent to the Health Companion directly from experts to provide habit suggestions and evaluation of the user's lifestyle and results.

4   System Integration

This section briefly presents the main aspects that will be considered in the PEGASO Project with respect to interconnecting all the software applications and computing systems, so that a whole platform will be obtained.

The envisioned mobile, social and networked platform will be a collaborative one, providing cloud-based services.

From a hardware point of view, the PEGASO platform will integrate different mobile devices (smartphones, bracelets, etc.), computing systems and database systems, by using specific communication protocols. These aspects are beyond the scope of this paper but they will obviously constitute the foundation for cloud Infrastructure as a Service (IaaS).

In terms of software, PEGASO will have to offer several mobile applications and also at least one web application. While the mobile apps are essential to linking teenagers with devices and sensors, the web application will serve as a central point that will allow for "working together". This is the defining characteristic of a Collaborative Platform. The PEGASO web application will allow its users to network. Sensor data will be available to users from the first moment they started using PEGASO. They will be able to track their progress, to share some of their data with others, to discuss, to compare, to receive advices (from friends, from experts), to collaborate in general.

The PEGASO Project will have to manage a cloud-based system integration because the platform will be provided as a service (PaaS – Platform as a Service). This kind of system integration is required for Software as a Service (SaaS) applications.

Some of the main characteristics of cloud-based system integration are: (1) deploying in an elastic cloud infrastructure, (2) no software development (every piece of software is available and ready to be connected to another one), (3) users do not manage the platform and (4) system management and monitoring services.

From a software engineering point of view, the PEGASO system will adopt the commonly used Continuous Integration technique. It is part of the extreme programming, agile methodology, and it essentially involves: test-driven development, maintaining a code repository, automating the build process and automating the deployment process. While this technique demands well defined test cases and a significant initial setup time, the idea is to offer continuous delivery and quality assurance.

Software tools like [21,22,23] will help towards PEGASO system integration. The orchestration will have to be managed properly as PEGASO will encompass a multitude of hardware devices (smartphones, tables, sensors, etc.), operating systems, communication protocols, web browsers, software applications and servers.

As described above, system integration is will assemble and package manufactured parts in successive phases in order to obtain more complete and more optimized systems allowing them to work together in the PEGASO scenarios.

In order to guarantee modularity and scalability, the integration framework will be made up by Open Source technologies in order to make the PEGASO ecosystem a real open platform, easy to up-grade and able to self-adapting very quickly both to technical progress and future mobile devices.

The integration framework will be structured by the following layers:

- *Prototypes integration layer*: this layer will integrate the prototypes such serious game, smart life companion, social network, bracelets, wearable sensors;
- *Integration software layer*: this is the main core framework software. It will provide libraries and programs to be employed by the devices and mobile/web prototypes in order to interface externally and with the API of the *common communication interface layer* ;
- *Common communication interface layer*: it will define a common language in order to make the prototypes able to communicate, through Open Data protocol, with the different software modules of PEGASO ecosystem.

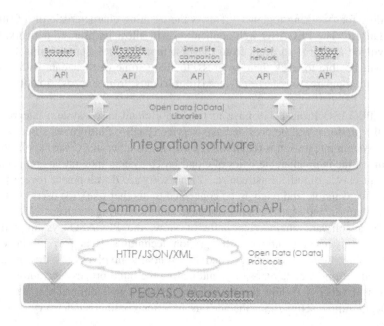

Fig. 6. System Integration

A complete definition of the common communication interface (API), having into account existing standards and interoperability with other components, will be performed and developed.

Interfaces' modules will be:

- *Open Data Libraries:* will provide information exchange among devices serious game, smart life companion, social network, bracelets, wearable sensors prototypes;
- *Open Data Protocols:* HTTP / JSON /XML;
- *Web services:* provide devices to interface with PEGASO ecosystem.

Communication interfaces of developed prototype will be connected with the whole PEGASO ecosystem through actual existing standards communication (3G or Wi-Fi network) providing both synchronization and data interchange. The architecture that will be developed will be modular in order to provide, during the prototype development, to fit efficiently to PEGASO system needs.

5   Conclusion and Discussion

In this paper, the PEGASO system Architecture has been presented. The PEGASO project is aimed at the development of a mobile-based platform whose aim is to generate awareness in teen agers about healthy behaviour in nutrition and lifestyles, and to create a social-based platform to motivate and engage the users to learn healthy habits. The progresses proposed by the PEGASO systems are related to the integration of different approach to education, such as the use of mobile media and technologies in healthcare, serious gaming approaches and location based services. The system architecture will be defined during the first year of the project and a UCD approach will be conducted to define the Users' requirements. The system integration definition will guarantee the reliability of the ICT platform and the technological frames.

References

1. WHO, http://www.euro.who.int/en/health-topics/noncommunicable diseases/obesity/obesity
2. Reilly, J.J., Methven, E., McDowell, Z.C., et al.: Healthconsequences of obesity. Archives of Disease in Childhood 88(9), 748–752 (2003)
3. Freedman, D.S., Khan, L.K., Dietz, W.H., Srinivasan, S.R., Berenson, G.S.: Relationship of childhood obesity to coronary heart disease risk factors in adulthood: The Bogalusa Heart Study. Pediatrics 108(3), 712–718 (2001)
4. Weiss, R., Caprio, S.: The metabolic consequences of childhood obesity. Best. Pract. Res. Clin. Endocrinol. Metab 19(3), 405–419 (2005)
5. Swartz, M., Puhl, R.: Childhood obesity: A societal problem to solve. Obesity Reviews 4(1), 57–71 (2003)
6. Baranowski, T., Frankel, L.: Let's Get Technical! Gaming and Technology for Weight Control and HealthPromotion in Children, Childhood Obesity 34–37 (February 2012)
7. Wright, J.D., Wang, C.Y., Kennedy-Stephenson, J., Ervin, R.B.: Dietary intake of ten key nutrients for public health, United States: 1999–2000. Advance Data no. 334, 1–4 (2003)
8. Patrick, K., Calfas, K.J., Norman, G.J., et al.: Randomized controlled trial of a primary care and home-based interventionfor physical activity and nutrition behaviors: PACE+ for adolescents. Archives of Pediatrics & Adolescent Medicine 160(2), 128–136 (2006)
9. World Health Organization. Population-based prevention strategies for childhood obesity: Report of a WHO forumand technical meeting, Geneva, 15–17 (December 2009)
10. Timmons, B.W., Leblanc, A.G., Carson, V., et al.: Systematic Review of physical activity and health in the early years (Aged 0 -4). Appl. Physiol. Nutr. Metab. 37, 773–792 (2012)
11. Chaput, J.-P., Lambert, M., Mathieu, M.-E., Tremblay, M.S., O'Loughlin, J., Tremblay, A.: Physical activity vs. sedentary time: Indepent associations with adiposity in children. Pediatric Obesity 7, 251–258 (2012)
12. Baranowski, T., Davis, M., Resnicow, K., Baranowski, J., Doyle, C., Lin, L.S.,... Wang, D.T.: Gimme 5 Fruit, Juice, and Vegetables for Fun and Health: Outcome Evaluation. Health education & behavior 27(1), 96–111 (2000)
13. Bonato, P.: Wearable Sensors and Systems. IEEE Engineering in Medicine and Biology Magazine 29 29(3), 25–36 (2010)
14. http://www.fitbit.com
15. http://kickinkitchen.tv
16. http://appsforhealthykids.challengepost.com
17. http://www.escapefromdiab.com
18. Sanders, E.B.: From User-Centered To Participatory Design Approaches. Design, 1–7. Taylor &Francis (2002)

19. Clark, N.M., Patridge, M.R.: Strengthening Asthma Education to Enhance Disease Control. Chest 121(5), 1661–1669 (2002)
20. Fogg, B.J.: A Behavior Model for Persuasive Design. In: Proceedings of the 4th International Conference onPersuasive Technology Persuasive (2009) ISBN:9781605583761
21. Hudson, http://hudson-ci.org/
22. Jenkins, http://jenkins-ci.org/
23. Rational Team Concert, https://jazz.net/products/rational-team-concert/

The Semantics of Refinement Chart

Dominique Méry[1] and Neeraj Kumar Singh[2]

[1] Université de Lorraine, LORIA, BP 239, Nancy, France
Dominique.Mery@loria.fr
[2] McMaster Centre for Software Certification, McMaster University, Hamilton, ON, Canada
singhn10@mcmaster.ca

Abstract. Refinement techniques play a major role to build a complex system incrementally. Refinement is supported by several modelling techniques in the area of system designing. These modelling techniques are either in textual notation or in graphical notation. This paper focuses on refinement chart (RC) that is based on graphical notations. The refinement chart is a graphical representation of a complex system using layering approach, where functional blocks are divided into multiple simpler blocks in a new refinement level, without changing the original behaviour of the system. The main contribution is to provide a formal semantical description of the refinement chart. The refinement chart offers a clear view of assistance in "system" integration that models complex critical medical systems. Moreover, it also sketches a clear view of different operating modes and their associated components. To realize the effectiveness of this approach, we apply this refinement based graphical modelling technique to model the grand challenge: *cardiac pacemaker*.

Keywords: Refinement, modelling, semantics, verification.

1 Introduction

Highly complex systems related to the medical domain are susceptible to error due to complex nature of the system operability and complexity of the system [1,2]. Software or hardware failure of a medical device can lead to injuries and loss of life. Design errors are considered as a main source of defects that can be introduced during the development process. There are several techniques available in the area of testing and formal verification to verify the correctness of system. However, existing techniques are not sufficient to prevent from the failure cases. Some additional techniques are required to handle the complexity of critical medical systems, and to make sure that the developed system is safe. The common notation of an existing technique is either textual or graphical. We know that a picture speaks louder than text, therefore graphical notations are much popular than textual notations. Nowadays graphical modelling techniques like Simulink, LabView and UML are main applications for developing the complex systems.

Despite all the efforts of the community, critical medical system designers still need a new way for modelling the systems, and to analyse the correctness of system behaviour. A set of requirements is given below that is mandatory for an efficient modelling solution:

V.G. Duffy (Ed.): DHM 2014, LNCS 8529, pp. 415–426, 2014.

- Integration of various modules of the medical critical systems and formal analysis of the inter-operations among the modules.
- Introspection features for identifying anomalies.
- Incremental model-based development.
- System integration of the critical infrastructure.
- Formalization of operating modes and associated components.
- Decomposition of a complex medical system into multiple subsystems.

This paper draws the attention towards a refinement-based graphical technique known as refinement chat for modelling the complex critical medical systems. This graphical technique provides an easily manageable representation for different refinement subsystems and offers a clear view of assistance in system integration. This graphical modelling technique may help for simplifying specification, synthesis, and validating the system requirements. Moreover, this technique enables an efficient creation/customization of the critical systems at low-cost and development time.

The main contribution of this paper is the semantical description of refinement chart [3,4], which provides automata of refinement chart including mode transitions, and operational semantics for a system refinement to carry out the sound and rigorous reasoning for developing the critical systems. Automata and operational semantics assist a designer to understand the mode transition and correct system behaviour of the different subsystems. The proposed approach of refinement chart captures all the above enumerated requirements. Moreover, this technique is not limited to medical systems only, but can be used to model highly critical systems like avionics, and automotive systems to identify the incorrect transitions or abnormal system behaviour.

This paper is organized as follows. Section 2 presents related work. Section 3 describes the refinement chart, and Section 4 presents the semantics of refinement chart. Section 5 presents assessment of the proposed technique using cardiac pacemaker case study. Finally, Section 6 concludes this paper along with future works.

2   Related Work

A *modal system* is a system characterized by *operation modes*, which coordinates system operations. Many systems are *modal systems*, for instance, space and avionic systems [5,1], steam boiler control [2], transportation and so on. Operation modes explore the actual system behaviour through observation of a system functioning under the multiple conditions according to the system environment. In this approach, a system is considered as a set of operating modes, where each operating mode is categorised according to the system functionality over different operating conditions. Each operating mode expresses the different functionality of the system.

Modecharts [6] is a graphical technique, which is used to handle mode and mode switching behavior of a system. This paper addresses the state space partition, and various working conditions of a system in order to define the controlling behaviour of the large state machines. However, the modecharts has lack of adequate support for specifying and reasoning about the functional properties.

Few papers [7,8] have also addressed the problem of mode changing in the real-time systems. Jorge et al. [7] present a survey on mode changing protocol for the real-time systems and propose several new protocols for schedulability analysis and configuration methods. The changing mode is based on delay and initiation of a new mode with consistently sharing the resources during mode change. Fohler et al. [8] discuss the issues of handling mode changes and requirements for their application for a real-time system, where they explore the specification of mode changes, sechedubility for modes and transitions, and run time execution of the mode changes including decomposition of the system into disjoint modes.

Dotti et al. [9] have proposed both formalization and a refinement notion for a *modal system*, using existing support for the construction of *modal system*. The paper presents the requirements for an Event-B model to realise a modal system specification using an industrial case study.

According to our literature survey, none of the existing approaches discuss a refinement-based technique for handling the complexity of a system. We propose a technique of refinement chart for presenting various operating modes for different subsystems. Each subsystem represents an independent function according to the operating modes. This refinement chart helps to design a complex system, system integration through code structuring, and to establish a relationship between two subsystems using operating modes.

3   Refinement Chart

3.1   Motivation

The development of embedded software for a critical medical system requires significant lower level manual interaction for organizing and assembling the different parts of system. This is inherently error-prone, time-consuming and platform-dependent. To detect the failure cases in a software is not an easy task. Manually reviewing the source code is the only way to trace the cause of a failure. Due to the technological advancement and modern complexity of the critical medical system software, this is an impossible task for any third party investigator without any prior knowledge of the software. Consequently, we propose a simple methodology of system decomposition and integration using the refinement chart, that seeks to minimize the effort and overhead.

Refinement chart can be used during the decomposition and integration phases of a complex medical system that can help to analyse the complex behaviors. The purpose of refinement chart is to provide an easily manageable representation of a complex medical system in multiple refinements. The refinement chart offers a clear view of assistance in system integration. This is an important issue not only for being able to derive the system-level performance and correctness guarantees, but also for being able to assemble components in a cost-effective manner. Moreover, It can also help to a code designer to improve the code structures, code optimization, and code generation techniques. Every incremental refinement presents additional functionalities. This refinement-based structure may improve the safety, hardware integration and guidelines to develop the critical medical systems. This approach also helps in code integration and to test the different subsystems of a system independently.

A refinement-based system development has a different cost structure than the traditional development life-cycle. The cost of building models and related other required

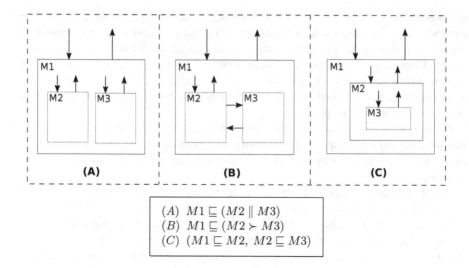

$$(A) \quad M1 \sqsubseteq (M2 \parallel M3)$$
$$(B) \quad M1 \sqsubseteq (M2 \succ M3)$$
$$(C) \quad (M1 \sqsubseteq M2, \; M2 \sqsubseteq M3)$$

Fig. 1. Refinement charts

design knowledge may be higher for producing the first system. However, these costs are amortized when reuse these models and designs for developing the other systems in future. Thus, the cost of producing first program may be higher, but the cost of development for reproducing advanced version of the products and reuse same codes in other products should be less than the conventional programming [10,11]. The cost of handling of proof obligations of specifications and refinements should be less than the cost of analyzing the final product.

3.2   Overview

Main objective of the refinement chart [3] is to specify the modal system requirements in a form that is easily and effectively implementable. During the modelling of modal system, several styles of specification are usually adopted for handling the complex operating modes. Functional blocks are divided into multiple simpler blocks in a new refinement level, without changing the original system behaviour. The final goal is to obtain a specification that is detailed enough to be effectively implemented, but also to describe correctly the requirements of a given system.

As the nature of critical medical systems is often characterizable as *modal systems*, we follow a state-based approach to propose suitable abstractions. We consider that the state of a model is detailed enough to allow one to distinguish its different operating conditions and also to characterize required mode functionality and possible mode switching in terms of state transitions.

Each subsystem that forms the specification is represented into a block diagram as a refinement chart. Fig. 1 presents the diagrams of the most abstract modal system. The diagrams use a visual notation loosely based on Statechart [12]. A mode is represented by a box with a mode name; a mode transition is an arrow connecting two modes.

The direction of an arrow indicates the previous and next modes in a transition. Refinement is expressed by nesting boxes. A refined diagram with an outgoing arrow from an abstract mode is equivalent to the outgoing arrows from each of the concrete modes. It is also similar to the ingoing arrows. In a refinement, nesting box can be arranged hierarchically and can be represented by basic rules of our refinement chart (see Fig. 2). The basic rules of refinements are: parallel refinement $[M1 \sqsubseteq (M2 \parallel M3 \parallel \ldots\ldots \parallel M_{n-1} \parallel M_n)]$, sequential refinement $[M1 \sqsubseteq (M2 \succ M3 \succ \ldots\ldots \succ M_{n-1} \succ M_n)]$ and nested refinement $[(M1 \sqsubseteq M2, M2 \sqsubseteq M3, \ldots\ldots, M_{n-1} \sqsubseteq M_n)]$. Furthermore, refinement charts, which appear in the hierarchical form can be expressed by any one rule, or several rules. A complex system can be represented by using refinement laws iteratively, means each subsystem can be refined by any rule (sequential, parallel or nesting) iteratively until to get the final model [3,4].

$$M1 \sqsubseteq (M2 \parallel M3 \parallel \ldots\ldots \parallel M_{n-1} \parallel M_n)$$
$$M1 \sqsubseteq (M2 \succ M3 \succ \ldots\ldots \succ M_{n-1} \succ M_n)$$
$$(M1 \sqsubseteq M2, M2 \sqsubseteq M3, \ldots\ldots, M_{n-1} \sqsubseteq M_n)$$

Fig. 2. Basic rules of Refinement Chart

Fig. 1 presents for only three modes (M1, M2 and M3) with different kinds of refinements. The parallel relationship among several refinement boxes states that a system operates simultaneously in the subsystems. For instance, Fig. 1(A) represents an abstract mode $M1$ and two parallel refinements are represented by nesting mode boxes $M2$ and $M3$. Transition between these two refinements $M2$ and $M3$ are not allowed. Entry into a parallel refined subsystem requires entry into all of its immediate child refinement. A transition out of one refinement requires an exit out of all the refined subsystems in parallel to it. The sequential relationship among several refinement boxes states that the system operates in at most one of these subsystems at any time. For example, Fig. 1(B) represents an abstract mode $M1$ and two sequential refinements are presented by the nesting mode boxes $M2$ and $M3$ in two levels of hierarchy, where $M2$ and $M3$ are embedded in $M1$. The transitions between $M2$ and $M3$ allows the system to go from one refinement to another refinement according to the operating modes. The nesting relationship among several refinement boxes states that the system operates in any subsystems. For example, Fig. 1(C) represents an abstract mode $M1$ and the subsystems refinement by a nesting box $M2$ and the subsystem $M2$ is refined by a nesting box $M3$ in three levels of hierarchy, where $M2$ is embedded in $M1$ and $M3$ is embedded in $M2$. A transition is allowed to next level of refined subsystem. A transition out of one refinement requires an exit out of all the refined sub level of refined subsystems.

3.3   Semantics of Refinement Chart (RC)

Automata RC. RC automata is similar to the classical automata, except that its modes can be of any RC type, and its transition function can refer to the concrete modes of automaton. Let $Automaton \triangleq (\Sigma, M, \delta, \theta, M_0)$ is a set of RC of type automaton. We have the following typing constraints on each elements of the automaton.

- Σ is a list of alphabets.
- M is a set of automaton modes.
- $\delta \subseteq \langle \mu, \sigma \rangle$ is an input transition relation, where:
  - μ denotes an input arrow.
  - σ an event of the transition.
- $\theta \subseteq \langle \nu, \sigma \rangle$ is an output transition relation, where:
  - ν denotes an output arrow.
  - σ an event of the transition.
- M_0 is an initial mode.

Operational Semantics. There are eight inference rules, written in the usual form $\frac{premiss}{conclusion}$. The first rule describes a transition between local modes using an input arrow. $\delta((m_1, m_2), \sigma)$ presents an input transition relation, where σ expresses an event of transition between two modes m_1 and m_2.

$$\frac{\delta((m_1,m_2),\sigma)}{m_1 \xrightarrow{\sigma} m_2} in$$

The second rule describes a transition between local modes using an output arrow. Similar to the input transition relation. $\theta((m_1, m_2), \sigma)$ presents an output transition relation, where σ expresses an event of transition between two modes m_1 and m_2.

$$\frac{\theta((m_1,m_2),\sigma)}{m_1 \xrightarrow{\sigma} m_2} out$$

Rule three provides the parallel operational semantics of an input transition relation, where parallel input transitions are presented by input arrows. $\delta((m_1, m_2, \cdots, m_n), (\sigma_1, \sigma_2, \cdots, \sigma_{n-1}))$ presents an input transition relation, where $(\sigma_1, \sigma_2, \cdots, \sigma_{n-1})$ expresses a set of transition events, and $(m_1, m_2, \cdots, m_n)$ presents a set of modes of the refinement chart.

$$\frac{\delta((m_1,m_2,\cdots,m_n),(\sigma_1,\sigma_2,\cdots,\sigma_{n-1}))}{m_1 \xrightarrow{\sigma_1} m_2 || \cdots || m_1 \xrightarrow{\sigma_{n-1}} m_n} ||in$$

Rule four shows the parallel operational semantics of an output transition relation, where parallel output transitions are presented by output arrows. $\theta((m_1, m_2, \cdots, m_n), (\sigma_1, \sigma_2, \cdots, \sigma_{n-1}))$ presents an output transition relation, where $(\sigma_1, \sigma_2, \cdots, \sigma_{n-1})$ expresses a set of transition events, and $(m_1, m_2, \cdots, m_n)$ presents a set of modes of the refinement chart.

$$\frac{\theta((m_1,m_2,\cdots,m_n),(\sigma_1,\sigma_2,\cdots,\sigma_{n-1}))}{m_1 \xrightarrow{\sigma_1} m_2 || \cdots || m_1 \xrightarrow{\sigma_{n-1}} m_n} ||out$$

Rule five shows the sequential operational semantics of an input transition relation, where sequential input transitions are presented by input arrows. $\delta((m_1, m_2, \cdots, m_n), (\sigma_1, \sigma_2, \cdots, \sigma_{n-1}))$ presents an input transition relation, where $(\sigma_1, \sigma_2, \cdots, \sigma_{n-1})$ expresses a set of transition events, and $(m_1, m_2, \cdots, m_n)$ presents a set of modes of the refinement chart.

$$\frac{\delta((m_1,m_2,\cdots,m_n),(\sigma_1,\sigma_2,\cdots,\sigma_{n-1}))}{m_1\xrightarrow{\sigma_1}m_2\succ\cdots\succ m_{n-1}\xrightarrow{\sigma_{n-1}}m_n}\succ in$$

Rule six shows the sequential operational semantics of an output transition relation, where sequential output transitions are presented by output arrows. $\delta((m_1,m_2,\cdots,m_n),(\sigma_1,\sigma_2,\cdots,\sigma_{n-1}))$ presents an output transition relation, where $(\sigma_1,\sigma_2,\cdots,\sigma_{n-1})$ expresses a set of transition events, and $(m_1,m_2,\cdots,m_n)$ presents a set of modes of the refinement chart.

$$\frac{\theta((m_1,m_2,\cdots,m_n),(\sigma_1,\sigma_2,\cdots,\sigma_{n-1}))}{m_1\xrightarrow{\sigma_1}m_2\succ\cdots\succ m_{n-1}\xrightarrow{\sigma_{n-1}}m_n}\succ out$$

Rule seven defines the nested operational semantics of an input transition relation, where nested input transitions are presented by input arrows. $\delta((m_1,m_2,\cdots,m_n),(\sigma_1,\sigma_2,\cdots,\sigma_{n-1}))$ presents an input transition relation, where $(\sigma_1,\sigma_2,\cdots,\sigma_{n-1})$ expresses a set of transition events, and $(m_1,m_2,\cdots,m_n)$ presents a set of modes of the refinement chart.

$$\frac{\delta((m_1,m_2,\cdots,m_n),(\sigma_1,\sigma_2,\cdots,\sigma_{n-1}))}{m_1\xrightarrow{\sigma_1}m_2\sqsubseteq\cdots\sqsubseteq m_{n-1}\xrightarrow{\sigma_{n-1}}m_n}\sqsubseteq in$$

Rule eight shows the nested operational semantics of an output transition relation, where nested output transitions are presented by output arrows. $\theta((m_1,m_2,\cdots,m_n),(\sigma_1,\sigma_2,\cdots,\sigma_{n-1}))$ presents an output transition relation, where $(\sigma_1,\sigma_2,\cdots,\sigma_{n-1})$ expresses a set of transition events, and $(m_1,m_2,\cdots,m_n)$ presents a set of modes in the refinement chart.

$$\frac{\theta((m_1,m_2,\cdots,m_n),(\sigma_1,\sigma_2,\cdots,\sigma_{n-1}))}{m_1\xrightarrow{\sigma_1}m_2\sqsubseteq\cdots\sqsubseteq m_{n-1}\xrightarrow{\sigma_{n-1}}m_n}\sqsubseteq out$$

Kleene Closure RC. This operator is borrowed from regular expressions. It allows an arbitrary number of iterations (including zero) on RC. An iteration is completed when the component RC has reached at the concrete level or final mode. Formally, let $Closure \triangleq \langle\bigstar,m\rangle$ is a set of Kleene closure RC, where $m \in M$ is a mode of the closure. It is essentially used to determine if a closure can immediately exit without any iteration.

There are two inference rules related to the input and output arrows. $\bigstar_{in}$ allows for zero or infinite iterations using input arrows from an initial mode of the RC until to reach at the concrete mode or final mode. Similarly, $\bigstar_{out}$ allows zero or infinite iterations using output arrows from an initial mode to the concrete mode or final mode. However, Kleene closure RC allows any operation from the parallel, sequential and nested in any order.

$$\frac{\delta((m_1,m_2),\sigma)}{(\langle||,\succ,\sqsubseteq\rangle\bigstar,m_1)\xrightarrow{\sigma}(\langle||,\succ,\sqsubseteq\rangle\bigstar,m_2)}\bigstar in$$

$$\frac{\theta((m_1,m_2),\sigma)}{(\langle||,\succ,\sqsubseteq\rangle\bigstar,m_1)\xrightarrow{\sigma}(\langle||,\succ,\sqsubseteq\rangle\bigstar,m_2)}\bigstar out$$

4   Case Study : Cardiac Pacemaker

4.1   Informal Description of Cardiac Pacemaker

A pacemaker is an electronic device implanted in the body to regulate the abnormal heart rhythm. The primary functions of pacemaker are *pacing* and *sensing*. The pacemaker actuator is used to pace by delivering a short, intense electrical pulse into the heart. The pacemaker sensor senses an intrinsic activity of the heart. The pacing and sensing activities are synchronized with natural rhythm in both chambers right atria and ventricle. The basic elements of pacemaker are as follows:

1. **Leads:** One or more flexible metal wires, that transmit electrical signals between the heart and a pacemaker, and the same wires are also used to detect the intrinsic heart activities.
2. **The Pacemaker Generator:** It contains an implanted battery for power source and a controller as a brain of pacemaker for pacing and sensing activities.
3. **Device Controller-Monitor (DCM):** An external device that controls the functionalities of pacemaker remotely through wireless connection.
4. **Accelerometer (Rate Modulation Sensor):** An electromechanical device inside a pacemaker that measures an acceleration of a body in order to allow modulated pacing during various physical activities like running, sleeping, walking etc.

4.2   Bradycardia Operating Modes

Table 1 presents the generic code of a cardiac pacemaker. The codes are in a sequential order of letters that provides a description of pacemaker pacing and sensing functions. The first letter of the code indicates which chambers are being paced; the second letter indicates which chambers are being sensed; the third letter of the code indicates the response to sensing and the final letter, which is optional indicates the presence of rate modulation in response to the physical activity measured by the accelerometer.

Table 1. Generic code of cardiac pacemaker

Category	Chambers Paced	Chambers Sensed	Response to Sensing	Rate Modulation
Letters	O-None	O-None	O-None	R-Rate Modulation
	A-Atrium	A-Atrium	T-Triggered	
	V-Ventricle	V-Ventricle	I-Inhibited	
	D-Dual(A+V)	D-Dual(A+V)	D-Dual(T+I)	

4.3   Development of Cardiac Pacemaker Using Refinement Chart

This section presents the development of cardiac pacemaker using refinement chart. Each subsystem of the pacemaker is modelled incrementally to capture all the operating modes. Fig. 3 and Fig. 4 present the abstract models for one and two-electrode pacemaker (A), and the resulting models of three successive refinement steps (B to D). The diagrams use a visual notation to indicate the bradycardia operating modes of pacemaker under functional and parametric requirements. One or multiple operating modes are presented by a box; an operating mode transition is an arrow connecting two operating modes. The direction of an arrow indicates the previous and next operating modes in a transition. Refinement is expressed by nesting boxes to show an integration of new behaviour of the system.

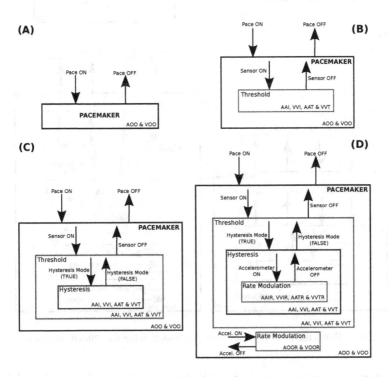

Fig. 3. Refinements of one-electrode pacemaker using the refinement chart

A refined diagram of an abstract mode is equivalent to a concrete mode. At the most abstract level, we introduce *pacing* activity into single and both heart chambers. In Fig. 3(A) and Fig. 4(A), *pacing* is presented by transitions *Pace ON* and *Pace OFF* for single chamber or both chambers. It is the basic transitions for all bradycardia operating modes.

In the next refinement (Fig. 3(B), Fig. 4(B)) step *pacing* is refined by *sensing*, corresponding to the activity of the heart, when sensing period is not under the refractory period (RF^1). In the first refinement of two-electrode pacemaker, sensors are introduced in both chambers. In Fig. 3(B) of one-electrode, sensing is represented by transitions *Sensor ON* and *Sensor OFF*, while in Fig. 4(B) of two-electrode, sensing is represented

---

[1] RF : Atria Refractory Period (ARP) or Ventricular Refractory Period (VRP).

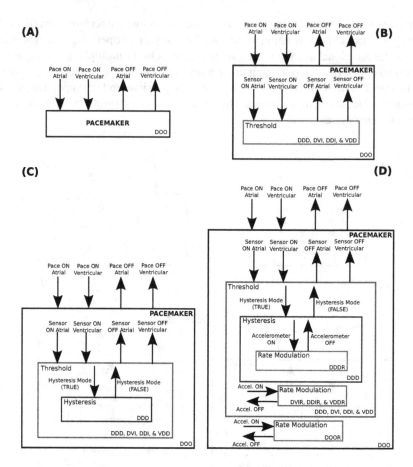

Fig. 4. Refinements of two-electrode pacemaker using the refinement chart

by transitions *Sensor ON Atria, Sensor ON Ventricle, Sensor OFF Atria* and *Sensor OFF ventricle*. The pacemaker's actuator and sensor are synchronizing to each other under the real-time constraints. The block diagrams (Fig. 3(B), Fig. 4(B)) represent the *threshold* refinement, that is a measuring unit which measures a stimulation threshold voltage value of the heart and a pulse generator for delivering stimulation pulses to the heart. The pacemaker's sensor starts sensing after the refractory period (RF) but pacemaker's actuator delivers a pacing stimulus according to the response of the sensor. Sensor-related transitions are available in all operating modes except AOO, VOO and DOO modes.

Third refinement step (Fig. 3(C), Fig. 4(C)) introduces different operating strategies under *hysteresis* interval: if the *hysteresis* mode is TRUE, then the pacemaker paces at a faster rate than the sensing rate to provide consistent pacing in one chamber (atrial or ventricle) or both chambers (atrial and ventricle), or prevents constant pacing in one chamber (atrial or ventricle) or both chambers (atrial and ventricle). In case of FALSE state of *hysteresis* mode, the pacemaker's sensor and actuator works in normal state and does not try to maintain the consistent pacing. Hysteresis mode is represented by transitions *Hysteresis Mode TRUE* and *Hysteresis Mode FALSE*. The main objective of hysteresis is to allow the patient to have his or her own underlying rhythm as much as possible.

According to the last refinement step (Fig. 3(D), Fig. 4(D)), it introduces the rate adapting pacing technique in the bradycardia operating modes of pacemaker. The rate modulation mode is represented by transitions *Accel. ON* and *Accel. OFF*. The rate modulation operating modes are available in all pacemaker operating modes which are given under multiple refinements. The pacemaker uses the accelerometer sensors to sense the physiologic need of the heart and increase or decrease the pacing rate. The amount of rate increases is determined by the pacemaker based on maximum exertion is performed by the patient. This increased pacing rate is sometimes referred to as the "sensor indicated rate". When exertion has stopped the pacemaker will progressively decrease the pacing rate down to the lower rate [3].

Refinement chart helps to model the system integration, which also complies with refinement based formal development. The block diagrams of the refinement chart help to build the complete system and used to handle the complexity of the whole system through decomposing in multiple independent parts. Here, refinement chart models different kinds of operating modes, and decompose the whole system based on operational modes. Decomposing using the refinement chart helps to analyse individual component and interaction or switching from one operating mode to other operating modes.

5   Conclusion

Today, in order to respect the certifiable assurance and safety, time to market and strict cost constraints, critical system designers need some new modelling and simulation solutions. The solutions must also permit software component modelling, component integration in a distributed environment, easier debugging of complex specifications, and mitigated connection with other, existing or new systems.

In this paper, we would like to stress the original contribution of our work through providing the automata and semantical operations of the refinement chart, where this technique can be used to model the desired system using layering approach in graphical block diagrams. The functional blocks are divided into multiple simpler blocks in a new refinement level, without changing the original behaviour of the system. Moreover, this technique offers decomposition, integration, and synchronization of the system components using incremental refinements. This approach helps in code integration and to test the different subsystems independently.

However, the refinement chart presents a block diagram for each subsystems and provides a structure in various refinements to build a complete system. The concrete refinement charts provide system integration information in the form of compose and decompose of software codes according to the blocks diagrams. Composition and decomposition help to improve the code structure and code optimization. To find a minimum set of events for each independent subsystem is known as code optimization. The refinement chart specially covers component-based design frameworks and decomposition, integration of critical infrastructure and device integration. The complexity of design is reduced by structuring systems using modes and by detailing this design using refinement.

System integration methodology using refinement charts are also used for system development, which helps a code designer to improve the code structure, code optimization, code generation for synthesizing, and synchronizing the software codes of a critical medical system like pacemaker. In the pacemaker case study, system has different kinds of functional requirements, and all the possible operating modes are decomposed in the refinement chart using multiple refinements related to the state flow models. Therefore use of the refinement chart, and formal specifications state the correctness of the system design and implementation. As a result, we have used manual development of the refinement chart in our pacemaker case study. In the future, we will develop an integrated development environment (IDE) for designing the medical critical systems using refinement chart and then automatic formalization from the developed models.

References

1. Miller, S.P.: Specifying the mode logic of a flight guidance system in CoRE and SCR. In: Proceedings of the Second Workshop on Formal Methods in Software Practice, FMSP 1998, pp. 44–53. ACM, New York (1998)
2. Abrial, J.-R., Börger, E., Langmaack, H. (eds.): Formal Methods for Industrial Applications, Specifying and Programming the Steam Boiler Control. LNCS, vol. 1165. Springer, Heidelberg (1996)
3. Singh, N.K.: Using Event-B for Critical Device Software Systems. Springer, Heidelberg (2013)
4. Méry, D., Singh, N.K.: Formal specification of medical systems by proof-based refinement. ACM Trans. Embed. Comput. Syst. 12(1), 15:1–15:25 (2013)
5. Butler, R.W.: An Introduction to Requirements Capture Using PVS: Specification of a Simple Autopilot. NASA Technical Memorandum 110255, NASA Langley Research Center, Hampton, VA (May 1996)
6. Jahanian, F., Mok, A.K.: Modechart: A specification language for real-time systems. IEEE Trans. Softw. Eng. 20(12), 933–947 (1994)
7. Real, J., Crespo, A.: Mode change protocols for real-time systems: A survey and a new proposal. Real-Time Syst. 26(2), 161–197 (2004)
8. Fohler, G.: Realizing changes of operational modes with a pre run-time scheduled hard real-time system. In: Proceedings of the Second International Workshop on Responsive Computer Systems, pp. 287–300. Springer, Heidelberg (1992)
9. Dotti, F.L., Iliasov, A., Ribeiro, L., Romanovsky, A.: Modal systems: Specification, refinement and realisation. In: Breitman, K., Cavalcanti, A. (eds.) ICFEM 2009. LNCS, vol. 5885, pp. 601–619. Springer, Heidelberg (2009)
10. Smith, D.R.: Generating programs plus proofs by refinement. In: Meyer, B., Woodcock, J. (eds.) Verified Software 2005. LNCS, vol. 4171, pp. 182–188. Springer, Heidelberg (2008)
11. Walters, H.: Hybrid implementations of algebraic specifications. In: Kirchner, H., Wechler, W. (eds.) ALP 1990. LNCS, vol. 463, pp. 40–54. Springer, Heidelberg (1990)
12. Harel, D.: Statecharts: A visual formalism for complex systems. Sci. Comput. Program. 8(3), 231–274 (1987)

Pegaso: A Serious Game to Prevent Obesity

Lucia Pannese[1], Dalia Morosini[1], Petros Lameras[2], Sylvester Arnab[2],
Ian Dunwell[2], and Till Becker[3]

[1] Imaginary srl, Milan, Italy
{lucia.pannese,dalia.morosini}@i-maginary.it
[2] Serious Games Institute, Coventry University, Coventry, United Kingdom
{PLameras,SArnab,Idunwell}@cad.coventry.ac.uk
[3] Bildungsberatung Till Becker & Co. GmbH, Waiblingen, Germany
till.becker@lernkultur-online.de

Abstract. The problem of obesity in the world has grown considerably in recent years. Between 16% and 33% of children and adolescents are obese. Even if obesity is among one of the easiest medical conditions to recognize, it is one of the most difficult to treat. The issue of individuals' motivation to change is the most significant obstacle in promoting positive health behaviours. Games' ability to reach and engage large number of players for long periods of time provides an opportunity for them to be used as a pedagogical tool. This paper describes how serious games and 'gamified' daily life processes appear to be a suitable means for supporting persuasion towards healthful behaviour within the frame of the Pegaso project that aims to develop a multi-dimensional cross-disciplinary ICT system to prevent overweight and obesity in the younger population.

Keywords: serious games, obesity, adolescents, healthy nutrition, game based learning.

1 Introduction

Obesity has become a worldwide public health problem but the most alarming fact arrives from the childhood obesity. In the past 30 years, this has more than doubled in children and tripled in adolescents [1], [2]. Further, childhood obesity is a global phenomenon affecting all socio-economic groups, irrespective of age, sex or ethnicity. Obesity is caused by many factors: genetic, psychological, environmental, socio cultural, lifestyle and person's habits. Usually adolescent obesity is determined by the co-presence of all these factors, or at least by some of them.

In this context, analysing the different roles that food and nutrition have within the adolescents' life can be really interesting [3]. Due to the cultural and social changes, parents today have less time to plan and prepare healthy meals, which results in adolescents opting for more processed and fast foods that are usually less healthy than home-cooked meals. Furthermore, the food sold in supermarkets is processed, high in fats and is containing too much sugar.

Eating habits are also adapted to the different contexts. For instance, in contrast to the communal eating habits within a family context, teenagers' eating habit tends to

V.G. Duffy (Ed.): DHM 2014, LNCS 8529, pp. 427–435, 2014.

be influenced by their social circles. In this case, food has become part of the identity development process, which allows teens to create or reinforce their peer relationships. It is not important what they are eating but with whom they are. In fact, the teenager's environments (family, friend, schools, etc.) reinforce lifestyle habits regarding diet and activity. For example if a parent is overweight and has poor diet and exercise habits, the child is likely to adopt the same habits.

Life style also depends on specific leisure interests, which influence the eating behaviour. For example, junk food is valued differently and is more rarely consumed by fitness-oriented individuals compared to those who spend their free time playing computer games.

Eating habits are also related to the specific gender differences. In general boys are less influenced by the social pressure about the body stereotypes than girls. Especially during adolescence girls exercise and do sports for modelling their figure. They experience their body mainly as a threat, unlike boys, in which the changing fat-muscle ratio meets the body needs [3].

Many girls encounter the natural change processes therefore with restrictive eating behaviours. These reduced-energy diets are sometimes performed as early as elementary school age. With increasing aging the older girls often leave meals (preferably breakfast), relinquish the so-called fattening foods, and other food items.

This happens also because for most of the teens and their parents it is not clear which amount of nutrients is adequate [4]. Another example portrays the trained unhealthy nutrition that has been observed in some families. In general, infants and young children are very good at listening to their bodies' signals of hunger and fullness. They stop eating as soon as their bodies tell them they had enough. But sometimes a parent or grandparents encourages children to finish everything on their plate. This forces them to ignore their fullness and to eat everything that is served to them. The way we eat when we are children may strongly affect our eating behaviours as adults. These habits may affect what we eat, when we eat, and how much we eat.

In conclusion, it is possible to argue that teens' eating habits are an expression of their lifestyle, are used for social positioning and allow teenagers to create their individual and social identity. Most of the time teenagers really don't know what they are eating and they are even not really aware of the consequences of their bad food habits. As adolescences are not easy to manage, especially by parents or other adults, it is really hard to convince and motivate them to change their life style in order to prevent obesity. In fact, the issue of individuals' motivation to change is the most significant obstacle in promoting positive health behaviours. The serious games' ability to reach and engage large number of players for extended periods of time provides an opportunity to motivate teens in terms of understanding the importance of a healthy life-style. As technology evolves to support an increasingly diverse range of complementary demands, various forms of technology-driven intervention have already been integrated into teaching and learning methods, including digital games. In such a context, games must be able to demonstrate effective learning (to be pedagogically-driven) whilst also remaining engaging and entertaining (to be fun driven). The engaging element of game technologies has been proven effective in formal and informal learning experiences in both blended and standalone contexts [5]. Gaming literature states several positive learning outcomes of using games: the development of social skills, cognitive abilities and motivation towards learning, social and emotional development [6], strategic decision making [7], logical and critical thinking [8], problem solving and collaboration [9], as well as communication and team-building skills [10].

This paper describes which characteristics a game should have in order to prevent obesity and overweight in the younger population. In particular, in section 2 the pedagogical role of serious games will be discussed. In section 3, some serious games, developed within the Mirror project, will be presented, as an example of games able to trigger reflection in order to make users more aware about their behavior. Finally, in section 4 the main features that a game should have in order to prevent obesity will be presented and discussed.

2   Serious Games: A New Pedagogical Approach

Over the past few years, with the widespread use of commercial games the domain of game-based learning has received increasing attention. However, until very recently, strategies for supporting the more efficacious methods of learning with games were uncertain. Research has shown that teachers were unsure which games to use, which context to use games and how they could be evaluated and validated.

Learning is mostly a process that leads to a change in behavior or understanding, rather than a quantitative increase in knowledge or storing information that can be reproduced. Learning is about internalization [11], i.e. about making sense or abstracting meaning, about being able to relate parts of the subject matter to each other and to the real world. Several methods and approaches exist to learning (e.g. collaborative, cooperative, contextual, inquiry-based, problem-based etc), each with its strengths and weaknesses, which make it more or less suitable for specific application settings.

Studies that compared traditional learning and game-based learning [12] found significant difference in favor of game-based learning. Studies in the US have also confirmed this finding [13]. Empirical studies reflecting the efficacy of game-based learning providing greater support for developing effective games for learning, and addressing user expectations of high fidelity games and 'immersive experiences' [14].

Some of the main hits of game-based learning include motivation and engagement as well as the ability to provide activity-led approaches to be modelled for individual users and user groups [15]. However, studies have opened up the importance of games as tools for supporting socially based learning, or social interactive learning [13].

The benefits of effective use of game-based learning are considerable, but as studies have shown use is often most effective with particular learners who enjoy learning with games. Therefore the optimal adoption of serious games may need to be considered to learners' specific ways of learning for achieving increase in nutritional knowledge and physical activity as means to prevent obesity.

There is a shift in the use of games to support delivery of formal and informal education. The application of pedagogically-driven digital games often seeks to capitalize on growing trends amongst a wide range of target audiences who engage with digital media recreationally. A frequent question in serious games design is how to best embed pedagogically-driven learning activities and learning content. A common argument is that this content integration must not obstruct the engaging aspects of the game [16], though in areas where the subject matter does not immediately lends itself to an entertainment gaming analogy, this may prove challenging. One solution might be to exploit a blended approach to apply extrinsic motivation on learners to play, though this can be at-odds to the frequently cited benefits of game-based approaches in stimulating intrinsic motivation. Isolating individual pedagogical elements and examining their relationship to game design is an obvious route [17], though one complicated by the reliance of these elements on other factors such as learner demographic, representational medium or learning context. Consolarium, a game-based learning (GBL) initiative of Education Scotland focuses on exploring and disseminating the efficacy of using computer games in terms of their positive impact on teaching and learning. The use of games as a pedagogical tool is also demonstrated by other initiatives such as the Institute of Play's Quest to Learn Middle School in New York, North West Learning Grid's DiDa program in England and Futurelab's Teaching with Games project.

Further, over the past few years there has been an increased use of digital technologies including games to initiate and sustain engagement across the healthcare sector, where the focus on tackling the attitudes and behaviours that may lead to complicated health conditions has seen games deployed to wide audiences [18], [19], [20].

As a tool to engage and educate young people, games such as 'Privates' have been commissioned by UK's Channel 4 TV Company to address sex health issues. Other entities, such as the Parliamentary Education Group, DEFRA and the US government (who held a competition around games for health) are increasingly commissioning games for learning purposes [20]. Some important scientific and empirical studies have also been undertaken towards establishing the scientific validity of a game-based approach. Controlled trials for game-based interventions such as Re-Mission demonstrates effectiveness in the support for medication adherence in children with cancer [21], and PR:EPARe shows positive outcomes in changed attitudes towards the issue of sexual coercion and pressure in adolescence relationships [22]. The issue of individuals' motivation to change is the most significant obstacle in promoting positive health behaviour. Games' ability to reach and engage large number of players for long periods of time provides an opportunity for them to be used as a pedagogical tool. Activities related to healthy living require individuals to embrace delayed satisfaction, where the reward may be as obscure as the prevention of a chronic condition [18]. The use of game mechanics and concepts to facilitate participation in such activity i.e. gamification, will commonly benefit from rewards and incentives to be used to sustain positive engagement. Behavioural change may be initiated by extrinsic sources of motivation, or external factors that influence how we behave [23]. The long-term goal will include nurturing intrinsic motivation and positive habit through sustained engagement, where individuals could discover their personal incentives and rewards for healthy behaviour. An example of a gamification ecosystem includes the Monster Manor gamification programme, which involves parents and clinicians in the 'playful' and 'incentivized' ecosystem. The aim is to encourage children with Type 1 Diabetes to check their blood sugar regularly. The HealthSeeker game promotes a healthy and social community by utilising on competitions and recognition, where peer-driven health challenges are issued through Facebook. Both the use of digital games and the concept of gamification present an opportunity for better understanding of individuals' knowledge, attitude and behaviour and assessment of their progresses, the provision of more personalised feedback and support towards a healthier lifestyle. Gamification as an enabling platform may provide a solution that will promote behavioural transformation towards healthier individuals.

In the next section the Mirror project will be presented. In particular the serious games developed within this project will be described as an example of games able to trigger reflection in order to make users more aware of behavior.

3   Learning by Reflection: An Example from the Mirror Project

As described in the previous section, the primary purpose of most existing IT-based health and daily life support tools is to enable users to generate novel solutions to problems. From a problem solving perspective there is a very limited support for learning per se in immersive and personalized environments. Nevertheless, when a role-play game that encourages users to solve tasks, make decisions and adopt behaviours is carefully designed to enhance reflection, it supports awareness building and learning in the given context.

The topic of 'reflective learning' has been deeply investigated in the Mirror project[1]. 'Mirror-Reflective learning at work' is a FP7 project with the aim of encouraging human resources to reflect on previous experiences at the workplace and learn from them. The focus of the project is the creation of a set of applications ('Mirror apps') that enable employees to learn lessons from their own experiences (as well as from the experiences of others) and thereby improve their future performance. A prerequisite for exploring innovative solutions in this context is the reliance on human ability to efficiently and effectively learn directly from tacit knowledge, without the need for making it explicit. Among all the techniques explored by Mirror, serious games have a special role as they provide virtual experiences to reflect upon. In particular in the Mirror project it has been studied how serious games can support learning by reflection and how support in form of a virtual tutor can be added to a game without breaking the flow. Three different games for three different business sectors (health, social care and emergency) were developed to empower and engage employees to reflect on past work performances and personal learning experiences in order to learn in 'real-time' and to creatively solve pressing problems. In particular, in order to support learning by reflection some specific tools were added into the games:

- in-game notebook functionality (the possibility to take notes during the game allows users to stop the flow of the game for a while and reflect on what they have done in the game until that moment);
- feedback (the possibility to receive a tutor's feedback after each choice of options helps users to better understand how they are performing);

---

[1] www.mirror-project.eu

- scores (the possibility to see their personal scores on the play-screen increases users' awareness that each of their actions has a consequence);
- wizard tool (the possibility to insert own content and experiences in the games allow users to reflect on what they have done in their work until that moment);
- individual reflection session (the possibility to self-evaluate own behavior during the virtual experience and to see all the activities that learners have carried out during the game helps users to reflect and to create a bridge to transfer what they have learnt in the virtual, safe environment into the real world).

Further, within the Mirror project, it has been studied a method to enlarge the gaming environment introducing a Virtual Tutor, starting from the Vygotskian theory[2][24], for supplying tutorial help to make learners more autonomous and confident. In particular some key aspects for the development of a Virtual Tutor inside a game were identified. In order to be able to maximize a users' 'Zone of Proximal Development'[3] a tutor to a peer must be able to:

- act as co-learner;
- provide a cognitive model of competent performance;
- have no position of authority with respect to the learner, because this creates relationship based on trust that facilitates self-disclosure of ignorance and misconception;
- add new capabilities and extend current capabilities (accretion), modify current capabilities (re-tuning), and build new understanding (restructuring in areas of completely new learning or cases of gross misconception or error) [25].

According to this theoretical framework the figure of the Virtual Tutor was designed inside the games to provide the user with:

- additional relevant information on demand;
- frequent, rapid and clear feedback completed by deep final reports showing a clear link between acts and consequences;
- specific help when repetitive errors or patterns are detected by the game system;
- adequate tools to take a step back and collect one's own thoughts.

The various gaming characteristics and supports offered by the Virtual Tutor create favourable conditions so as to allow learners to adopt a reflective attitude towards their own past/present acts and experiences, learning to take place and eventually to maximize the Zone of Proximal Development of the learner.

The games were tested with more than 100 users with different tools (questionnaire, focus group and interview) and the preliminary analysis of this set of evaluations have shown that games were perceived positively, and were evaluated as a useful tool to support learning by reflection.

---

[2] Vygotsky (1978) is one of the main authors of the Socio-Cognitivism theories. According to his perspective learning occurs within a social context, and that interaction between learners and their peers is a necessary part of the learning process.

[3] Vygotsky (1978) describes those capabilities that are beyond the learner on their own, but are able to be carried out with the assistance of more knowledgeable peers, as capabilities in the Zone of Proximal Development (ZPD).

The lessons learned, insights and scientific results derived from the Mirror project will be exploited and applied on the teen-agers target group of Pegaso in the given health scenario to prevent obesity.

4   Conclusions

According to what has been discussed in this paper, obesity is a worldwide public health problem that increasingly affects the younger population. Motivate teenagers to modify their bad food habits in favour of a healthy lifestyle seems to be one of the possible solution in order to prevent overweight and obesity in the younger population. Serious games and 'gamified' daily life processes appear to be a suitable means for supporting persuasion towards healthful behaviour within this frame: however there are some important characteristics that a serious game should have in order to prevent obesity in adolescents.

Although effective in delivering pedagogical contents, serious games in fact offer limited explicit support for adaptation and personalization in daily life motivational processes. One reason for this is the need to encode all of the required behaviours of a game in response to all possible player choices. In simple terms, the capability of a game to respond to nonlinear, non-standard thinking and problem-solving by a player is heavily constrained by what the game designer has predefined. Currently available serious games fail to adapt and evolve in response to dynamic and flexible thinking. Hence, the specification, design and development of the Pegaso game will ensure that these issues will be addressed both individually and collaboratively. In addition, users should be empowered to customize their game, for instance the level of a cognitive challenge, the frequency of a specific activity.

Further, the game's fruition should be essentially conceived as an activity on-the-move, in order to avoid teenagers sitting for hours in front of a PC thus jeopardising the prevention of obesity. With the aim of increasing users' mobility the exploitation of augmented reality as well as 'real virtuality' (i.e. the intervention of a moderator within real life technology-supported gaming scenarios) will be explored. The game should be dynamically aggregated within a virtual highly-interactive and personalised environment, which should offer a very engaging and stimulating daily experience by taking into account both individual needs as well as the promotion of socialization, networking and inclusion, thus in turn contributing to users' motivation to interact with the game.

The game-based environment should be conceived as a reactive tutoring system, enriched through the integration of a smart virtual companion, as a non-playing character is able to support users in their daily life and in the system usage. Therefore, besides being a continuous support in more general non-gaming daily activities, the virtual intelligent companion should also flexibly act and react within the gaming environment according to the users' personal profiles, their behavior and the surrounding context at that moment. The solutions by which awareness is raised, attitudes and behaviours are transformed and positive habits are nurtured should therefore be improved, which could potentially reduce pressure on public health expenditure in the long run.

References

1. Ogden, C.L., Carroll, M.D., Kit, B.K., Flegal, K.M.: Prevalence of Obesity and Trends in Body Mass Index Among US Children and Adolescents. Journal of the American Medical Association 307, 483–490 (2012)
2. National Center for Health Statistics. Health, United States, 2011: With Special Features on Socioeconomic Status and Health. Hyattsville, MD; U.S. Department of Health and Human Services (2012)
3. Bartsch, S.: Jugend isst anders. UGB-Forum 5/2011, S. 214-217, ISSN 0936-1030
4. Reinher, Kersint, van Teeffelen, Widham: Pädiatrische Ernährungsmedizin: Grundlagen und Praktische Anwendung, Stuttgart (2012)
5. Morgan, A., Kennewell, S.: The Role of Play in the Pedagogy of ICT. Education and Information Technologies 10, 177–188 (2005)
6. Hromek, R., Roffey, S.: Promoting Social and Emotional Learning with Games. Simulation & Gaming 40, 626–644 (2009)
7. Linehan, C., Lawson, S., Doughty, S., Kirman, B.: Developing a serious game to evaluate and train group decision making tools. In: 13th Interntional MindTrek Conference: Everyday Life in the Ubiquitous Era, pp. 106–113 (2009)
8. Watson, W.R., Mong, C.J., Harris, C.A.: A Case Study of the In-class Use of a Video Game for Teaching High School History. Computers in Education 56, 466–474 (2011)
9. Sanchez, J., Olivares, R.: Problem solving and collaboration Using Mobile Serious Games. Coputers in Education 57, 1943–1952 (2011)
10. Ellis, J.B., Luther, K., Bessierre, K., Kellogg, W.A.: Games for virtual team building. In: Proceedings of the 7th ACM Conference on Designing Interactive Systems, New York, pp. 295–304 (2008)
11. Nonaka, I.: The Knowledge Creating Company. Harvard Bussines Review (1991)
12. Jarvis, S., de Freitas, S.: Evaluation of an Immersive Learning Programme to support Triage Training. Paper presented at the 1st IEEE International Conference in Games and Virtual Worlds for Serious Applications, Coventry, UK (2009)
13. Mautone, T., Spiker, V., Karp, D.: Using Serious Game Technology to Improve Aircrew Training. Paper Presented at the Interservice/Industry Training, Simulation & Education Conference (I/ITSEC), Orlando, FL (2008)
14. Lameras, P., Petridis, P., Dunwell, I., Hendrix, M., Arnab, S., de Freitas, S., Stewart, C.: A Game-based Approach for Raising Awareness on Sustainability Issues in Public Spaces. Paper presented at the The Spring Servitization Conference: Servitization in the Multi-organisation Enterprise, Aston Business School Birmigham, UK (2013)
15. Lameras, P., Petridis, P., Torrens, P., Dunwell, I., Hendrix, M., Arnab, S. (2014). Training Science Teachers to Design Lesson Plans thtough an Inquiry-Based Serious Game. Paper accepted for Publication at the The Sixth International Conference on Mobile, Hybrid, and Online Learning, Spain, Barcelona (2014)
16. Zyda, M.: From Visual Simulation To Virtual Reality to Games. IEEE Computer 8, 25–32 (2005)
17. Wilson, K., Bedwell, W., Lazzara, E., Salas, E., Burke, C., Estock, J., Orvis, K., Conkey, C.: Relationships Between Game Attributes and Learning Outcomes. Simulation & Gaming 40, 217–266 (2009)
18. Arnab, S.: Hobby to habits. Public Service Review: Health and Social Care (35), 105-105 (2013)
19. Arnab, S., Dunwell, I., Debattista, K.: Serious Games for Healthcare: Applications and Implications, Hershey, PA (2013)

20. Ulicsak, M.: Games in education: Serious games. A Futurelab literature review (2010), http://media.futurelab.org.uk/resources/documents/litreviews/Serious-Games_Review.pdf
21. Kato, P.M., Cole, S.W., et al.: A Video Game Improves Behavioral outcomes in Adolescents and Young Adults With Cancer: A Randomized Trial. Pediatrics 122, 305–317 (2008)
22. Arnab, S., Brown, K., Clarke, S., Dunwell, I., Lim, T., Suttie, N., Louchart, S., Hendrix, M., de Freitas, S.: The Development Approach of a Pedagogically-Driven Serious Game to support Relationship and Sex Education (RSE) within a classroom setting. Computers & Education 69, 15–30 (2013)
23. Seifert, C.M., Chapman, L.S., Hart, J.K., Perez, P.: Enhancing Intrinsic Motivation in Health Promotion and Wellness. Am. J. Health. Prom. (2012)
24. Vygotsky, L.S.: Mind in Society: The Development of Higher Psychological Processes. Harvard University Press, Cambridge (1978)
25. Rumelhart, D.E., Norman, D.A.: Analogical Processes in Learning. In: Anderson, J.R. (ed.) Cognitive skills and their acquisition. Erlbaum, Hillsdale (1981)

Virtual Knee Arthroscopy Using Haptic Devices and Real Surgical Images

Shahzad Rasool[1], Alexei Sourin[1], Vladimir Pestrikov[2], and Fareed Kagda[3]

[1] Nanyang Technological University, Singapore
{shahzadrasool,asourin}@ntu.edu.sg
[2] Moscow Institute of Physics and Technology, Russia
vipestr@gmail.com
[3] Alexandra Hospital, Singapore
fareed_kagda@juronghealth.com.sg

Abstract. Knee arthroscopic surgery is performed on the knee joint by making small incisions on the skin through which an endoscopic camera (arthroscope) is inserted along with miniature surgical instruments. It demands from the surgeons to acquire special motor-skills. A few commercial simulators are available for arthroscopic surgery training however the area is still very open for research and development. In contrast to the common fully-3D way of simulation of knee arthroscopy, we propose a hybrid image-based approach where real arthroscopic videos are converted to panoramic images which are augmented with 3D deformable models of the tissues as well as 3D models of surgical instruments. The motions of the virtual arthroscope and the instruments are controlled by two desktop haptic devices. The hybrid virtual scene is visualized through a moving circular window, which follows the motion of the virtual arthroscope.

Keywords: virtual arthroscopy, haptics, image-based.

1 Introduction

Arthroscopic surgery procedures are performed on joints in a minimally invasive way by making small incisions on the skin through which a miniature endoscopic camera (arthroscope) is inserted along with special surgical instruments. The arthroscope is a wide-angle oblique-viewing camera with view angles of 30°, 70° or 90° and a light source attached to its end. Arthroscopy demands from the surgeons to acquire special motor-skills while learning complex stepwise tasks including positioning (triangulation) of the instrument in front of the surgical camera (arthroscope), examination of the tissues in the surgical area, and using different instruments for cutting away and removing damaged parts of the tissues. The major challenge for the trainee surgeons is that the surgical area is observed as a 2D image on the video monitor which is physically displaced from the remotely controlled instruments. The specifics of the side-looking arthroscope creates further challenges in its manipulation to be able to see the surgical instruments inserted through the incision made a few centimeters

V.G. Duffy (Ed.): DHM 2014, LNCS 8529, pp. 436–447, 2014.

away from the camera incision point. To achieve these skills, the surgeons have to go through special training programs.

Simulation of arthroscopic surgery for training purposes can be done in virtual reality environments using common personal computers and haptic devices. It is very feasible because the surgeons are detached from the actual three-dimensional surgical scene, see it as a two-dimensional image on a video monitor, which can be replaced by a computer monitor, and operate within the scene with remotely controlled instruments, which can be quite realistically simulated with desktop haptic devices.

In this paper we first survey the works related to virtual arthroscopy done with haptic devices and camera models for oblique-viewing endoscopes (Section 2). Then we address the problem of modeling virtual arthroscopic cameras controlled by desktop haptic devices in a hybrid image-based virtual environment (Section 3). We consider /1/ how to simulate the constraint camera motion which is characteristic for minimally invasive surgery, and /2/ how to simulate photorealistic views corresponding to the actual arthroscopic cameras. The paper is concluded in Section 4.

2   Related Work

Haptics-based simulation has become a growing research topic in arthroscopy simulation. Thus, Sherman et al. [1] developed a virtual environment knee arthroscopy training system where a custom-made force feedback device is attached to the mock instruments to provide haptic feedback to the user. Gibson et al. [2] used volumetric object representations and smoothed these models before surface normal calculation to ensure stability of the haptic algorithm presented. Bayona et al. [3] presented a low-cost arthroscopic simulation system where a commercial laparoscopic interface is employed as the surgical instrument for delivering haptic feedback. Mabrey et al. [4] used commercial haptic devices to interact with the underlying volumetric representation of the knee. Pinto et al. [5] presented an orthopedic surgery simulator with a mixed surface and volumetric models were used for calculating the force feedback. Wang et al. [6] proposed a surgical procedure simulation system for training of arthroscopic anterior cruciate ligament reconstruction, where two specially designed force feedback models were used for the haptic rendering of probing and drilling operations. A few commercial simulators for arthroscopic surgery training have been developed. Among them are ArthroS from VirtaMed [7], ArthroSim from TolTech [8], ARTHRO-Mentor from Simbionix [9], and SIMENDO arthroscopy from SIMENDO [10].

A few camera models have been proposed to incorporate oblique-viewing property of endoscopic cameras. Yamaguchi [11] was the first to formulate a camera model and calibration method for such cameras to be used in an augmented reality system. Based on Tsai's camera model, it establishes the extrinsic parameters of the camera as a function of rotation about the arthroscope axis. Calibration is performed by attaching optical markers to the camera and tracking them. Rotation parameters are measured using a rotary encoder. In [12], the calibration was simplified by tracking the arthroscope rod instead of camera head hence reducing the number of parameters to be estimated. However, two additional optical trackers were used in an attempt to eliminate the need for the rotary encoder. Buck et al. [13] generalized Yamaghuchi's method by incorporating the changes to camera intrinsic parameters and a radial distortion component. Optical trackers are used for calibration but the calibration result is slightly less accurate. A real-time method for calibration and removal of radial distortion is proposed in [14], along with a formulation of relative rotation between endoscope axis and camera head. These methods provide calibration procedures for endoscopic camera so that a mapping between the 3D scene and the resulting 2D image can be extracted.

In this paper, we propose modeling of arthroscopic camera in hybrid image-based virtual environments where 3D reconstruction of the anatomical structures is mostly avoided. Instead, real arthroscopic videos are converted to panoramic images which are augmented with 3D deformable models of the tissues as well as 3D models of surgical instruments as in [15]. The location and orientation of the virtual camera are derived from the combined constraint motion of the arthroscope rod. A new formulation of the camera view direction in terms of arthroscope axis rotation is presented with physical simulation of the incision (pivot) point for the arthroscope and the instrument rods.

3   Modeling the Arthroscopic Camera in Hybrid Image-Based Virtual Environment

We propose a hybrid image-based approach for arthroscopy simulation where real arthroscopy images are mostly used for visual and haptic rendering rather than 3D models of the surgical area. At the preprocessing stage, a panoramic image of the entire knee cavity has to be created by stitching some frames of a real arthroscopy video. This image file then is visualized through a moving circular window which follows the motion of the virtual arthroscopic camera (Fig. 1).

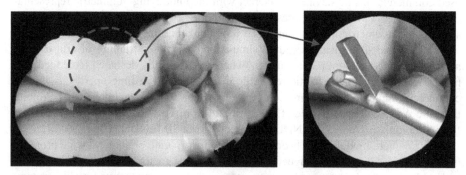

Fig. 1. Panoramic image created by stitching images obtained from the actual surgical video and the hybrid simulated view

The image displayed should correspond to what can be seen for any given location and orientation of the arthroscope. The panoramic backdrop image is then augmented with a few 3D models of deformable tissues as well as models of the surgical instruments which will be seen by the camera. The images displayed on the virtual monitor are then very close to those displayed during the actual surgery.

To haptically render the backdrop image as if it were the actual 3D scene, a depth map is then extracted from the intensity values of its pixels while some noise removal filters are applied to improve the approximation of depth map from pixel intensities, as it was previously reported in [16-17]. This approach can produce believable interaction with much shorter turnout time than that of the full 3D modeling approach provided there is a reliable and quick pipeline for making panoramic images from the surgical videos taken during the operation. A straight-forward but tedious way of doing it is to manually make an image by adding the matching parts from the consecutive images. We have come up, however, with a method allowing for automatic making of panoramic images from the surgical videos. In the rest of this section we will consider the novel issues related to making the panoramic images and the specifics of simulating the arthroscopic camera in this hybrid virtual environment.

3.1   Automatic Generation of Panoramic Images

There are a few software tools commonly used for making panoramic images of streets and nature scenes from video clips, such as, Arcsoft Panorama Maker [18], SoftOptics Panoptica [19], and Microsoft Image Composite Editor [20]. However, they cannot be used in case of the arthroscopic videos since their individual frames are lacking clear feature points [21] which can be compared and used for finding the stitching transformations. To identify such feature points in the individual arthroscopic images, we propose to use the methods based on analysis of the gradient of brightness. However, this gradient is rather low in the arthroscopic images. Hence, we increase the image contrast by using image histogram of brightness. To improve the precision of calculations, we need to first equalize the illumination of the objects. For this task, we used SSR (Single Scale Retinex) algorithm. We then use SURF (Speeded-Up Robust Features) algorithm [22] for extracting feature points from the images, while library FLANN (Fast Library for Approximate Nearest Neighbors) [23] was used for comparing the features. The selection of SURF was based on the surveys done in [24] and [25]. Next we have to find a homographic transformation of source images to match the corresponding singular points belonging to different images. We used RANSAC (RANdom SAmple Consensus) method to find the initial approximation. The computed homographic transformation matrix is further refined with the Levenberg-Marquardt method in order to reduce the re-projection error even more. After this, automatic finding of the matching features becomes more reliable, and individual images can be automatically stitched into the panoramic image. However, while applying this algorithm to individual video frames, we noticed that the central parts of the images stich better than the peripheral parts. This happens due to the fish-eye distortions in the individual images. The distortions can be eliminated from each contributing video frame before they are processed for stitching. This requires taking with the arthroscopic camera a calibration image of the Cartesian grid. Knowing the parameters of the camera and the fish-eye projection transformation, the function mapping the original pixels to non-distorted image can be obtained (Fig. 2).

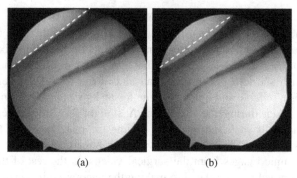

(a)   (b)

Fig. 2. Removal of equisolid fisheye distortions for the images taken with "LINVATEC HD4300 4mm" with the focal length 18.5 mm and the angle of view 30°. (a) A Frame from the actual surgical video (b) The respective corrected frame. Notice the differences at the outlined parts.

The final panoramic image obtained from a short arthroscopic video which was first corrected to eliminate fish-eye distorted and then processed by the proposed algorithm followed by additional blending, as in [26], is shown in Fig. 3.

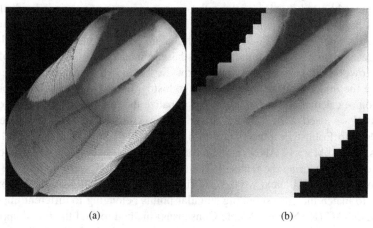

(a)   (b)

Fig. 3. Automatic stitching and blending of the whole arthroscopic video (a) into the panoramic image (b)

3.2   Modeling Arthroscopic Camera and Surgical Instruments

Two desktop haptic devices are used to control the virtual arthroscopic camera and the surgical tools. To constrain their motion as that of the surgical camera and instruments pivoting about the point of insertion into the joint, we modified the haptic devices by extending them with actual surgical tools, as shown in Fig. 4. The handle of each device moves in and out and rotates about its fixed pivot point as in the actual surgery. As a result, the constrained motion of the haptic devices reflects the insertion of the camera and the tool through the incisions on the body of the patient.

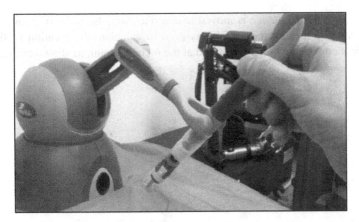

Fig. 4. Geomagic Touch haptic device modified for minimally invasive surgery simulation

The relative positions of the haptic interface point (HIP), the incision point and the virtual camera are shown in Fig. 5.

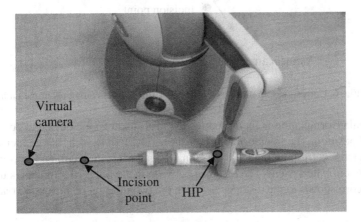

Fig. 5. Location of HIP, virtual camera and incision point on the modified haptic device

First, the virtual camera must be calibrated which refers to the calculation of the incision point coordinates in the device coordinate system. This is implemented by moving the device handle and pressing the primary stylus button at two different handle positions. The HIP position and position of the virtual camera, which is at a specific distance from the HIP defined by the length of the device extension, are recorded at the two instances when the stylus button was pressed. The intersection between the two lines defined by these two pairs of points gives the coordinates of the incision point. Note that the incision point can be located anywhere between the HIP and the virtual camera based on the calibration.

For a fixed distance between the HIP and the incision point, the movement of the HIP is restricted to a virtual spherical surface centered at the incision point. For such motion, the virtual camera traverses along another spherical path, also centered at the incision point. As the device is moved in and out, the radii of the two spherical paths are altered. The location of the HIP is used to calculate the location of the virtual camera in a coordinate system centered at the incision point, as shown in Fig. 6.

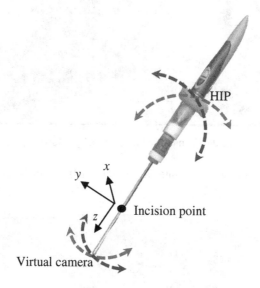

Fig. 6. Corresponding motion of HIP and virtual camera along spherical paths

A similar formulation is then used for the instrument haptic device to compute virtual tool position. The transformation for the virtual tool is such that its incision point and hence the corresponding local coordinate system has its origin on the x-axis of the camera coordinate system. The distance between the two insertion points is user tunable and corresponds to the distance between the two incision points on the real joint.

3.3   Visualization of the Surgical Area

A special method has to be used to model visualization with the oblique-viewing arthroscopic camera. Here, we need to display the relevant part of the existing panoramic image following the motion of the virtual camera controlled by the haptic device mimicking the actual surgical camera. Hence, we have to solve a problem of displaying various parts of the image as if they were seen by the actual surgical camera.

To this end, the position of the virtual camera is mapped onto the image coordinates. Let's first consider the case of a forward looking camera. As mentioned previously, the virtual camera moves along a virtual sphere. Hence, for each position of the camera on the sphere, a pixel P in the image is selected as the center pixel of the camera view. This is done by using the latitude and longitude angles formed by the virtual camera with the local coordinate system defined at calibration. Notice that the inward or outward movement of the camera would not alter the pixel at the center of the view as the latitude and longitude angles are constant for such motion. Any rotation of the arthroscope about its axis is then a rotation of the image about this pixel. However, since the actual arthroscopic cameras are usually oblique-viewing, therefore the selected pixel cannot be used as the center pixel of the view. Instead, a pixel P' at a distance r from P is used as the center of the view. Any rotations of the arthroscope about its axis will then translate into the rotation of pixel P' about pixel P. Thus, the rotation of the arthroscope about its axis results in a set of center pixels that form a circle with radius r on the image. The distance r between pixels P and P' is controlled by the inward or outward movement of the device. Thus, as expected, such motion brings the offset pixel P' closer to P.

In order to validate the motion of the virtual camera, we use a regular grid image and plot the pixels at the center of the camera view for a few frames when the camera device handle is rotated about its axis at different depths of insertion. This is shown in Fig. 7 where the location of these pixels is outlined as the camera device rotates. Figs. 7 (c-d) show the same for a panoramic arthroscopic image stitched together from the frames of the actual surgical video.

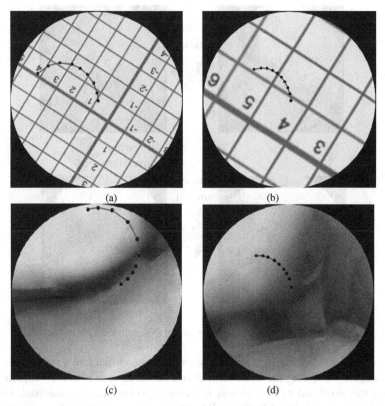

(a)   (b)

(c)   (d)

Fig. 6. Pixels at center of the camera view as the camera device is rotated about its axis at different depths of insertion

3.4   Depth Estimation for Haptic Rendering

To haptically render the backdrop image as if it were the actual 3D scene, the depth
for collision detection is calculated from the image with pixel precision. Since arthroscopic images are frontally illuminated, image intensity has a direct correspondence
to scene depth. However, in order to account for different contributions of various
color components to the grayscale value of each pixel, some colors must be filtered.
This is because certain muscle and tissue parts may have a higher dominance of one
color component as compared to the white bones. We know that the knee cavity does
not usually have green or blue colored areas but rather either have white bones, me-
nisci or cartilage, or have some muscle parts with a dominant red component. The
original RGB image is thus color-filtered to reduce the dominance of red component
and converted to grayscale to use its intensity values as depth map, which is normalized to occupy the entire depth range of the scene. A second filtering pass, for example using a median filter, is applied to remove noise in the extracted depth map as
shown in Fig. 8.

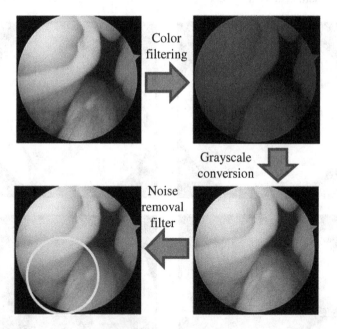

Fig. 7. Extraction of depth information from arthroscopic images

As mentioned in Section 3.2, for each position of the virtual tool a pixel is identified
on the image by mapping the instrument device coordinates to image coordinates. The
depth for this pixel and its 8-neighbors is then used to calculate the feedback force, as
previously proposed in [15-17]. When 3D objects are augmented to the scene for modeling editable tissues in the form of either implicitly defined functions or polygon
meshes, collision detection is performed as with fully 3D scenes. The haptic rendering

algorithm then branches to common 3D force feedback algorithms for force calculation. Various scenes illustrating simulated surgical procedures are shown in Fig. 9.

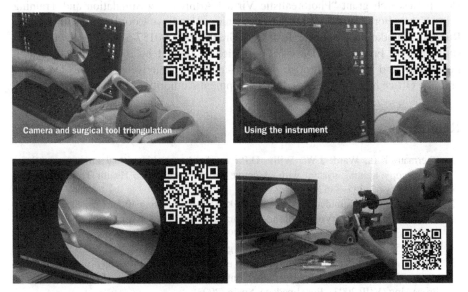

Fig. 8. Various simulations with the QR codes linking to the respective YouTube videos

4   Conclusion

We have presented a way of modeling arthroscopic camera views using haptic devices in hybrid image-based virtual environments. Based on the specifics of the wide-angle oblique-viewing arthroscopic camera, a virtual camera model was presented by formulating the viewing direction as a function of the rotation of the arthroscope axis. Camera position and up vector are two other parameters that define the virtual camera for which physical constraints are proposed to restrict the motion by making extensions of the haptic device. Thus, the haptic device handle mimics the displacements and rotations of the actual surgical camera.

In contrast to the full 3D modeling, in the hybrid image-based virtual environments the problem of simulating views of the virtual camera is rather unusual and more complicated since the challenge is to properly deliver the actual surgical images while navigating the simulated virtual camera. It also involves special methods of making panoramic images from the surgical videos. The challenge in making such panoramas is that common methods and tools cannot be immediately used here since the arthroscopic images are lacking clear feature points needed for automatic image stitching. We therefore proposed our own approach to solve this problem, and it allowed us to achieve very acceptable results that can be used straight away in virtual arthroscopy. The use of a moving hemisphere is proposed to generate undistorted photorealistic views of the surgical area. The proposed approach has been validated by the professional surgeon to be used in the surgical training system.

Acknowledgements. This project is supported by the Singapore MOE Grant "Collaborative Haptic Modeling for Orthopaedic Surgery Training in Cyberspace", Jurong Health Research grant "Photorealistic Virtual Arthroscopy Simulation and Training using Haptic Force Feedback Devices to Achieve Hand-eye Coordination", and by the Russian Foundation for Basic Research Grant 12-07-00157-a. The project is also supported by Fraunhofer IDM@NTU, which is funded by the National Research Foundation and managed through the multi-agency Interactive & Digital Media Programme Office hosted by the Media Development Authority of Singapore.

References

1. Sherman, K.P., Ward, J.W., Wills, D.P., et al.: A portable virtual environment knee arthroscopy training system with objective scoring. Studies in Health Technolgies and Informatics 62, 335–336 (1999)
2. Gibson, S., et al.: Simulating Arthroscopic Knee Surgery using Volumetric Object Representations, Real-Time Volume Rendering and Haptic Feedback. In: Troccaz, J., Grimson, E., Mösges, R. (eds.) CVRMed-MRCAS 1997, CVRMed 1997, and MRCAS 1997. LNCS, vol. 1205, pp. 367–378. Springer, Heidelberg (1997)
3. Bayona, S., Espadero, J., Pastort, L., et al.: A low-cost arthroscopy surgery training system. In: The IASTED International Conference on Visualizatoin, Imaging and Image Processing (VIIP 2003), Benalmadena, Spain (2003)
4. Mabrey, J.D., Gillogly, S.D., Kasser, J.R., et al.: Virtual reality simulation of arthroscopy of the knee. Arthroscopy: The Journal of Arthroscopic & Related Surgery: Official Publication of the Arthroscopy Association of North America and the International Arthroscopy Association 18(6), 28e (2002)
5. Pinto, M.L., Sabater, J.M., Sofrony, J., et al.: Haptic simulator for training of Total Knee Replacement, pp. 221–226.
6. Wang, Y., Xiong, Y., Xu, K., et al.: vKASS: A surgical procedure simulation system for arthroscopic anterior cruciate ligament reconstruction. Computer Animation and Virtual Worlds 24(1), 25–41 (2013)
7. VirtaMed, VirtaMed ArthroS - Virtual Reality training for arthroscopy, VirtaMed AG (2012)
8. TolTech. ToLTech - ArthroSim Arthroscopy Simulator (2013),
   http://www.toltech.net/medical-simulators/products/
   arthrosim-arthroscopy-simulator
9. Simbionix, Arthro Mentor - VR training simulator for knee and shoulder arthroscopic procedures, Simbionix Corporation (2012)
10. Simendo, B.V.: SIMENDO Arthroscopy (May 2011),
    http://www.simendo.eu/products/
11. Yamaguchi, T., et al.: Camera Model and Calibration Procedure for Oblique-Viewing Endoscope. In: Ellis, R.E., Peters, T.M. (eds.) MICCAI 2003. LNCS, vol. 2879, pp. 373–381. Springer, Heidelberg (2003)
12. Chenyu, W., Jaramaz, B.: An easy calibration for oblique-viewing endoscopes. In: Proceedings of the IEEE International Conference on Robotics And Automation, pp. 1424–1429 (2008)

13. De Buck, S., Maes, F., D'Hoore, A., Suetens, P.: Evaluation of a Novel Calibration Technique for Optically Tracked Oblique Laparoscopes. In: Ayache, N., Ourselin, S., Maeder, A. (eds.) MICCAI 2007, Part I. LNCS, vol. 4791, pp. 467–474. Springer, Heidelberg (2007)

14. Melo, R., Barreto, J.P., Falcao, G.: A New Solution for Camera Calibration and Real-Time Image Distortion Correction in Medical Endoscopy Initial Technical Evaluation. IEEE Transactions on Biomedical Engineering 59(3), 634–644 (2012)

15. Rasool, S., Sourin, A.: Image-driven virtual simulation of arthroscopy. The Visual Computer, pp. 1-12 (2012)

16. Rasool, S., Sourin, A., Kagda, F.: Image-driven haptic simulation of arthroscopic surgery. Studies in Health Technology and Informatics 184, 337–343 (2013)

17. Rasool, S., Sourin, A.: Tangible images. In: SIGGRAPH Asia 2011 Sketches, Hong Kong, China (2011)

18. ArcSoft. ArcSoft Panorama Maker, http://www.arcsoft.com/panorama-maker/ (September 26, 2013)

19. SoftOptics. panOptica, http://www.panopticas2.softoptics.co.uk/ (September 26, 2013)

20. Microsoft. Microsoft Research Image Composite Editor (ICE), http://research.microsoft.com/en-us/um/redmond/groups/ivm/ICE/ (September 26, 2013)

21. Brown, M., Lowe, D.G.: Automatic Panoramic Image Stitching using Invariant Features. Int. J. Comput. Vision 74(1), 59–73 (2007)

22. Bay, H., Tuytelaars, T., Van Gool, L.: SURF: Speeded Up Robust Features. In: Leonardis, A., Bischof, H., Pinz, A. (eds.) ECCV 2006, Part I. LNCS, vol. 3951, pp. 404–417. Springer, Heidelberg (2006)

23. Muja, M., Lowe, D.: Fast approximate nearest neighbors with automatic algorithm configuration, pp. 331-340

24. Bauer, J., Sünderhauf, N., Protzel, P.: Comparing Several Implementations of Two Recently Published Feature Detectors. University of Pennsylvania Law Review 154(3), 477 (2006)

25. Juan, L., Gwon, O.: A Comparison of SIFT, PCA-SIFT and SURF. International Journal of Image Processing (IJIP) 3(4), 143–152 (2009)

26. Brown, M., Lowe, D.G.: Automatic Panoramic Image Stitching using Invariant Features. Int. J. of Computer. Vision. 74(1), 59–73 (2007)

Using Ontologies and Semantic Web Technology on a Clinical Pedigree Information System

João Miguel Santos[1], Beatriz Sousa Santos[1,2], and Leonor Teixeira[2,3]

[1] Dep. Electrónica, Telecomunicações e Informática, Universidade de Aveiro, Aveiro, Portugal
[2] Instituto de Engenharia Electrónica e Telemática, Universidade de Aveiro, Aveiro, Portugal
[3] Dep. Economia, Gestão e Engenharia Industrial, Universidade de Aveiro, Aveiro, Portugal
{miguelsantos,bss,lteixeira}@ua.pt

Abstract. Clinical family histories, in the form of clinical pedigrees, are recognized as valuable tools in the diagnostic, risk assessment and treatment of patients and their family members. The lack of adequate tools in present health information systems (HIS) is one of the factors that currently deter practitioners from making full use of these tools. In this paper we present OntoFam, an ontology-based clinical pedigree information system that can be integrated with existing HIS. We focus on the usage of ontologies and semantic web technology in the context of this information system and present a practical scenario of integration with hemo@care, a HIS designed for hemophilia care.

Keywords: ontology-based information system, clinical family history, clinical pedigree, semantic web technology.

1 Introduction

It has long been observed that certain diseases are more prevalent in some families than in others. Since ancient times, medical practitioners have been complementing patient symptoms with their respective family history to better understand disease manifestations [1]. Advances in Genetics have unveiled dozens of medical conditions that are linked to genetic factors, including common illnesses such as diabetes, Alzheimer, schizophrenia and depression, among many others [2-4]. It is therefore becoming increasingly important to record patients' clinical family histories to aid in the diagnostic, risk assessment and treatment of patients and their family members [4, 5]. Risk assessment is particularly important, as the timely detection of at-risk individuals may allow preventive medicine to delay, diminish or avoid illnesses or symptoms [6].

There are several ways to record clinical family histories, in either text form (checklists, forms, descriptive text) or graphic form (genograms, ecomaps, clinical pedigrees) [2, 7]. Clinical pedigrees are a particularly well-accepted tool for recording and presenting clinical family histories, as they are relatively easy to generate and understand – a basic hand-drawn pedigree can be constructed in minutes and, because it is a graphical representation, important information such as disease heredity

V.G. Duffy (Ed.): DHM 2014, LNCS 8529, pp. 448–459, 2014.

patterns, penetrability, mortality and risk can be quickly assessed by observers [1, 2, 8]. Standard symbols and rules are available to graphically represent family structure, patient symptoms, environmental factors, test results, genetic traits and other relevant information on a pedigree, thanks to the efforts of the Pedigree Standardization Work Group (PSWG) [9, 10]. Fig. 1 represents an example clinical pedigree using PSWG notation: circles and squares represent females and males, respectively; spouses are joined at the sides by horizontal lines from which a vertical line may depart, denoting the existence of offspring; in the case of multiple children, siblings are grouped below an horizontal line that connects to their parents' vertical offspring line; filled shapes represent medical conditions and dotted shapes denote carriers; diagonal strokes symbolize deceased individuals and arrows point to individuals that have been studied; roman numerals denote generations, and arabic numerals enumerate and distinguish individuals within a generation.

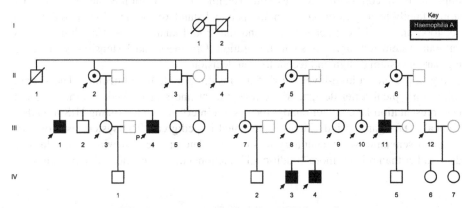

Fig. 1. A clinical pedigree using PSWG notation

Even though the usefulness of clinical pedigrees has been proven in several studies, they are still not as widely used as would be desirable [1, 6, 11]. We believe the reasons for this are twofold: on the one hand, practitioners may not be fully aware of the advantages of keeping clinical family histories of patients; on the other hand, many Healthcare Information Systems (HIS) do not provide adequate tools for keeping family history information or representing clinical pedigrees [3, 4, 11, 12]. Some practitioners solve the latter problem by resorting to external pedigree-drawing tools or generic graphic design software, but this approach results in pedigrees that are "disconnected" of current clinical information and are therefore difficult to keep up-to-date. It appears evident that the use of an information system to effectively manage clinical family histories and pedigrees, and that integrates with existing HIS, will remove many of the hurdles that currently deter practitioners from adopting and taking full advantage of clinical family histories and pedigrees.

In this paper we present OntoFam – an ontology-based information system that facilitates the creation and management of clinical pedigrees and that can be integrated with existing Health Information Systems. This is, to the best of our knowledge, the first open system to use ontologies and semantic data to represent knowledge about clinical family histories and pedigrees.

We begin by describing the design goals and resulting system architecture in section 2. Section 3 focuses on ontologies and semantic web technology, briefly describing the relevant concepts before detailing the chosen ontology and exemplifying the resulting semantic data. The expected benefits of choosing these technologies are also presented. Section 4 summarily describes a practical application of the system and section 5 presents our conclusions and suggestions for future work.

2   Overview of System Architecture

We aimed at designing a system that could be used either in standalone form or, more importantly, in conjunction with existing Healthcare Information Systems (HIS); that stored family history information in an open and standard format which could be understood and used by other systems; and that could adapt to specific clinical areas without system redesign. As such, Integration, Openness and Extensibility played a big part in system design and technological decisions.

Fig. 2 presents a high-level view of the resulting system architecture. The system follows a typical n-tier design, where a central business layer mediates the data and user presentation layers. Optionally, the system interfaces with existing HIS to gather clinical data regarding individuals represented in pedigrees. The system uses ontologies and semantic web technology to store, validate and reason with family history data, rather than rely on more "traditional" relational database-oriented approaches.

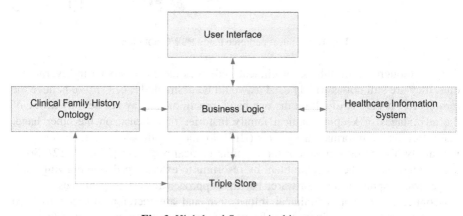

Fig. 2. High-level System Architecture

The **user interface layer** consists of a web application that uses Scalable Vector Graphics (SVG) to represent pedigrees in PSWG notation (refer back to Fig. 1 in section 1 for an example). The Madeline 2.0 Pedigree Drawing Engine [13, 14] is used internally to generate the predigree SVGs, as we have found that this engine produces the most standard-compliant clinical pedigrees, out of several open-source and freeware tools that were considered (Cranefoot, Haplopainter, Hughes RiskApps

Pedigree Module, Kinship package in R, PedHunter, PedigreeQuery, Pelican, and My Family Health Portrait). The pedigree representation is interactive – users can add and remove family members and edit their clinical information – therefore the same graphical representation is used for input and output of information. This contrasts with some pedigree-generation systems that use tables and forms to gather pedigree information and produce a graphical pedigree as a result (for example, the My Family Health Portrait tool [15]). While tables and forms may be sufficient for household consumers and simple family structures, we believe that a more direct "What You See Is What You Get" (WYSIWYG) graphical approach is preferable for practitioners' use and for representing complex families, as seen on professional systems such as Progeny Clinical [16]. We have considered the latter as a reference on the sort of interaction to achieve on our system.

The **business logic layer** coordinates data exchange between the user interface and data layers. It resides on the server-side component of the web application and essentially acts as a translator between the visual and ontological representations of clinical family histories. It uses ontologies to validate and reason with data, ensuring that it is semantically correct and inferring new information from existing data, when possible. The dotNetRDF library [17] is used internally to connect to the triple store and to process semantic data and ontologies.

The **triple store** acts as the data layer of the system. Thanks to the flexibility offered by the dotNetRDF library, many different triple stores can be used to store data, such as AllegroGraph, 4store, Fuseki, Virtuoso, Stardog or any Sesame-based store. Most of these stores are capable of understanding ontologies and can therefore infer information from stored triples, a task that the dotNetRDF library is also capable of. At present, we are experimenting with several triple stores in order to determine the best fit, but this will most likely be a choice delegated to the deployment stage, allowing an organization to choose whichever store is more appropriate for its environment.

The optional **interface to existing Health Information Systems** allows patient data to be gathered and refreshed automatically from the HIS, so that the clinical information on the pedigree is always up-do-date. Internally, the system uses a plug-in architecture to allow communication with different HIS. The task of the plug-in is to translate patient data from HIS to ontological representations. At present, we are utilizing plug-ins that import data in custom HIS formats, but are also working on a plug-in that consumes Health Level Seven International (HL7) standards, namely SECTION 1 Primary standards, which appear to be the most popular for integration and interoperability purposes [18].

3 Usage of Ontologies and Semantic Web Technology

This section focuses on OntoFam's usage of ontologies and semantic web technology. The most relevant concepts are briefly described before presenting the ontology and example semantic data used by the system. The expected benefits of choosing these technologies conclude this section.

3.1   Introduction to Ontologies and Semantic Web Technology

Originally a philosophical term related to the study of reality and existence, in computer science an ontology can be briefly described as the representation of an area of knowledge in a way that machines can understand [19]. Built on World Wide Web Consortium (W3C) standards such as eXtensible Markup Language (XML), Resource Description Framework (RDF) and Web Ontology Language (OWL), among others, ontologies use classes, attributes, relations, restrictions and rules to describe a knowledge domain in a consensual, shared and formal manner [19, 20]. These technologies were initially aimed at building the Semantic Web, Tim Berners-Lee vision of a "web of data" where the World Wide Web would no longer consist of a series of unrelated documents but rather a web of interrelated knowledge usable by humans and computers agents alike [21]. However, semantic web technology found its way into information systems not directly related to the Web, such as the system described in this paper. The BioMedical field appears to be particularly proficient in ontology construction and usage, with applications employing ontologies for knowledge and workflow management, data integration and interoperability, decision support and computer reasoning [22].

3.2   Representation of Semantic Data

As previously mentioned, an ontology defines a set of classes, properties and rules that describe a knowledge domain. Actual semantic data, that is, data that conforms to a certain ontology, is represented in *triples*: statements describing that an entity (subject) has a certain relation (predicate) with another entity (object). The ontology dictates what subjects can relate in what way to what objects. It can also further describe that relation by imposing restrictions and rules.

At the beginning of any ontology-oriented project, a choice must be made whether to build new or reuse existing ontologies. Given that interoperability is one of the goals of ontologies, and indeed of our information system, reuse of existing ontologies, when available, is advisable. A third option is to extend an existing ontology that is a "close fit" by adding the elements that are missing. For example, new classes and properties can be added, or derived from existing entities, to fill gaps and further describe the knowledge domain.

To facilitate share and reuse of ontologies, several repositories exist on the Web, with Unified Medical Language System and BioPortal being two of the largest [23]. Using these tools, we were hoping to find genealogy and clinical ontologies that we could combine to represent clinical family histories. Instead, we have found that work had already been done on an ontology to specifically represent clinical family histories [24, 25], resulting in the Family Health History Ontology (FHHO)[1]. This ontology defines 240 classes and 290 properties that allow representation of family relations and illnesses, including non-biological relations such as adoptive, foster and

---

[1] Available at http://bioportal.bioontology.org/ontologies/FHHO
(accessed 2012-10-30)

emotional. It also includes rules to automatically compute 3 generations of family relations. The ontology has been instance-tested and found adequate for representing most, though not all, of the relevant information for the tested families [26]. Fig. 3 represents FHHO's conceptual model, demonstrating how persons relate to each other and to their health states in this ontology.

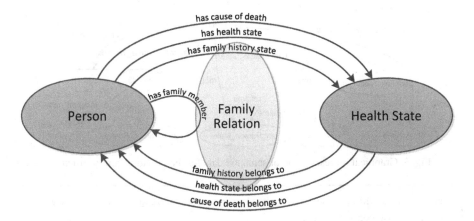

Fig. 3. Family Health History Ontology conceptual model, adapted from [25]

Given that FHHO closely matched the needs of our system, we chose to use it as the foundation for knowledge representation about clinical family histories, extending it where necessary, such as further detailing health conditions, symptoms and health risk behaviors (which we found to be lacking in completeness).

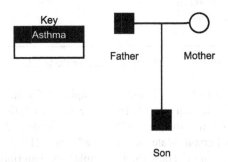

Fig. 4. Clinical pedigree representation of a simple family structure

As an example of what semantic data that follow this ontology looks like, Fig. 4 presents a simple clinical pedigree (3 individuals, two of which suffer from asthma) and Fig. 5 contains a graphical representation of the semantic data involved (simplified for brevity). Directed edges represent predicates, nodes from which edges depart represent subjects and remaining nodes represent objects. Subjects and objects which are instances of classes are represented as ellipses, while simple objects, such as plain strings, are represented as rectangles. Fig. 6 presents the same semantic data in Turtle syntax (a terse alternative to XML-based RDF representation). The "fam:" prefix is used to shorten the full path to classes and properties and the "a" shortcut is used to define that a subject is of a certain type (i.e., is an instance of a certain class). Consecutive triples that refer to the same subject are separated by semi-colons and omit the subject from the second statement onwards.

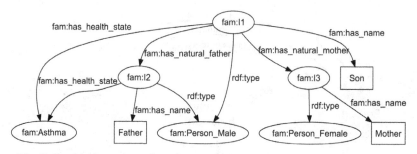

Fig. 5. Graphical representation of semantic data for the previous family structure

```
@prefix fam: <http://www.owl-ontologies.com/Ontology1172270693.owl#>.
fam:I1 a fam:Person_Male;
     fam:has_natural_father fam:I2;
     fam:has_natural_mother fam:I3;
     fam:has_name "Son";
     fam:has_health_state fam:Asthma.
fam:I2 a fam:Person_Male;
     fam:has_health_state fam:Asthma;
     fam:has_name "Father".
fam:I3 a fam:Person_Female;
     fam:has_name "Mother".
```

Fig. 6. Turtle representation of semantic data for the previous family structure

The semantic data from figures 5 and 6 is simplified for brevity. Because of inference and ontology rules, many more triples are used to fully describe this family history. For example, the fact that I1 is a Person_Male implies that it is also a Person, the class from which Person_Male derives. And since I1 has I2 for a father, that implies that I2 is_father_of I1. These inferred triples are materialized and stored in the triple store, in order to allow powerful and flexible queries to be quickly performed.

3.3   Benefits of Using Ontologies and Semantic Web Technology

The decision to design OntoFam around ontologies and semantic web technology, rather than use more traditional approaches such as relational databases, was largely based on a series of benefits that contribute towards our goal of designing an open, extensible and interoperable information system.

Interoperability: XML, RDF, OWL and other semantic web technologies are W3C standards, which means that the clinical family history data generated by our system is inherently interoperable with other systems. Data integration and interoperability are indeed two of the main reasons why ontologies are used in biomedical information systems [22]. Furthermore, because semantic data and ontologies can be represented in plain text format, recorded family histories are relatively safe from obsolescence and will be readable in the future, even if the original software used to create them is no longer available.

Flexibility: Family histories can be quite complex. While a basic ancestor tree can be organized around a simple Person class, with recursive relations for Mother and Father properties, a clinical family tree needs to handle not-so-obvious relations between individuals such as twins, adoption, fostering, interbreeding and interrupted pregnancies, among others. Furthermore, clinical information regarding individuals must also be stored. Rather than depend on relational data tuples, semantic data relies on simple subject-predicate-object triples as units of information. This simplicity offers great flexibility, as any entity characteristic or relation can ultimately be decomposed into triples. This means that complex relations that would imply intricate relational database schemas can be easily represented in a series of related triples.

Extensibility: Existing ontologies can be extended, further describing certain aspects of a knowledge domain. A basic clinical ontology describing high-level diseases and symptoms can be extended to handle more specific information, by branching existing classes into subclasses or by adding new attributes and classes. Unlike relational databases, subclassing or adding properties to an ontology does not break the existing "schema" and does not invalidate existing data [27]. This means that the information system is able to adapt to particular or evolving scenarios with little or no code changes and without raising incompatibilities with existing data.

Computer Reasoning and Inference: Ontologies include relations, restrictions and rules, which can be used to validate input, reason with data and infer new information from existing data. Family structures are a good example of where inference may be helpful, indeed FHHO includes a set of rules that allow the system to automatically infer family relations up to the third generation (for example, the fact that A is mother of B and B is mother of C implies that A is grandmother of C). More importantly, rules can be used to automatic perform risk analysis and detect at-risk individuals.

Queriability: Semantic data can be queried using SPARQL (a recursive acronym for SPARQL Protocol and RDF Query Language). This query language builds on the triple nature of semantic data to allow very flexible queries. Fig. 7 presents an example SPARQL query for obtaining the names of the persons whose great-grandparent have asthma.

```
PREFIX fam:<http://www.owl-ontologies.com/Ontology1172270693.owl>
SELECT ?name
WHERE {
  ?person a fam:Person.
  ?person fam:name ?name.
  ?person fam:has_great_grandparent ?ggp.
  ?ggp fam:has_health_state fam:Asthma.
}
```

Fig. 7. Example SPARQL query to obtain persons whose great-grandparent have asthma

4   Prototype Integration with a Health Information System

Hemo@care is a HIS built specifically for hemophilia care. It was initially deployed at the Hematology Service of Coimbra Hospital Center, in Portugal, and has since been extended to provide a nationwide registry of hemophiliac patients [28, 29].

While hemo@care stores electronic health records (EHR) that contain most of the information pertinent to the treatment and health condition of patients, the system had limited family history capabilities. Fig. 8 presents a clinical family history as presented by hemo@care prior to OntoFam integration. This representation uses background colors to distinguish hemophiliacs (pink) and carriers (blue) from non-carriers (white). Studied individuals are denoted with a red outline, known family members are represented in full color icons which contrast with unknown family members, represented in grayscale. Family members that have EHRs have their family relation written in bold, while those without EHRs are strikethrough.

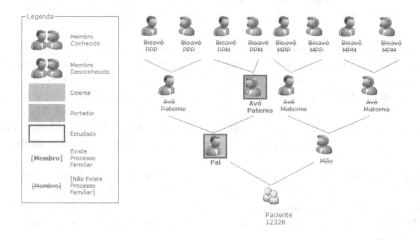

Fig. 8. Hemo@care's representation of a clinical family history (user interface in Portuguese)

The main problem with this representation is that it only includes information regarding ancestors (parents, grandparents and great-grandparents) of patients. Because of this, practitioners that wanted to study the full family history resorted to using external drawing tools to represent clinical pedigrees. As mentioned before, this practice produces "disconnected" pedigrees that are difficult to keep up-to-date.

Seeing as an integrated clinical pedigree information system would benefit users, hemo@care's team welcomed a prototype integration with OntoFam, which is currently being implemented. This involved extending the FHHO to incorporate concepts of hemophilia, as it was limited in that respect. Subclasses of Health_State were created to describe patients with Haemophilia A, B, C and asymptomatic carriers. A specific plug-in was developed to allow OntoFam to acquire patient data from hemo@care. Fig. 1, in section 1, provides an example of a clinical pedigree in PSWG notation applied to the hemophilia field, resulting from the integration of OntoFam and hemo@care. In the process of standardizing the pedigree representation, hemo@care's notation was replaced with the corresponding PSWG symbols, maintaining all relevant information on the pedigree.

Even though the hemo@care ⇔ OntoFam integration is currently at a prototype stage, the preliminary results and user feedback are promising. Practitioners are now able to build and study the complete family histories of patients in context and without resorting to external, disconnected tools.

5   Conclusions and Future Work

Several authors have identified the need for family history-aware Health Information Systems (HIS), yet presently most systems have little or no such capabilities. We believe that an open clinical pedigree information system, which can be integrated with existing HIS, may provide an immediate solution. OntoFam represents our efforts in designing and implementing such a system. We chose to design the system around ontologies and semantic web technology in order to achieve the degrees of Openness, Interoperability and Extensibility that we find necessary for its successful integration with existing HIS.

Though the system is currently at a prototype stage, integration with an existing HIS dedicated to hemophilia care yielded positive and encouraging feedback. In the near future, we expect to finalize the system implementation and begin performance and user acceptance tests to confirm the system's viability and adequacy. In the longer term, we intend to further explore inference and computer reasoning capabilities inherent to semantic web technology in order to enable automatic risk analysis and decision support in OntoFam.

Acknowledgments. This work is funded by National Funds through FCT - Foundation for Science and Technology, in the context of the project PEst-OE/EEI/UI0127/2014.

References

1. Hinton Jr., R.B.: The Family History: Reemergence of an Established Tool. Crit. Care Nurs. Clin. North. Am. 20, 149–158 (2008)
2. Bennett, R.L.: The Practical Guide to the Genetic Family History, 2nd edn. Wiley-Blackwell (2010)
3. Kmiecik, T., Sanders, D.: Integration of Genetic and Familial Data into Electronic Medical Records and Healthcare Processes (2009),
   http://www.surgery.northwestern.edu/docs/KmiecikSandersArtic le.pdf (November 13, 2012)
4. Rich, E.C., Burke, W., Heaton, C.J., Haga, S., Pinsky, L., Short, M.P., Acheson, L.: Reconsidering the Family History in Primary Care. Journal of General Internal Medicine 19, 273–280 (2004)
5. Morales, A., Cowan, J., Dagua, J., Hershberger, R.E.: Family History: An Essential Tool for Cardiovascular Genetic Medicine. Congestive Heart Failure (Greenwich, Conn.) 14, 37–45 (2008)
6. Frezzo, T.M., Rubinstein, W.S., Dunham, D., Ormond, K.E.: The Genetic Family History as a Risk Assessment Tool in Internal Medicine. Genet. Med. 5, 84–91 (2003)
7. American College of Obstetricians and Gynecologists, "Committee Opinion No. 478: Family History as a Risk Assessment Tool," Obstet Gynecol, vol. 117, pp. 747-750 (Mar 2011)
8. Wattendorf, D.J., Hadley, D.W.: Family History: The Three-Generation Pedigree. Am. Fam. Physician 72, 441–448 (2005)
9. Bennett, R.L., Steinhaus, K.A., Uhrich, S.B., O'Sullivan, C.K., Resta, R.G., Lochner-Doyle, D., Markel, D.S., Vincent, V., Hamanishi, J.: Recommendations for Standardized Human Pedigree Nomenclature. J. Genet. Couns. 4, 267–279 (1995)
10. Bennett, R.L., French, K.S., Resta, R.G., Doyle, D.L.: Standardized Human Pedigree Nomenclature: Update and Assessment of the Recommendations of the National Society of Genetic Counselors. J. Genet. Couns. 17, 424–433 (2008)
11. Feero, W.G., Bigley, M.B., Brinner, K.M.: New Standards and Enhanced Utility for Family Health History Information in the Electronic Health Record: An Update from the American Health Information Community's Family Health History Multi-Stakeholder Workgroup. Journal of the American Medical Informatics Association 15, 723–728 (2008)
12. Scheuner, M.T., de Vries, H., Kim, B., Meili, R.C., Olmstead, S.H., Teleki, S.: Are Electronic Health Records Ready for Genomic Medicine? Genet. Med. 11, 510–517 (2009)
13. Trager, E.H., Khanna, R., Marrs, A., Siden, L., Branham, K.E.H., Swaroop, A., Richards, J.E.: Madeline 2. 0 PDE: A new program for local and web-based pedigree drawing. Bioinformatics 23, 1854–1856 (2007)
14. Trager, E.H., Khanna, R., Marrs, A.: Madeline Pedigree Drawing Engine, version 2.0 rev. 99 (2011),
    http://eyegene.ophthy.med.umich.edu/madeline/index.php
15. U.S. Department of Health & Human Services. My Family Health Portrait (2009),
    http://familyhistory.hhs.gov/ (November 11, 2012)
16. Progeny Software, "Progeny Clinical", version 8.0 (2011),
    http://www.progenygenetics.com/clinical/
17. Vesse, R., Zettlemoyer, R.M., Ahmed, K., Moore, G., Pluskiewicz, T.: Dotnetrdf - Semantic Web, RDF and SPARQL Library for C#/.Net, version 1.0.3 (2014),
    http://www.dotnetrdf.org/

18. Health Level Seven International. HL7 Standards - Section 1: Primary Standards (2013), http://www.hl7.org/implement/standards/product_sectioncfm?section=1 (January 09, 2013)
19. Boulos, M.N.K., Roudsari, A.V., Carson, E.R.: Towards a semantic medical Web: Health-CyberMap's tool for building an RDF metadata base of health information resources based on the Qualified Dublin Core Metadata Set. Medical Science Monitor: International Medical Journal of Experimental and Clinical Research 8, MT124 (2002)
20. Antoniou, G., Van Harmelen, F.: A semantic web primer. MIT Press (2004)
21. Berners-Lee, T., Hendler, J., Lassila, O.: The Semantic Web. A new form of Web content that is meaningful to computers will unleash a revolution of new possibilities. Scientific American 284, 1–5 (2001)
22. Bodenreider, O.: Biomedical ontologies in action: Role in knowledge management, data integration and decision support. Yearb. Med. Inform. 47, 67–79 (2008)
23. Fung, K.W., Bodenreider, O.: Knowledge representation and ontologies. In: Richesson, R.L., Andrews, J.E. (eds.) Clinical Research Informatics, pp. 255–275. Springer, Heidelberg (2012)
24. Peace, J., Brennan, P.F.: Ontological representation of family and family history. AMIA Annu. Symp. Proc. 1072 (2007)
25. Peace, J., Brennan, P.F.: Formalizing nursing knowledge: from theories and models to ontologies. Stud. Health Technol. Inform. 146, 347–351 (2009)
26. Peace, J., Brennan, P.F.: Instance testing of the family history ontology. AMIA Annu. Symp. Proc., 1088 (2008)
27. Segaran, T., Evans, C., Taylor, J.: Programming the semantic web. O'Reilly Media, Incorporated (2009)
28. Teixeira, L., Ferreira, C., Santos, B.S.: User-centered requirements engineering in health information systems: A study in the hemophilia field. Computer Methods and Programs in Biomedicine 106, 160–174 (2012)
29. Teixeira, L., Ferreira, C., Santos, B.S., Saavedra, V.: Web-enabled registry of inherited bleeding disorders in Portugal: Conditions and perception of the patients. Haemophilia 18, 56–62 (2012)

Formalizing the Glucose Homeostasis Mechanism

Neeraj Kumar Singh, Hao Wang, Mark Lawford,
Thomas S.E. Maibaum, and Alan Wassyng

McMaster Centre for Software Certification, McMaster University
Hamilton, Ontario, Canada
{singhn10,wanghao,lawford,wassyng}@mcmaster.ca, tom@maibaum.org

Abstract. The failure of hardware or software in the medical domain can lead to injuries and loss of life. Design errors are a major source of the defects that are introduced during the system development process. Traditional validation and verification techniques such as simulation and testing are effective methods for detecting these defects, but are seriously limited in that they cannot guarantee to find all existing defects. Formal methods provide a complementary alternative to testing and simulation, and, although we do not yet have a 'theory of coverage' when combining formal validation and verification techniques with testing and simulation, the combination provides better coverage than any one of them on its own. The insulin infusion pump (IIP) is a critical system that is used by millions of people around the world. IIP failures are responsible for a large number of serious illnesses and deaths. This paper presents the formalization of the glucose homeostasis mechanism that provides an environmental model for the IIP. We can then use this model to validate the appropriateness and correctness of system behaviours at an early stage of development.

Keywords: Homeostasis, Diabetes, Event-B, Formal methods, Proof-based development, Refinement.

1 Introduction

Glucose is the main source of energy for humans, and the glucose-insulin regulatory system maintains an appropriate blood plasma glucose concentration level within the body. The *glucose homeostasis* (GH) system has to maintain a very narrow range of plasma glucose concentration in the blood. The normal range of glucose concentration for most humans after fasting is 70-100 mg/dL. Levels lower than 70 mg/dL are likely to cause a state of hypoglycemia, which is life threatening. Levels higher than 100 mg/dL cause hyperglycemia, and chronic elevated hyperglycemia would normally be diagnosed as *diabetes*. Several diabetic diseases occur when the GH system is not able to maintain the glucose concentration in the blood within the normal range [1–3].

The *Insulin Infusion Pump* (IIP) is an advanced medical device that is designed to maintain normal levels of glucose for people diagnosed with diabetes or some other failure of the GH system. The IIP is a small computerized system that delivers insulin in order to maintain an appropriate level of glucose. Over the past few years, IIPs have been used more and more to control diabetes. However, over these years, the failure rate of the IIP due to malfunctions also has increased tremendously. The failure of the IIP

V.G. Duffy (Ed.): DHM 2014, LNCS 8529, pp. 460–471, 2014.

is responsible for a large number of serious illnesses and deaths. For instance, during 2006-2009, 17,000 adverse-events were reported by the U.S. Food and Drug Administration (FDA), including 41 deaths due to malfunctioning of an IIP [4]. FDA officials have found that many deaths and illnesses related to the devices are caused by product design and engineering flaws, and these are considered to be firmware (software) problems [5, 6].

Since software plays such an important role in the medical domain, certification standards and regulators like the FDA, need to make sure that the developed health care systems or related devices are safe and reliable [7, 6, 8]. Regulatory agencies have been striving for a rigorous engineering-based review strategy that could provide this assurance. Many people believe that formal techniques have the potential to provide us with the assurance we need in developing and certifying safe and dependable medical systems. Formal techniques have been successfully used in several applications of health systems and medical devices [9–11, 8]. However, we caution that formal techniques need to be much better targeted at practical software development and certification than they seem to be at present [12].

1.1 Motivation

Biological environment modelling, used for simulating/testing the functional behaviour of devices or drugs, is an extremely challenging problem. There are several clinical models [3] based on complex mathematical equations, that require high computation and a large memory to simulate the expected behaviour. There is a lack of simulation of biological environment, which can be used at an early stage of the system development during system design and development. For example, an IIP requires an interactive glucose homeostasis environment to verify the correctness of system behaviour (see Fig. 1). Medical devices are tightly coupled with the biological environment in which they are designed to work. They use actuators and sensors to respond to abnormal behaviours in the biological environment, and we can observe the resulting behaviour in the biological environment (by observing the behaviour of the model) to ensure that the system behaves correctly under the required conditions.This approach is clearly dependent on the fidelity of the model of the biological environment. If the model is accurate, this approach can help to provide us with assurance that the behaviour of the device is safe within that environment, and will effectively achieve its purpose.

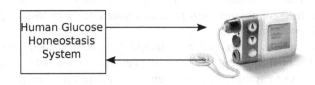

Fig. 1. Interaction between IIP and Human Glucose Homeostasis System

To model a biological environment (the GH) for an IIP, we propose a method for modelling a mathematical GH model based on simple logic. This environment model is based on continued monitoring of the glucose-insulin regulatory system [1]. We believe that for our purpose, we can model the GH system under normal and diabetic conditions, by using α-cells and β-cells, and rising or dropping plasma glucose level to model pancreatic behaviour, and blood test levels for diagnosis of diabetes/prediabetes. This model is developed through an incremental refinement, which helps to introduce several properties in an incremental way and to verify the correctness of the glucose homeostasis model. The key feature of this model is that it exhibits all possible normal or abnormal (hyperglycemia or hypoglycemia) conditions, which characterize a patient model. The environment model also demonstrates the failure of the GH system. There are several motivations behind this approach, which are given as follows:

1. The use of simple logic to understand the complex behaviour of the GH system.
2. Formalization of the GH system to provide a biological environment for verification and validation.
3. Verification and validation of the required behaviour of an IIP under a patient model using closed-loop modelling.
4. To analyze the interaction between the biological homeostasis model and an IIP, and use this to obtain the necessary certification for the IIP.

The mathematical GH model based on standard logic is verified through the Rodin [13] proof tool and model checker ProB [14].

2   Related Work

Clinical models are used for identifying and predicting the various stages of diseases like diagnostics, control, progression, complication etc. Bolie et al. [2] presented the first mathematical model based on differential equations to model the glucose and insulin concentration, illustrating the dynamics of insulin-glucose for diagnostic purpose and evaluating several parameters of the diabetic and pre-diabetic conditions. Silber et al. [15] proposed an integrated insulin-glucose model for analyzing the diabetic condition using a bidirectional insulin-glucose feedback mechanism. Chay et al. [16] proposed the theoretical treatment of the effect of external potassium on oscillations in the pancreatic β-cells, which can be used to demonstrate that insulin infusion may be useful for mimicking pancreatic insulin secretion. Several other models have been developed that incorporate different physiological processes associated with insulin-glucose dynamics and different variations [3, 17–19].

The literature suggests that existing models, with their mathematical constraints and higher order differential equations, are not easy to express in first order logic, and thus make it difficult to express the system requirements for verification purpose. However, we were motivated and encouraged by our previous work on heart modelling [10] that presents an abstract notion of complex heart behaviours. We have adopted the same methodology to design an efficient and optimum environment model for the GH system using formal techniques. To our knowledge, there does not exist any environment model for homeostasis system based on formal methods that can be used for validation/verification at the early stage of system development. Our approach is based on formal techniques for modelling the GH system through analysis of the glucose regulation mechanism. In this article, we propose a methodology to develop an environment model for the GH system, based on *logico-mathematical* theory enabling the validation/verification of system requirements [10]. The model is developed using an incremental refinement approach that helps to introduce several properties in a progressive way, and to verify the correctness of the GH model under normal and abnormal behaviours (hyperglycemia, hypoglycemia or diabetic complications).

3   The Glucose Homeostasis System

Glucose is the major metabolic fuel of the human body. To maintain an appropriate level of glucose in the body and to provide normal functionality, we need a regular supply of glucose to the body. Failure of the glucose level causes several diseases such as diabetes mellitus, galactosemia and glycogen storage diseases [3].

Fig. 2 depicts the normal GH system[1], which presents the structural flow of the hormones and a functional behavioural pattern of the different organs. It is vital for the body to maintain an appropriate glucose concentration, so both low and high glucose levels are serious, life-threatening problems. The body regulates its glucose concentration using the pancreas and liver. The pancreas produces two main hormones *insulin* and *glucagon* to control the GH system. The body cells use the available glucose whenever the body receives glucose from the infusion or hepatic function. There are two different type of cells that use the glucose. For instance, the brain and nervous system cells use glucose without insulin, while other type of cells like muscle and fat use glucose with the help of insulin. The glucose concentration level fluctuates in the body, and is maintained in the plasma through the pancreatic secretion of glucagon and insulin. In general, the body attempts to maintain an appropriate level of glucose in the body, but there are some natural stable oscillations that occur in the glucose and insulin concentrations [1].

Low and high glucose levels are the two main biological responses that the body uses to maintain an appropriate plasma glucose concentration. When the glucose level drops, then the α-cells in the pancreas produce glucagon, which is transformed into glucose with the help of the liver. This process helps to increase the glucose concentration in the body. Similarly, when the plasma glucose level goes higher than expected, then the β-cells in the pancreas are stimulated to lower the glucose concentration [3]. This stimulation process can be completed within 5 to 15 minutes, and during this period the insulin is produced by β-cells of the pancreas. The secreted insulin can be used by insulin dependent cells to utilize the available glucose, and to stop the natural hepatic glucose production for reducing the glucose concentration in the blood. The liver is the central organ for regulation of glucose and glycogen and behaves as a distributor of nutrients through blood to other tissues. The presence of insulin inhibits the transformation of glucagon to glucose.

---

[1] The 'normal GH system' is when the GH system functions as it should, i.e., there are no abnormal behaviours exhibited by the system.

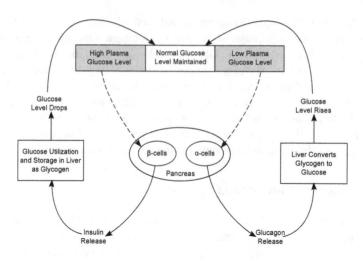

Fig. 2. The GH System (adopted from [3])

4   Proposed Idea

Our proposed method describes a GH model based on logico-mathematics to help the formal community verify the correctness of IIP models. The GH model is mainly based on the glucose regulation system of the body. This method uses advance capabilities of the combined approach of formal verification and behavior simulation, in order to achieve considerable advantages for GH system modelling. Fig. 2 shows the main components of the GH system. The system comprises different states of the glucose level in the blood and biological organs, in order to control the glucose level. To formalize the GH system, we consider eight significant landmark nodes (*Hi, No, Lo, Ac, Bc, Li, St, Tr*) in the homeostasis functional network as shown in Fig. 3, which can control the GH system. We have identified these landmarks through a literature survey [3, 1, 2, 15], and use them to express an abstract functionality of the system. We introduce the necessary elements to formally define the GH systems as follows:

Definition 1 (The GH System). *Given a set of nodes N, a transition T, is a pair (i, j), with $i, j \in N$. A transition is denoted by $i \rightsquigarrow j$. The GH system is a tuple GHS = (N, T, N_0) where:*
- *$N = \{$ Hi, No, Lo, Ac, Bc, Li, St, Tr $\}$ is a finite set of landmark nodes in the GH network;*
- *$T \subseteq N \times N = \{Hi \mapsto Bc, Lo \mapsto Ac, Bc \mapsto Li, Ac \mapsto Li, Li \mapsto St, Li \mapsto Tr, St \mapsto No, Tr \mapsto No, St \mapsto Hi, Tr \mapsto Lo, Tr \mapsto Hi$, is a set of transitions to present data flow between two landmark nodes. It should be noted that the last three transitions are possible when we consider the case of failure of the GH system;*
- *$N_0 = No$ is the initial landmark node (normal glucose level);*

The automata shows the flow of the GH system, where by default the GH system is considered to be in its normal state (*No*). The normal state indicates that there is

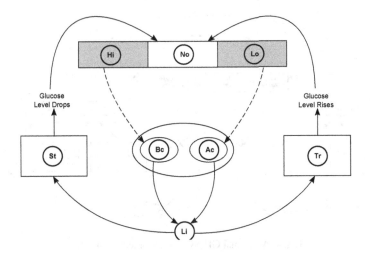

Fig. 3. The GH Automata

an appropriate glucose level in the blood. Whenever the glucose level fluctuates in the blood, resulting in a high or low glucose level, the GH system controls the fluctuated glucose level with the help of the pancreas and liver. The high and low states are presented by Hi and Lo nodes (see Fig. 3). The pancreas has two type of cells: α-cells and β-cells, which are indicated by the Ac and Bc nodes, respectively. The liver is denoted by the Li node that is used to convert the glycogen to glucose using glucagon, and to store the glucose as glycogen in the liver with the help of insulin. If the liver is well behaved, then the glucose level either rises or drops according to whether there is a low or high glucose level in the blood, respectively. Eventually, the glucose level returns to an appropriate level.

4.1   Diabetes or Abnormal Homeostasis System

Fig. 4 presents abnormal behaviours of the GH system. The liver plays a central and crucial role for regulating the glucose level in the blood. The main task of the liver is the continual supply of required glucose energy sources to the body. Failure of the GH system causes several diseases, and in particular, diabetes. There are two type of diabetes: *insulin-dependent diabetes* (also know as *type 1 diabetes*) and *non insulin-dependent diabetes* (also know as *type 2 diabetes*). Insulin-dependent diabetes may be caused by insufficient or no insulin secreted due to β-cells defects. In non insulin-dependent diabetes, insulin is produced, but the insulin receptors in the target cells do not work due to insulin resistance in the cells, so the insulin has no effect. In both cases there can be a very high glucose level in the blood. Low glucose level can be caused by α-cell defects or abnormal glucagon release, which can be further classified as insufficient or no glucagon secretion, excess insulin, and excess glucagon secretion. Excess glucagon secretion and defects in β-cells may also indicate a persistent high glucose level, which can be classified as hyperglycemia-induced diabetes complications [3].

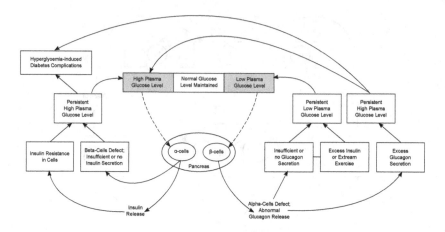

Fig. 4. Abnormal GH System (adopted from [3])

4.2 Blood Sugar Concentration

The blood sugar concentration or blood glucose level is an amount of glucose (sugar) present in the blood of the body. The body naturally regulates blood glucose levels as a part of metabolic homeostasis. The glucose level fluctuates many times in a day. In general, the glucose level is always low in the morning, and it can rise for about an hour after having a meal. There are two types of tests used to detect abnormal behaviours: FPG (Fasting Plasma Glucose) Test and the OGTT (Oral Glucose Tolerance Test) [20]. The FPG test is used to detect diabetes and prediabetes. The FPG test measures blood glucose in a person who has fasted for at least 8 hours and is most reliable when given in the morning. The OGTT can be used to diagnose diabetes, prediabetes, and gestational diabetes. This test is applied when a person has fasted for at least 8 hours and 2 hours after the person drinks a liquid containing 75 grams of glucose dissolved in water. The normal glucose level should be within the range of 70 mg/dL to 99 mg/dL for a non-diabetic person using the FPG test, while the glucose level should be within the range of 70 mg/dL to 139 mg/dL for a non-diabetic person using the OGTT [20]. In the case of low glucose level, for both FPG and OGTT tests the glucose level should be within the range of 0 mg/dL to 70 mg/dL. Similarly, for a high glucose level, readings should be greater than 126 mg/dL in the FPG test, and greater than 140 mg/dL using the OGTT. A blood sugar level outside of the normal range indicates an abnormal glucose concentration. A high level of glucose is referred to as hyperglycemia and a low level of glucose is referred to as hypoglycemia.

Property 1 (Blood Glucose Level). *The blood glucose level defines different stages, such as hyperglycemia, hypoglycemia and normal. We say that the glucose level is low (hypoglycemia) if $FPG \in 0 .. 69$ or $OGTT \in 0 .. 69$, and the glucose level is high (hyperglycemia) if $FPG \geq 126$ or $OGTT \geq 200$, and the glucose level is normal if $FPG \in 70 .. 99$ or $OGTT \in 70 .. 139$. We classify prediabetes to be the range where $FPG \in 100 .. 125$ or $OGTT \in 140 .. 199$.*

5   Formalization of the GH System

To develop a biological environment of the GH system based on formal techniques, we use the Event-B modelling language [21] that supports an incremental refinement to design a complete system in several layers, from an abstract to a concrete specification. Firstly, the initial model captures the basic behaviour and biological requirements of the GH system in an abstract way. Then subsequent refinements are used to formalize the concrete behaviour for the resulting GH biological environment that covers normal and abnormal behaviours (hyperglycemia, hypoglycemia or diabetic complications).

5.1   The Context and Abstract Model

To model a biological environment for diabetes, we choose the standard GH mechanism. An abstract behaviour of the GH system is depicted in Fig 5. This figure shows an automata that models the changing state of the glucose in the body. When the glucose level is normal then it can either stay in the same state or can switch to any other state (high or low). If the glucose level is in either the high or low state, it will stay in the same state or it will switch back to the normal state. To model the GH system, we identify necessary biological behaviour under various glucose levels. In the context of the initial model, we define two enumerated sets *Glucose_level* to indicate the different type of glucose levels in the body using *Normal*, *High* and *Low*, and *GHS* to indicate the glucose level status using *OK* and *KO*. *OK* presents the normal glucose level, while *KO* presents an abnormal level of the glucose in the body.

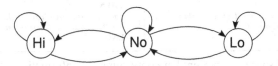

Fig. 5. Automata of an Abstract Model

$$axm1 : Glucose\_level, \{Normal\}, \{High\}, \{Low\})$$
$$axm2 : partition(GHS, \{OK\}, \{KO\})$$

An abstract model is used to indicate the normal or abnormal condition through observing the glucose level in the body. The machine model formalizes the dynamic behavior of the GH system. To define the dynamic properties, we introduce two variables *Current_Glucose_Level* and *Diabetic_Condition*. The variable *Current_Glucose_Level* represents the current state of the glucose level in the body, and the other variable *Diabetic_Condition* represents diabetic conditions *OK* or *KO*. A list of interesting safety properties is given in invariants (*inv3-inv4*). Invariant (*inv3*) expresses that the current glucose level is either high or low if and only if the diabetic condition is *KO*. The last safety property states that the current glucose level is normal if and only if the diabetic condition is *OK*.

$$
\begin{aligned}
&inv1: Current\_Glucose_Level \in Glucose\_level \\
&inv2: Diabetic\_Condition \in GHS \\
&inv3: Diabetic\_Condition = KO \Leftrightarrow \\
&\qquad Current\_Glucose\_Level = High \lor Current\_Glucose\_Level = Low \\
&inv4: Current\_Glucose\_Level = Normal \Leftrightarrow Diabetic\_Condition = OK
\end{aligned}
$$

In this abstract model, we introduce three events *Normal_Glucose* to present a normal state of the GH system, *High_Glucose* to indicate a high glucose level, and *Low_Glucose* to show a low glucose level.

The event *Normal_Glucose* specifies a set of required conditions for the GH system to be in the normal state. The guard of this event shows that the current glucose level can be in any state (Normal, High or Low). The action of this event assigns the current GH state to Normal, and the diabetic condition is set to OK.

```
EVENT Normal_Glucose
  WHEN
    grd1 : Current_Glucose_Level = Normal∨
           Current_Glucose_Level = Low∨
           Current_Glucose_Level = High
  THEN
    act1 : Current_Glucose_Level := Normal
    act2 : Diabetic_Condition := OK
  END
```

The next event *High_Glucose* is used to set the current glucose level to High, and the diabetic condition to KO, when the current glucose level is normal or high. Similarly, the last event *Low_Glucose* is also used to set the current glucose level to Low, and the diabetic condition to KO, when the current glucose level is normal or low. All these events behave similar to the given abstract level automata (see Fig. 5).

```
EVENT High_Glucose
  WHEN
    grd1 : Current_Glucose_Level = Normal∨
           Current_Glucose_Level = High
  THEN
    act1 : Current_Glucose_Level := High
    act2 : Diabetic_Condition := KO
  END
```

```
EVENT Low_Glucose
  WHEN
    grd1 : Current_Glucose_Level = Normal∨
           Current_Glucose_Level = Low
  THEN
    act1 : Current_Glucose_Level := Low
    act2 : Diabetic_Condition := KO
  END
```

Due to limited space, we present here only summary information about each refinement of the homeostasis mechanism, and omit detailed formalization and proof details. The following outline is given about every refinement level to understand the basic formal notion of the GH model.

First Refinement (Introduction of α-cells and β-cells of the Pancreas). The pancreas is a gland organ that is a part of the digestive system, which produces enzymes and hormones for food processing. The α-cells, and β-cells are generated by the pancreas. The α-cells produce glucose and the β-cells produce insulin that is secreted into the bloodstream in order to regulate the glucose or sugar level of the body. This refinement step introduces the α-cells and β-cells and their release functions to enrich the GH mechanism, and to identify the normal or diabetic conditions corresponding to the releasing functions of the α and β-cells. Moreover, this refinement level specifies the behaviour required to maintain the normal glucose level in order to release the required level of insulin by β-cells, and glucagon by α-cells in situations in which the glucose level is fluctuating, formalizing high and low glucose levels when the diabetic condition is abnormal, and the behaviour of the α-cells and β-cells is abnormal.

Second Refinement (To convert or to store glucose by the Liver). This refinement introduces the liver functionalities to regulate the glucose level in the body. The glucose is used by muscle and other cells, and an excessive amount of glucose is stored by liver as glycogen. Whenever the glucose level drops, the liver converts stored glycogen into glucose and releases it. The biological process of converting glucose into glycogen and converting it back from glycogen into glucose helps to maintain the appropriate glucose level. In this level of refinement, we formalize the liver functions for storing and converting glucose, including abnormal behaviour of the liver to address the variation in the glucose levels.

Third Refinement (Abnormal Condition of the Pancreas, Diabetic Conditions, and Diabetes Complications). This refinement formalizes the abnormal conditions of the pancreas, persistent low or high glucose level, and hyperglycemia-induced diabetes complications. All these abnormal conditions are captured to formalize required behaviour of the GH mechanism.

Fourth Refinement (Blood Sugar Concentration for Assessing Diabetes and Prediabetes). The final refinement introduces the process for assessing the blood sugar concentration or blood glucose level in the blood, thus determining the actual amount of glucose. The body naturally regulates blood glucose levels as part of the metabolic homeostasis. As we saw earlier, there are two types of tests: FPG and OGTT. To formalize the assessment of blood glucose concentration, we introduced the relevant mathematical properties (see Property 1). Assessment of glucose concentration using standard testing techniques FPG and OGTT is included in the formalization process for modelling the GH system.

5.2 Model Validation and Analysis

This section presents validation of the developed model through animation, using a model checker tool ProB [14], and the generated proof obligations. Validation, in this context, is a process that shows consistency between formal models and requirements. This tool enables us to validate the GH model according to the glucose fluctuation in the body. We have validated different kinds of scenarios of normal and abnormal glucose levels. In order to test the abnormal behaviour of the GH system, we have also validated the diabetics, prediabetics, and diabetics complication conditions. The ProB tool is not only used for animation, but it also verifies an absence of error, for example (no counter example exists) and no deadlocks at each level of developed model from abstraction to the final concrete model.

Table 1. Proof Statistics

Model	Total number of POs	Automatic Proof	Interactive Proof
Abstract Model	16	16(100%)	0(0%)
First Refinement	13	6(46%)	7(54%)
Second Refinement	7	6(86%)	1(14%)
Third Refinement	25	24(96%)	1(4%)
Fourth Refinement	62	60(97%)	2(3%)
Total	123	112(91%)	11(9%)

Table 1 shows the proof statistics of the development in the RODIN tool. In order to guarantee the correctness of the system behaviour, we established various invariants in the incremental refinements. This development results in 123(100%) proof obligations, in which 112(91%) are proved automatically, and the remaining 11(9%) are proved interactively using the Rodin prover. These proofs are quite simple, and can be achieved with the help of simplifying predicates. An incremental refinement of the GH system helps to achieve a high degree of automatic proof.

6   Conclusion and Future Challenges

There are several existing clinical models that are too complex to use for verification purpose. The existing models use differential equations and higher order polynomial equations, which require significant computation and a large memory to simulate the expected behaviour of the clinical models. However, in our approach, the GH model is presented in an abstract way to simulate the desired behaviour to avoid the mathematical complexity.

This paper presents a methodology for modelling a biological environment of the GH using simple logical mathematics. This is the first computational model based on logical concepts to simulate the GH behaviour in order to analyze the normal and diabetic conditions. The developed model highlights a different aspect of the problem, making different assumptions and establishing different properties concerning the variation in glucose levels, normal and diabetic conditions, and malfunction of biological organs like the liver and pancreas. This is a promising simulated biological environment model that can be used to develop a closed-loop model of the biological environment and IIP. Formalizing the GH system, we used the Event-B modelling language to develop the proof-based formal model in several layers of refinements. Incremental refinement based development allows us to achieve a high degree of automatic proof using the Rodin tool. Our incremental development reflect not only many facets of the problem, but also that there is a learning process involved in understanding the problem and its ultimate possible solutions.

Our most important goal is that this formal model helps to obtain certification for the medical devices related to the homeostasis system, such as IIP. This environment model can also be used as a diagnostic tool to diagnose or understand patient requirements. This has been the first attempt to our knowledge in GH modelling based on logico-mathematical theory. In the future, our goal will be to integrate IIP and the GH system to model the closed-loop system for verifying the desired behaviour under relevant safety properties, and guarantee the correctness of the functional behaviour of IIP.

References

1. Li, J., Kuang, Y., Mason, C.C.: Modeling the glucoseinsulin regulatory system and ultradian insulin secretory oscillations with two explicit time delays. Journal of Theoretical Biology 242(3), 722–735 (2006)
2. Bolie, V.W.: Coefficients of normal blood glucose regulation. Journal of Applied Physiology 16(5), 783–788 (1961)

3. Ajmera, I., Swat, M., Laibe, C., Novère, N.L., Chelliah, V.: The impact of mathematical modeling on the understanding of diabetes and related complications. CPT: Pharmacometrics & Systems Pharmacology 2, e54 (2013)
4. Chen, Y., Lawford, M., Wang, H., Wassyng, A.: Insulin pump software certification. In: Gibbons, J., MacCaull, W. (eds.) FHIES 2013. LNCS, vol. 8315, pp. 87–106. Springer, Heidelberg (2014)
5. Center for Devices and Radiological Health: Safety of Marketed Med. Devices, FDA (2006)
6. A Reseach and Development Needs Report by NITRD: High-Confidence Medical Devices: Cyber-Physical Systems for 21st Century Health Care, http://www.nitrd.gov/About/MedDevice-FINAL1-web.pdf
7. Keatley, K.L.: A review of the fda draft guidance document for software validation: Guidance for industry. Qual. Assur. 7(1), 49–55 (1999)
8. Lee, I., Pappas, G.J., Cleaveland, R., Hatcliff, J., Krogh, B.H., Lee, P., Rubin, H., Sha, L.: High-confidence medical device software and systems. Computer 39(4), 33–38 (2006)
9. Bowen, J., Stavridou, V.: Safety-critical systems, formal methods and standards. Software Engineering Journal 8(4), 189–209 (1993)
10. Singh, N.K.: Using Event-B for Critical Device Software Systems. Springer, Heidelberg (2013)
11. Méry, D., Singh, N.K.: Real-time animation for formal specification. In: Aiguier, M., Bretaudeau, F., Krob, D. (eds.) Complex Systems Design & Management, pp. 49–60. Springer, Heidelberg (2010)
12. Wassyng, A.: Though this be madness, yet there is method in it? In: Proc. FormaliSE, pp. 1–7. IEEE (2013)
13. Project RODIN: Rigorous open development environment for complex systems (2004), http://rodin-b-sharp.sourceforge.net/
14. Leuschel, M., Butler, M.: ProB: A Model Checker for B. In: Araki, K., Gnesi, S., Mandrioli, D. (eds.) FME 2003. LNCS, vol. 2805, pp. 855–874. Springer, Heidelberg (2003)
15. Silber, H.E., Jauslin, P.M., Frey, N., Gieschke, R., Simonsson, U.S.H., Karlsson, M.O.: An integrated model for glucose and insulin regulation in healthy volunteers and type 2 diabetic patients following intravenous glucose provocations. The Journal of Clinical Pharmacology 47(9), 1159–1171 (2007)
16. Chay, T.R., Keizer, J.: Theory of the effect of extracellular potassium on oscillations in the pancreatic beta-cell. Biophysical Journal 48(5), 815 (1985)
17. Han, K., Kang, H., Kim, J., Choi, M.: Mathematical models for insulin secretion in pancreatic β-cells. ISLETS 4, 94–107 (2012)
18. De Gaetano, A., Arino, O.: Mathematical modelling of the intravenous glucose tolerance test. Journal of Mathematical Biology 40(2), 136–168 (2000)
19. Drozdov, A., Khanina, H.: A model for ultradian oscillations of insulin and glucose. Mathematical and Computer Modelling 22(2), 23 (1995)
20. Siperstein, M.D.: The glucose tolerance test: A pitfall in the diagnosis of diabetes mellitus. Adv. Intern. Med. 20, 297–323 (1975)
21. Abrial, J.R.: Modeling in Event-B: System and Software Engineering (2010)

ENT Disease Diagnosis Using an Expert System

Duwaraka Yoganathan and Sangaralingam Kajanan

Department of Information Systems, School of Computing,
National University of Singapore,
13 Computing Drive, Singapore 117417
duwaraka@comp.nus.edu.sg, skajanan@comp.nus.edu.sg

Abstract. The field of medicine has witnessed a dramatic growth. However, the accurate and timely diagnosis of disease continues to be a serious clinical problem. This is particularly important for Otolaryngology/Ear-Nose-Throat (ENT) disease because ENT disorders can affect hearing, speaking, learning and many other important activities. Further, certain untreated ENT diseases can be fatal. Therefore, early diagnose of ENT diseases is vital. While ENT specialist's service is not always readily accessible, computer aided smart technologies that can assist general physicians or junior medical officers in diagnosing ENT diseases and subsequently refer complicated cases to senior ENT experts can enhance the efficacy of healthcare system. Despite the significance of computer aided ENT disease diagnosis systems, the research related this subspecialty is limited. Therefore, in this paper, we describe the research project about an ENT diagnosis expert system that can assist physicians in diagnosing ENT diseases. In particular, we will discuss in detail the development, evaluation and potential benefits of an ENT disease diagnosis expert system.

Keywords: ENT Expert System, Otolaryngology Disease Diagnosis, Expert System, Inferencing.

1 Introduction

Today, the field of medicine has improved immensely due the advancements in computing technology. Computers are involved in almost all the clinical practices. Artificial intelligent (AI) technologies assist both healthcare practitioners and patients in numerous ways. AI is a branch in computer science that can analyze complex medical data and identify meaningful relationships that can be used for clinical diagnosis and treatment.

Despite the latest advancements in healthcare, it does not always reach out to those most in need. Enormous difficulties have been faced by ordinary people in seeking medical assistance. Particularly, access to medical specialist is a critical problem(Van Doorslaer, Masseria, & Koolman, 2006). Due to the limited availability of specialist, ordinary people find it difficult to channel specialist frequently. i.e. specialist attend only critical cases and are only available in metropolitan hospitals. Thus, the accurate and timely diagnosis of disease continues to be a serious clinical problem.

V.G. Duffy (Ed.): DHM 2014, LNCS 8529, pp. 472–483, 2014.

Therefore, smart technologies that can assist in early diagnosis and prevention of serious health problems can be a great relief for many patients and healthcare system in general. This is particularly important for Otolaryngology/Ear-Nose-Throat (ENT) disease because ENT disorders can affect hearing, speaking, learning and many other important activities. Further, certain untreated ENT diseases can be fatal. Therefore, early diagnose ENT diseases is vital. As discussed above specialist access is not always available. While Otolaryngology specialist's service is not always readily available, computer aided smart technologies that can assist general physicians or junior medical officers in diagnosing ENT diseases and subsequently refer complicated cases to senior ENT experts can enhance the efficacy of healthcare system.

Despite the significance of computer aided ENT disease diagnosis systems, the research related this subspecialty is limited. Therefore, in this study we have developed a research based ENT (Ear-Nose Throat) Disease Diagnosis Expert System that can assist physicians or junior doctors in diagnosing ENT diseases. In particular, we will discuss "how an ENT disease diagnosis system can be designed and evaluated?" Furthermore we discuss the potential benefits of the system. The proposed system uses rule-based inferencing in diagnosis process and adopted an approach similar the one followed by ENT experts in their diagnosis process. Therefore, this system can not only used by physicians but also to train medical students towards ENT diseases diagnosis process and patient centered healthcare systems.

The rest of the paper is organized as follows. The immediately following section provides a background on existing medical expert systems. Then we describe our ENT disease diagnosis system- Virtual Doctor followed by the implementation details of the system. Subsequent sections provide discussion and finally conclusion.

2   Background

Artificial intelligent systems in medicine, started to emerge during late 1960s and many experimental systems were developed by research laboratories. Early AI based medical applications have laid the foundation for many new, recent applications. MYCIN(Edward Hance Shortliffe, 1976), is one the popular early rule-based expert system to diagnose and treat infectious disease. INTERNIST(Miller, Pople Jr, & Myers, 1982), is also rule-based expert system designed for the diagnosis of complex problem in internal medicine. The system was capable to cover 80% of the knowledge in internal medicine. CASNET(Weiss, Kulikowski, & Safir, 1978), is an expert system based on causal-associational network and was used for the diagnosis and treatment of glaucoma. Based on the concepts of MYCIN, expert systems such as ONCOCIN(Edward H Shortliffe, 1986) and PUFF(Aikins, Kunz, Shortliffe, & Fallat, 1983) were designed to assist physicians in treating cancer and lung diseases respectively.

These first generation expert systems laid the foundation for the next generation expert systems. In recent years expert systems have integrated multimedia technologies, machine learning, artificial neural networks and fuzzy logic and genetic algorithms to enhance the diagnosis. Examples of such systems are AI/RHEUM(Athreya, Cheh, & Kingsland III, 1998), ESTDD(Keleş, 2008) and ODPF(Chi, Street, & Katz, 2010).

AI/RHEUM(Athreya et al., 1998) is an expert system designed to diagnose, rheumatic diseases. The results from AI/RHEUM reveal 92% accuracy. The authors claim that this expert system can assist in both consultation and education. The AI/RHEUM uses criteria table paradigm for reasoning and provides conclusions at three levels of certainty- definite, probable and possible. Melek et al(Melek, Sadeghian, Najjaran, & Hoorfar, 2005) developed a neuro fuzzy based expert system for disease diagnosis. This system aims to assist physicians in their daily practices.

Expert System for Thyroid Disease Diagnosis (ESTDD)(Keleş, 2008), is a fuzzy rules based expert system for diagnosing thyroid diseases. The results reveal that the tool is able to predict a thyroid diseases diagnosis with 95.33% accuracy. Optimal Decision Path Finder (ODPF)(Chi et al., 2010) is a machine learning based expert system, which can expedite the diagnosis process and reduce the cost of diagnosis by reducing the number of diagnostic tests ordered. It is a decision support system that provides information on the disease probability, based on patient's available information. The system dynamically estimate minimum set of tests that are likely to confirm a diagnosis. The ODPF algorithm mainly uses lazy learning classifiers, confident diagnosis and, locally sequential feature selection (LSFS).

According to the literature review, medical expert systems have been developed for coronary artery diseases , thyroid diseases (Keleş, 2008), bone diseases (Hatzilygeroudis, Vassilakos, & Tsakalidis, 1997), rheumatic disease (Athreya et al., 1998), dengue (Karim, Suryaningsih, & Lause, 2009), cancer (Edward H Shortliffe, 1986), lung disease (Aikins et al., 1983), infectious diseases(Edward Hance Shortliffe, 1976) and glaucoma(Weiss et al., 1978). However, research on expert system that diagnoses ENT diseases is limited. Besides, the diagnoses of ENT diseases are based on symptoms which are often difficult identify. Many sophisticated examinations may be necessary in the diagnosis process. Thus, we aim to fill this gap by building an expert system to diagnose ENT diseases.

3   Virtual Doctor – ENT Disease diagnosis System

"Virtual Doctor" is an artificial intelligence (AI) based expert system, designed to assist physicians or junior doctors in the diagnosis of ENT related disease in the absence of ENT experts. Thus, this system can reduce the backlog created due to the busy schedules of ENT experts and enhance the effectiveness and efficiency of healthcare system. Virtual Doctor - ENT diagnosis uses rule based system for knowledge representation and has five core sub-systems which would enhance the physician's ability in reaching a diagnosis decision with confidence. Initially the symptoms are captured through the user interfaces as inputs. Then these symptoms are matched with inference rules in the knowledge base and finally a diagnosis is made by the inference engine. If the system is unable to diagnose the disease with the given symptoms or if the system is unable to identify the exact ENT disease the expert system recommends for some laboratory tests. Subsequently when these test results are provided, diagnosis will be carried out with more accuracy. If the system is unable to diagnose the disease even after producing the laboratory test results, the system will recommend for an ENT specialist consultation. The following sections describe the five main functionalities in detail. Figure 1(a) shows the main interface of Virtual Doctor, with references to each sub-module. For example when user (i.e. physician) clicks on disease diagnosis (see figure 1(b)) he/she will be directed to disease diagnosis sub-module.

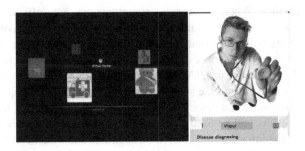

Fig. 1. (a) Virtual Doctor Main –with a 3D rotation menu for each of the sub-modules (b) Disease diagnosis sub system

Disease Diagnosis. Disease diagnosing sub-system prompts the physician to gather set of preliminary medical investigation related information, such as body temperature, blood pressure from patient. Based on this information, the system will intelligently prompt more related questions, in order to acquire detailed information of the disease. After analyzing the given information, the system derives conclusions accordingly. i.e. (1) the system may either report the decision about the disease and prescribe medication (i.e. when the disease is diagnosed with higher certainty) or (2) when clinical symptoms are not sufficient to come up with a diagnosis decision, the system recommends appropriate laboratory tests in order to help further diagnosis of the disease with more accuracy. Besides, the system stores all the data related to the patient for future references.

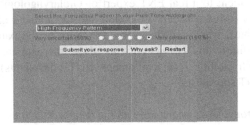

Fig. 2. Analyzing the objective evidence

Prescribing. During the disease diagnosis process, if the disease is accurately identified with higher level of certainty, the disease information (ENT disease) will be transferred to 'Prescribing' sub-system. Before prescribing medication, this sub-system would inquire about the patient's allergic conditions (to drugs or food), and patient's current medication details (such as whether the patient is currently being administered any other drugs, for some other disease). Based on this information the system would prescribe appropriate medication (i.e. system takes into account the interaction or contradiction between drugs). Moreover, this sub-system also stores the information for future reference.

Recommend Testing. When the clinical symptoms are not sufficiently enough to decide on the diagnosis with certainty, appropriate and comprehensive clinical tests and supporting tests will be recommended in order to decide on the diagnosis with higher level of certainty. Laboratory testing, X-ray or other relevant checkups will be recommended. If the patient provides details of the clinical and supporting tests, the test results will be entered into the system or scanned image will be uploaded into the system. Image processing techniques will identify patterns. Details of the clinical and supporting tests results will be used for detailed diagnosis with greater level of accuracy. In addition, the information gathered through this sub-system will also be transferred to database for future references. Table 1 provides a list of tests that can assist in ENT disease diagnosis. Table 2 provides details of the test results and possible diagnoses.

Table 1. Types of specific tests

Category	Test
Hearing Tests	Pure Tone Audiometry, Tympanometry, Speech & Voice Analysis
Nasal Tests	Finger-nose test, Standard Smell Test, Nasal endoscopy
Throat Tests	Throat Culture, Rapid Strep Test

ENT Specialist Referral. With the given symptoms and test results if the 'Virtual Doctor' expert system is unable to diagnose the ENT disease with certainty, the system will refer the patient to a real ENT expert or Otolaryngologist. The system will request for patient's current residence location and recommend an appropriate ENT expert (i.e. consultant), who is in the close proximity to the patient. Based on the seriousness of the illness this sub-system can advise the patients to get admitted to closer hospitals with facilities (i.e. equipment, ENT consultants) and facilitate appointments with ENT specialists.

Track Patient History. The system store all the details related to the patients, including symptoms, test results, diagnosis details, medicine prescribed, etc. The information gathered will be used for further analysis and will be used as an input for the self-learning learning system.

Table 2. Specific Tests for objective evidence

Test	Test Result	Possible Diseases
Pure Tone Audio-gram	High Frequency Pattern	Age Related Hearing Loss
		Vesticular Neuronitis
	Low Frequency Pattern	Meneire's Syndrome
	Part Frequency Pattern	Age Related Hearing Loss
	Unilateral Hearing Loss	Acoustic Neuroma
CT Scan	Tumor affecting the VC Nerve	Acoustic Neuroma
X Ray - Sinuses	Thickening of lining in Mucosa, Fluid in the Sinus	Sinusitis
	Thickening of lining in Mucosa, Fluid in the Sinus, Post Nasal Space	Epitasis
Blood Test (Full Blood Count)	Hemoglobin level outside the base lines. WBC > 12000	Infection
	Hemoglobin level outside the base lines. Platelet < 80000	Dengue

4   Virtual Doctor Design and Implementation

Virtual Doctor is intended to be used by physicians who are not advanced computer users. Therefore the user interfaces were designed to be more user-friendly. Following sections describe the details of implementation.

Knowledge Engineering for the E.N.T. Disease Diagnosis Expert System. Several different AI techniques were considered for the design of 'Virtual Doctor', including multi-agent systems and expert systems to solve the diagnosis problem. After discussing with knowledge engineer, AI expert, medical professionals and analyzing the existing literature, we decided to choose rule-based expert system, as it would best represent the diagnosis process of an ENT expert. Once the AI technique was chosen, discussions with a panel of ENT experts were carried out in order to gather relevant data. We gathered all necessary information, including a list of important ENT diseases, their symptoms, diagnosis procedures, treatment options, clinical and laboratory tests (see Figure 4). In addition, ENT related publications and books were analyzed as an additional source of information. Once the required knowledge was gathered, the details were organized and presented to ENT specialist for verification. Certain items were removed and few items were added based on the advice from ENT specialists. Once the items were finalized the acquired knowledge was encoded into rules in the knowledge base.

Table 3. Knowledge Acquisition – ENT disease and their symptomps

	Disease	Diagnosis investigation
Ear Diseases	Presbyacusis	1. Is the patient having difficulty in speech discrimination? 2. Is the patient having difficulty in phone conversation? 3. Has the patient had any trauma? 4. Has the patient got any infection? 5. Does the patient get fits? 6. Does the patient get Tinitus?
	Mener's Syndrome	1. Is the patient having hearing loss? 2. The hearing loss is sudden onset or Episodic? 3. Does the patient have associated Tinitus or Virtigo? 4. Is the patient having fever?
	Vestibular Neuronitis	1. Does the patient have hearing loss? 2. The hearing loss in patient in sudden onset or Severe? 3. Does the patient have Vertigo or tinnitus 4. Does the patient have fever?
	Acoustic Neuroma	1. Does the patient have Hearing loss? 2. Does the hearing loss gradually progressing form months to years? 3. Does the patient have initially Tinitus then Vertigo? 4. Does the patient has unilateral (one sided hearing) loss?
Nose Diseases	Allergic Rhinids/Catarrh	1. Does the patient have nasal discharge? 2. Is the nasal discharge clear or watery? 3. Does nasal discharge increases during morning or night? 4. Does the patient have sneezing? 5. Does the patient have itching in eyes, nose, or throat? 6. Does the patient have tearing of eyes? 7. Does the patient have fever?
	Sinusitis	1. Does the patient have nasal discharge? 2. Is the Nasal discharge thick or yellow discharge? 3. Does the patient have nasal block? 4. Is the nasal block is bilateral? 5. Does the patient have headache? 6. Does the patient have bleeding from nose?
	Nasal Discharge	1. Does the patient have discharge from the nose? 2. Is the nasal discharge is unilateral or bilateral? 3. Is the discharge from the nose is yellow or clear? 4. Is the discharge watery or thick? 5. Does the patient have Post Natal Drip (PND)? 6. Is the PND yellow or clear? 7. Does the patient have nasal block? 8. Is the nasal block unilateral or bilateral? 9. Is the nasal block episodic or persistent? 10. Does the patient have fever?

Table 3. (*Continued.*)

		11. Does the patient have headache? 12. Does the patient have sneezing? 13. Does the patient have itching in nose, eyes, and in palate or throat? 14. Does the patient have bleeding in nose or throat?
Nose Diseases	Foreign body in nose	1. Does the patient have nasal discharge? 2. Is the nasal discharge initially clear and then yellow?
	Bloody discharge or Epistaxis	1. Does the patient have bloody discharge or phlegmy discharge? 2. Did the patient have a trauma? 3. Does the patient have any infection? 4. Does the patient take any medication to thin the blood? 5. Does the patient involved in Drug abuse (Cocane)?
Throat Disease	Pharyngitis	1. Does the patient have sore throat? 2. Does the patient have fever? 3. Does the patient have hoarse voice? 4. How long the patient has hoarse voice is it a sudden onset (days) or long time (months to years)? 5. Does the patient have cough? 6. Does the patient have breathing difficulty? 7. Does the patient used to smoke or beetle chewing or alcohol use?
	Tonsulitis/ Oesophagitis	1. Does the patient have sore throat? 2. Does the patient have fever? 3. Does the patient have hoarse voice? 4. How long the patient has hoarse voice (is it a sudden onset (days) or long time (months to years))? 5. Does the patient have cough? 6. Does the patient have pain in swallowing or obstruction is swallowing?
	Laryngitis	1. Does the patient have Sore throat? 2. Does the patient have hoarse voice for a short duration? 3. Does the patient have fever?
	Cancer of Larynx/ Vocal code	1. Does the patient have fever? 2. Does the patient smoke? 3. Does the patient exposed to second hand smoking? 4. Does the patient have the habit of Betel Chewing?

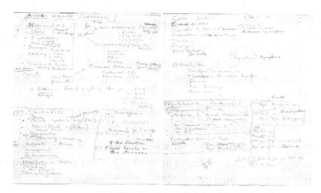

Fig. 3. Knowledge Acquisition

Knowledge Base Design. An expert system shell was used to create the knowledge base. Gathered information (such as symptoms, disease) was converted into a table format in order to implement the knowledge base (See Table 3). The rules were then written into expert system shell.

Inferencing. Once the knowledge is encoded into rules inferencing mechanism would diagnose the disease. Virtual Doctor – ENT diagnosis uses forward chaining mechanism to implement the inferencing logic using java classes. That java class logic takes user inputs (such as symptoms) through applets and subsequently the symptoms are matched with the knowledge base rules. Based on the match it will prompt further questions for clarification through applet and eventually diagnose the disease accordingly.

Reasoning with Uncertain Data. While the physician has to be certain about his/her assessment of patient's symptoms, the Virtual Doctor - ENT diagnosis system allows the user (i.e. physician) to provide confidence factor along with his/her response, which offers flexibility when he/she is not so sure about the symptoms (see Figure 3). Confidence measurements are usually called certainty factors or confidence factors (or CF). Similarly, based on the inputs' certainty, Virtual Doctor provides the diagnosis with a corresponding level of certainty or confidence.

Implementation and Integration. 'Virtual Doctor – ENT Diagnosis' comprises several sub-systems, which are built on top of an inference engine and knowledge base. All the sub-systems that are connected to the inference engine have the ability of communicating with each other using web services. The backend knowledge base (i.e. rule - based) together with the inference engine was implemented using java (e.g. forward chaining algorithms). The database server (i.e. Microsoft SQL Server) stores knowledgebase data and patient information. The front-end interfaces are built using Visual Studio & XAML, which provides a better look and feel for the user interfaces. Applets have been used to get the inference to the front end which is displayed with in XML web page. The XML web page uses Silver light to make it more attractive with the animations. ASP.NET was used for the development of web application. Java scripts were used to capture user interaction with the systems and all the interactions are stored in the database. Moreover, C#.NET was used implement algorithms to update the knowledge base, with new acquired knowledge about disease or symptoms. This enables the self-learning capability of our system. The system as a whole combinedly provides assistance for physicians in ENT diseases diagnosis, prescribing, recommend clinical laboratory tests and refereeing patients to real ENT experts when necessary. To deploy the system one needs a web server (IIS) and an application server (java) to host the application, All the modules in this system use the common software and hardware interfaces as they have been connected together.

5   Evaluation and Validation

Evaluation of Virtual Doctor- ENT Diagnosis includes addressing issues related to accuracy and usefulness. The system we have developed is being evaluated by ENT experts and specialists. The aim of our system is to emulate ENT specialist. Thus, several reliability and validity checks are warranted. The process of evaluation is described below.

Initially a team of ENT specialist created a set of test cases based on real patients' histories and symptoms, who visited the hospital for ENT diseases diagnostic consultation. These test cases were chosen to be complex enough that physicians would be likely to request a diagnostic assistance from an ENT specialist. Ten ENT specialists were assigned 30 diagnosis cases (each three). The same test cases will be diagnosed by set of ten ENT specialists as well as by Virtual Doctor-ENT disease diagnosis system. This phenomenon is similar to Turing Tests which have been used in validating expert systems (such as MYCIN and ONCOCIN). Same test will be repeated with general physicians, so that we will be able to know how far Virtual Doctor-ENT disease diagnosis system can help physicians in diagnosing ENT diseases in the absence of ENT expert. In order to compare the real diagnosis with virtual doctor – ENT system, the physician and ENT specialist will be requested to produce a list of possible diagnoses, and rank the order of each diagnosis. Currently the system is being evaluated by ENT experts and general physicians. Once this process is completed Kappa scores(Cohen, 1960) will be calculated to evaluate the agreement beyond chance. Higher Kappa score will be perceived as greater accuracy of the system and thus confirming the validity of Virtual Doctor – ENT diagnosis system (i.e. Diagnosis similarity between real ENT specialist and Virtual Doctor Expert system). In addition, the tests will be repeated twice with another set of ENT specialist and physicians to ensure reliability of diagnosis.

Once the accuracy and reliability of the system is ensured, the usefulness aspect of 'Virtual Doctor' expert system will be validated based on the following key aspects: (1) Structure - How well the 'Virtual Doctor' ENT disease diagnosis expert system would fit into its environment(i.e. healthcare system), do doctors find it helpful? (2) Process – What effects does the 'Virtual Doctor' have disease diagnosis process, such as accuracy of decision(as discussed above) (3) Outcome – Are the effects on healthcare process reflected on patient outcomes i.e. does the patient feel the same satisfaction that he/she would feel while diagnosed by an ENT expert? (how far it is similar to that of a real ENT expert) (Donabedian, 2005).

6 Discussion

The Virtual Doctor expert system was designed in a similar manner that an ENT consultant would approach an ENT disease diagnosis. The diagnosing processes includes steps such as initial gathering of subjective information(i.e. knowledge acquisition of symptoms related to ENT disease), generation of probable diagnosis list, gathering objective evidence(i.e. evidence from scan reports and laboratory tests), and hypothesis evaluation (i.e. finalize the disease based on subjective and objective information). Thus, Virtual Doctor ENT diagnosis system has important contributions for research and practice.

The major contribution of Virtual Doctor - ENT diagnosis system is to the healthcare domain. As the research on computerized diagnosis of ENT disease is limited, this study has an important contribution for ENT sub-specialty. Virtual Doctor - ENT diagnosis system can help general physicians in the diagnosis of ENT diseases in the absence of ENT expert. Thus, it can help in short listing the critical patients who can be referred to ENT specialists and reduce the backlog created due to busy schedules of limited accessibility of ENT experts. Hence our Virtual Doctor-ENT diagnosis can improve the efficiency, effectiveness of the healthcare system and improve the quality of patient care. With effective extensions, 'Virtual Doctor' can also be used in ENT education to train healthcare professionals and medical students to get a better understanding on ENT diseases and diagnosis processes. Besides this artifact (Virtual Doctor – ENT diagnosis system) has important implication for Design Science paradigm. This artifact is created to solve the problem faced by the healthcare community due lack of ENT experts. We demonstrate this artifact through experiment with real users of the system.

Despite the several contributions, Virtual Doctor has its limitations too. Even though the Virtual Doctor is designed mimic the diagnosis approach of an ENT specialist, certain aspects were not feasible to implement. First, complete expertise of an expert is difficult to extract and encode, because the knowledge of the specialist cannot be fully explained. Therefore, sometimes the required knowledge may not be available through the system. Second, ENT experts may sometimes use common sense, which cannot be programmed. Third, our system may also have problems in recognizing issues outside the knowledge domain. However, we overcome these limitations by referring the patient to consult real ENT specialists when the physician is unable diagnose the disease with the aid of 'virtual doctor' or by his/her medical knowledge. Fourth, the expert system have limited sensory experience compared to human ENT specialist, however our system try to overcome this issue to some extent by using image processing techniques that would process the webcam images of patients with abnormal conditions(e.g. swollen eye) and map it to the given patterns of normal and abnormal conditions. Besides, physicians can also record their observations manually, if the system is unable to recognize the patterns or image.

7 Conclusion

In this paper, we described the development of a rule based ENT diseases diagnosis expert system the 'Virtual Doctor', which can be used by physicians in their daily practice. The proposed system closely follows the steps followed by ENT specialist in diagnosing ENT diseases, therefore it is highly likely that this system would be accepted and adopted by physicians to assist them in the ENT disease diagnosis. However, extensive field trials need to be carried out in order to overcome the legal and ethical concerns, in order to incorporate such tools into healthcare systems.

References

1. Aikins, J.S., Kunz, J.C., Shortliffe, E.H., Fallat, R.J.: PUFF: An expert system for interpretation of pulmonary function data. Computers and Biomedical Research 16(3), 199–208 (1983)
2. Athreya, B.H., Cheh, M.L., Kingsland III, L.C.: Computer-assisted diagnosis of pediatric rheumatic diseases. Pediatrics 102(4), e48–e48 (1998)
3. Chi, C.-L., Street, W.N., Katz, D.A.: A decision support system for cost-effective diagnosis. Artificial Intelligence in Medicine 50(3), 149–161 (2010)
4. Cohen, J.: A coefficient of agreement for nominal scales. Educational and Psychological Measurement 20(1), 37–46 (1960)
5. Donabedian, A.: Evaluating the quality of medical care. Milbank Quarterly 83(4), 691–729 (2005)
6. Hatzilygeroudis, I., Vassilakos, P.J., Tsakalidis, A.: XBONE: A hybrid expert system supporting diagnosis of bone diseases. Networks (ANNs) 5(6), 2 (1997)
7. Karim, S., Suryaningsih, H., Lause, A.: Expert System for Diagnosing Dengue Fever. Seminar Nasional Aplikasi Teknologi Informasi, SNATI (2009)
8. Keleş, A.A.: ESTDD: Expert system for thyroid diseases diagnosis. Expert Systems with Applications 34(1), 242–246 (2008)
9. Melek, W.W., Sadeghian, A., Najjaran, H., Hoorfar, M.: A neurofuzzy-based expert system for disease diagnosis. In: 2005 IEEE International Conference on Systems, Man and Cybernetics, vol. 4, pp. 3736–3741. IEEE (2005)
10. Miller, R.A., Pople Jr, H.E., Myers, J.D.: Internist-1, an experimental computer-based diagnostic consultant for general internal medicine. The New England Journal of Medicine 307(8), 468 (1982)
11. Shortliffe, E.H.: Update on ONCOCIN: a chemotherapy advisor for clinical oncology. Informatics for Health and Social Care 11(1), 19–21 (1986)
12. Shortliffe, E.H.: Computer-based medical consultations: MYCIN, vol. 388. Elsevier, Amsterdam (1976)
13. Van Doorslaer, E., Masseria, C., Koolman, X.: Inequalities in access to medical care by income in developed countries. Canadian Medical Association Journal 174(2), 177–183 (2006)
14. Weiss, S., Kulikowski, C.A., Safir, A.: Glaucoma consultation by computer. Computers in Biology and Medicine 8(1), 25–40 (1978)

Application of Bayesian Networks in Consumer Service Industry and Healthcare

Le Zhang[1], Yuan Gao[1], Balmatee Bidassie[3], and Vincent G. Duffy[1,2]

[1] School of Industrial Engineering
[2] School of Agriculture and Biological Engineering, Purdue University,
47907 West Lafayette, IN, USA
{zhan1255,gao186,duffy}@purdue.edu
[3] Department of Veteran Affairs, Center for Applied Systems Engineering,
Detroit, MI, USA
balmatee.bidassie@va.gov

Abstract. Bayesian networks are powerful in data mining and analyzing causal relationships of an uncertain-reasoning problem. The implementation of Bayesian networks in industry and healthcare diagnosis can facilitate the process of locating causations in complex issues. This study conducted two case studies by BayesiaLab in consumer service and healthcare domain. Case Study One used unsupervised learning and supervised learning on the individual data set of county road traffic volume in Indiana State and concluded that road type has the most significant impact on daily vehicle miles traveled. In Case Study Two, only supervised learning was used to observe the aggregated data of adverse mental health effect on civilians, deployed veterans and nondeployed veterans of different genders. Both types of veterans showed higher probability to have adverse mental health compared to civilians. In conclusion, Bayesian networks provided valid results to support prior research. Further research is needed to investigate the differences between using individual data and aggregated data, and to apply Bayesian networks in meta-analysis.

Keywords: Bayesian Networks, BayesiaLab, Traffic Volume, Mental Health.

1 Introduction

Data mining is the automated or convenient extraction of patterns representing knowledge implicitly stored or captured in large databases and other storage media. It assists human in data collection, instead of the traditional method which relies on manual analysis and interpretation [1, 2]. Among data mining techniques, Bayesian networks, based on Bayes' Theorem, is a powerful technique to work with probabilities rather than relying on factual observations, especially for complicated issues involving association and causal relationships yet to be discovered.

A Bayesian network is an annotated directed graph that encodes probabilistic relationships among distinctions of interest in an uncertain-reasoning problem [3]. Its graphic presentation provides an exceptional demonstration of the relationships (arcs)

V.G. Duffy (Ed.): DHM 2014, LNCS 8529, pp. 484–495, 2014.

among all the factors (nodes) in a complex problem. Since the model deals with dependencies among all variables, it can cope with incomplete and uncertain data, and especially uncertain rules of reasoning, strengthening the power of diagnosis and prediction [4]. Bayesian networks also support learning abilities, allowing automatic application of this methodology in complex problems [5]. Another important feature is "omnidirectional inference" - while traditional statistical models usually contain one dependent and many independent variables, all variables can be treated equivalently in a Bayesian network, which is interesting for exploratory research [6].

In the last decade, many fields, from the traditional industries to new areas, have seen applications of Bayesian networks. Bayesian networks have risen to prominence as the preferred technology for probabilistic reasoning in artificial intelligence, with a proliferation of techniques for fast and approximate updating and also for their automated discovery from data [7]. In the management of complex industrial systems, it is used for dependability, risk analysis and maintenance areas [8]. In finance and banking, it can be used for fraud detection and credit scoring. In marketing, it is used for consumer survey analysis, market segmentation and simulation. In healthcare, it's used in diagnostic systems. Other applications include quality management, operational safety simulation, etc [9].

Mental health disease diagnosis is a field with many factors involved and interacting with each other. Clinical diagnosis of mental disorders is more complicated and more difficult compared to other sectors in primary care, with more risk factors involved, including personal profile, residential and work environment, cultural and sociological settings, etc [10]. For veterans, the challenges are even bigger due to additional factors, such as their military service experience, higher chances of physical injuries and disabilities, and the need to get readjusted to life out of the armed forces [11]. Bayesian networks can be introduced as a holistic approach to monitor and evaluate mental health risks from patients' perspective, and further facilitate early diagnose and prevention of implicit mental conditions.

In this study, we propose an application in consumer service to identify key factors and causal relationships, used as strategic guidelines in consumer satisfaction improvement and cost saving. Following the case studies of traffic volume analysis of the road system of the state of Indiana, an analysis of mental health risk factor among veterans and civilians will be showed to illustrate Bayesian networks implementation in industry and health care. This research demonstrates how to find out the hidden ties through BayesiaLab [12], and how it can benefit early diagnosis and prevention of mental health problems among veterans.

2   Methodology and Tool

The tool used in both case studies was BayesiaLab, a modeling software developed and supported by Bayesia, a designer of decision aid software packages in Bayesian networks for data mining [12]. BayesiaLab provides a complete laboratory for handling Bayesian networks to develop, communicate with and use readable illustrated decisional models that are strictly faithful to reality. Among its many features, the most appreciable ones for this case study include: highly intuitive graphical network presentation, learning capability, and the Bayesian power of inference.

In Data mining, unsupervised learning is defined as when a learning human, animal or man-made system observes its surroundings and, based on observations adapts its behavior without being told to associate given observations to given desired responses, as opposed to supervised learning, which has a targeted classifier whose value is analyzed based on the influences of the other factors [13]. With its learning function, individual data can be translated into Bayesian networks. Both learning techniques are supported by BayesiaLab with various algorithms, among which Naive Bayesian algorithm is based on the assumption (known as class-conditional independence) that the effect of an attribute value on a given class is independent of the values of the other attributes [14]. It simplifies the computations involved and, in this sense, is considered "naive".

Bayesian networks can be developed based on individual data or aggregated data. Individual data presents the parameter of every factor on each subject. In contrast, aggregated data presents the percentages of each factor on every subject. Based on the learning capability of BayesiaLab, Case Study One used individual data to develop a model. Case Study Two showed how aggregated data can be used to conduct meta-analysis [15] on mental health.

3   Case Study One: Traffic Volume Analysis of the Road System of the State of Indiana

Daily Vehicle Miles Traveled (DVMT) is a measure of the traffic volume flowing along a roadway during an average 24 hours period [16]. It is calculated by multiplying the Average Annual Daily Traffic (AADT) by the length of the road. This data is an important indicator used to assess transportation needs, system performance and highway planning and program recommendations [17]. In this case study, we looked into the DVMT data of each county's highway system in the State of Indiana from 2006 to 2010, and use learning capability of Bayesian networks to build a simply model to explore the risk factors affecting DVMT.

3.1   Hypothesis

Based on the definition, DVMT is directly affected by the average daily traffic volume and the length of roads. In Indiana, traffic volume raw data are collected by permanent continuous count stations, as well as portable traffic counters, and then adjusted and seasonally factored [17]. Road traffic volume is affected by many factors, ranging from road conditions, gasoline prices and toll, weather, and social and demographic factors such as age of the population, household size, labor force participation and car ownership [18]. This case study was designed based on the hypothesis that a certain extent of relationship exists between county populations and DVMT. Compared to other factors like vehicle ownership and labor force, the total population of a county is not known to have an explicit causal relationship with traffic volume, but it is logical to assume that the more people reside nearby, the higher traffic volume the area is likely to have. Therefore, it was chosen for the case study to test and demonstrate Bayesian networks' ability to explore unknown relationships.

3.2   Modeling and Analysis

DVMT data came from the Historic Vehicle Miles Traveled (VMT) by County & Systems data published by Indiana Department of Transportation (INDOT) [19]. For the 92 counties of Indiana, each of them includes some or all of 4 types of routes: City and County Roads, Interstate Roads (I), State Roads (SR) and U.S. Highways (US). County population is based on data published by STATS Indiana [20].

The source data were prepared so that each type of road in each county is listed as an individual data point. County population is duplicated for multiple road types. In the model, county names are omitted because name itself doesn't affect the traffic volume in any way. And a new parameter was calculated by dividing DVMT with the length of road. In theory, it should be equal to AADT. However, without the original AADT data from INDOT, or the exact method of calculating DVMT, it is named "Usage Rate" to indicate the extent of usage of the road. By doing this, the bias caused by the multiplying effect of road length in traffic volume is removed. Table 1 shows an example of the data of Allen County in 2006 (Note that the column "County" was removed during actual modeling).

Table 1. Data Example of Allen County in 2006

Year	County	Road Type	Length (Miles)	DVMT	Usage Rate	Population
2006	Allen	City and County Roads	2686.94	6061000	2255.73	345976
2006	Allen	I	98.8	2104000	21295.55	345976
2006	Allen	SR	87.24	936000	10729.02	345976
2006	Allen	US	65.87	1017000	15439.5	345976

During data import, KMeans was used as the discretization method for its benefits in removing the effect of outliers [21]. An initial analysis using BayesiaLab's unsupervised learning feature and distance mapping layout is shown in Fig. 1. In this model, BayesiaLab automatically connected nodes (factors) based on the mutual information and correlation between each two, and the amount of information each node can provide to reduce the uncertainties of other nodes, given the value of the specific node itself. The node "Year" is greyed out with no connection due to its insignificance. Using the feature Distance Mapping, the model is presented in a two-dimensional form where the length of arc between any two nodes indicates the Mutual Information as in information technology [22]. The closer two nodes are, the higher mutual information value they have in between. The color and figures of each arc reflect the relationship between two nodes in Pearson Correlation coefficient [23]: red color means negative correlation and blue means positive.

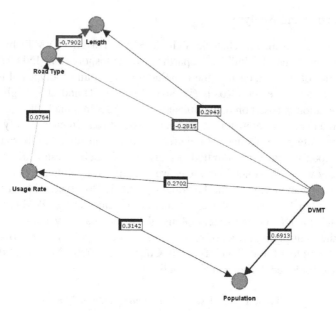

Fig. 1. Unsupervised Model in Mutual Information Distance Mapping Layout

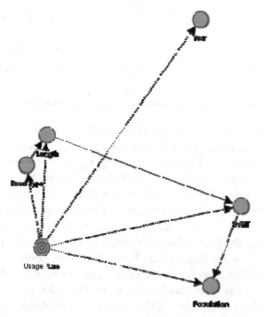

Fig. 2. Supervised Model with Usage Rate as Target Node

DVMT and Road Type are the two most information-rich parameters in this diagram, and Road Type has strong mutual information ties with Length and Usage Rate, while DVMT is related to county Population. It's noteworthy that Road Type is treated as discrete data and ranked in alphabetic order by default: City and County Road first and U.S. last. This helps understand the positive/negative correlation.

Next, a targeted analysis using BayesiaLab's Supervised Learning feature was performed with Usage Rate set as target node. Using Augmented Naïve Bayes learning algorithm [14], the system is modeled as in Fig. 2. The predefined Naive Bayes structure is highlighted with the dotted arcs, while the augmented arcs (from the additional Unsupervised Learning) are shown with solid arcs.

3.3   Results

Fig. 3 illustrated the posterior probability analysis on the supervised model, showing that Road Type has a significant impact on DVMT, Usage Rate and other variables. Comparing the left and right sides conditioned on different road types, it's obvious that in Indiana, City and County Roads are most likely to have the longest lengths, but lowest average traffic volume, and they are most likely to exist in counties with smaller populations. While Interstate roads are the shortest in length, but have higher volume and are more likely to exist in counties with larger populations. We only present the comparison result of these two types of roads because they demonstrated the largest divergence. The other two road types, US and SR, are in the middle, with SR showing relatively higher probability of lower usage rate than US. Overall, from 2006 to 2010, time didn't play a big role in the amount of road traffic or usage rate.

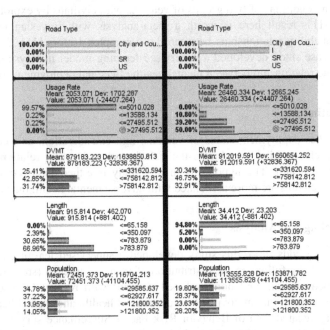

Fig. 3. Comparison of Impact of Road Type

4   Case Study Two: Analysis of Mental Health Risk Factor among Veterans and Civilians

Veterans' mental health problems are considered related to war experience for military service [24]. The numbers of mental health diagnosis are increasing and often coexisting with other medical problems, causing a "downward spiral" as stated by Secretary Eric K. Shinseki: "unseen" psychological wounds interplaying with biological and physical ailments, resulting in personal isolations and even more serious issues like homelessness and suicide [11]. Meanwhile, experience from military services could put veterans into long term struggles caused by brain injuries, disabilities and chronic diseases such as diabetes, obesity and hypertension, which are found to contribute to mental disorders, making their self-management more difficult and causing suicidal ideation [25]. Posttraumatic Stress Disorder (PTSD) is a psychiatric disorder that can occur after someone goes through a traumatic event like war, assault, or disaster [26]. To understand the adverse mental health effect within veterans, a large amount of studies focus on risk factors like gender, age, race, combat exposure, and war zone deployment, and PTSD [27, 28]. However, veterans who hadn't served in a war theater were also considered associated with war zone deployment and combat exposure in researches [29].

Hoglund [29] summarized in his study that adverse mental health effect was associated with veterans who had military service in a combat and war zone (deployed veterans) and female veterans who didn't have military service in a combat or war zone (nondepoyed veterans). Calculated the odds ratio of risk factors, he compared mental health conditions of two groups of veterans with civilians by exploring gender differences. This result here is worth a meta-analysis with Bayesian networks to explore probability relationships between those complex factors [15]. Based on his results, this case study developed a supervised learning model in BaysiaLab [12] to investigate the relationship between mental health effect and deployment status.

4.1   Hypothesis

This study takes deployment status of veterans into consideration, as well as social demographic characteristics to locate the risk factors and causal relationships with adverse mental health. The hypothesis in this study is either deployed veterans or nondeployed veterans are more associated with adverse mental health than civilians.

4.2   Modeling and Analysis

Instead of using odds ratio, this study developed a supervised learning model with BayesiaLab [12] by following the distribution of men and women (stratified by civilian, developed veteran, and nondeveloped veteran) with respect to race/ethnicity, marital status, education, employment status, general health, and mental health. This study used aggregated data of Behavior Risk Factor Surveillance survey which was summarized by Hoglund [29]. Table 2 showed the data set for deployed veterans.

The data set included the race/ethnicity, marital status, education, employment status, general health, and a self-report of the number of days when mental health was not good during the previous 30 days (14 days or more indicated adverse mental health).

Table 2. Aggregated Data from Behavior Risk Factor Surveillance Survey [29]

| | | Deployed Veterans (N=978) | |
		Male (N=846)	Female (N=132)
Race/Ethnicity	Nonwhite and/or Hispanic	0.20	0.33
	White Non-Hispanic	0.80	0.67
Marital Status	No Spouse or Partner	0.25	0.41
	Spouse or Partner	0.75	0.59
Education	High School or Less	0.27	0.08
	Some College or More	0.73	0.92
Employment	Not Employed	0.12	0.13
	Employed	0.88	0.87
General Health	Fair-to-Poor	0.12	0.15
	Good-to-Excellent	0.88	0.85
Mental Health	14+Poor Mental Health Days	0.09	0.17
	13 or Fewer Poor Mental Health Days	0.91	0.83

Eight factors (nodes) were created and mental health was set as the target factor in supervised learning. The probability for the effects of each factor were given by aggregated data from Behavior Risk Factor Surveillance survey [29]. As showed in Table 2, deployment and gender had relation to other factors. Thus, we manually connected arcs between deployment and gender with other factors. The model was presented with radial layout as Fig. 4. In probability mode, the probability of deployment and gender can be changed to 100% or 0. In this way, the probability of adverse mental health effect for each combination of deployment and gender can be observed. The probabilities were presented in histogram as Fig. 5.

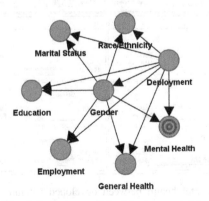

Fig. 4. Bayesian model of deployment data

4.3   Results

The histogram from Fig. 5 showed a higher probability of adverse mental health effect on veterans (9% and 11% for male deployed veterans and nondeployed veterans, 17% and 19% for female deployed veterans and nondeployed veterans) than on civilians (8% for male civilians, 13% for female civilians), which evidently support the hypothesis. Hoglund's research [29] indicated deployed veterans were associated with adverse mental health for men and possibly women; nondeployed veterans were associated with adverse mental health for women, but not for men. This study provided similar results on male deployed veterans, female deployed veterans, and female nondeployed veterans. However, male nondeployed veterans also showed a high probability on having adverse mental health.

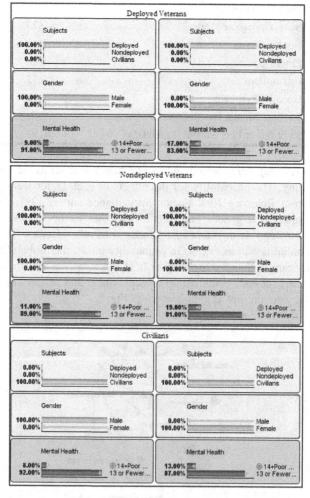

Fig. 5. Comparison of mental health between developed veterans, nondeveloped veterans, civilians by gender

5   Discussions

The findings of Case Study One are in line with existing literature. The interstate highway system has a much higher density of use than other components of U.S. surface transportation system. A 1996 report [30] shows interstate highways take up 23% of the market share of America's surface transport, and is 26 times as many person miles per route mile as all other roads (including low usage rural roads). Another more recent report in 2008 [18] shows that the rate of growth in VMT (Vehicle Miles Traveled) has fallen sharply since 2000, with a miniscule 0.6% in 2006. And this leveling off in VMT growth may be a long-term trend due to various socio-economic factors. This report also points out that regional population has a minor influence on VMT, though specific age/occupational groups have a more significant role in the growth of VMT, such as car owners, female labor force and working age population.

The Bayesian networks model of Case Study Two was developed from aggregated data, which had been translated into the probability of effect on each factor. Aggregated data also defines the relation between each factor. In such condition, only supervised learning can be applied on this data. Similar results from Hoglund's research [29] were provided. However, this model showed male nondeployed veterans (11%) presented a higher probability on having adverse mental health than male deployed veterans (9%), which differs from Hoglund's conclusion that male nondeployed veterans has insignificant association with adverse mental health effect. Since Bayesian networks provide probability relationships of each event rather than significant influence, even if adverse mental health effects present insignificant influence on nondeployed veterans, it still has probability to happen on nondeployed veterans and this probability is higher than deployed veterans.

This paper demonstrated the strength of Bayesian networks in discovering relationships in systems involving multiple risk factors, and the validity of this method through verification by existing literature and comparative study. The second case study showcased a new application area of this methodology in diagnosis of mental health issues among veterans. Compared to traditional statistics analysis methods, Bayesian networks enable modeling in intuitive graphic views for analysts to identify the key factors and relationships at a glance. Modern software such as BayesiaLab have incorporated advanced visualization features and learning algorithms to further utilize the probabilistic predictive and diagnostic power of Bayes' theorem. However, it must be pointed out that the direction of the arc should not be interpreted as causal relationship, but statistical association. The existence of causation should be verified by further study and literature.

The difference in data processing between the two cases reflect different scenario in real world research. Sometimes, data of each individual subject is available. However, in some cases, such data is not directly accessible, or will take enormous time and efforts to collect, especially in the health care field where the subjects are usually patients and clinical experiments are expensive. The concept of meta-analysis advocates leveraging existing researches on similar topics in a systematic view [15]. To further verify the validity of modeling with aggregated data, a comparative study was performed based on data set of Case Study One to sum up individual data into percentages and obtained similar results: road type affects DVMT and usage rate most. But the results are not exactly the same with minor variance (e.g. the probability for DVMT to be greater than 657,000 with aggregate data is higher than individual date by 1.47 percentage point). This may be due to the integration effect during aggregation. It is also noteworthy that different discretization methods will affect the presentation of results. Therefore, using aggregated data should be based on a good knowledge of the type and distribution of the data set, and a good understanding of the research subject, content are and context. While this study shows the potential of using Bayesian networks in the context of meta-analysis, further study should be conducted to investigate the detailed application in different areas.

Acknowledgements. The author would like to acknowledge the support of the Department of Veteran Affairs, VA-Center for Applied Systems Engineering, Clinical Partnerships in Healthcare Transformation (CPHT), as well as the Detroit Veteran Affairs Medical Center.

References

1. Fayyad, U., Piatetsky-shapiro, G., Smyth, P.: From Data Mining to Knowledge Discovery in Databases. 17, 37–54 (1996)
2. Han, J., Kamber, M., Pei, J.: Data Mining Concepts and Techniques, 3rd edn. (2011)
3. Heckerman, D., Mamdani, A., Wellman, M.P.: Real-world applications of Bayesian networks. Commun. ACM. 38, 24–26 (1995)
4. Stassopoulou, A., Petrou, M.: Obtaining the correspondence between Bayesian and Neural Networks. Int. J. pattern Recognit. Artif. Intell. 12, 901–920 (1998)
5. Santander Meteorology Group: Data mining and artificial intelligence: Bayesian and Neural networks, http://www.meteo.unican.es/research/datamining
6. Conrady, S., Jouffe, L.: Vehicle Size, Weight, and Injury Risk High-Dimensional Modeling and Causal Inference with Bayesian Networks Table of Contents (2013)
7. Korb, K.B., Nicholson, A.E.: The Causal Interpretation of Bayesian Networks. In: Holmes, D.E., Jain, L.C. (eds.) Innovations in Bayesian Networks. SCI, vol. 156, pp. 83–116. Springer, Heidelberg (2008)
8. Weber, P., Medina-Oliva, G., Simon, C., Iung, B.: Overview on Bayesian networks applications for dependability, risk analysis and maintenance areas. Eng. Appl. Artif. Intell. 25, 671–682 (2012)
9. Neapolitan, R.E.: Learning Bayesian Networks. Pearson Prentice Hall Upper Saddle River (2004)
10. Laufer, N., Zilber, N., Jecsmien, P., Maoz, B., Grupper, D., Hermesh, H., Gilad, R., Weizman, A., Munitz, H.: Mental disorders in primary care in Israel: Prevalence and risk factors. Soc. Psychiatry Psychiatr. Epidemiol. 48, 1539–1554 (2013)
11. Department of Veteran Affairs: Strategic Plan Refresh, FY 2011-2015., Washington, DC 20420 (2011)
12. Bayesia: Bayesia, http://www.bayesia.com/en/about-us/index.php
13. Huang, T.-M., Kecman, V., Kopriva, I.: Unsupervised Learning by Principal and Independent Component Analysis. In: Huang, T.-M., Kecman, V., Kopriva, I.: Kernel Based Algorithms for Mining Huge Data Sets. SCI, vol. 17, pp. 175–208. Springer, Berlin (2006)

14. Han, J., Kamber, M., Pei, J.: Classification: Basic Concepts. In: Data Mining Concepts and Techniques. pp. 327–391 (2012)
15. Borenstein, M., Hedges, L.V., Higgins, J.P., Rothstein, H.R.: Introduction to meta-analysis. Wiley.com (2011)
16. Division of Planning, Office of Technical Services, O.D. of T.: Daily Vehicle Miles Traveled Report (DVMT),
    http://www.dot.state.oh.us/Divisions/Planning/TechServ/traff
    ic/Pages/DVMT.aspx
17. Autumn Young: Latest INDOT Traffic Adjustment Factors., Indianapolis (2013)
18. East-West Gateway: Trends in Regional Traffic Volumes Signs of Change (2008),
    http://www.ewgateway.org/pdffiles/library/trans/trafficvolum
    es/vmtrpt.pdf
19. Indiana Department of Transportation: Historic VMT by County & Systems (2006-2011),
    http://www.in.gov/indot/files/TrafficStastics_HistoricIndian
    aVMTByCounty2006-2011.pdf
20. STATS Indiana: Population,
    https://www.stats.indiana.edu/topic/population.asp
21. Hautamäki, V., Cherednichenko, S., Kärkkäinen, I., Kinnunen, T., Fränti, P.: Improving K-means by outlier removal. In: Kalviainen, H., Parkkinen, J., Kaarna, A. (eds.) SCIA 2005. LNCS, vol. 3540, pp. 978–987. Springer, Heidelberg (2005)
22. Cellucci, C.J., Albano, A.M., Rapp, P.E.: Statistical validation of mutual information calculations: Comparison of alternative numerical algorithms. Phys. Rev. E. 71, 66208 (2005)
23. Lee Rodgers, J., Nicewander, W.A.: Thirteen Ways to Look at the Correlation Coefficient. Am. Stat. 42, 59–66 (1988)
24. Jakupcak, M., Hoerster, K.D., Blais, R.K., Malte, C.A., Hunt, S., Seal, K.: Readiness for Change Predicts VA Mental Healthcare Utilization Among Iraq and Afghanistan War Veterans. 165–168 (2013)
25. Bossarte, R.M., Blosnich, J.R., Piegari, R.I., Hill, L.L., Kane, V.: Housing instability and mental distress among US veterans. Am. J. Public Health. 103(suppl.), S213–6 (2013)
26. Buckley, T., Tofler, G., Prigerson, H.G.: Posttraumatic Stress Disorder as a Risk Factor for Cardiovascular Disease: A Literature Review and Proposed Mechanisms. Curr. Cardiovasc. Risk Rep. 7, 506–513 (2013)
27. Maguen, S., Ren, L., Bosch, J.O., Marmar, C.R., Seal, K.H.: Gender differences in mental health diagnoses among Iraq and Afghanistan veterans enrolled in veterans affairs health care. Am. J. Public Health. 100, 2450–2456 (2010)
28. Metraux, S., Clegg, L.X., Daigh, J.D., Culhane, D.P., Kane, V.: Risk factors for becoming homeless among a cohort of veterans who served in the era of the Iraq and Afghanistan conflicts. Am. J. Public Health. 103(suppl.), S255–61 (2013)
29. Hoglund, M.W., Schwartz, R.M.: Mental health in deployed and nondeployed veteran men and women in comparison with their civilian counterparts. Mil. Med. 179, 19–25 (2014)
30. Cox, W., Love, J.: 40 Years of the US Interstate Highway System: An Analysis, The Best Investment A Nation Ever Made (1996)

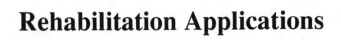

Rehabilitation Applications

Design and Ergonomics of Monitoring System for Elderly

Giuseppe Andreoni[1], Fiammetta Costa[1], Alberto Attanasio[2], Giuseppe Baroni[3],
Sabrina Muschiato[1], Paola Nonini[3], Andrea Pagni[4], Roberto Biraghi[4], Roberto Pozzi[5],
Maximiliano Romero[1], and Paolo Perego[1]

[1] Design Department, Politecnico di Milano, via durando 38/a, 20158 Milan, Italy
[2] La Meridiana, Società Cooperativa Sociale, Via G. dei Tintori 18, 20900 Monza, Italy
[3] Flextronics Design srl, via B. Gerolamo 27, 20052 Monza, Italy
[4] STMicroelectronics srl, via C. Olivetti 2, 20864 Agrate Brianza, Italy
{giuseppe.andreoni,fiammetta.costa,paolo.perego,
maximiliano.romero}@polimi.it, alberto.attanasio@gmail.com,
{roberto.biraghi,andrea.pagni}@st.com,
{giuseppe.baroni,SabrinaMuschiato,
Paola.Nonini}@it.flextronics.com, roberto.pozzi@datamedsrl.com

Abstract. This paper presents the study and the development of a tele-monitoring system with the aim to support elderly people living alone. The intent of our new system is to permanently connect the elderly with their relative and caregivers. The tele-monitoring system allows to continuously monitoring the subjects as they were in a hospital and, in case of anomalies in the health state, automatically share and alarm to caregivers and relatives. The continuous monitoring is done using two different sub-systems: wearable sensors for biomedical data collection and infrared video cameras for fall detection. The main goal of this study is to develop and test the system prototype not only from a functional point of view, but also from the user acceptability and usability point of view. For this reason this studies was based on a parallel development of acceptability and technical issues; this allows to create an ad-hoc tele-monitoring system for elderly,

Keywords: Tele-medicine, Tele-monitoring, Elderly, Wearable devices, Optical monitoring devices.

1 Introduction

Data from Eurostat estimations [1] shows that European population is constantly and progressively aging; in 2012 there are four people in working age for every over 65s; and the prediction shows that they become two in 2060; in 260 the overs-65s is predicted to reach more than 42% of population [2]. These aspects cause an increase in the cost the National Sanitary System has to face; in the last 15 years, the health spending has grown more than twice the Gross Domestic Product (GDP), with an average hospitalization cost for one day which amount to 674€ [3]. With this trend in aging population and costs rising, it is easy to expect a collapse of the National Sanitary System. For these reason many countries are trying to find alternatives and

V.G. Duffy (Ed.): DHM 2014, LNCS 8529, pp. 499–507, 2014.

strategies based on early de-hospitalization and tele-medicine with the aim to reduce costs. Thus many applied research projects focused on home care services based on Information Communication Technology (ICT) systems have been carried out [4][5][6]. Contrarily to other studies, this work targets to develop and test few prototypes not starting from the technology point of view, but from the users.

This kind of systems have the goal of monitoring people, for this reason the human component is fundamental and can not be forgotten during the design of the project; moreover accessibility and acceptability issues of technological system in healthcare are mandatory for success. As Norman [7] said we are now in a mature phase of technology where product has to shift from a technology centered to a user perspective.

Design can offer several tools to develop technological systems which can be handle by users with special needs; furthermore, if the systems include house interactive environment for non-invasive support, an ergonomic approach to design domestic context integrated by technology can solve several problems related to the use of that kind of system by people for whom technology could be a big barrier (social inclusion).

Therefore, the MAMMA (Multimodal Ageing Monitoring and Assistance) project, co-founded by Lombardy Region (Italy) and involving companies, university and health care provider, develops a tele-monitoring system for elderly people to support autonomously living at their homes with a top-down approach starting from acceptability and usability evaluation of the system, the products and the interfaces between humans and devices.

We can summarize the project objective with the following points:

- Low invasively; the measurement has to be efficient and reliable, but it has to be invisible in order to be easily used during daily activity;
- High accuracy in order to read all the possible anomalies (cardiac problem and fall event);
- Plasticity; the system can be adapted to different environment configuration (space flat, two-rooms flat…) and different users;
- Easy to use and learn;
- Connected; the system has to be connectable with different communication system in order to send alarm to caregivers and relatives.
- Low cost.

2   The Monitoring System

The project starts with the aim of monitoring elderly people in their home environment. Many studies show that elderly are subjected to many risk [8][9], from fall to heart complication. In order to record all this different situation, the system needs to be a multi-parametric filter. Our system is so composed by two main parts:

- Videocameras for fall detection;
- Wearable garment or patch for biomedical data recording.

The first subsystem was developed by Flextronics Design srl and it is composed by a patch which collects biomedical data (ECG, body movement, respiration) with the aim to detect heart complications.

The biomedical wearable device, as shown in fig. 1, is composed by four parts:

- ECG Patch
- Bluetooth Sensor Node
- Gateway receiver
- Server

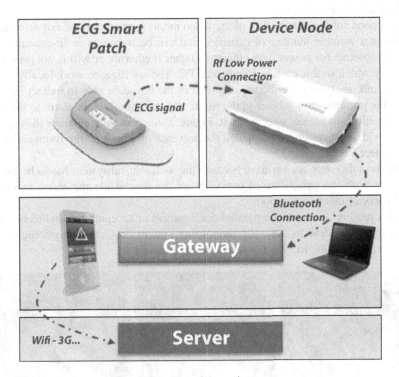

Fig. 1. Diagram of the entire system

The first part consists in the sensitive part: it is composed by the wearable conductive adesive patch and the ECG amplifier. The patch has two electrodes and an adesive part and can be easily attached to the skin as a normal plaster. The amplifier is made by flexible circuit in order to have high wearability and comfort, and it is connected to the patch with four snap button which allow for securely fit the device avoiding noise and interference during ECG signal recording due to device unintended movements.

The acquired ECG signal is transmitted to the second part which consist of the Device Node. The Device Node, because of the dimension, has a bigger battery than the ECG smart patch so that can be used to transmit the entire acquired signal to the gateway via bluetooth. As shown in figure 1, the ECG smart patch communicate with de Device Node via RF connection that is low power in order to save battery consumption; the Device Node instead communicate with the gateway with standard Bluetooth™ 2.0. The node has to be dressed trough a band or has to be placed at a maximum distance of two meters from the Smart Patch. The gateway, depending on whether the elder is in the house or outside, can be a computer or a bluetooth enabled smartphone. The Gateway process signals in order to extract features that can be used by the local intelligence to generate alarms that will be sent to the remote assistant & health management.

The gateway provides also access to data and sanitary services through an ad hoc console with different interaction levels according to the different users: elderly people, relatives, caregivers...

The second subsystem consists of the video monitoring system for fall detection. It consists in a variable number of cameras (that can be webcams or IP-cameras) connected to ethernet (or power over ethernet adapter if ethernet or wifi is not present) to a gateway which in this case is a dedicated PC. The intelligence work locally on this gateway and, analyzing the picture recorded in the house, is able to extract information on the presence of a subject in the room, and communicate an alarm to the assistant & health management over internet. Figure 2 shows in three pictures the capability of the video subsystem to recognize the presence of a body in the room and verify if the subject has fallen.

Both the subsystem are invasive because the wearable subsystem has to be directly in contact with the skin, dressed everyday all the day, while the video subsystem record every instance in the room.

Fo this reason, we conduct a parallel development of acceptability and technical issues in order to allow to tune tele monitoring system on elderly physiological and social needs according to User Centered Design principles.

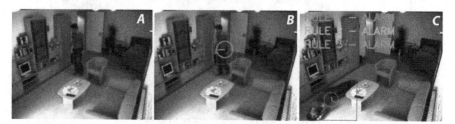

Fig. 2. A. Input image of the camera, B. Processed image, C. Processed image in case of fall detection and generated alarm.

3   Methodology

As described in the previous chapter, the parallel development has been conducted with the aim of a user centered design. In our hypothesis, if it is possible to provide technologies to elderly people and if they accept them, then it will be easy to use it for environment and social improvements. For this reason we focus the first part of the research on usability [10] and acceptability [11] evaluation.

The first study has been conducted on elderly people in small protected apartments in the Oasi San Gerardo, located in Monza (Italy).

The study goal is to collect information about the real user needs and at the same time, check acceptability. Since this study as been conducted in the first stage of the development, the products did not exist yet; for this reason the first ergonomic study has been conducted using Wizard of Oz techniques [12]. Mock-up of the products have been manufactured and provided to the elderly people. A first Focus Group has been carried out before the acceptability test with the aim to explain the project to elderly, relatives and care givers. The mock-up consist into four products:

- Smart patch product;
- Smart t-shirt product [13];
- Camera monitoring system;
- Forniture with embedded video monitoring system.

These fake products, organized in two subsystem (t-shirt with smart forniture and smart patch with camera) have been used by two male elderly (respectively 85 and 89 years old) both for five days. Figure 3 shows the two subsystem tested.

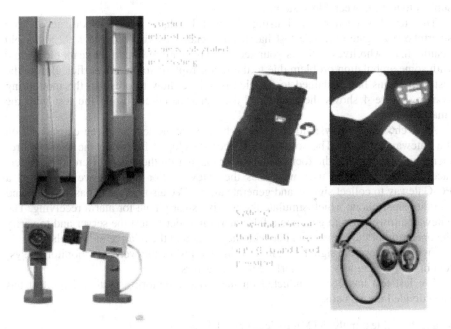

Fig. 3. The two subsystems Mock-up for monitoring test of elderly at home

After two weeks another Focus Group has been performed to collect information about the test experience highlighting pros and cons. Using the methodology of Focus Group it was possible to gain informations also from elderly who haven't used the system. The configuration of the two monitoring products and devices has been designed according to the result of this previous ergonomics analysis.

The parallel development allowed ST Microelectronics and Flextronics to define systems' architecture and the base of user interface. After this phase, using the data acquired during focus groups, a strong laboratory activity was developed in order to optimize the performances and the reliability of the wearable platform, improving RF communication, power consumption and the usability of the relevant sensors (smart patch and device node). A dedicated activity has been performed on ID/User Interface with the aim of choosing the most comfortable material and the best technology to be used for better wearability and end user usability.

During the hardware and software development, algorithms for signals and video analysis have been design; these algorithms extract some features from signals and video which can be used to generate alarms. The alarms are generated by the gateway locally (both on personal computer if the aged subject is in the home, and on android based smartphone if the subject is outside). The generated alarms are than sent to the Server that is part of the remote assistant & health management service.

After this development phase, the project has been carried out through three different functional tests.

The first one has been conducted by technicians in the Oasi San Gerardo on two subject to test the wearable system.

This test has been realized using a Smart Patch, a Device Node, an android smartphone as gateway, The test has been attended by two elderly, a 92 years old healthy male who lives with his younger wife take care of him; a 82 years old widow with some ambulation problem due to the femur rupture six month earlier. Before the test technicians has explained to the elderly subject how to dress up the monitoring system. Figure 4 shows the quality of the signal acquired during the test with the smart patch.

After checking the system work properly, the second test has been carried out on the gateway software. The software has been developed following the user requirements collected during the focus groups. For this reason there is a different user interface depending on the user who uses the gateway. For this test we have used a PC-Gateway to collect signals and generate alarm. We also use a PC-based server and an other smartphone which simulate the relative smartphone for alarm receiving. The gateway allowed also to generate a false alarm in order to test the server and to verify the operation of the connection between the server and the relative mobile phone.

Figure 4 shows the signal acquired during the test of the wearable monitoring system in the PC-Gateway user interface for care givers.

The last test has been conducted on the video monitoring system. This test has been divided in two parts:

- a technical test in the STMicroelectronics laboratory;
- a test in the Oasi San Gerardo with real user.

The first test had the aim to verify the capability of the system, algorithm and intelligence to generate alarm in case of fall detection. The test has been done using 34 video files at a resolution of 1024x768 px and with a frame rate of 15 fps of fall occurred in controlled environment. The files come from the Hannover Database [14]

The algorithm and local intelligence in the PC-gateway has an accuracy of 93%. Table 1 reports the results of this test.

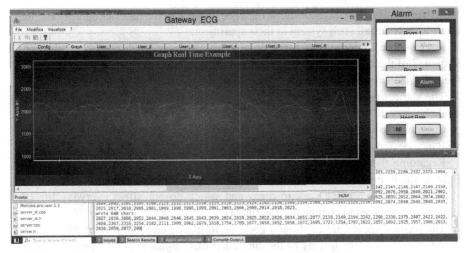

Fig. 4. PC-Gateway user interface

Table 1. Test results on fall detection algorithm

Numbers of falls in the used video	15
True positive fall detected	14
False positive fall detected	2
False negative fall not detected	1
Precision of the fall detection algorithm	93.3%

The test on real users has been carried out in three rooms of the Oasi San Gerardo. The three room are respectively a studio flat, a two-room flat and a big common room. Testing the system in this three different room allow us to try different type of cameras (Webcam Logitech C905, Network STMicroelectronics Camera and Axis M1011 Network camera) with different configuration. In the studio flat we use a single two Logitech Webcam cameras (because forniture hide a part of the room). Figure 5 shows the image from the image camera configuration.

4   Results

As shown in previous chapter in this studies two different kind of research have been carried on: an ergonomic study and a technological studies.

The results after the ergonomic study show a reluctance on the part of elderly to adopt a system that can help them to prevent accident and call for help. If the subject have no cardiac problem, he/she refuses to use wearable monitoring system; the same thing happens for fall monitoring, it the aged subject never had falling episode, they don't want to install such system in their apartment.

For example, after the final focus group, only two over 20 elderly accept the entire system, 7 of the could accept the system only if personalized (wearable device wearable in a different way, different monitoring eg. temperature...).

The subject prefer normal videocamera because the adoption of special forniture could be very difficult because of house's different configurations.

Contrarily to what was expected, all the subject show no problems using video surveillance devices that record images of their daily life.

Regarding the wearable system, the answer reported during the focus group highlight a small preference for the smart patch respect to the smart t-shirt/bra; the subjects prefer something easy to dress and which do not affect everyday life (the subjects do not need to change their garment).

The technological studies show a good performance an reliability of the wearable monitoring system; the quality of the single led ECG signal is good enough to extract HR easily. The subjects who tested the wearable device had no difficulty wearing the patch. However the test lasted only few days was and the wearability should be verified also on a longer time period.

Regarding the tele-monitoring system we verified that one camera per room is generally enough, through more cameras it is possible to reach higher precision since the algorithm has detection difficulties when the subject falls in front of the camera.

An accelerometer integrated in the wearable device and connected with the camera could be applied to improve the accuracy of the system and could be used to detect falling accidents also outside the home.

5   Conclusion

The technical goal regarding the capability of the camera system to detect falling accidents and the capability of the patch to collect and send biomedical data has been reached and verified in real environment, although the caparison and integration of the two different data sets is much more difficult.

We also verified that elderly people preferences cannot be given for granted and it is very important to apply specific user research techniques in each project involving this user group.

The integration of early acceptability tests and subsequent technical development allowed to chose adequate solutions and tune the tele-monitoring system on elderly physiological and social needs according to User Centered Design principles realizing prototypes fully accepted by users.

Further researches will be needed to scale the system in modular parts according to users specific need and to face practical problem as the integration of ICT in existing home.

References

1. Report on demography. In: 2012, for every person aged 65 or older, there were 4 people of working age in the EU27. Eurostat (2013)
2. Marsili, M., Sorvillo, M.P.: Previsioni della popolazione residente per sesso, età e regione dal 1.1.2001 al 1.1.2051, Istituto Nazionale di Statistica, ISTAT, Roma (2002)
3. European Commission. Directorate-General for Economic, and Economic Policy Committee of the European Communities. The impact of aging on public expenditure: projections for the EU-25 Member States on pensions, healthcare, long-term care, education and unemployment transfers (2004-50). Office for Official Publications of the European Communities (2006)
4. Mahmud, K., Lenz, J.: The personal telemedicine system. A new tool for the delivery of health care. Journal of Telemedicine and Telecare 1(3), 173–177 (1994)
5. Brownsell, S.J., Bradley, D.A., Bragg, R., Catlin, P., Carlier, J.: Do community alarm users want telecare? Journal of Telemedicine and Telecare 6(4), 199–204 (2000)
6. Jenkins, R.L., McSweeney, M.: Assessing elderly patients with congestive heart failure via in-home interactive telecommunication. Journal of Gerontological Nursing 27(1) (2001)
7. Norman, D.A.: The invisible computer: why good products can fail, the personal computer is so complex, and information appliances are the solution. MIT Press (1999)
8. Tinetti, M.E., Williams, T.F., Mayewski, R.: Fall risk index for elderly patients based on number of chronic disabilities. The American Journal of Medicine 80(3), 429–434 (1986)
9. Lloyd-Jones, D., et al.: Heart disease and stroke statistics—2010 update A report from the American Heart Association. Circulation 121(7) (2010)
10. Jeffrey, R., Chisnell, D.: Handbook of usability testing: how to plan, design, and conduct effective tests. Wiley. com (2008)
11. Jordan, P.: Designing pleasurable products: An introduction to the new human factors. CRC Press (2000)
12. Maulsby, D., Greenberg, S., Mander, R.: Prototyping an intelligent agent through Wizard of Oz. In: Proceedings of the INTERACT 1993 and CHI 1993 Conference on Human Factors in Computing Systems (1993)
13. Perego, P., Moltani, A., Andreoni, G.: Sport Monitoring with Smart Wearable System. In: PHealth 2012: Proceedings of the 9th International Conference on Wearable Micro and Nano Technologies for Personalized Health, Porto, Portugal, June 26-28, vol. 177. IOS Press (2012)
14. Debard, G., et al.: Camera-Based fall detection on real world data. In: Dellaert, F., Frahm, J.-M., Pollefeys, M., Leal-Taixé, L., Rosenhahn, B. (eds.) Real-World Scene Analysis 2011. LNCS, vol. 7474, pp. 356–375. Springer, Heidelberg (2012)

A Low Cost Haptic Mouse for Prosthetic Socket Modeling

Giancarlo Facoetti[1], Andrea Vitali[2], Giorgio Colombo[3], and Caterina Rizzi[2]

[1] BiGFLO s.r.l. (BG), Dalmine, Italy
bigflo@bigflo.it
[2] Department of Engineering, University of Bergamo (BG), Dalmine, Italy
{andrea.vitali1,caterina.rizzi}@unibg.it
[3] Department of Mechanical Engineering, Polytechnic of Milan, Milan, Italy
giorgio.colombo@polimi.it

Abstract. This paper refers to the design of prosthetic socket adopting a computer-aided approach. The main goal is to make available a modeling tool, named SMA-Socket Modeling Assistant, which permits to replicate/emulate manual operations usually performed by the prosthetist. Typically, s/he also relies on the sense of touch; therefore the underlying idea has been to develop and experiment haptic devices. The paper presents a haptic mouse at low-cost to make it affordable also by small orthopedic labs. It is essentially a traditional mouse device enhanced with a servomotor and a pressure sensor pad integrated with Arduino board and SMA. The application within SMA is described as well as the haptic interaction with physically-based model of the residual limb. Finally preliminary tests are illustrated.

Keywords: prosthesis socket modelling, haptic devices, low cost haptic mouse, Arduino.

1 Introduction

Nowadays, lower limb prosthesis design is a hand-made process and the final results depend on the technician skills. The lower limb prosthesis is composed by standard components (foot, knee, tubes, adaptors) and custom parts (socket and sometimes the liner). The socket is the most important component and has to be realized starting from the shape of the patient's residuum, since it has its own specific and unique geometry. Moreover, the socket is the interface with the human body and the final comfort of the whole prosthesis mostly depends on its quality. The traditional design process starts with the realization of negative and positive plaster casts of the residual limb. The prosthetist pushes and manipulates the residual limb in order to create the right plaster cast and to understand how to modify correctly the geometry and obtain a comfortable socket. Then, the prosthetist manually modifies the positive cast by adding and removing material to reach the optimal shape. This operation is meaningful and necessary to provide the right fitting and lower pressure in sensitive anatomical zones. For example, where there are bony protuberances or tendons the socket does

V.G. Duffy (Ed.): DHM 2014, LNCS 8529, pp. 508–515, 2014.

not have to press the limb, and at the same time not to be too wide because it could cause other physical problems. Figure 1 shows two examples of residual limb/plaster cast manipulation.

Even if the prosthetist is well skilled, the traditional process follows a trial and error approach and often iterations and socket physical prototypes are required.

In order to optimize the entire process and decrease psychological impact on patients, we have developed an innovative software platform to design and test the prosthesis totally in a virtual environment [1].The platform includes a 3D CAD module, named SMA-Socket Modeling Assistant, which provides a virtual laboratory where the orthopedic technician can replicate all the traditional operations to define the socket shape. The system embeds technicians' knowledge, best practices and rules that drive the traditional process, so the user is guided through the process. Finally, SMA has been integrated with a FE solver to study the interaction between the socket and the residual limb and check pressure distribution over the residuum critical zones.

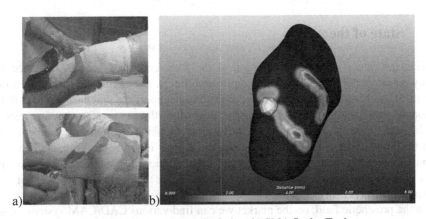

Fig. 1. a) Hand-made manipulation; b) SMA Sculpt Tool

The user can modify the socket shape using several tools that help and guide the user to create the right socket shape around the geometry of the residual limb. Some tools work in automatic mode (e.g., circumference reduction), on the base of the design rules embedded in the system. Others are interactive and simulate traditional operations performed by the prosthetist. Among these, the most important is the Sculpt Tool that permits to freely modify the surface geometry. A sphere cursor can be moved over the residuum or socket models and the vertexes inside the sphere are pulled or pushed along their normal axis in order to create the required deformation (Figure 1). It is also possible to change the ray of the sphere in order to set the area of deformation. This operation emulates the operation of adding or removing material from the plaster cast.

However, as mentioned before, along the traditional design process, the prosthetist uses his/her hands to manipulate the residuum and/or socket shape (Figure 1a) and often relies on the sense of touch. S/he uses hands to evaluate residual limb tonicity and manipulate/modify accordingly the socket shape. Haptic interaction could help the technician to regulate better the entity of the deformation: the more the user presses on the haptic device, the greater is the depth of the deformation. Adopting a physic-based model makes possible to simulate the behavior of a real limb subjected to the manipulation.

To replicate this operation using sense of touch within SMA (at least partially), we investigated the possibility to adopt haptic device for managing the interaction with the 3D model of the residual limb. Devices available on the market, possible at low cost, have been analyzed, since costs could be a key issue for small orthopedic labs. From the analysis and first tests carried with Novint Falcon device (http://www.novint.com/) [2], we have decided to develop a prototype of a haptic mouse, that can provide the user, at low cost, an haptic interaction with the residuum or socket virtual models.

In this paper we first introduce the scientific background in considered field; then the developed haptic mouse. Finally the application within the SMA module and preliminary results are presented.

2   State of the Art

During last years, computer emulation of the five senses has been investigated by many researchers [3-5] for different applicative fields. For example, [4] describes the use of 3D technologies and stereoscopic vision to support the diagnosis and rehabilitation of low-vision related pathologies. Regarding the sense of touch, interesting applications are related to surgery simulators to emulate real hand-made operations and train practitioners [6-11].Other important aspects involved in the sense of touch simulation are the feeling of temperature, pain, friction and vibration [11]. To this end, many haptic devices have been designed in order to simulate these different tactile perceptions [12-14].

In the prosthetic field, on the market we can find various CAD/CAM systems (e.g., Seattle ShapeMaker, Rodin4d, Bioshape, and Vorum Canfit™). They use reference model templates as starting point to build positive chalks. However, but they do not include any simulation tools, even if we can find in literature several research works that consider finite element analysis to simulate and analyze interaction between the socket and the residual limb[15-17].

In this context, the kind of interaction provided by the existing systems refers to the traditional mouse-keyboard paradigm. Only Rodin (www.rodin4d.com) proposed a CAD system (Rodin4Design software) that utilized the haptic 3D arm Phantom to provide the user force-feedback during virtual carving and sculpting of the 3D models.

Phantom devices are used also in the dental CAD/CAM applications (www.sensabledental.com) and as a general-purpose 3D haptic modeler (http://www. dentsable.com/products-freeform-systems.htm).

For the prosthetic field, haptic gloves, such as the CyberGrasp, from CyberGlove System LLC [18] could be adopted since they permit to replicate the behavior of the hands interacting with a real object. On the other hand, they are complex, expensive and not affordable for small orthopedic labs. Therefore, we decided to consider low-cost haptic devices and, in particular, to develop a haptic mouse specifically conceived and tested for our application.

3   Haptic Mouse Prototype

To build low-cost and easy to use device, we considered, at this stage, sufficient the possibility to interact with one finger, by which the user can feel the softness/hardness of the residuum surface and perceive better the virtual object.

The haptic mouse prototype is basically a traditional mouse device enhanced with a servomotor and a pressure sensor pad (Figure 2).The servomotor is the Hitec HS-225BB high speed model, with 0.14 sec/60 deg. transit time; while, the pressure sensor is the Flexiforce piezoresistive force sensor built by Tekscan. If pressed, its resistance changes from infinite to about 50.000 Ohm. Figure 3 shows the haptic prototype.

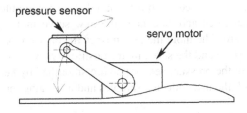

Fig. 2. Haptic mouse operating principle

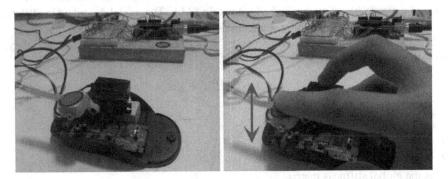

Fig. 3. Haptic mouse prototype

The pressure sensor pad works as input device, measuring the force the user applies with her/his finger. The servomotor works as output actuator setting its position according the physic-based model computations.

To get data from the pressure sensor pad and to drive the servomotor, we exploited the Arduino board linked to the computer running the Socket Modeling Assistant (Figure 4). The communication between Arduino board and the computer is through USB port, with serial protocol.

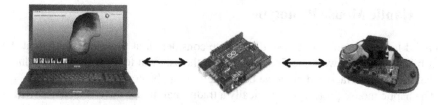

Fig. 4. Computer - Arduino - Haptic mouse workflow

The user can move the sphere cursor of the Sculpt Tool by moving the mouse, as s/he would do with a traditional mouse. Putting one finger on the pressure pad, the user can push the pressure sensor and the pressure value is read by Arduino and transmitted to SMA. The embedded physic-based model computes the deformation created by the applied force and calculates the new servo motor position, which is moved by Arduino board. The more the user pushes the pressure pad, the deeper is the deformation of the surface and the servo motor position is lowered.

The input data from the pressure sensor pad are smoothed by keeping a FIFO (first in first out) buffer with the last collected samples and averaging them.

3.1   Physics-Based Model of the Residuum

In order to compute the deformation of the surface according to the user input, we developed a physic-based model, embedded within SMA. The model described in [19]and developed for surgical simulation applications has been taken into consideration.

The mathematical model is composed by a mesh of tetrahedral elements and obeys the following equation:

$$f = Mu'' + Du' + Ku$$

where:

M is the mass matrix.

D is the damping matrix.

K is the global stiffness matrix.

f is the vector of the external forces applied to the model and obtained by reading the pressure sensor pad.

u is the vector of nodes displacements due to the deformation.

The equation is solved with an explicit approach [19]. In order to give the user a consistent simulation of the sense of touch, the haptic loop has to be rendered at least with a frequency of 1000 Hz and the equation has to be resolved in real time. Therefore SMA uses GPU computation that permits to obtain about 10x faster computation speed.

For simplicity, we considered lumped masses at nodes; so, M and D are diagonal matrices and this can simplify computations. To reduce computational time, a pre-processing phase performs condensation of the K matrix: we eliminate rows and columns corresponding to the fixed nodes (e.g., those belonging to the bone). For materials characterisation (bones and soft tissues) we considered data found in literature [15-16].

After the pre-processing and matrix condensation phase, the part of the equation having high computational times is only the Ku multiplication. This kind of computational problem is well addressed by GPU computation. As K is a sparse matrix, we perform the Ku multiplication with the CUSPARSE library (a sub-library of CUDA) that has fast and optimized matrix-vector multiplication features.

4   Preliminary Testing

We experimented the haptic mouse to create the shape of the socket starting from the residual limb model and to emulate the operation of adding and removing material from the plaster cast.The 3D model of the residual limb of a transtibial (amputation below knee) patient has been acquired by MRI (Magnetic Resonance Imaging) and automatically reconstructed using a hoc module embedded within SMA [1]. The 3D model, represented by NURBS surfaces, includes bones soft tissue geometry.

To evaluate how the haptic mouse replicates the curves and slopes of the residuum virtual surface, we first tested it only with the servomotor and without the pressure sensor. By moving the mouse on the table plane, the servomotor sets its height position according to the height of the surface of the virtual model. In case of fast movements, we noted a small delay to update the servomotor position due its speed limits. However, in case of normal movements in a limited area, the servomotor follows the virtual surface with good approximation. Afterwards, we tested the complete system including the pressure sensor pad. We found some fake peaks in the detection of applied forces; however the filtering software routine limited the problem.

Prosthetist considered interesting these first tests, even if the haptic device permits to emulate only the interaction of one finger. Figure 5 shows some example of the shape modeling using the haptic mouse. Anyway, the haptic force feedback can help the technician to manipulate the geometric model as s/he usually acts using hand.

As mentioned before, in previous research activities, the commercial low cost device, namely the Novint Falcon, has been tested. From a preliminary comparison of results reached so far, we noted that the haptic mouse seems to be more intuitive and easy to use. For example, sometimes, the first testers were not able to correctly understand the position of the cursor respect to the virtual model of the residual limb.

We have planned to test the prototype with real cases in collaboration the ortho-pedic lab involved in the project, in order to test if this kind of devices could be included in the real workflow. We have also planned to evaluate other input sensors and output actuators with better performances.

5   Conclusions

In this paper, the authors presented the first prototype of a haptic mouse integrated with a prosthetic modeling tool, i.e., SMA, to interact with the 3D model of the residual limb or of the socket. This should make more natural the interaction especially for those users, such as orthopedic technicians, without specific skills on computer-aided tools. The main features are one-finger haptic interaction and ease of use. The haptic mouse works like a traditional mouse, permitting to control a virtual cursor with the movement of the hand on a plane; moreover, it's possible to interact with a virtual object and feel its surface with the added haptic feature. Preliminary results have been considered promising; however, we need to evaluate hardware (servo motor and pressure pad) with better performance while maintaining the working principle.

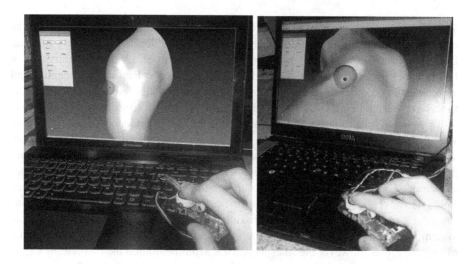

Fig. 5. Use of the haptic device to interact with the 3D model of the residuum or of the socket

The haptic device can be improved and used in other application fields. For example, we can add more couples of servomotor and pressure sensor to provide haptic force-feedback with multiple fingers. This should permit to perceive better curves and slopes of the surface. Another potential field of application the authors are going to investigate is the use of the haptic mouse for visual impaired people to help them to feel a virtual surface. Finally, it would be interesting to test this kind of device with general purpose or artistic modeling software, such as Pixologic Zbrush (pixologic.com).

References

1. Colombo, G., Facoetti, G., Rizzi, C.: A digital patient for computer-aided prosthesis design. Interface Focus. 3(2) (2013)
2. Colombo, G., Facoetti, G., Rizzi, C., Vitali, A.: Socket virtual design based on low cost hand tracking and haptic devices. In: Proceedings VRCAI 2013 - 12th ACM SIGGRAPH International Conference on Virtual-Reality Continuum and Its Applications in Industry, pp. 63–69. ACM SIGGRAPH (2013)
3. Narumi, T., Kajinami, T., Tanikawa, T., Hirose, M.: Meta cookie. In: Proceedings SIGGRAPH 2010 ACM SIGGRAPH 2010 Emerging Technologies. Article n.18 (2010)
4. Facoetti, G., Gargantini, A., Vitali, A.: An environment for contrast-based treatment of amblyopia using 3D technology. In: Proceedings ICVR 2013 International Conference on Virtual Rehabilitation (2013)
5. Bordegoni, M., Ferrise, F., Covarrubias, M., Antolini, M.: Haptic and sound interface for shape rendering. Presence: Teleoperators and Virtual Environments 19(4), 341–363 (2010)
6. Hutchins, M., Adcock, M., Stevenson, D., Krumpholz, A.: The design of perceptual representations for practical networked multimodal virtual training environments. In: Proceedings of the 11th International Conference on Human-Computer Interaction (2005)
7. Katsura, S., Iida, W., Ohnishi, K.: Medical mechatronics - An application to haptic forceps. Annual Reviews in Control 29(2), 237–245 (2005)
8. Sela, G., Subag, J., Lindblad, A., Albocher, D., Schein, S., Elber, G.: Real-time haptic incision simulation using FEM-based discontinuous free-form deformation. Computer-Aided Design 39(8), 685–693 (2007)
9. Perez-Gutierrez, B., Martinez, D.M., Rojas, O.E.: Endoscopic endonasal haptic surgery simulator prototype: A rigid endoscope model. In: Virtual Reality Conference (VR). IEEE (2010)
10. Coles, T.R., Meglan, D., John, N.W.: The role of haptics in medical training simulators: A survey of the state of the art. IEEE Transactions on Haptics 4(1), 51–66 (2011)
11. Riener, R., Harders, M.: Virtual Reality in Medicine. Springer, London (2012)
12. Colombo, G., De Angelis, F., Formentini, L.: Integration of virtual reality and haptics to carry out ergonomic tests on virtual control boards. International Journal of Product Development 11(1), 47–61 (2010)
13. Ohnishi, K., Katsura, S., Shimono, T.: Motion control for real-world haptics. IEEE Industrial Electronics Magazine 4(2), 16–19 (2010)
14. Ninu, A., Dosen, S., Farina, D., Rarray, F., Dietl, H.: A novel wearable vibrotactile haptic device. In: ICCE 2013 IEEE International Conference on Consumer Electronics (2013)
15. Portnoy, S., Yizhar, Z., Shabsin, N., Itzchak, Y., Kristal, A., Dotan-Marom, Y., Siev-Ner, I.: Gefen: Internal mechanical conditions in the soft tissues of a residual limb of a transtibial amputee. Journal of Biomechanics 41(9), 1897–1909 (2008)
16. Colombo, G., Facoetti, G., Morotti, R., Rizzi, C.: Physically based modelling and simulation to innovate socket design. Computer-Aided Desing and Applications 8(4), 617–631 (2011)
17. Sewell, P., Noroozi, S., Vinney, J., Amali, R., Andrews, S.: Static and dynamic pressure prediction for prosthetic socket fitting assessment utilising an inverse problem approach. Artificial Intelligence in Medicine 54(1), 29–41 (2012)
18. Abu-Tair, M., Marshall, A.: An empirical model for multi-contact point haptic network traffic. In: Proceedings of the 2nd International Conference on Immersive Telecommunications (2009)
19. Meier, U., Lòpez, O., Monserrat, C., Juan, M.C., Alcaniz, M.: Real-time deformable models for surgery simulation: a survey. Computer Methods and Programs in Biomedicine 77(3), 183–197 (2005)

Evaluating Work Disability of Lower Limb Handicapped within a Human Modeling Framework

Yan Fu[1], Xingsheng Chen[2], Shiqi Li[1], Jacob Gwenguo Chen[3], and Bohe Zhou[4]

[1] School of Mechanical Science & Engineering,
Huazhong University of Science & Technology, Wuhan, Hubei Province, 430074, China
[2] School of Physical Education, Wuhan Institute of Physical Education,
Wuhan, Hubei Province, 430074, China
[3] Foxconn (Hong Hai) Technology Group, Shenzhen, 518159, China
[4] National Key Laboratory of Human Factors, China Astronaut Training & Research Center,
Beijing, 100094 China
Laura_fy@mail.hust.edu.cn

Abstract. An accurate disability evaluation provides good basis for job place-ment of the handicapped and corresponding accommodations. In this study a work disability analysis model is firstly developed to predict human perfor-mance in certain task scenarios and the disability index is finally correlated to DOF of joints, the inner joint moments, the muscle pressure around the stump. The model is made of three levels. The outcome of the third level algorithm will be reflected in digital human in simulated task scenarios. To simulate handi-capped behavior, the study further presents a simulation framework to realize the above three-level model, which integrate the two kinds of constraints: task constraints and physical function constraints, reflecting on posture and motion of the digital man. To validate the modeling framework, the study used material handling task as an ex-ample. Ten male BKAs were recruited in Chinese elec-tronic manufacturing companies. The model calculated the optimization angles and moments of knee, hip, elbow joints of healthy and unhealthy parts. The cal-culated results are put to biomechanical-disability spectrum to generate a weighted disability index, compared to evaluation results by an occupational therapist. Meanwhile, results were put in Jack environment and a manikin was created and compared to another manikin created by motion capture data. The matching results will validate the applicability of the proposed framework to modeling handicapped behavior.

Keywords: Limb handicapped, work disability, human modeling, evaluation.

1 Introduction

Work disability is a term, which occupational therapists use to evaluate the suitability of those handicapped in daily time and occupational situations. Human performance is the final result of disability interacting with task scenarios. Many tools have been developed to perform human behavior analysis in virtual environments, such as Jack[1], SAMMIE[2], MANERCOS[3] and SAFEWORK[4]. These tools are

V.G. Duffy (Ed.): DHM 2014, LNCS 8529, pp. 516–526, 2014.

commonly used by designers to perform occupational ergonomic analysis on a virtual mock-up by immersing a virtual human controlled by direct or inverse kinematics in the task environment. Within the above applications, the human models account for about 90% of the population, but not the handicapped population. A new approach, called "design-for-all" [5,6] aims to perform accessibility tests on an even wider range of the population.

Many Work disability evaluation methods directly apply function disability variables to predict the handicapped work capacity in different kinds of task contexts. but cannot predict accurately the interaction effect of body disability with task factors. In other words, function disability of may correspond to different level of work disability in different task contexts. A task-related work disability evaluation is critical for accurate prediction of handicapped performance. It is necessary to specify the characteristics of the operator, the machine, the environment and the operator's interaction with machine and environment.

In the virtual environment, functional description can be used to simplify the interaction between the humanoid and the objects in the simulated scenario [1]. To simulate the functional ability, there are varying notions such as anthropometric data, functional ability, admissible joint angles as well as physiological data such as maximum strength, recovery time and fatigue [7-10]. Badler et al[11] proposed a framework named PAR (Parameterized Action Representation) to simulate the interaction between human and machine in the dimension of movement. Kallmann [12] used the Smart Object framework as the physical simulator to reflect the interaction of humanoid with the environment. Safonova[13] proposed a framework simulating the anthropometric characteristics in task-specific workspaces spaces. Rodriguez[9] modeled and simulated fatigue associated with joint movement. The above methods provide good insights into how to simulate functional ability of the human interacting with machine, tool and environment system.

To simulate the functional ability of the physical handicapped, Porter [2] set up a database con-taining the movements of physically disabled people. Using this data, it is possible to display the problems that each recorded individual is expected to experience. However, recorded behaviors cannot easily be applied to new tasks or individuals. Reed et al [10] reviewed a variety of ap-proaches to find that most posture and motion prediction methods have been focused on relatively narrow range of tasks and thus introduced a new methodology, the Human Motion Simulation (HUMOSIM) Framework that is intended to be extensible to most human movements of interest for ergonomics. By HUMOSIM framework, the motion and posture can be predicted based on the constraints derived from the end-effectors.

To consider the functional interaction of the disabled with the product system, the constraints not only lies in the tasks but also the variance in functional disability of the handicapped body part. The integration of physical constraints with task constraints is far more complex because of func-tional disability and its extended influence on adjacent body parts. This study presents a frame-work dedicated to integrate the two kinds of constraints and thus model the specific behavior of the physical handicapped in the virtual environment generated by the product specifications. Based on 3 levels of constraints, the model can predict the physical capacity in the dimension of joint kinematics associated with product use. The model can calculate the posture and motion of the physical handicapped based on the optimization of strength and torque under physical and dynamic constraints of physical disability. To validate the model itself, the study used material handling task (squatting and reaching) as an example and compared the modeled result with that from the motion capture.

2   Modeling Method

Generally speaking, the functional performance in the task interaction can be evaluated at three main levels: task level, occupational level and physiological level [11]. This study presents a disa-bility constrained model to evaluate all the three levels of the functional performance when human interacts with the product system (See Fig1). At task level, human biomechanical laws concluded by empirical studies are required. For example, NIOSH[12] can compute the strength maneuvering on a certain handle by the input of anthropometric parameter and handle size. Occupational analysis can be conducted in the simulation scenario. The physiological analysis deals with the forces associated with the motion, implying the information of fatigue and musculoskeletal pain. The main problem with the physiological method is the requirement of complex models to simulate the muscle function. However, to add the physiological analysis into the simulation system can help retrieve the kinetic parameters such as forces and torques, which is a critical factor evaluating the usability index of the product At the occupational level, the motion data collected can be connected with the individual, which makes the analysis realistic.

The constraints led to functional disability can be categorized as 3 groups: appearance (effecter) constraints such as broken arm or amputation, kinematics constraints such as inaccurate pointing and less degree of freedom (DOF) of the joints and the physical constraints such as strength limits. Fig. 1 shows how the controllers operate with the interaction of the 3 kinds of constraints.

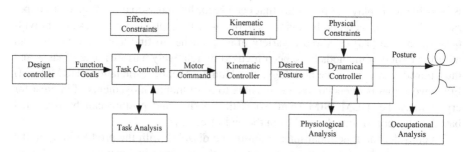

Fig. 1. Constraint-driven Model of Physical Handicapped Motion/Posture

There are 4 controllers in this model. Human, task and environment variables entered into the interaction controller with the constraints result in variations of the virtual humanoid's posture until the posture is achieved. First, the design controller conveys the human function in the interaction as a goal. The data flowing into the task controller are from the task specifications. For instance, hold on a hand tool can be translated as grasping the hand tool handle and the grasp can be transmitted to the task controller. The task controller will be constrained by the physical disability, named by effecter constraints (E). For example, if the right hand of the user is dysfunctional and has weak grip strength, E is the disabled right hand. Then the resulting motor commands will be passed to the kinematics controller. This controller is responsible for generating a posture requiring for grasping the hand tool. Kinematics constraints are passed as parameters of the controller and together generate the resulting posture. The algorithm behind this controller may be function of the motor command, which will be discussed in the following sections. The resulting posture will be controlled by the dynamic controller, which can generate forces required for this posture, and produce the final posture when the user holds the hand tool. A physical simulator is enabled to generate the dynamic physics like forces and torques on the humanoid to achieve the desired posture. The physical constraints such as the strength limits are the parameters to the controller. The algorithm of dynamic controller constrained by the physical factor will be discussed in Section 3. At last the posture obtained is given back to the task controller to determine whether the function goal is achieved. When new changes were made to the task controller, the process shall go on through the kinematics controller and dynamic controller. New postures can be generated by changed kinematics controller and dynamic controller. The constraints are the key to the physically handicapped model and motion synthesis visualizes the functional capacity of the physically disabled. And the work disability can be reflected as physiological and occupational parameters.

3   Motion and Posture Generation Method

To generate the motion/posture, the motion element is dispatched to each body component. 4 modules (gaze module, upper-extremity module, torso module and lower-extremity module) related to the body dimensions are built up to manipulate the controller based on different DOF kinematics skeletal model. (See Fig.2).

Constrained by the task variables, kinematics variables and dynamic variables, the values are to be ad-justed based on function optimization. The generation process consists of 3 main parts: (1) a set of de-sign variables, which are joint profiles (i.e., joint angles as a function of time) and the torque profiles at each of joint; (2) multiple cost functions to be optimized, which are human performance measures that represent functions that are important to accomplishing the motion (e.g., energy, speed, joint torque); (3) constraints on the motion (e.g., collision avoidance, joint ranges of motion, strength limits). The motion accomplishment requires optimization of multiple cost functions such as energy, speed and joint torque. The optimization is under the constraints such as ranges of motion and force requirement. In this study, both joint angle and torque file are generated by optimizing cost function in kinematics and dynamic dimensions.

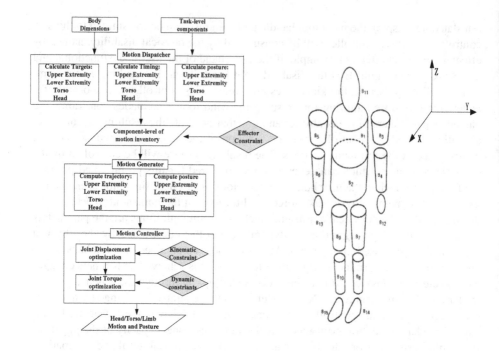

Fig. 2. Motion Generation Process   **Fig. 3.** Human Body of 15 Segment Links

3.1   Kinematics Skeletal Model

Hanavan's [13] fifteen finite segment model of the human body is applied to represent a simplified model of physical handicapped body (See Fig. 3). This model consists of upper arm, forearm, hand, torso, upper leg, lower leg, foot and head. 15 segment links are the maximum and number of the links is deducted based on the availability of body parts. For a right under-knee prosthesis wear, the human body can be described by 14 finite segment model, combining right lower leg and right foot as one finite segment.

Degrees of freedom (DOF) of each link representing the fidelity of the human modeling. Determining an appropriate level of fidelity is critical. Not every DOF for the human body is considered, especially with respect to the spine and neck. For example, a complete spine (24 vertebrae with 72 DOF) may not be necessary when we consider how the spine affects the overall motion of the body. The method defines degrees of freedom by specific components in difference scenarios. In the lift task scenario, an upper-extremity segment of torso-spine-shoulder-arm is built on 15 DOF while in reaching task scenario the same body segment is built on 14 DOF without considering the one DOF of torso [14].

3.2   Joint Kinematics Optimization

Various human performance measures provide the objective functions of the optimization formulation. The most popular function is concerned about joint displacement, energy, and effort. Factored by the kinematics constraints, the optimization is firstly based on joint displacement, which is given as follows:

Joint Displacement Profile:

$$F(q) = \sum_{i=1}^{n} w_i \left(q_i - q_i^N \right) \tag{1}$$

$$\text{St: } q_i^L \leq q_i \leq q_i^U$$

Where q_i^L is neutral position of joint i, and is selected as a relatively comfortable posture, a standing position with arms at one's side. w_i is the deviation caused by the kinematics constraints for joint i and can be determined later by feed-forward network training based on motion capture data of subjects. q_i^L, q_i^U represents the upper and lower limits of ith joint angle, derived from physical constraints of human motion. They are measured by medical tests or defined by the occupational test inventory of specific tasks.

As stated above, the end-effectors' vector can be defined by specific task variables. The inverse kinematics is used to calculate q. For the serial chain and tree-structured system, the joint velocity vector within the operation space can be described as

$$\varepsilon = J(q_i)\dot{q}_i \tag{2}$$

Where, ε is the m dimension of position vector of the end-effecter and is defined by the design controller and task controller. $J(q_i) \in T_{m \times n}$, $T_{m \times n}$ is the $m \times n$ Jacobian matrix of velocity vector, m is the dimension of the end-effecter and n is DOF of joint i. $T_{m \times n}$ can be obtained by partially differentiating to the joint speed through Eqn (3)

$$\dot{q}_n^0 = R_n^0 \dot{q}_n = R_0^0 R_2^1 \cdots R_{i-1}^i \cdots R_n^{n-1} \dot{q}_n \qquad i = 1,2,\ldots\ldots, n \tag{3}$$

The Denavit and Hartenberg Representation Method (DH method) was used to sketch the coordination system of each segment link. The DH method is based on characterizing the configuration of joint i with re-spect to joint i-1 by a (4×4) homogeneous transformation matrix representing each joint's coordinate system as shown by Eqs (4).

$$R_{i-1}^i = \begin{bmatrix} \cos\theta & -\cos\alpha\sin\theta & \sin\alpha\sin\theta & a\cos\theta \\ \sin\theta & \cos\alpha\sin\theta & -\sin\alpha\cos\theta & a\sin\theta \\ 0 & \sin\alpha & \cos\alpha & d \\ 0 & 0 & 0 & 1 \end{bmatrix} \tag{4}$$

Where α, θ, d and a denote the values indicated in Fig. 4

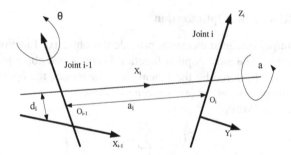

Fig. 4. The relation between two coordination systems with four parameters (α, θ, d and a)

q and $\ddot{q}$ can be obtained separately by integration and deviation to $\dot{q}$,

$$\dot{q}_i = J^+(q_i)\varepsilon \tag{5}$$

$$\ddot{q}_i = J^+(q_i)[\dot{\varepsilon} - \dot{J}(q_i)\dot{q}_i] \tag{6}$$

Where, $J^+(q_i)$ is the pseudo inverse of $J(q_i)$.

3.3   Joint Dynamic Optimization

Energy is the drive force of joint displacement while effort is a substitute to the changing posture from one point to another. Further optimization formulation is conducted to compute the factor of dynamic constraint for multi-DOF body segments.

Joint Displacement Profile:

$$F(q') = \sum_{i=1}^{n} w_i'(q_i' - q_i)^2 \tag{7}$$

To minimize:

$$\min F(\tau) = \sum_{i=1}^{n} w_i'|\tau_i| \tag{8}$$

St : $F(q_i') \in F(q_i)$

$$\tau^L \le \tau_i \le \tau_i^U$$

w_i' is the deviation caused by the physical constraints. τ_i can be calculated through Eqn (9) according to Kim et.al.[15]

$$\tau_i = M_{ik}(q_i)\ddot{q}_i + \sum J^+(q_i)m_{ik}g + \sum J^+(q_k)F_k \qquad i = 1, 2, \dots, n. \tag{9}$$

m_{ik} is the mass of link (i,k), F_k is the external force on the joint k. Joint i and k are the two joints on each side of the link (i,k). $M_{ik}(q)$ is the mass inertia of link (i,k) and can be calculated by Eqn (10):

$$M_{ik}(q) = \sum_{j=\max(i,k)}^{n} R_j \left\{ \frac{\partial T_j(q)}{\partial q_k} I_{ik} \left[\frac{\partial T_j(q)}{\partial q_i} \right]^T \right\} \qquad i,k,j = 1,2,3,...n \qquad (10)$$

I_{ik} is the mass inertia of link (i,k), $I_{ik} = \dfrac{m_{ik}l^2}{3}$.

4   Example

To validate the calculation model, the paper sets up an experiment of reaching and lifting task. Five under-knee prosthesis wearers on the right sides with varying body dimensions, age, and strength participated in the study. The task was bending the torso, reaching for a target in front of the subjects on the ground and lifting it up to overhead level (45 deg). The object is 2kg. In the Siemens Jack 6.0 human modeling was made based on the motion captured by VICON system (Qualysis MacReflex) with six cameras at 50 Hz. Twenty-one markers were attached to the subjects at pre-defined body landmarks. The landmarks were used to estimate joint center locations using custom software (VICON BodyBuilder). And the matching human modeling is made by defining the joint angle and displacement calculated based on the proposed model and realized in Jack environment as well.

Feed-forward neural network was built up to calculate the relative importance of each joint w_i and w'_i. The example extracted the values w_i and w'_i from recorded movements. The skeleton used to reproduce arm motion has 12 joints joints (neck, L/R wrist, L/R elbow, L/R shoulder and a virtual joint on the spine, L/R hip and L/R knee). Each of 12 joints has different DOF. For each DOF of every joint, a weight is computed in the dimension of time. In the scenario of lifting and overreaching task, there are 20 weight groups for all joints. The learned weights of 2-DOF knee joint (healthy side) across the task time are shown in Fig 5. The limit values of each joint on different dimensions of freedom were measured. In practice, they can also be defined by medical and occupational tests.

Task simulation of subject 5 was used to explain the validity of the model. The anthropometric data of subject 5 (See Table 1) was the input of the optimization model. Subject 5 wears prosthesis on the right side.

The study chose five postures during the task to represent the whole task process. Manipulated by the weights at each corresponding time point, the model calculated the optimization angles of 12 joints. The calculated results were put into Jack environment and a manikin was created, and compared to another manikin created by motion capture data. The prosthesis foot (right) is marked with black and white. The matching results were shown in Fig. 6. In Fig. 7, the person with yellow shirts represents the observed posture by motion data capture while blue shirt stands for the posture predicted by the model.

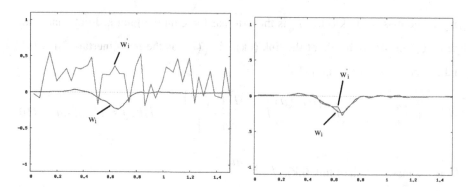

Fig. 5. The weights (a: X direction and b: Y direction) of the knee's degrees of freedom over time. The red curve represents the value of W_i and the green represents the value of w_i'.

Table 1. Anthropometric Data and Mass Properties of Subject 5

Link	Hand	Forearm	Upper arm	Torso	Upper leg	Sound leg part	Amputee
Length (m)	0.214	0.402	0.405	0.712	0.387	0.421	0.386
Mass (kg)[1]	0.55	2.02	1.46	28.88	10.32	10.64	3.92
$M(q_i)(kg \cdot m^2)$	0.001	0.012	0.011	0.294	0.172	0.184	0.210

[1] Was calculated based on the length of each link across the same mass density except for the disabled side of leg.

As Fig. 7 shows, the yellow shirt is almost overlapped with blue shirt. The most obvious mismatching between the yellow shirt and blue shirt lies in the two extreme postures: squatting and bending to the lowest and reaching overhead. Thus, further calculations were made on the two extreme postures of all five subjects. The mismatches are shown in Fig.6. The similar mismatching can also be observed on other 4 subjects. There might be at least two reasons to explain the mismatching. The variation might lie in the weight obtained from neural network training of small number of subjects. Or physical disa-bility causes big variance in modeling the task when the disabled body parts exert great effort to im-plement the task. Further study should be conducted to train weight neural network to diminish the variance across different subjects.

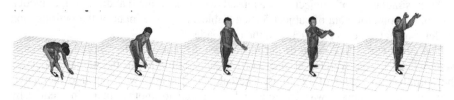

Fig. 6. Comparison of observed (yellow shirt), and predicted (blue shirt) task postures for subject 5

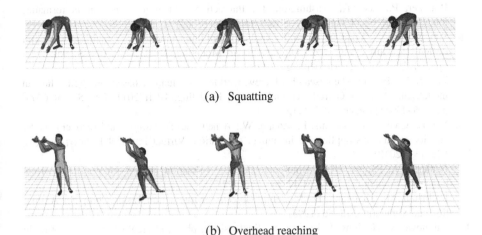

(a) Squatting

(b) Overhead reaching

Fig. 7. Comparison of captured (yellow shirt) and modeled (blue shirt) postures of all five subjects

5 Conclusion

This paper aimed to present a framework to evaluate work disability. By reproducing disabilities at three levels: effectors, kinematic and physical, the proposed model can optimize the position of the physical handicapped through motion and posture controller. Using object transferring as an example, the calculated results and observed results are simulated in Jack 6.0 to give a visual comparison. The unsatisfactory part of the results lies in the validity of the weights and simplified kinematics model with roughly estimated DOF for each joint. The future work can focus on the enhancement of our weight based constraint model by train the neural network with more samples and set up a kinematics skeleton based on careful observation of the real motion which definitely require more DOF for each body link and joint.

References

1. Badler, N.J.: Virtual Humans for Animation, Ergonomics, and Simulation. Non-rigid and Articulated Motion Workshop, pp. 28–36 (1997)
2. Porter, J.M., Case, K., Marshall, R.: Beyond Jack and Jill: designing for individuals using HADRIAN. International Journal of Industrial Ergonomics, 249–264 (2004)
3. Gomes, S., Sagot, J.C., Koukam, A.: MANERCOS, a new tool providing ergonomics in a concurrent engineering design life cycle. In: Euromedia, pp. 237–241 (1999)
4. Safework, http://www.safework.com
5. Case, K., Porter, M., Gyi, D., Marshall, R.: Virtual fitting trials in design for all. Journal of Materials Processing Tech. 117, 255–261 (2001)
6. Baek, S.-Y., Lee, K.: Paramettic human body shape modeling frame-work for human-centered product design. Computer-Aided Design 44(1), 56–67 (2012)

7. Bounker, P., Lee, T., Washington, R.: Interactive vehicle level human performance modeling. Intelligent Vehicle Systems Symposium (2003)
8. Sun, X., Gao, F., Yuan, X., Zhao, J.: Application of human modeling in multi-crew cockpit design. In: Duffy, V.G. (ed.) Digital Human Modeling, HCII 2011. LNCS, vol. 6777, pp. 204–209. Springer, Heidelberg (2011)
9. Zheng, Y., Fu, S.: The research of crew workload evaluation based on digital human model. In: Duffy, V.G. (ed.) Digital Human Modeling, HCII 2011. LNCS, vol. 6777, pp. 446–450. Springer, Heidelberg (2011)
10. Ma, L., Chablat, D., Bennis, F., Zhang, W.: A new muscle fa-tigue and recovery model and its ergonomics application in human simulation. Virtual Physical Prototyping 5(3), 123–137 (2010)
11. Badler, N.I., Palmer, M.S., Bindiganavale, R.: Animation control for real-time virtual humans. Communication ACM 42, 64–73 (1999)
12. Kallmann, M., Thalmann, D.: Modeling Objects for Interaction Tasks. Computer Animation and Simulation, 73–86 (1998)
13. Safonova, A., Hodgins, J., Pollard, N.: Synthesizing physically realistic human motion in low-dimensional behavior-specific spaces. ACM Transactions on Graphics 23(3), 514–521 (2004)
14. Rodriguez, I., Boulic, R., Meziat, D.: A Joint-level model of fatigue for the postural control of virtual humans. Journal of 3D Forum, 70–75 (2003)
15. Reed, M.P., Chaffin, D.B., Martin, B.J.: The HUMOSIM Ergonomics Framework: A New Approach to Digital Human Simulation for Ergonomic Analysis. Human Factors and Ergonomics in Manufacturing 17, 4–475 (2007)

Development of a Tendon-Driven Dexterous Hand for Fine Manipulation

Jamie Galiastro, Hao Zhang, David Ribeiro, Anthony Mele,
William Craelius, and Kang Li

Rutgers University, Piscataway, NJ 08854, USA
jdogg614@gmail.com

Abstract. This paper presents a tendon-driven dexterous hand capable of object manipulation. This dexterous hand is anatomically sound and mimics the musculoskeletal structure of human fingers including the passive mechanism, bone geometry, tendon network. One of the key features of this prosthetic hand is the ability to perform fine finger manipulation motions such as holding a pen with two fingers and rotating the pen. With this feature the user of the prosthesis will be potentially capable of performing a wider range of motions and tasks, which is the key feature missing from current commercially prosthetic hand available today. Some of these tasks can include holding utensils, performing fine manipulation movements in manufacturing settings, as well as many other tasks to greatly assist the user of the prosthesis.

Keywords: Tendon-Driven, Fine Manipulation, Dexterous Hand.

1 Introduction

Limb loss presents a serious healthcare problem in the United States. It was estimated that every year 185,000 persons had an limb amputation [1]. In 2005, around 1.6 million people with limb loss were living within this country and half a million had the loss of an upper limb. The number of persons living with limb loss is expected to be doubled over the next forty years. These amputees are desperate to restore their upper limb functions and improve the quality of life.

Dexterity of the human hand is a fundamental attribute that enables one to touch, press, or manipulate objects, and to convey information through gesture. The arm is a complex biomechanical system consisting of 27 bones, 39 muscles, and over 30 degrees of freedom (DOF's), possessed mostly by the fingers [2]. The fingers are so vital that amputation at the metacarpophalangeal (MCP) joints is considered to be 54% impairment of an entire person [3]. The number of possible motions and positions that can be created by the hand is vast, [4] yet individuals are able to control this complex system with amazing ease and efficiency.

The loss of manual dexterity from amputation limits fundamental activities of daily living (ADL) such as eating, dressing, driving a car, writing or typing, playing music, telephone usage, equipment operation, and self-care.

V.G. Duffy (Ed.): DHM 2014, LNCS 8529, pp. 527–534, 2014.
© Springer International Publishing Switzerland 2014

Present-day prostheses can restore relatively limited functionality to upper limb amputees, primarily grasping with a prehensile hand and elbow function. Manipulation and intuitive versatile control are still beyond the reach of current prostheses. In fact, the most commonly used UL prosthesis today uses a split hook for grasping, a device which was first patented in 1912 [5]. A more advanced control option is available, using 'myoelectric' control, but this too only offers a prehensile (open-closing) function. Restoring normal upper-limb functionality thus remains a major challenge for the prosthetic field.

In this paper, we presented a novel prosthetic hand, which mimics the tendon and bone structure information of the index finger and simplifies the thumb and middle, ring, and little fingers. It has realistic bone segments, realistic tendon network and is easily modifiable and maintained. We also developed a structure to mimic the passive properties, which has been demonstrated to play a major role in control of hand movement [6]. In addition, we developed a Kinect sensor-based gesture recognition system enabling the artificial hand to follow human gestures. We demonstrated that this artificial hand was able to perform a wider range of tasks.

2   Design

The structure of our artificial hand consists of three essential components consisting of the fingers, palm, and forearm. Each component is responsible for serving various operations in the building of the hand. Figure 1 is an overall view of the hand structure:

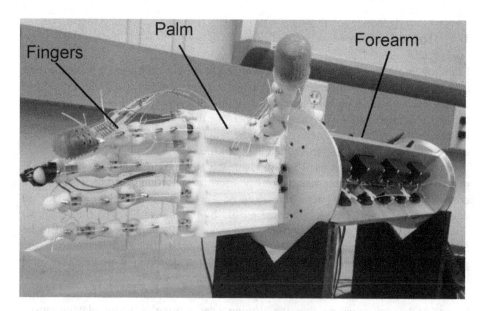

Fig. 1. Overview of the prosthetic hand

The fingers are the most essential component of this artificial hand, which are made of a poly-plastic using 3D printing (Figure 2). The segments of each finger are connected together with custom made sub-miniature hinges. The hinges are custom manufactured in order to set the correct degrees of freedom, allowing the finger segments to be the correct distance apart, and allowing the fingers to move in a realistic manner.

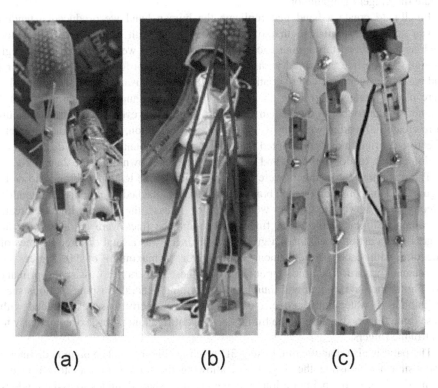

Fig. 2. Muscle tendon structure of the artificial fingers: (a) thumb (b) index finger (c) middle, ring, and little fingers

In order to create fingers that accurately represent the human hand three additional factors needed to be taken into consideration including degrees of freedom, passive property, and tendon webbing configuration.

The index finger was produced to accurately mimic the human hand. The index finger was given four degrees of freedom, with the exclusion of movement backwards, because 15 degree movement towards the back of the hand added very little to the capabilities to the hand. By having four degrees of freedom the index finger is capable of accurately replicating the movement of the human index finger. The thumb had the same number of degrees of freedom as a human thumb would have.

Additionally, the passive property of these two fingers was taken into consideration. In order to obtain fine finger control, the human hand deploys a mechanism called the passive property. This property ensures when a finger moves in any direction that it will return to a neutral position once the tendons and muscles pulling on it have become in a relaxed state. To replicate this process and obtain fine finger control we implemented a system of elastic cord strategically located within four different spots on each finger. The four pieces of elastic cord were located on the front, back, and both sides of the bone segment closest to the palm. By implementing the passive property into our system, we were capable of obtaining further control of these two fingers to create fine finger manipulation.

Finally, to create a hand that replicate the human hand we produced a tendon driven actuation, similar to that of the human hand with replication of how the tendons are webbed throughout each finger. The tendons were recreated using high strength fishing line that could withstand a large amount of force through the pulling and passive property needed to control the fingers. Also, custom manufactured guides were placed strategically along all sides of the finger to guide the fishing line in a manner similar to that of the human hand. The thumb, however, is extremely difficult to re-create the tendon webbing so through experimentation, a simple but extremely effective configuration was adapted that provided the amount of control desired. The tendon guides, tendon webbing, and passive property is shown in Figure 2a and 2b.

The remaining three fingers were controlled with simple tendon webbing shown in Figure 2c. This consisted of each bone segment being attached to an individual tendon directly to a servo motor that would pull or release the fishing line to create movement. Similar to the index finger and thumb the lines were guided along the fingers with custom made tendon guides. Each finger was a total of three degrees of freedom, with each bone segment being given a maximum of 90 degrees of movement forward. The sole responsibility of these fingers is to assist the primary two digits (the index finger and thumb) in performing general grasping motions such as grabbing a water bottle, cube, etc. The passive property was not included with these three fingers; because of the limited degrees of freedom it was extremely easy to control the fingers.

The palm is also manufactured using 3D printing (Figure 1). The palm is distinctly responsible for assisting the fingers and allowing the routing to smoothly operate. Along the front of the palm are long rectangular tube shaped guides to assist tendons in a linear path. The back of the palm has a similar configuration as the front to also assist those tendons in running along a linear path. Also along the back of the palm knuckles are present to limit the degrees of freedom that each finger is capable of moving. Holes are strategically placed along the knuckles to assist in tendon routing, as well as custom made screws with miniature holes manufactured to along guidance of the tendons. On the front of the palm there is a platform set at a 60 degree angle to place the thumb to accurately resemble a human thumb.

Although the palm that is used does not appear to look like a human palm, it does consist of parts that are present to replicate the actions and limitations of a human hand. Unlike, a human hand, our palm is completely stationary, however, the movement of the palm is very difficult to replicate, and does not offer enough to warrant attention and budget when aiming for the achievement of fine finger manipulation.

The forearm is responsible for hosting the servos that produce the movement of the fingers. There are four separate plates found between the two lids of the forearm shown in Figure 1. Two plates are manufactured to host smaller and less powerful servos that control the middle, ring, and little fingers and two host the powerful servos for controlling the index finger and thumb. The servos were placed directly in the servo of each of the plates to ensure that a casing could fit onto the structure without running into the servo arms. By placing the servos where they are placed it allows us to compact our structure while keeping our design extremely organized and easy to perform maintenance on any tendons or improperly working servos if needed. The entire forearm is built to be encased with an acrylic case to protect the servos and tendons from being manipulated in any manner.

The servos are controlled with a Mini Maestro 24 channel micro controller (MM). Each pin set in capable of individual pulse width modulation (PWM) and can be issued commands via serial communications.

An inverse kinematics based method is used for finger control. Given an effector position, we determine the excursions of all the tendons and then convert them to the angles the servos should move.

As the artificial hand interacts with objects, the necessary finger positions to negotiate the particular shape as well as are saved as a learned motion pattern and can be reloaded if a similar object is encountered.

For the artificial hand to hold an object without damaging it, the hand needs to be able to sense the amount of pressure it exerts on the object. Two pressure sensors which are able to sense between 1 and 100psi of pressure, are layered into latex finger tips of the index finger and thumb. In addition, force requirements and limits can also be stored so that appropriate values are used in future encounters with the same object.

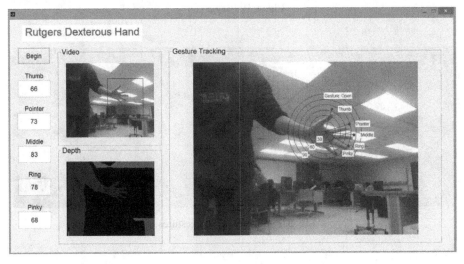

Fig. 3. Manual Control GUI

In order to generate different hand gestures, we also create a gesture library including Rock&Roll, Fist, Open, Peace, Trident, Fork, and Thumbs up signs. To demonstrate the gesture generation capability, we also develop a manual control GUI (Figure 3) to recognize the hand gesture of a human being using the Kinect Sensor so that our artificial hand can follow the movement of a real hand movement. To quickly identify gestures, the algorithm uses the number extended fingers and the distances between each finger and the centroid.

3   Result

The prototype has fine digit control, including pinching, gripping and twirling between thumb and index finger. In Figure 4, it is shown that this hand is rolling a pen. Figure 6 shows this hand following human gestures. Figure 5 shows that the hand can pick a screw driver, cube, and hold a cylinder.

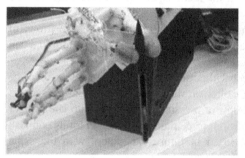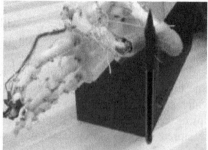

Fig. 4. Rolling a pen

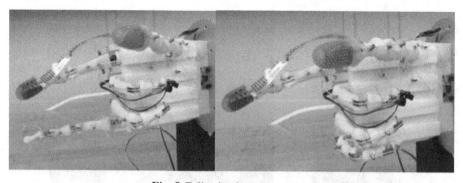

Fig. 5. Following human gestures

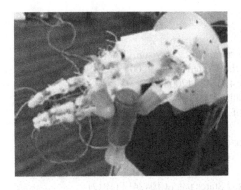
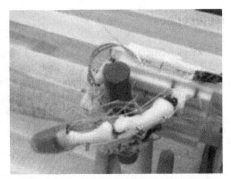
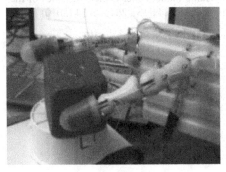

Fig. 6. Picking a screwdriver, cube and grasping a cylinder

4   Conclusion

We have developed a dexterous hand capable of performing fine finger manipulation. Currently on the market and research laboratories across the world there is an inability to perform fine finger manipulation with individual control of each finger making our hand extremely unique. This hand has the ability to significantly improve the quality of life for amputees by allowing them to perform common daily tasks much easier.

We plan to develop more rigorous control schemes to drive the movement of this artificial as well as the control interface between the hand and a real amputee.

Acknowledgements. This work was supported in part by the Department of Industrial and Systems Engineering of Rutgers University, the NASA-New Jersey Space Grant Consortium (NJSGC), and the NSF (CNS 1229628 and NSF CMMI 1334389).

References

1. Ziegler-Graham, K., MacKenzie, E.J., Ephraim, P.L., Travison, T.G., Brookmeyer, R.: Estimating the prevalence of limb loss in the United States: 2005 to 2050. Archives of Physical Medicine and Rehabilitation 89(3), 422–429 (2008)
2. Tubiana, R.: The Hand. Saunders, Philadelphia (1981)
3. Engelberg, A.: Guides to the evaluation of permanent impairment, 3rd edn. American Medical Association, Chicago (1988)
4. Soechting, J.F., Flanders, M.: Flexibility and repeatability of finger movements during typing: Analysis of multiple degrees of freedom. Journal of Computational Neuroscience 4(1), 29–46 (1997)
5. Dorrance, D.: Inventor Artificial Hand. United States patent 1042413 (1912)
6. Li, K., Zhang, X.: A probabilistic finger biodynamic model better depicts the roles of the flexors during unloaded flexion. Journal of Biomechanics 43(13), 2618–2624 (2010)

Mobile Navigation for Limited Mobility Users

Bettina Harriehausen-Muhlabauter

Computer Science Department, University of Applied Sciences
Darmstadt, 69121, Germany
bettina.harriehausen@h-da.de

Abstract. Modern information technology can improve life in many places and situations in our society. This includes the improvement and simplification of life for people with special needs. We have developed a mobile navigation tool called Wheel Scout, which combines modern mobile information technology, such as smartphones and their programming, with existing navigational technology, meeting the goal to serve specific needs for people with special needs. In comparison toexisting tools, we concentrate on barrier-free routes rather than barrier-free buildings and our enhancements include: (a) the marking of barriers on a chosen route, (b) an intelligent computation of a detour in case the chosen route contains barriers, (c) the customization of the app by defining your personal profile(s), (d) the opportunity to include both static as well as temporary barriers, and (e) a high degree of interactivity which enhances the app steadily.

Keywords: Mobile navigation, Calculation of barrier-free walkways, Customization based on degree of impairment, Mobile insertion of static and temporary barriers, Enhancement through interactivity.

1 Introduction

Steep ramps, stairs, bouldering and other uneven footpath surfacing are often insurmountable barriers for the mobile handicapped or wheelchair users. On the basis of the geographical data of OpenStreetMap [4], we have developed a mobile navigation app which enables mobility impaired people to navigate from A to B on a barrier-free route. In addition to commonly known features of navigation systems, we are using the points of interest (POI) feature and their geo dataset to add barriers to the maps. Therefore, according to our definition, POIs are not tourist sights, gas stations or restaurants, but rather geographical positions that mark barriers for the mobile handicapped, such as steep ramps, narrow passages, staircases or uneven surfaces, or temporary barriers, such as fallen trees or construction sites.

2 Research and Related Work

During our initial research, we started by investigating commonly used GPS navigation systems with regard to their functionalities as well as their open interfaces

V.G. Duffy (Ed.): DHM 2014, LNCS 8529, pp. 535–545, 2014.

to add individual enhancements. We found that recent developments for the computing of a route have extended the choice of transportation to pedestrians but none of the popular systems (TomTom [1], Garmin [2], Google Maps [3] or OpenStreetMap [4] currently support features for wheelchair users or handicapped people.

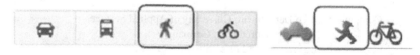

Fig. 1. Choice of pedestrian routing in GOOGLE maps and OpenStreetMap

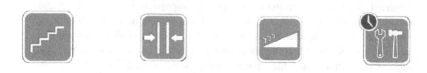

Fig. 2. Icons for barriers (stairs, narrow passage, incline, temporary construction site)

Besides looking at those popular navigation systems, we investigated several wheelchair navigation and support systems and found that they all differ heavily in their functionalities as well as their product status. Excellent tools, such as WheelMap [5], focus on barrier-free buildings rather than routes, and systems with a similar focus to ours, such as Rollstuhlrouting.de [6] or EasyWheel [7] haven't left their prototype-status yet or do not cover all of the features that we have focused on. After a general research regarding related work, we concentrated our research and the following design of the system on direct contact and interviews with wheelchair users. This led us to the definition of the following barriers, which can be added to the map by the users interactively: stairs, narrow passages, ramps, and various insurmountable surfacing. We have developed self-explanatory icons for all of those barriers. In addition to statics barriers, users can also add temporary barriers (marked by a red clock symbol), such as fallen trees or temporary construction sites. Presently, these temporary POIs are being automatically removed from the map after 2 days, unless another user renews its existence.

3   Design

We are using the traffic light metaphor to mark the selected paths according to the feature of being passable or not, i.e. whether they are barrier-free or not. In our app, "passable" is either defined by a standard profile or can individually be defined by the user, as certain barriers may cause difficulties for some users but not others; i.e. several members in our testing group were able to climb staircases with several stairs, whereas others would not be able to mount low steps. In case the path is barrier-free, it is marked as a green route from S (start) to Z (goal, German: Ziel). A path marked yellow contains barriers, which may cause difficulties for certain people but not others, i.e. the user can individually decide whether or not s/he wants to select that route.

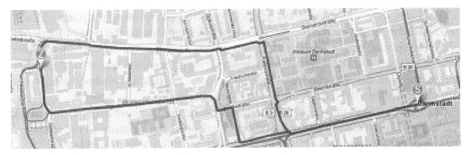

Fig. 3. Marking of routes (green: barrier-free, yellow: route includes surmountable barriers, red: route includes barriers)

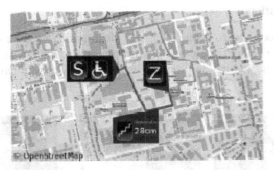

Fig. 4. Display of a barrier (staircase with steps of 28cm height) along a selected route (red) and computed barrier-free detour (green)

In case the app detects a barrier along the shortest route, that route will be marked red and a barrier-free (green) alternative will be computed automatically.

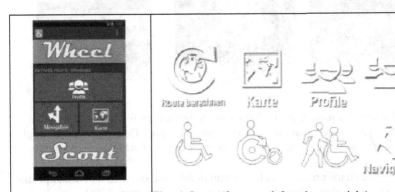

Fig. 5. Wheel Scout GUI

Fig. 6. Icons (from top left to bottom right): compute a route, show map, show profile, add a profile, active wheelchair, electric wheelchair, wheelchair with companion, navigation

In all cases, the user can always select to view the barrier along the route and will be shown the details for the barrier, which includes the icon on the type of barrier as first information, but in addition also text which specifies the barrier, such as the number of stairs and the height of the stairs. In case a photo was added for the barrier before, the user can also choose to view that photo. All this information helps to decide whether or not the barrier can be surmounted or not.

The look & feel of the app is designed so it can be used without major explanations and each GUI is held very simple without overloaded functionalities. The icons we developed for the barriers (see ch. 2) and the functionalities are self-explanatory:

4   Functionalities

4.1   Customization

For users who choose not to define their individual profile, we have predefined three standard profiles (Fig.7a), one for active wheelchair users, the second one for users of electric wheelchairs, and the third one for wheelchair users who have a companion, who helps them to move.

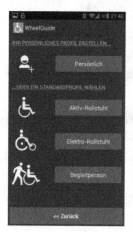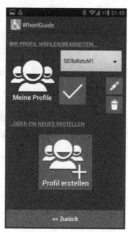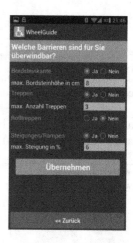

Fig. 7. (a) Selection of a profile, (b) Definition of an addition profile, (c) Customization of individual profile, here: Which barriers are surmountable for you? Curbstone with its height, stairs with the number of steps, escalators, ramps and their degree of incline

Beyond these standard profiles, each user can define one or more individual profile (Fig.7b). Our users' feedback has shown that not only do the individual profiles vary on a daily basis, but the range of what is regarded as a barrier can vary tremendously among wheelchair users of the same type of wheelchair. Some users were able to climb staircases with a relative high number of steps, others would already consider low steps unsurmountable. Our app guides the user through the definition of an individual profile (Fig.7c).

4.2   The Marking of Barriers

We distinguish between two types of barriers: permanent and temporary barriers. Examples for permanent barriers are staircases and ramps, temporary barriers can be temporary construction sites which make a passage unpassable, fallen trees or surface conditions due to temporary weather conditions, e.g. icy roads. Once a temporary barrier is included into the map, it will be automatically removed after two days, unless it is re-entered by the same or another user.

Permanent Barriers. There are three possibilities for permanent barriers to appear in the app:

1. they are predefined by OSM,
2. we include them into the OSM maps before distribution by using the POI feature and current GPS position to include a "point of interest", i.e. one of our barriers, or
3. the second option is performed by one of our users interactively, i.e. the app and its correctness of barriers will grow by using it.

Temporary Barriers. There are two possibilities for temporary barriers to appear in the app:

1. they are interactively included by users when they see or experience a temporary barrier, or
2. they are included by the road traffic licensing departments of cities which decide to use the app as a means to receive and distribute data about temporary barriers.[1]

4.3   Interactivity

The marking of barriers, and thus the correctness and completeness of the app, depends to a high degree on the interactivity of the users. When experiencing or seeing a permanent or temporary barrier that is not included in the app yet, the user can include it by using the GUI shown in Fig.9, which asks to report and include a barrier (German: Barriere melden), to specify the type of barrier (German: Barrierenart), here: ramp, to specify more detailed information on the barrier (German: Steigung in %), here: the degree of incline, and to optionally take a picture of the barrier, so future users can decide upon the picture whether or not the barrier will cause difficulties. In case of a ramp, the user may decide, and later see, the image in Fig.8.

After the new barrier is added to the app, its position is marked on the map with the corresponding icon. Upon selection (touch or roll-over) the additional textual information is given, as well as a thumbnail image of the barrier, in case a picture was previously added. In that case, the image can be enlarged.

---

[1] Note: In Germany, temporary barriers, such as temporary construction sites, have to be reported to the city's road traffic licensing department before the barrier is set up. But of course, barriers such as fallen trees cannot be reported beforehand.

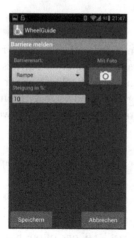

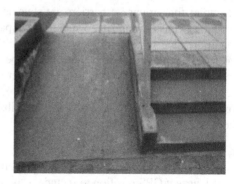

Fig. 8. Reporting and adding a new barrier-information

Fig. 9. Image of a ramp taken by a user and added to the POI-barrier

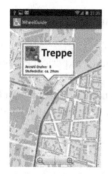

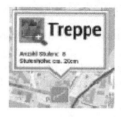

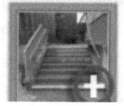

Fig. 10. Information that is displayed for each barrier upon request (here: staircase with the number and height of stairs, as well as image)

4.4   Computation of Individual, Barrier-Free Routes

The basis of our route computation is provided by the free navigation tool Open-StreetMap (OSM), which provides map data for locations worldwide. Independent of Wheel Guides functionalities, users can use OSM to compute an individually chosen route, depending on their means of transportation (e.g. by car, by bicycle, by foot). As Wheel Guide users will never choose highways or big country roads without foot-paths along the side as their routes, those are blocked in our algorithm. We use OSM's information on barriers as well as our added barriers to computer the shortest possible path for each user depending on his profile. In case an unsurmountable barrier is detected on the shortest path, that path will be marked red, the barriers will be displayed and a barrier-free detour will be computed and shown as a green route. In case barriers are detected which may cause difficulty, but the user should decide whether or not they can be handled, the routes will be displayed in yellow color and the barriers are displayed with all information that is available in our database.

5   Implementation and Technology

5.1   HTML5

In a first step, we started developing the app for Android platforms, but soon found that this was an unacceptable limitation, as the mobile market is much too diverse and dominated by at least 4 "key players": Android phones, Apple's iPhones with iOS, RIM's Blackberry and Windows Phones. And apart from the mobile market, we also wanted to offer our navigation tool to users without smartphones and to those in general who want to compute their routes from their homes. Therefore, we have chosen to develop an HTML5 website which makes it possible to inform users without smartphones about barriers and to plan routes from home. In addition, it saved us development time, which we would have had to invest if we had chosen to develop the app for all available platforms natively. By having chosen HTML5, all users can access our app, even if their smartphone is not natively supported, as they can use the browser alternative instead. This way, the web version of our app can be used via browsers on hardware which we do not explicitly support.

5.2   Open Street Map

We have chosen OpenStreetMap (OSM) [4] as the underlying map, as its interfaces enable us to add data to the existing maps, i.e. our barriers as "points of interest", and we can access its data, which enables us to extract the information that we need to compute ideal routes for our individual wheelchair user. The data that we extract from OSM includes ways and their nodes, as well as all barriers, such as steps, inclines, curbstones and the nature of the ground, such as soil conditions. All these data are needed to check which ways and nodes exist and which ones are passable according to the user's profile. The ways and nodes include feature-value pairs, called tags. Examples of such tags are: `surface=cobblestone`, `surface=grass`, `smoothness=intermediate`, `incline=*`, and `width=*`, including the gradient of the incline in percent or the width of a passage in meters[2]. The tags are accessed via the Overpass API [8], which returns custom selected parts of the OSM map data. It acts as a database over the web: the client sends a query to the API and gets back the data set that corresponds to the query [9].

An XML file is being returned which is loaded by the server and used in the next processing step in which the single nodes and ways from the file are translated into Java objects which contain the ID of the objects and their information about barriers as a key-value-pattern. An example for an entry for a staircase could be highway[3] = steps and step_count = 5 for 5 steps. When a user sends a route computation query,

---

[2] The complete list of tags we use from OSM can be looked up here:
http://wiki.openstreetmap.org/wiki/DE:Rollstuhlfahrer-
Routing#Tags_f.C3.Bcrs_Routing

[3] The OSM attribute *highway* is used for any way that is developed, as opposed to dirt tracks or trails.

these data are compared with the user's profile by the route computation algorithm in order to check which ways and nodes are passable or not.

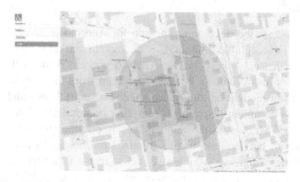

Fig. 11. Marking of the position based on the IP address only

5.3   GPS

The entire computation of the routes, the detours and the barriers is based on GPS data which is provided by HTML5's geolocation functions, which include functions for error handling, the availability of the location functions, and the query of the position. When the latter is called from the mobile device, the current GPS data is sent. In case the app is used via a browser, the position is estimated by means of the device's IP address and the possibly existing WLAN signal. In cases where only the IP address is known, the accuracy of the position is not very exact and can only be shown for a general region, e.g. metropolitan area of a city, meaning an accuracy of approximately 25-150 km.

In cases where we have a WLAN signal known by Google, an accuracy of approximately 0.5 m is theoretically possible. Our experience and tests have shown that the accuracy in a large city is usually between 30 and 75 m. But because we only need to access these possibilities when no GPS signal is available, this scenario is limited to stationary computers in residential homes. In these cases a vague positioning doesn't cause problems, as the user doesn't need to find or locate his position on a map, as he knows where he lives, but it's rather used to simplify the use of the map.

When using the web-version of Wheel Guide, the browser will ask for permission, each time the position is being computed. With the mobile version this step happens automatically, as the app will be permanently authorized to access the GPS function upon download.

5.4   Computation of Routes and Barrier Handling

The most prominent feature of our app is the handling of barriers and the resulting computation and drawing of a barrier-free route. In order to check whether the chosen route contains barriers, we compare the list of tags and values which exist for each node and way with the individual profile of the user (shown on the left of Fig. 13). This will tell us whether the route is passable and barrier-free (drawn as a green route) or not.

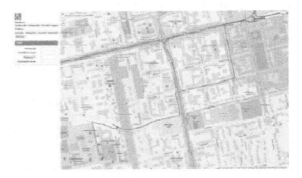

Fig. 12. Computing and drawing a route based on a profile which allows 1 step (German: Stufenanzahl), widths of 735 cm (German: Rollstuhlbreite in mm), an incline gradient of 6% (German: Steigung in %), and curb heights of 30 mm (German: Bordsteinhöhe in mm

We are using the Dijkstra-algorithm [10] to compute the optimal route for our users. This algorithm computes the shortest path for a given start-node and one (or more) target-nodes, in our case the goal or location the user wants to travel to.

In OSM and our database an intersection is called node and a street or path is called way.

First, the start- and target-nodes are determined by selecting the nodes from our database which are closest to the selected start- and target-nodes. Starting from these (database) nodes, the algorithm will check for the next nearest nodes. These will be connected by ways. In case the connecting way is impassable for wheelchair users due to barriers, this node will be ignored. For all nodes that can be reached on a barrier-free way, the distance between the nodes will be computed and stored for further computation.

Once the distances between the start node and all reachable nodes are stored in the reachable nodes, the start node will be marked off as „visited" and will be ignored until the goal node is reached. The following steps will then be processed in this order:

1. Look for the node with the shortest distance and which hasn't been visited yet.
2. Compute the distances to all reachable nodes and record the distance in case no value has been entered yet or the distance is shorter than the previous value.
3. Return to step 1. until the node with the lowest value and which hasn't been visited yet, is the target-node.

This process will be repeated twice in order to compute a green and a yellow or red path. After first trying to find a green path, the process will be repeated for a yellow or red route. The yellow route will include the user's profile data for yellow routes, i.e. barriers, which are surmountable for some users or under certain circumstances. In case barriers are detected along the chosen route, they will be buffered in the data for that route in order to be retrieved and included in the app later upon request of the user. At that stage, the user can decide individually, whether the barriers are surmountable for him or not. When computing and drawing a red route we do not include profile data, as those routes are not surmountable under any circumstances and the app will always draw the shortest route.

```
public void pathDraw() {

    StrictMode.ThreadPolicy policy = new
    StrictMode.ThreadPolicy.Builder().permitAll().build();
    StrictMode.setThreadPolicy(policy);

    road = new Road(pRouteGet());
    PathOverlay pathOverlay = RoadManager.buildRoadOverlay(road,
    mapView.getContext());

    pathCalculate();

    switch (pType.charAt(0)) {
        case 'G':
            pathOverlay.setColor(Color.GREEN);
            break;
        case 'T':
            pathOverlay.setColor(Color.YELLOW);
            break;
        case 'R':
            pathOverlay.setColor(Color.RED);
            break;
    }
    Paint pPaint = pathOverlay.getPaint();
    pPaint.setStrokeWidth((float) (pPaint.getStrokeWidth() + 2.0));
    pPaint.setAntiAlias(true);
    ;
    pathOverlay.setPaint(pPaint);

    mapView.getOverlays().add(pathOverlay);
    mapView.invalidate();
}
```

Fig. 13. Pathdraw function – drawing routes in different colors according to the computed passability for the individual user

Depending on the result of this computation process, the function *pathdraw* [see Fig. 13] will draw the computed route in the appropriate color:

6   Testing

During the entire process of the design and development, we worked closely together with a group of wheelchair users. Their constant feedback enabled us to find bugs and optimize the app appropriately.

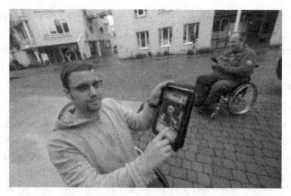

Fig. 14. Wheelchair users testing the Wheel Guide app

7   Conclusions and Next Steps

The initial feedback from users after the app was launched showed us that we were on the right track. The community of Wheelchair users responded very positively and together we have defined more functionalities, which we have started to build into Wheel Scout. These include: barrier-free toilets along the routes and specific locations (e.g. pharmacies, bakeries, banks), which the user may individually choose to be included and shown along the chosen route.

References

1. TomTom, TomTom Navigation app für Android (2014),
   http://www.tomtom.com/de_de/products/car-navigation/tomtom-navigation-for-android/ (last access June 02, 2014)
2. Garmin, Garmin Straßennavigation (2014),
   http://www.garmin.com/de-DE/explore/ontheroad (last access June 02, 2014)
3. Google Maps, Google Maps für Android, http://www.google.de/mobile/maps/ (last access June 06, 2014)
4. OpenStreetMap, http://www.openstreetmap.org/ (last access August 6, 2013)
5. Wheelmap, Wheelmap project, http://wheelmap.org/ (last access August 6, 2013)
6. Rollstuhlrouting, Rollstuhlrouting project (2013),
   http://www.rollstuhlrouting.de/ (last access August 6, 2013)
7. Menkens, C., et al.: EasyWheel - A Mobile Social Navigation and Support System for Wheelchair Users. In: Proceedings 2011 Eighth International Conference on Information Technology: New Generations, Las Vegas, Nevada USA, April 11-13 (2011)
8. Overpass API, http://overpass-api.de/ (last access December 6, 2013)
9. Overpass API, http://wiki.openstreetmap.org/wiki/Overpass_API (last access December 6, 2013)
10. Dijkstra Algorithm last access (2013),
    http://en.wikipedia.org/wiki/Dijkstra%27s_algorithm (December 6, 2013)

Analysis of Luria Memory Tests
for Development on Mobile Devices

J.A. Hijar Miranda[1], Erika Hernàndez Rubio[1], and Amilcar Meneses Viveros[2]

[1] Instituto Politécnico Nacional, SEPI-ESCOM, México D.F.
[2] Departamento de Computación, CINVESTAV-IPN, México D.F.

Abstract. Specialist in mental health and neuropsychology apply tests
to patients to evaluate impairment level of people cortical functions.
Luria tests are designed to treat defects caused by local lesions that
may affect the higher functions of the man. In particular, Luria test
study the memory and intellectual processes. An application of Luria test
is determinate the level of memory impairment. An example of suffers
of memory impairment are older adults. The application efficiency of
Luria memory tests in older adults decreases owing to biological factor
such as inability moving to place of performance testing. In addition,
there are a great demand for health services compared with the number
specialist capable of addressing mental deterioration. This increases the
complexity of control and monitoring patients. A solution for the problem
of application efficiency of Luria tests is a digital implementation of the
Luria tests on mobile devices, taking advantages of the characteristic
of mobile computing. This solution requires an analysis of the Luria
memory tests considerate the HCI factors, the different mobile interfaces,
the elements of interaction of mobile devices and in the case study of older
adults, the special considerations for this kind of people.

Keywords: Luria memory test, mobile devices, older adults, mobile interfaces, HCI factors, collaborative systems.

1 Introduction

Specialists in mental health apply many test to patients to evaluate impairment
level of people cortical functions [1]. Luria tests aim to find the fundamental
defects that are caused by local lesions in the brain. According to the general
approach of A. R. Luria in [2], Luria tests are directed to the study of motor functions, visual functions, hearing functions, functions of language, writing,
reading, calculus operations and memory and intellectual processes. There are
variants of the Luria tests, such as WAIS test, used to measure the IQ, and Neuropsi test, which proposes a scale to interpret results of evaluations of cognitive
functions [3].

An application of Luria tests is determinate the level of memory impairment
in patients who have decreased their memory functions [4]. For example, suffers
of memory impairment are older adults. Ageing causes physical limitations that

V.G. Duffy (Ed.): DHM 2014, LNCS 8529, pp. 546–557, 2014.

affect quality of life of people, such as decreased visual and hearing abilities, reduced mobility of hands and fingers, decreased attention and reasoning abilities and memory impairment. [5] [6] [7]. For example in Mexico, approximately, 8.6% of older adults have memory impairment [8]. Therefore, it's possible apply the Luria tests to older adults to determinate their level of memory impairment.

The application efficiency of Luria memory tests decreases in older adults owing to biological factors that are pertaining to the human body such as genre, age, and race [1] [9]. For example, inability or difficulty moving to the place of performance of testing, or difficulty in solving the test due to visual deterioration or motor skills. Another problem that has been detected is the coverage to meet the demand for health services. Few health centres and specialists capable of addressing mental deterioration. Each specialist can have a significant number of patients who must apply the tests, which increases the complexity of monitoring patients. In particular, specialists apply the tests and take control and monitoring traditional and face shape (pencil, paper and paper files). One solution is to provide a software tool to assist in this process and have the flexibility to take advantage of mobile technologies.

A solution to the problem of the application efficiency of Luria tests is a digital implementation of the Luria tests on mobile devices. Taking the mobility advantages of this devices, with a mobile system the users can use this tool every time and every place, only if they have an internet connection [10]. This solves the problem of patients mobility. In addition, mobile devices have interaction elements such as touchscreen, microphone, speaker and camera, etc, which providing usability to user [10].

In this paper, we focus in an analysis of Luria tests applied in the research of memory processes and the feasibility of implementation on mobile devices. In addition, it's considerate the analysis for case study of older adults including the terms of interface design and usability for these kind of people [11] [12].

2 Related Work

Currently, there are software tools oriented to treating memory impairment. For example, in the *Sistema Interactivo de Ejercitación de Memoria para Personas Mayores de 50 años*, an implementation of an interactive system was perform, which present Beta-IIR and WAIS test for treating the memory impairment. The system is composed for a web application and a local application in a PC [13]. Another example is *ACTIVAMENTE*, it's a stimulation of cognitive activity software developed to prevent or intervene the memory impairment. *ACTIVA-MENTE* has 4800 different exercises and use multimedia elements such as text, sounds and images. It was developed by *Neuroinnovation* enterprise, dedicated to cognitive functions research. Today, it's a system only for PC [14].

3   Luria Tests in the Research of Memory Processes

In neurology and psychology research related with disturbances of the higher cortical functions caused by local lesions of the brain, cognitive, motor or symbolic impairments stand frequently [2].

According with A. R. Luria, the fundamental task of the study of cortical functions is to highlight the fundamental flaw of local brain lesions. From this defect, resulting secondary systematic alterations, thus closer to the explanation of the syndrome that is the result of the primary defect. By this way, the clinical-psychology research can help to brain lesions diagnosis and form and essential part in the general system of clinical research patient. Exist many methods focused to the accomplishment of this task, which constitute the appearance of research neuropsychology methods of patient. In this methods, there are the Luria tests sets directed to the study of motor functions, visual functions, hearing functions, functions of language, writing, reading, calculus operations and *memory and intellectual processes* [2].

In particular, the study of memory processes is one of the most developed parts of the clinical-psychology research and has a particularly great significance for the analysis of the pathological alterations of the psychic processes [4] [2] [9]. The research method of memory processes, that has a particularly importance for the clinical study, are presented in this analysis [2].

4   Interfaces in Mobile Devices

Today, use of mobile devices has increased significantly with the appear of many kind of smartphones and tablets which operate with different platforms oriented to mobile computing [15].

Use of mobile devices has also led to research in the Human Computer Interaction (HCI) area to improve the interaction and users experience on mobile devices, through the different elements of interaction and the types of interfaces that can be leveraged.

Some HCI researchers, are looking for ways to provide computer systems with natural forms of communication, in order to provide the human computer interaction. There are a wide range of development of techniques for mobile devices interaction, which seek to make better use of user capabilities. When the users interact with mobile applications have a limited number of interaction styles available that can take advantage [16]. This interactions is shown below [17]:

- *Hearing interfaces*: From the point of view of mobile interaction design, the audio input and output between the user and device is very attractive and provides a more natural user experience.
- *Haptic interfaces*: The mobile phones have haptic interfaces that are very simple, such a "vibration mode" or touchscreen technologies that allow users to interact directly on the device screen with different finger movements that are interpreted as signals to perform some action.

– *Gestural interfaces*: Research on gesture goes from simple to complicated movements of the device head movement (Augmented Reality), which provide a practical way to enter information.

An important characteristic of mobile devices that are involves in the creation of interfaces is the display [19] According with [20], mobile devices are used under a wide range of environmental conditions with different lighting, which is usually brighter than the brightness of the mobile device display, and this causes that the user cannot visualize correctly what is on the device screen. The tablets and smartphones tend to be held by users at different angles that collect more light from the natural environment unlike desktop computers and laptops that have a vertical orientation. The contrast, the visibility and legibility of the screen depend on the combination of display brightness and reflection on the screen. As greater is the brightness and lower is the screen reflection the better visualizes the contents of the screen [20].

Exist different sizes and resolution for mobile displays [15] [19]. The table 1 shows the classification resolution of Android mobile devices since smartphone to tablet [20]. In this paper, the display considerations are based on the classification shown in the table 1 because the Android platform is open.

Table 1. Resolution of Android mobile devices. From [20].

Screen size	Resolution
Small	426 x 320
Normal	470 x 320
Large	640 x 480
Extra-Large	960 x 720

5 Analysis of Luria Memory Tests for Mobile Devices

According with Steve Love, Human Computer Interaction (HCI) refers to the study of interaction between users and computer systems and applications of everyday life. From this HCI study, exist the concept of Human Centered Design (HCD), which seek the greater usability in an application. Usability refers if an applications is easy to learn, easy to use and friendly to use for final users. Usability is a essential factor in the design of different products, including applications for mobile devices [16] [18].

The analysis of Luria memory tests is performed for the purpose of granting an alternative general implementation of these tests on mobile devices, from point of view of HCI and HCD, considering elements of interaction and the interfaces of mobile devices such as smartphones, tablets, laptops, etc. In addition, the analysis considers each test within an application scenario with general functions, such as send to and data receive from server and storage and query database if the test needed.

The test involved in the memory processes research shown below. For each test under analysis, First briefly describe the test procedure and after presented the implementation analysis for mobile devices. In general, the instructions of every test should be able to show in a pop-up with legible text before the applications solicited an action. A button in the interface must have the functionality to open the current instructions pop-up.

5.1 Words Learning

Description: Are presented to the person many words or numbers, not linked to each and whose number exceeds the amount that can remember. Usually the series consist of 10 to 12 words o 8 to 10 numbers. The patient is asked to recall and repeat the series in any order. After recording the number of items retained, presents to the patient again the series and re-record the results. This process is repeated 8 to 10 times and the data obtained are shown in graphical form called "memory curve". After complete all repetitions and spent 50 to 60 minutes, the specialist must ask to the patient the series of words without mentioning it to the patient again.

The application must download the series of words in a database containing common series for this test. Must have a variety of these series, so that no repetition between tests. The test shows that words can be read to the patient or in the form of text. In this analysis we consider two cases.

- For the case in which the words are presented in the form of text, must take the general considerations of a text in this analysis. The words are displayed on screen with an appearance time for the user to have a chance to read the word and hold it. In this analysis it is proposed that the time of occurrence for word is 5 to 10 seconds.
- For the case in which the words are presented in the form of audio, playback of sound files is required in the mobile devices. This represents a higher data download and use more features. This form is recommended for this test, because it's similar to testing experience between the patient and the specialist.

Once the series of words presented to the patient, the application indicates that the patient must enter the words that were presented above. These instructions can be displayed as text on screen. The test suggests that the reproduction of the words to be spoken instead of being written. This requires a hearing user interface. The implementation of a speech recognition algorithm for mobile devices solves this problem. When the user pronounce the words that recalls, the application transform the received audio into text, allowing to store as a string the words the patient recalls. Once record a word, the application must request more words until the user indicates that they no longer remember more words or reached the total words. The application should display a button to indicate that the user does not remember more words and will terminate the test process. Currently, there are dedicated speech recognition research on mobile devices can be applied in this solution [21]. A simpler way to implement this phase of the test is to apply the words through a text input, that is, the user will write the words remember and these strings register for the test. Incorrect orthography is a problem when validating a user input word belongs to the series of words.

After all the repetitions, an automatic task in the application, must indicate to patient spend for 50 to 60 minutes to repeat the words of the series presented in the same way that in each repetition. The results of this test, it should be stored in a database that subsequently can generate the curve on the memory.

5.2   Mediate Memory

Description: It is proposed the subject to remember a series composed of 12 to 15 words, using appropriate images that will serve as support for memorization. The images doesn't must directly represent the meaning of the words, the patient selects the images by setting a certain relationship between the meaning of the word and image. The number of images must be of 15 to 20. Once the patient has chosen an image to associate with a word, specialist must ask the patient why chose that image, this relationship should be considered and the patient must remember this association. After 40 minutes, the specialist should show to the patient the selected pictures and asked to mention the word that associate with that image.

In this test we must considerate the size of the images because their represent objects or everyday items, therefore this images must be distinguishable. The test indicates that the patient should be able to see all the images at once. If we consider that the largest number of images in the test are 20, it is clear that they can not be displayed properly on devices with small and medium screen size. Therefore, the suitable screen size is large or extra-large and it is recommended, if possible, use the smallest number of images allowed (15 images). For ease, the patient should be able to select an image to view larger.

Once the images shown, the application must show the patient the series of words to associate with images. The words can be presented in audio or text form. For this test we take the considerations mentioned early in *words learning* test. After the applications present a word, the user must select the image that he related with the word, this association is saved and the application will request the patient to indicate why he choose that image for the current word. In this phase of the test, there are two solutions again: audio or text input. In the audio input case, a file audio will be generated by the mobile device and send to a database so that the specialist can play it later and get results. However, the audio input represents complexity because can be generate a file too big and this implies a problem with the storage of results. A solution for this problem in this case is stablish a time limit to the patient for record his explanation about the association, thus the size of the audio file always be the same. A time limit of 1 to 2 minutes is enough for the patient and won't generate a file too big. In the text input case, the application will display a text entry box for the patient to enter a long string giving the explanation of the association that will subsequently be consulted by the specialist.

After 40 minutes, the application will display in the screen the selected images one by one asks the patient to enter the word that he associate with the current image. The words can be introduced, again, via audio or text input. At this stage, the application should display a button that allows the patient to indicate that he do not remember the word that is asked. The data obtained in the reproduction must be storage in the database.

5.3   Pictogram

Description: This test is a variant of the *mediate memory* test. The test consists of presenting to the patient a series of 12 to 15 words. For each word the patient should draw any sign or figure that can be used to remember the word.

To present the words in this test, we can use the analysis in the *words learning* test. For each word, the application request to the patient draw a figure that associate with the current word. For this is needed a haptic interface. The touch-screen technology allow the user to do actions with the fingers, in this case the action is draw. The draws maked by the patient must be saved in a lightweight format such as JPEG. This images will be shown to the patient after 40 minutes just like the words reproduction in the *mediate memory* test.

5.4   Reproduction of Stories

Description: The reproduction of the contents of stories is a test considered a proposal for the recognition of hearing footprints. The specialist should read the patient any single story and is proposed to the patient who narrates. Then the same is done with a second story (which includes elements of the former). After the patient is asked to narrate the second story, the examiner asks the patient to remember the first story.

The application must provide both the patient stories in audio form. Audio files of the stories should be obtained from a repository. Remember that these stories have elements in common. The application displays a button to start playing the story. After the patient hear the story, the application should ask the patient to narrate the story. This is a audio input similar problem to the *mediate memory* test. We can use the same solution given in this test but with some modifications. The time limit on this test must be at least the time of the original story. Based on the examples described by A. R Luria, the playtime of the stories beyond the original story playtime. Therefore, the time limit of the audio input will be the duration of the original story by adding an additional time. In this analysis, the additional time will consist of half the time the original story. Another solution to this problem is to use text input. The application should display a text box where the user can type the reproduction of the story.

At the end of the test, we will have three sets of data, either text or audio, that the specialist would be responsible for analysing: the first reproduction of the first story, the reproduction of the second story, and the second reproduction of the first story. This information must be stored in the database.

5.5   Direct-Fixation Footprints Test

Its purpose is to establish to what extent the patient is able to maintain direct footprints (visual, hearing ans tactile) produced by different stimulus and clarify whether or not volume alterations and strength preserving footprints.

The research beginning with the analysis of the after-images, that are defined as the footprints that remain a certain time after a visual, hearing or tactile stimulus, and there are test for every type of after-images [2].

In this analysis, we don't including tactile test because it cannot be implemented on mobile devices yet.

Visual Afterimages Test. *Description:* Consists in presenting the patient with 3 or 4 bright red geometric figures over a heterogeneous background (white or gray) for 15 or 20 seconds each one. After this, the patient must be draw the figures that can remember.

For testing visual footprints, it is possible to present 3 or 4 random geometric figures (square, circle, pentagon, etc) bright red on the mobile device display, indicating that remain for 15 to 20 seconds and must be indicated in the instructions that the patient should remain viewing this pictures during this time. The application solicit to the patient to draw the figures that was showed before. As *mediate memory* test, in this test its needed a haptic interface that can be implemented with the touchscreen technology. The draws maked by the patient must be saved in a lightweight format such as JPEG and send to the database.

Hearing Afterimages Test. *Description:* To study the retention of hearing footprints, some methods for short-term memory are used, for example a three-step test is used: first series of three, four and finally five words is read to the patient, after listen the patient must repeat immediately. In the next step, a pause of 5-10 seconds between reading and reproduction is done. In final step, the reproduction of the series of words separated from its presentation by a break of 10 to 15 seconds, during which the patient is distracted talking. In all these cases, the patient must reproduce the words in the same order they were presented.

For this test, the interface can only be hearing. The series of words must be obtained from a repository as audio files that will be played on the mobile device. For the first phase, the words were presented in order and as the series has finished playing, the application should ask the patient to repeat soon. In subsequent phases, the indication is the same, just the break time to retry the number of words should be indicated. At the final step, the distraction in the break mentioned in the test can be an element of multimedia, like a video or a lyric selected by the specialist. The user interface should also indicate the stage at which it is and the necessary buttons to start the test at that stage. This test can use the same audio input method that was mentioned on *words learning* test. The words that the patient mentioned will be compared with the original series and storage that result.

5.6   Summary

In table 2, we can see the summary of the analysis of memory tests shown above and the suitable mobile device for the implementation of each test, generally. Also consider the input and output of each procedure involves testing, according to the proposed solution is also considered in the analysis.

Table 2. Summary: General analysis of memory Luria test

Test	Input	Output	Suitable device
Words learning	Audio or text	Audio or text	Smartphone/Tablet
Mediate memory	Text and images	Audio or text	Tablet
Pictogram	Text	Images	Tablet
Reproduction of stories	Audio or text	Audio or text	Smartphone/Tablet
Visual after-images test	Images	Images	Smartphone/Tablet
Hearing after-images test	Audio	Audio	Smartphone/Tablet

6   Case Study: Older Adults

As seen, Luria test are applied to patients to determinate the level of memory impairment. The older adults are a potential kind of people for application of Luria memory tests, because memory impairment are a common factor that affects quality of life of older adults [7] [9] [8]. However, the use of Luria memory tests by specialist to older adults decreases its efficiency due to limitations of individuals because of ageing, for example, inability to move to where the tests are performed.

A digital implementation of Luria tests on mobile devices is a solution to the problem of the application efficiency of the test and to the problem of patient mobility. In addition, in this case study, take into account the limitations of older adults caused by ageing.

The analysis of Luria tests made in this work provides an alternative implementation on mobile devices with HCI considerations in general. For this case study, the analysis must take a new approach: design interfaces with HCI considerations for older adults applied to mobile devices [5] [6].

Based in the general analysis showed before and design recommendations in [5] and [6], the next general design considerations are proposed for the case study of older adults:

- *Display*, with large or extra-large screen size to reduce visual limitations and with touchscreen technology.
- *Information*, the text showed, including instructions, must have Sans Serif font and contrast color with backgrounds for a grater understanding.

– *Buttons*, big dimensions and must use text instead icons to the user to determine the function of the button more easily.
– *Audio*, must exist a volume control for the user, preferably use female voices with a level of acuity below average. This is according with [5].

Table 3 shows a summary of the analysis of memory tests with HCI considerations for older adults. With the limitations of older adults as new factor in this case study and the new design considerations presented above, the input and output data and the suitable device for each test may change according with needs of this kind of users. Note that for this population the suitable device is a tablet, because the tablet dimensions and display characteristics help reducing visual and haptic limitations.

Table 3. Summary: Analysis of Luria memory tests for case study of older adults

Test	Input	Output	Suitable device
Words learning	Audio or text	Audio or text	Tablet
Mediate memory	Text and images	Audio or text	Tablet
Pictogram	Text or Audio	Images	Tablet
Reproduction of stories	Audio or text	Audio or Text	Tablet
Visual after-images test	Images	Images	Tablet
Hearing after-images test	Audio	Audio	Tablet

7   Conclusion

Based in the analysis made, this paper has identified a considerable Luria memory tests set that can be implemented on mobile devices. There are some tests that can't be implemented because the current technology in mobile computing doesn't offer the usability required for these tests, for example direct-fixation in tactile footprints test. Create a mobile application that containing greater part of Luria memory tests analysed in this paper, will assist significantly to neuropsychology specialist and patients when applying the tests to determinate the level of memory impairment, reducing the number of consultation meetings.

Luria tests, in particular those focused on memory processes, have a wide range of potential users for its application. The analysis made of case study of older adults in this paper, determined that also is possible to make an user-centred implementation taking account the different capacities and limitations of older adults and the usability factors of HCI which can be applied in mobile computing.

In the analysis of the tests, different implementation solutions that can be used for the same test were explored, considering the capabilities that users might have. This might result the beginning to create adaptable solutions which depends of the user capacities and abilities and the different characteristics of mobile devices that can be exploited. This refers to plasticity, a capacity of

interactive systems to adapt to context of use while preserving the usability
of the application [22]. This concept can be applied in the case study of older
adults. For example, the speech recognition algorithms for mobile devices may
replace the traditional input text in displays when people with health problems
that limit the haptics capabilities, for example arthritis. Therefore, in this case
the user needs a natural interface.

References

1. Papalia, D., Wendkos, S., Feldman, R.D.: Human Development, 9th edn.
   McGraw-Hill, New York (2003)
2. Luria, A.R.: Higher cortical functions in man. Springer, U.S.A (1995)
3. Ostrosky-Solís, F., Ardila, A., Rosselli, M.: NEUROPSI: A brief neuropsychological
   test battery in Spanish with norms by age and educational level. Journal of the
   International Neuropsychological Society, vol. 5 5, 413–433 (1999)
4. Herreras, E.B.: Study of Lurias learning curve in patients with injured brains.
   Enseanza e Investigación en Psicología, vol. 15, nm. 1, enero-abril, pp. 147-158,
   Consejo Nacional para la Enseanza en Investigación en Psicologá, México (2010)
5. Pak, R., McLaughlin, A.: Designing Displays for Older Adults. CRC Press, United
   States (2011)
6. Fisk, A.D., Rogers, W.A., Charness, N., Czaja, S.J., Sharit, J.: Designing for older
   adults. CRC Press, United States (2009)
7. Sotolongo, P., Casanova, P., Carrillo, C.: Deterioro cognitivo en la tercera edad.
   Rev. Cubana Medicina General Integral 20, 5, 6 (2004)
8. Instituto Nacional de Estadística y Geografía (INEGI). Estadísticas a propósito del
   día internacional de las personas de edad, Aguascalientes, Aguascalientes, (October
   2013)
9. Pérez, M.: Deterioro Cognoscitivo: Instituto de Geriatría. México D.F (2010)
10. Satyanarayanan, M.: Mobile computing: the next decade. SIGMOBILE Mob.
    Comput. Commun. Rev. 15(2), 2–10 (2011)
11. Swanson: What develops in working memory? A life span perspective. Developmental Psychology, 35 (4), pp. 986-1000 (1999)
12. Sharp, H., Rogers, Y., Preece, J.: Interaction design - Beyond human-computer
    interaction. John Wiley & Sons, Ltd. (2009)
13. Ledesma, R.F., Rosales, I., Vázquez, Y.O.G.: Sistema Interactivo de Ejercitación
    de Memoria para Personas Mayores, Trabajo Terminal 20090080, de la Escuela
    Superior de Cómputo del IPN. México, Mayo del (2010)
14. ACTIVAMENTE: Software de estimulación y actividad cognitiva, Neuroinnovation, Chile, http://www.activamente.cl/
15. Cerejo, L.: The elements of the Mobile User Experience; Mobile Design Patterns,
    Smashing eBook No.28, Freidburg Germany (September 2012)
16. Love, S.: Understanding Mobile Human-Computer Interaction. ISS, 1st edn.,
    Uxbridge, UK (2005)
17. Jones, M., Marsden, G.: Mobile Interaction Design. John Wiley and Sons, England
    (2006)
18. Jacko, J.A.: The Human-Computer Interaction handbook. CRC Press, 3rd Edition,
    United States (2012)
19. Lee, V., Schneider, H., Schell, R.: Mobile Applications: Architecture, design and
    development. Prentice Hall. New Jersey, United States (2004)

20. Sánchez, D.V., Rubio, E.H., Ledesma, E.F.R., Viveros, A.M.: Students roles functionalities towards LMSs as open platforms through mobile devices. In: Proceedings to Appear in 24th International Conference on Electronics, Communications and Computers, CONIELECOMP 2014, Universidad de las Amricas, Cholula Puebla, Mxico February pp. 26–28. IEEE (2014)
21. Castañeda, F.J.H., Gamez, B.E.C., Rubio, E.H., Viveros, A.M.: Discrete Wavelet Transform for mobile speech recognition; Preprint, Escuela Superior de Cómputo. Instituto Politécnico Nacional. Cd. de México, Distrito Federal, México
22. Tzovaras, D.: Multimodal User Interfaces: From Signals to Interaction. Springer Series on Signals and Communication Technology. Springer, Heidelberg (2008) ISSN 1860-4862

Research on Senior Response to Transfer Assistance between Wheelchair and Bed
EEG Analysis

Mikako Ito[1], Yuka Takai[2], Akihiko Goto[2], and Noriaki Kuwahara[3]

[1] Social Welfare Corporation KEISEIKAI
[2] Osaka Sangyo University
[3] Kyoto Institute of Technology
kantamikako@hct.zaq.ne.jp, takai@ise.osaka-sandai.ac.jp,
gotoh@ise.osaka-sandai.ac.jp, nkuwahar@kit.ac.jp

Abstract. As of October, 2012, the Japanese population was found to be aging at a rate of 24.1 %. The results determined that the rate of aging for this sector of the Japanese population makes Japan one of the most aged societies in the world.

As the aging population continues to increase in size, we anticipate that more nursing will be necessary to accommodate the future needs of seniors.

Due to the complex nature and challenging field of senior care, nursing homes experience high employee turnover rates. The shortage of skillful employees is problematic, so the option of training employees without a nursing background may be an integral part of the solution.

Proper "transfer assistance between wheelchair and bed" is a fundamental element of senior care. However, large gaps in how to perform a safe transfer are noticeable amongst skilled and non-skilled caregivers. To analyze and provide seniors a safe and comfortable transfer, we measured seniors' brain waves and facial expressions as transfers were performed by skilled and non-skilled caregivers. The experiment was not limited to the analysis of transfer techniques. Differences in brain waves, facial expressions, voice, tone and the requests of skilled and non-skilled caregivers were measured as well.

Keywords: patient safety, transfer assistance between wheelchair and bed, brain waves.

1   Introduction

1.1   Japan is a Super Aged Society

Japan is one of the most aged societies in the world, and the proportion of seniors (65years and up) occupies 24.1% of the entire Japanese population. Currently, the rate of aging is on the rise and more people are expected to receive nursing care. (1)

V.G. Duffy (Ed.): DHM 2014, LNCS 8529, pp. 558–566, 2014.
© Springer International Publishing Switzerland 2014

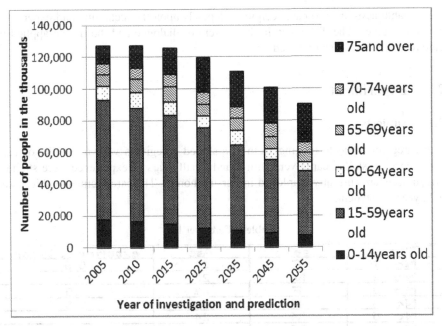

Fig. 1. Age-specific population of Japan

Due to the current wave of aging, senior care facilities are facing a number of difficulties. Despite the addition of new employees, a demand for a heavier workload is causing a higher employee turnover rate when compared to other professions. (2)

	2006(year)	2007	2008	2009	2010	201˙
All industry quitting a job rate	16.2%	15.4%	14.6%	˙6.4%	14.5%	14.4%
Care staff quitting a job rate	20.3%	21.6%	18.7%	˙7.0%	17.8%	16.1%

Fig. 2. Comparison of the quitting a job rate

1.2   The Purpose of This Study

The most difficult hurdle which senior care employees face is acquiring the necessary skills to be successful at their job. The transference of a senior between a wheelchair and a bed is one of the fundamental techniques required for senior care.

The transfer technique facilitates basic daily care, such as going to the toilet, and offering support in the bathroom for bathing.

It takes months for new employees to acquire a transfer technique skill.

In this study, while observing the changes that occur in the brain waves and facial expressions of care recipients, we verified the fact that in order to provide safe and comfortable assistance to care recipients depends upon the technique and experience of the caregiver. The difference in the content of dialogue and the timing applied to care recipients was also recorded.

2   Experiment

2.1   Subjects

Ten caregiver subjects ranging from non-skilled caregivers with 6 months of care experience, to skilled caregivers with 7 and a half years of experience were studied. All subjects are currently employed in nursing homes. The care recipient subject was a 22 year old student.

Table 1. Caregiver'list

	sex	Age	experience (year)
No. 1	F	21	0.5
No. 2	M	23	0.5
No. 3	F	22	1.5
No. 4	F	22	1.5
No. 5	M	24	1.5
No. 6	M	25	2.5
No. 7	F	25	2.5
No. 8	F	28	5.5
No. 9	F	27	6.5
No. 10	F	28	7.5

2.2   Conditions of Measurement

The experiment was conducted in a room at a nursing home. All trials were carried out in order from procedure (A) to procedure (B). The experimental subjects were employees from the nursing staff, and each employee was randomly selected to take part in the experiment regardless of their years of experience. The electroencephalograph (EEG) used for the care recipient subject was a portable EEG manufactured by Digital Medic Co.

2.3   Measurement Content

(A) The caregiver assisted in taking the care recipient in a wheelchair to the side of a bed. Then, the recipient was transferred from the wheelchair onto the bed, at the foot of the bed.

(B) The care recipient was transferred from a seated position on the bed to a wheelchair, which was positioned beside the foot of the bed.

The transfer assistance procedures conducted in (A) and (B) were classified into five steps based on the new employees' training manual (3) for this facility. The results are listed in the table below.

Table 2. Process of transfer

Process of transfer (A)		Process of transfer (B)	
A–1	B–ing one foot down from a footres:	B–1	Shallow reseat
A–2	Shallow reseat	B–2	Move handle aside
A–3	Move handle aside	B–3	Transfer assistance to wheelchair
A–4	Transfer assistance to bed	B–4	Deep reseat
A–5	Deep reseat	B–5	Place a foot on a footrest

3   Experiment Results

3.1   Scores for the Respective Steps

We focused on the verbalization of the caregiver subjects (from No.1 to No.10) during each of the five assistance steps. In order to determine how work experience influences the process; the time it takes to assist, the verbal approach to the care recipient, and the implementation of the basic operations for transfer assistance were recorded. The scores are listed and divided into the following three types. The score for each subject for (A) and (B) are shown in the table below.

- ○: The care giver acknowledged the care recipient's response after the care giver's verbalization, including a clear explanation for each procedure. (5points)
- △ : Began the transference assistance at the same time verbal communication with the care recipient was initiated. (3points)
- × : Lack of verbal communication with the care recipient, or a skipped step in the assistance process. (0points)

Table 3. Score list of the timing for the voice

	Evaluation of (A)					Evaluation of (B)					
	A–1	A–2	A–3	A–4	A–5	B–1	B–2	B–3	B–4	B–5	
No. 1	3	0	3	3	3	0	3	5	5	3	No. 1
No. 2	5	0	0	3	0	0	3	3	0	3	No. 2
No. 3	0	0	3	3	3	5	0	3	0	0	No. 3
No. 4	3	3	3	3	0	3	3	3	0	3	No. 4
No. 5	3	0	3	3	0	0	0	3	5	0	No. 5
No. 6	3	0	5	3	3	5	3	5	0	3	No. 6
No. 7	5	5	0	3	5	3	0	3	0	0	No. 7
No. 8	5	3	3	3	3	3	3	3	0	5	No. 8
No. 9	5	3	5	3	5	0	0	3	5	3	No. 9
No. 10	3	0	5	5	0	0	5	5	3	5	No. 10

(A)

No.1	No.2	No.3	No.4	No.5	No.6	No.7	No.8	No.9	No.10
12	8	9	12	9	14	18	17	21	13

(B)

No.1	No.2	No.3	No.4	No.5	No.6	No.7	No.8	No.9	No.10
16	9	8	12	8	16	6	14	11	18

3.2   Correlation between Brain Waves and Scores

We focused on the brain waves of the care recipient during the transfer assistance procedure (A) and (B).

On the assumption that the alpha-wave dominance rate of the care recipient while resting was 100%, we calculated the alpha-wave dominance rate during the transfer. The correlation between the alpha-wave value and the employees years of experience is shown in Figure 3,4. The correlation between the timing of initial verbalization and the employee's years of experience is shown in Figure 5,6. The correlation between

(A) Bed to wheel chair

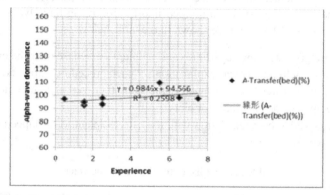

Fig. 3. Correlation between alpha-wave dominance and Experience of staff

(B) Wheel chair to bed

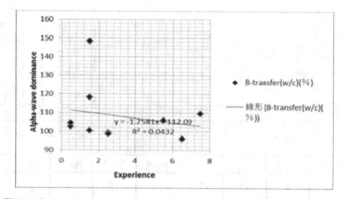

Fig. 4. Correlation between alpha-wave dominance and Experience of staff

the amount of verbalization and the years of experience is plotted in Figure 7,8. For procedure (A), employee verbalization was counted from the moment a wheelchair was placed beside the foot of the bed and the care recipient was transferred onto the bed, to the time when the caregiver left. For procedure (B), verbalization was counted from the moment a wheel chair was set beside the foot of the bed, followed by a transfer from the bed to a wheelchair, to the time when the caregiver released the brake and started moving the wheelchair.

(A) Bed to wheel chair

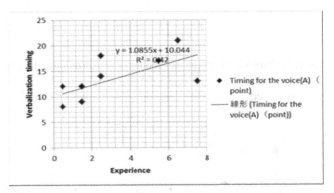

Fig. 5. Correlation between verbalization timing and experience

(B) Wheel chair to bed

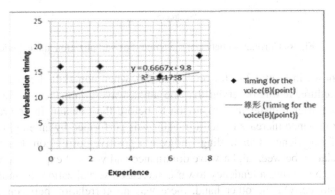

Fig. 6. Correlation between verbalization timing and experience

(A) Bed to wheel chair

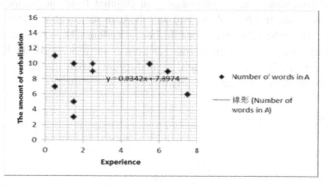

Fig. 5. Correlation between the amount of verbalization and experience

(B) Wheel chair to bed

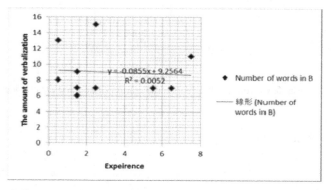

Fig. 6. Correlation between the amount of verbalization and experience

As shown in Figure 3,4, for procedure (A), when non-skilled caregivers performed the procedure, it was observed that the alpha-wave dominance of the care recipient decreased after transfer in comparison to before the transfer. In contrary, the alpha-wave dominance increased after a transfer was performed by an employee with many years of experience. Our findings indicate a positive correlation. For procedure (B), no correlation between alpha-wave dominance and years of experience was observed.

Figure 5,6 shows a tendency towards increased verbalization the more experienced the employee. On the other hand, there was no correlation between the amount of verbalization and the years of experience as shown in Figure 7,8.

4   Discussion

We observed a positive correlation in the increase of alpha-wave dominance corresponding to the length of employee experience for (A). This results suggest that the anxiety of the care recipient subject was alleviated when being assisted by skilled caregivers. No correlation was observed for (B), but the possibility exists that the uneasiness felt by the care recipient subject was decreased because the experiment was carried out in order, from (A) to (B).

Judging from the observation of the experiments, there were large individual gaps among non-skilled employees (No.1 and No.2) and mid level employees (No.3 – No.7) with 2 to 3 year- experience. The findings suggest that some employees relied on their physical strength and assisted the care recipient without proper communication. Other employees offered assistance following the basic procedure. This resulted in significant differences when it came to scoring. However, during procedure (B), both caregivers and care recipients seemed more relaxed because the pressure of performing as part of an experiment was alleviated.

As Figure 5,6 shows, we observed positive correlations between the years of experience and the scores of the timing of verbalization for both (A) and (B).

In fact, as shown in Table.3, it is obvious that the scores related to the timing of verbalization were stable for skilled employees with five or more years of experience (No.8 –No.10). Their scores were higher than 30 points. On the other hand, there were large individual gaps among non-skilled employees and mid level employees. At certain points during the process, skilled employees intentionally did not verbalize with the recipient, because they were able to make an instant assessment of the care recipient's condition. The lack of communication was an attempt to reduce the burden of the care recipient, and to save care assistance time in accordance to the employees' training manual.

As indicated in Figure 7,8, there was no correlation observed between the amount of verbalization and the years of employee experience for both (A) and (B). The non-skilled employees who consistently follow the steps in the basic care manual perform the transfer while acknowledging their technique and behavior during the process. Also, the employee frequently conversed with the care recipient in a short repetitive manner in order to gain cooperation from the recipient. Some mid-leveled employees verbalized in a short and frequent manner similar to the non-skilled employees. However, some of the mid-level employees concentrated mainly on assisting the recipient and proceeded, devoid of conversation. Skilled employees tended to verbalize less as they conducted their assistance procedure within the minimum time.

5   Conclusion

This study suggests that the proper timing of verbalization is cultivated according to the length of the employee's experience. Proper timing when conversing with a care recipient eases anxiety felt by the recipient. Observations reflect that there was no significant difference in the amount of verbalization between non-skilled employees and skilled employees.

This means that the amount of verbalization does not give the care recipient a sense of safety. The care recipient feels safe when they know "What the caregiver is going to do", or "How the caregivers' verbal content influences cooperation from the care recipient". The results also verified that the timing of verbalization in all care assistant procedures is an important factor in order to confirm and comprehend the status of the care recipient.

Currently detailed regulations do not exist in the employee training manual in reference to verbal communication between the caregiver and care recipient. Care givers acquire individual skills through their daily assistance experiences. The content of verbalization corresponds to the communication skill, and therefore differs based on the person and care site.

It is obvious that acquiring conversational skill is important. Therefore, it is suggested that further study is necessary to clarify how employees time verbalization, choose their wording carefully and alter their verbalization to suit the care recipient.

The experiment trial involved ten caregivers and was conducted in one day. The care recipient subject became accustomed to receiving care to a certain extent. Thus we observed that the student subject adjusted his body, such as relaxing the lower limbs, or keeping an upright position dependent upon the caregiver's method of assistance. For future experiments, the care recipient subject could wear clothing or equipment which immobilizes them to assume a paralytic condition. Also, the experiment should be conducted over several different days. We would like to adopt the above mentioned options to determine whether we will attain different results.

References

1. The, White Paper on Aged Society, in the page 2, Cabinet Office (2012)
2. "Turnover Rates of Nursing Care Staff and Home Visit Care Staff" from "Care Work Factual Investigation", Care Work Foundation
3. "New Employees' Training Manual", in the pp. 11–111, "Transfer and Move", Zuikoen Nursing Home

Effectiveness of Paper Coloring Recreation in an Elderly Persons Care Home

Shinichiro Kawabata

Graduate School of Kyoto Institute of Technology, Japan
arser3@gmail.com

Abstract. Aging poses a problem all over the world, and the numbers of dementias patients are increasing. In connection, number of elderly nursing home is also increasing. Accordingly, health care sector is facing a serious labor shortage. There are needs to create an recreational activity which can expect improvement of elderly people's dementia prevention and easing a care worker's burden. In this study picture colouring was carried out, as a result behavior problems of elderly people decreased dramatically and burden of care worker has also decreased.

Keywords: Recreation, Elderly care home, colour brush pen, picture coloring.

1 Introduction

The population of the world is aging at an accelerated rate and it has becoming a serious problem in wide area of the world. The number of elderly people increased more than threefold since 1950, from approximately 130 million to 419 million in the year 2000. The number of elderly people is now increasing by 8 million per year, and by 2030, this increase will reach to 24 million per year. The most rapid acceleration in aging will occur after 2010, when the large post World War II baby boom cohorts begin to reach age of 65. Declining fertility rates combined with steady improvements in life expectancy over the latter half of the 20th century have produced dramatic growth in the world's elderly population. People aged 65 and over now comprise a greater share of the world's population than ever before, and this proportion will increase during the 21st century. This trend has immense implications for many countries around the globe because of its potential to overburden existing social institutions for the elderly. As of October 1, 2010, the elderly population aged 65 and over became 29.6 million people to be the highest ever in Japan. Moreover the proportion of the population of the total population over the age of 65 was also recorded the highest of 23.1%. When this tendency continues, one person in four people comes to enter the age of senior citizen in 2015. Accordingly, health care sector is facing a serious labour shortage. That is largely due to the fact that those positions don't pay much more than minimum wage, even though they are incredibly demanding jobs. Furthermore the numbers of dementia patients are also increasing and various measures for dementia prevention are taken place. The recreational activities which has

V.G. Duffy (Ed.): DHM 2014, LNCS 8529, pp. 567–574, 2014.
© Springer International Publishing Switzerland 2014

possibilities to eases a care worker's burden and can also expect an effect also from prevention of dementia are required. Therefore picture colouring which is easily carried out for both elderly and care givers was paid to attention. When starting colouring, people needs to observe the original picture carefully. At this time, lobus occipitalis that take charge of the sight work. Moreover, to understand the original picture accurately, the temporal lobe that takes charge of the memory works to refer from the memory the shape and the colour sow in the past. The parietal lobe cooperates when the balance of the entire picture is gripped. As written above picture colouring has the effect to activate a widespread area of the brain. In this study picture colouring was taking place at the elderly nursing home for the aged resident as part of the recreation activity, and the influence given to the resident was verified.

2   Methodology

2.1   Selection of Writing Instrument for Picture Colouring

As for the first stage of this study, experiment to select the optimal writing instrument for picture colouring was carried out. The colouring experiment was carried out with four kinds of writing instruments, such as crayon pastel (SAKURA COLOUR PRODUCTS CORP), colour pencil(MITUBISHI PENCIL CO., LTD.), felt-tipped pen(Too Corporation.), and colour brush pen (soliton corporation CO. LTD.). Four writing instruments are shown in Figure 1. These four writing instruments are commonly used instruments for picture colouring at elderly nursing home. The brain activity in each case was measured.

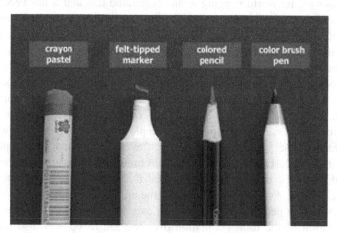

Fig. 1. Four kinds of writing instruments for picture colouring

Experimental Method. Electroencephalograph (EEG) of Digital Medic co.,Ltd, was used to measure the brain activity. Five postgraduates aged 21-31cooperated in this experiment as a test subject. To make experimental conditions impartial, each test with different writing instrument was conducted in the same time zone of a different day using the same laboratory with a tranquil environment. An interval of 7days was given between each experiment. The sequential order for colouring the grain of the grape was been determined to make equal condition between the subjects. After having installed the EEG, test subject will close eye for 1 minute to record the brain wave at the rest situation, subsequently after that picture colouring was taken place for three minutes to record the brain wave during colouring. By comparing brain wave of eye closure situation and colouring, we have tried to eliminate the rose of the body condition to the results. Assuming the brain waves at the time of eye closure as 100%, the brain waves of alpha wave and beta wave under colouring work in progress was compared.

2.2   Colouring Recreation Activity at Elderly Nursing Home

The Frequency of the Fall Accident and the Number of the Nurse Calls. Colouring recreation activity was taken place at the elderly nursing home to 56 residents using colour brush pen. The frequency of the recreation carried out was 2-3 times a week, and each recreation was about 1.5 hours. The frequency of the fall accident and the number of the nurse call (sensor mat type) before and after the recreation was recorded.

The Frequency of Wandering Around and Petition of Excretion. Five residents who have more behavior problems comparatively with other resident, such as wandering around, petition of excretion and unnecessary nurse calls were chosen as a test subject. Each colouring recreation was operated for approximately thirty minutes and the frequency of the colouring recreation was two or three times a week, changing according to physical condition of the residents. The experiment was conducted for three months and the frequency of wandering around, petition of excretion was recorded.

The Relationship between the Number of Nurse Calls at Night and Sleeping Hours. Additional experiment was carried out to one other test subject to find out the relationship between number of nurse calls and sleeping time of the resident after working on colouring. Checking of sleeping hour was operated once in every fifteen minutes. Furthermore, in order to verify the influence of stopping the colouring recreation, as for this test subject, picture colouring experiment was stopped after two month and follow up observations were carried out.

3   Results and Discussions

3.1   Selection of Writing Instrument for Picture Colouring

The results of the beta wave brain activity of four different writing instruments are shown in Figure 2 and the result of the alpha wave brain activity are shown in Figure 3. Colour brush pen and colour pencil showed the high value of Beta wave, which of 139% compared to rest condition. Beta wave is related with active thinking and concentration, therefore by using colour brush pen and colour pencil the user can achieve more concentration of the brain. The lowest value for the alpha wave was colour brush pen by 93% compared to rest condition. It is suggested that colour brush pen has softest tip compared to other writing instruments. Thereby the test subject had to be vividly aware to hand movement of not only the XY-axis of left to right, but also to the Z-axis of up and down movement, leading alpha wave to decline consequently. From these results colour brush pen is demonstrated as the writing instruments which gives most stimulation to the brain. The reason for testing with postgraduates was because the physical and mental load was too heavy for the elderly people to wear EEG. Therefore in this study the experiment was conducted to the postgraduates.

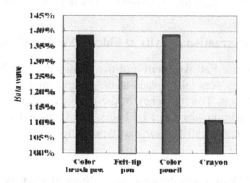

Fig. 2. Comparison of Beta wave between at rest and colouring using different writing instruments

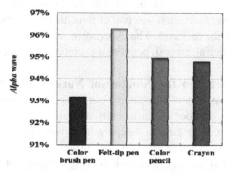

Fig. 3. Comparison of Alpha wave between at rest and colouring using different writing instruments

3.2   Colouring Recreation Activity at Elderly Nursing Home

The Frequency of the Fall Accident and the Number of the Nurse Calls. The number of the fall accident per month before and after the recreation activity is shown in Fig. 4 and the frequency of the nurse call is shown in Fig.5. The averages of fall accident per month at elderly nursing home decreased to 4.6 times from 10.7 times which in the percentage by 57% decrease. When the frequency of the recreation including colouring increased, the frequency of the nurse call decreased to average of 832 from 1469. The decreasing percentage was 35%.

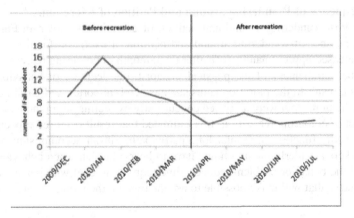

Fig. 4. The number of fall accident before and after recreation

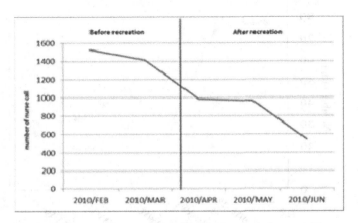

Fig. 5. The number of nurse call accident before and after recreation

There are usually a lot of nurse calls at nighttime when the helper's round is fewer compare to day time. When you increase the frequency of the recreation, the frequency of the nurse call decreased. It is suggested the possibilities of the brain and the body received stimulation and produce fatigue which might have led to enough and refreshing sleep at night. Additionally, though it is a result of only the woman, research results are reported that the fall accident risk is higher to an aged woman with short sleeping time. The result shows that good quality sleep was urged by the colouring recreation, and the possibility of causing a decrease of the fall accident was suggested. During this experimental period, other activities was also taken place in this nursing home, however, those activities has been carried out before this colouring experiment. Therefore it is suggested that these changes are influenced by picture colouring recreation.

The Frequency of Wandering around and Petition of Excretion. The result for the frequency of wandering around and petition of excretion is shown in Figure 6. The average number of wandering around and petition of excretion for five test subjects have decreased approximately 40% after three month of colouring recreation. According to the commentary of the physical therapist, the decrease of behavior problems occur as a result to the plural domains such as cerebral cortex and basal nuclei, cerebellum, the brainstem were activated concurrently by feeling strain increase caused by the effect of colouring recreation. It is estimated that result occurred especially by the change in the function of frontal lobe participating in an accomplishment function. The workers at elderly nursing home have to bear a burden when behavior problems occur. If the behavior problem reduces, time required to deal with behavior problems also reduces, that will make possible to use the time on the requisite care situation.

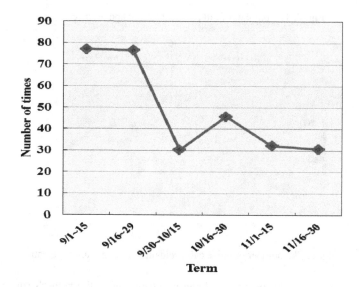

Fig. 6. Average frequency of wandering around and petition of excretion

The Result for Number of Nurse Calls and Sleeping Hour. The result for the relationship between the number of nurse calls and sleeping hours of the resident is shown in Figure 7. After starting the experiment, the number of nurse calls decreased dramatically. Due to this change, the hours of sleeping time has increased up to average of 4.5 hours per day to 7.9 hours per day in maximum. The number of the nurse calls increased up to 87 times and hours of sleeping time declined again to average of 4.8 hours per day after aborting the colouring experiment. Even thou this experiment is a provisional examination, it was very interesting to see correlation between the number of nurse call and sleeping hour of the residents. We would like to conduct the experiment using more subjects. From this result, as for the increase of nurse calls and decrease of sleeping hours after stopping colouring experiment, it is suggested that colouring should be carried out continuously to gain effective influence.

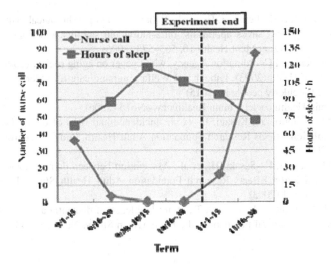

Fig. 7. Results for number of nurse calls and sleeping time

4   Conclusions

In this study, optimal writing instrument for colouring is suggested as colour brush pen. The number of nurse calls, fall accident, wandering around frequency and petition excretion of the resident at nursing home decreased due to working on colouring recreation. The number of test subject might be short as representive sample, however in the case which the aging society are placed, this research has the possibilities to give a positive impact to the health care sector. Colouring is easily done compared to painting and descriptions, also regardless to the needing care degree. Moreover a care worker's burden can also be reduced because the time for handling unnecessary nurse calls, wandering around and petition of excretion can be reduced. As the result shows, colouring is suggested as an activity that should be taken as one of the recreations at the elderly nursing home.

Acknowledgment. I would like to express my special appreciation and thanks to my advisor Professor Hiroyuki Hamada, you have been a tremendous mentor for me. I would like to thank you for encouraging my research and for allowing me to grow as a research scientist. Your advice on both research as well as on my career have been priceless.

References

1. Katie, L., et al Stone: Actigraphy-Measured Sleep Characteristics and Risk of Falls in Older Women. Archives of Internal Medicine 168, 1768 (2008)
2. Tanaka, H., et al.: Effect that memories colouring paper gives to slight dementia patient acknowledgment function, psychology function, and side of daily life. Journal of Rehabilitation and Health Sciences 7, 39–42 (2009), ESRC. 2009, Retrieved 19th October, 2010

3. Fauth, E.B., Zarit, S.H., Femia, E.E., et al.: Behavioral and psychological symptoms of dementia and caregivers' stress appraisals: intra-individual stability and change over short-term observations. Aging Ment Health 10, 563–573 (2006)
4. The Management and Coordination Agency, white paper on aging society (2005)
5. The Ministry of Health(2003), Labour and Welfare nursing care for elderly people society Nursing care for elderly people in (2015)
6. Japanese brain Health society, brain Health news No15 (2006)
7. Yamada, M., Mimori, Y., Kasagi, F., et al.: Incidence and risks of dementia in Japanese women: Radiation Effects Research Foundation Adult Health Study. J. Neurol. Sci. 283(1-2), 57–61 (2009)
8. Yamada, M., Kasagi, F., Sasaki, H., et al.: Association between dementia and midlife risk factors: the Radiation Effects Research Foundation Adult Health Study. J. Am. Geriatr. Soc. 51(3), 410–414 (2003)
9. Bachman, D.L., Wolf, P.A., Linn, R.T., et al.: Incidence of dementia and probable Alzheimer's disease in a general population: the Framingham Study. Neurology 43(3Pt 1), 9–515 (1993)

Risk, Safety and Emergency

Non-financial Factors of Job Satisfaction
in the Development of a Safety Culture Based
on Examples from Poland and Romania

Marcin Butlewski[1], Agnieszka Misztal[1], and Ruxandra Ciulu[2]

[1] Poznan University of Technology, Chair of Management and Computing Systems
{marcin.butlewski,agnieszka.misztal}@put.poznan.pl
[2] Al. I. Cuza University, Iasi, Romania
ruxandra.ciulu@mail.uaic.ro

Abstract. Job satisfaction is a very important criterion which cannot be overstated, and it is, therefore, the subject of a number of studies. Satisfied employees often determine that a success of an organization depends on the level of employees' perception in relation to which the workplace affects the attitude to the performed tasks. This model is the subject of an ongoing research by the authors of non-financial factors of job satisfaction in Polish and Romanian manufacturing (industry) companies. Among the studied factors affecting job satisfaction, there are issues related to occupational safety and ergonomics, and these in turn are main aspects of building a safety culture. The article describes the relationships between: ergonomic level and workplace safety perceived by the employee, safety culture, and the overall level of job satisfaction. The paper discusses the pilot studies carried out so far to verify research tools of questionnaires assessing the non-financial factors of job satisfaction. As a consequence of the interpretation of the results, the article presents the elements comprising safety culture in enterprises in Poland and Romania.

Keywords: job satisfaction, safety culture, ergonomics.

1 Introduction

Job satisfaction is known as a positive or a negative attitude towards work, company and co-workers, resulting from particular employees' comparisons between their expectations and what they received for their work. It is important that a term 'occupational satisfaction' is comprehensible not only as an aspect which satisfies material needs but it also considers many different factors, such as: a need of prestige, affiliation, self-fulfillment and constant development. The level of job satisfaction should be measured with a multi-faceted, multi-criteria approach. The concepts developed in relation to this assume the existence of such determinants as [15]: salary, promotions, conduct of supervision, nature of work, and the characteristics of co-workers, but also job design, level of empowerment, training, performance appraisal, incentives, and flexible working hours.

V.G. Duffy (Ed.): DHM 2014, LNCS 8529, pp. 577–587, 2014.
© Springer International Publishing Switzerland 2014

Job satisfaction is also connected with the way it is performed, with commitment and compliance with the rules that establish a job. These factors have mutual character since some of them, having a character of ergonomic factors, can simultaneously affect a company's safety culture, and at the same time being a factor influencing job satisfaction. Such factors are like double amplifiers that directly and indirectly increase safety culture. Job satisfaction examination allows for a subjective assessment of offered working conditions made by employees, and in further perspective, improving those conditions. The aim of this article is to present results of pilot studies considering non-financial criteria influencing job satisfaction in two countries: Poland and Romania in context of creating safety culture in companies.

2   Job Satisfaction Factors and Safety Culture

Job satisfaction factors are highly commented in the literature of the field. The most frequently discussed factor is that connected with economic issues and influence of the other factors, such as age, gender or education [14, 16]. The relationships between job satisfaction and engagement are being examined and discussed. [7] There is no doubt that, the economic factors have a huge influence on job satisfaction, since absolute and relative pay have been found to be important determinants of satisfaction [6]. However, there are some differences in this matter, especially those related to an employee's gender, but they do not disturb the general tendency. The relationship between the general job satisfaction and safety culture has been stated in a case of flying personnel. [4]. Similar arrangements have been carried out in nuclear energy industry where a low level of job satisfaction constituted a factor increasing carelessness and lack of interest in obeying safety procedures. [11]. There is still one matter to be established: is job satisfaction the result of high level of safety culture in a company, or is that relationship inverted or mutually connected? The problem here is a high level of differently related elements of ergonomic factors which could influence job satisfaction. An analysis of resultants of ergonomic factors, such as low back pain, allowed to state that they do not constitute a criterion of change in the level of job satisfaction. [12]. Therefore, measurable level of job satisfaction may not include factors which an employee could directly acknowledge as connected with work processes. [5]. As a consequence, there is a need for an assessment that could examine particular parameters of job satisfaction connected with work environment and to find its deviation from safety culture.

3   Influence of Working Conditions on Employee's Perception

Ergonomics covers all aspects of a job. It assesses an employee's perception of work conditions through an analysis of work environment adaptation to a worker. Ergonomics is not a simple science because it relies on many other branches of science, and at the same time, it considers variety of different factors. It happens very often that lack of knowledge about ergonomics leads to distortion of its rules, and something commonly named 'ergonomic' is not in fact ergonomic and very often it could be even dangerous. That is a management that should be responsible for implementation of ergonomic rules and ideas in a given company. They should also be responsible for efficiency of system's operation they are leading, and ergonomics allows increasing that efficiency.

Work is a component of everyone's life, thus should meet one's expectations and also needs that are not always conscious. We spend at work approximately one third of our daily time, excluding sleeping time. It means that the way we work, to a large extent will influence our psychophysical condition. That is why work cannot only be limited to fulfilling the workers' financial needs. Work causes some kind of impairment even if it theoretically does not seem to be strenuous and does not require considerable activity [10]. If the workers are aware of this fact, it will give them the chance to protect themselves from manifold diseases and give them an opportunity to consciously decide about their life. Guaranteeing workers physical activity in optimal scope, increases job fulfillment and helps to keep them in the state of wellbeing, protecting them at the same time from MSDs formation risk. In case of similar experiments, the researchers came to a conclusion that despite the fact that one year after training, no significant decreases in the prevalence of MSDs were found for any part of a body except the legs, training significantly increased safe behavior in work practices [18]. Similarly, different outcome proves that implementation of certain gymnastic exercises into work, caused a significant progress only after six months. As a result, there was a reduction of muscular tension which was a direct cause o MSDs formation.

The necessity to adjust working conditions in terms of ergonomics requirements for white-collar workers has been an object of study in the beginning of 80's in such countries as Sweden [1]. It is possible that people will soon realize that it is not enough to limit the possible risk at work. The preliminary stage of planning the work process should involve their prevention or even regression.

Investing in human resources proves to be very profitable, since the efficiency of management systems, right next to processes, is dependent to employees. [2, 3] Unfortunately, profitability from expanses made on employees sometimes is not directly visible, or it is a long term process that, at one point, people forget about its existence. However, if we provide better working conditions for employees it may lead to a situation where they would start doing their job more effectively and more preferably. At the same time we could have an opportunity to lower absence level connected with different illnesses, not only those professional illnesses but also those that are related to employee's tiredness which influences his/her general physical and psychological efficiency. Such actions are also taken to lower the level of occupational burnouts occurences through improving satisfaction from work. However, awareness of that fact is only supported by a few. The majority will not change their disposition in this matter, as long as there is not proper transfer of knowledge in this field.

Highly ergonomic quality of work environment favours improvement of work efficiency, decreasing biological costs of work, lowering a number of costs of lacks and numbers of errors made at work, decreasing absence levels connected to illnesses, and experiencing satisfaction from a contact with technical devices.[9, 17]. Consequently, inappropriate shaping of work environment leads to economic and moral losses in a company. Concluding, implementation of ergonomic basis into a workplace environment planning proclaims that the management not only follows rules and norms of ergonomics in case of safety and hygiene at work, but it also constitutes that supervision and management processes have been present from the very beginning in the process of planning a workplace that could perfectly fit its worker.

4   Assumptions and the Research Method

An initial assumption of carried studies was a relationship between employee's perception of the following aspects: occupational safety and ergonomics, the culture of safety, and job satisfaction. [13] (fig.1).

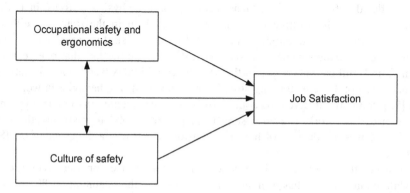

Fig. 1. Relationships between the occupational safety and ergonomics, the culture of safety and the job satisfaction (own preparation)

For the sake of a research a questionnaire was made. It consisted of a set of questions referring to general groups of factors which, according to authors, are important at workplace, and then factors assessing levels of workplace ergonomics in relation to:

— Importance of a factor for an employee in perception of job satisfaction.
— Presence of a factor at a given work post.

The inquired answered assessing validity and satisfaction in 4 groups of factors (General, Leadership, Technical environment, and Ergonomics of tech workplace). According to the authors, these groups of factors were considered as good determiners of a description of job satisfaction model. Questions were delivered as statements for which the inquired defined a level of fulfillment. E1. My work is adapted in terms of physical effort (I do not do activities beyond my physical strength).

— E2. My job provides me with sufficient physical activity (I do not suffer from lack of movement in my work).
— E3. Work activities and work environment allow for working in an unforced and comfortable body position (I do not feel pain because of body position).

- E4. Mental effort of my work is adapted to my needs (there is not it too much or too little).
- E5. The job is not monotonous; I am doing my work with pleasure.
- E6. Technical work environment is friendly (comfortable, understandable, easy to use and operate, allows to work efficiently).
- E7. I do not feel the negative impact of work environment factors such as inadequate temperature, humidity, light, radiation and noise.
- E8. The organization of work is appropriate (work pace, breaks, etc.).
- E9. I do not feel stress at work (work and its environment is not causing me any stress reactions).
- E10. I have good contact with colleagues and superiors (good atmosphere in workplace).
- G1. My work salary allows me to purchase luxury items, to have financial resources.
- G2. My work provides occupational development in a given position.
- G3. My work provides prestige, titles, awards.
- G4. My work provides positive relations with other people (friendship, safety, acceptance).
- G5. My work provides me with favorable tasks and a favorable environment.
- G6. My work provides influence on work results.
- G7. My work provides participation in decision-making processes.
- G8. My work provides me with a feeling of dignity (honesty, reliability, justice, courage, loyalty, solidarity, goodness, responsibility, truthfulness, generosity, patriotism, tolerance, impartiality, professionalism, independence, personal freedom).
- G9. There would have to exist serious reasons, for me to resign from the current workplace.

The first pilot questionnaires were directed to employees of three production enterprises in Poland and Romania. The following marginal conditions for election of enterprises and respondents were created:

- Productive character of activity.
- Size of an enterprise extending 50 people.
- Machinery park including not only small devices but also machines or assembly lines.
- Time of enterprise activity min. 5 years.
- Inquired worker employment min. 1 year in a given enterprise.

In every examined enterprise a special attention was given to the fact that assessment was delivered not only to productive but also administrative employees, and also to those accomplishing service processes in relation to main processes. Table 1. presents the structure of participants in particular enterprises.

Table 1. Data on respondents (own preparation)

Companies	Number regards the type of work		Number regards the age		Number regards the gender	
Company 1 (Poland)	Office	6	≤29	8	Women	8
	Production	20	30-39	11	Men	18
	Service	0	40-49	5		
			50-59	2		
			≥60	0		
Company 2 (Poland)	Office	5	≤29	15	Women	22
	Production	17	30-39	7	Men	4
	Service	4	40-49	4		
			50-59	0		
			≥60	0		
Company 3 (Romania)	Office	2	≤29	0	Women	19
	Production	27	30-39	4	Men	11
	Service	1	40-49	17		
			50-59	9		
			≥60	0		

Enterprise 1 is a medium Polish printing company. Its offer consists of such products like: brochures, leaflets, books, etiquettes, forms and wrappings. The company functions on market for 20 years and is still developing. As a proof of care of client's satisfaction, and also surrounding environment and other parties, the enterprise possesses implemented and certificated quality management and environmental management systems and basic elements of corporate social responsibility.

The second Polish enterprises which took part in a research is a producer and a supplier of comprehensive solutions for a BTL industry. It is a medium enterprise functioning on market for 26 years which clients are mainly large organizations. As the answer for customer's demands, the company possesses implemented and certificated quality management system ISO 9001 for 7 years. A rising role of environmental and social issues in business contacts with partners caused that the management of the company decided to include new element into organization management system. One year ago the enterprise started to build and implement a business social responsibility system. The basic reference documents which are used in the enterprises in this process are: norm ISO 14001, OHSAS 18001, chose elements of SA 8000.

Enterprise 3 is one of the Romanian factories of chemical products with a long tradition and it was established in the 1950s. Going through major changes (after the revolution of 1989), after renewing the technology and obtaining all international quality certificates in the industry, in 2013 the portfolio includes 150 products, out of which 70 are registered for export. The enterprise is the world leader for a bulk active substance (more than 40% market share for the product) and its products are distributed in 40 countries. The enterprise has about 1500 employees and most of the shares are detained by the Romanian government.

The assessment of levels of safety culture in particular enterprises was not delivered, however, in case of further study, an assessment of perfection level in this matter will be conveyed on the basis of the holon model.[8].

5   Results of Research of Non-financial Factors of Job Satisfaction

Results of the questionnaire were presented separately for every of the examined enterprise. The authors made a contrasting analysis of the results of a given enterprise. Contrasting the assessments of enterprises was not the aim of the study and due to that fact it was not performed. The main aim of the analysis of the results was to confirm the usefulness of the research tool and definition of its propriety towards enterprises of different branches and of differentiated levels of organizational culture.

Graphic interpretations of the results for the groups of factors relevant to the work were summarized in Table 2.

Table 2. Graphical interpretation of the overall evaluations of job satisfaction (own preparation based on research results)

The criteria rated on a scale: awful, very poor, poor, average, fair, good, excellent	Company 1 (Poland)	Company 2 (Poland)	Company 3 (Romania)
economic conditions			
interpersonal relationships			
method of supervision and leadership			
technical and IT environment			
work safety and ergonomics of my workstation (adjustment to my needs)			

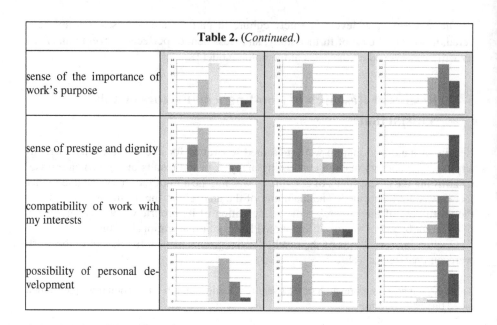

Table 2. *(Continued.)*			
sense of the importance of work's purpose			
sense of prestige and dignity			
compatibility of work with my interests			
possibility of personal development			

Table 3. Graphics visualization of positive ratings of the different factors at work (own preparation based on research results)

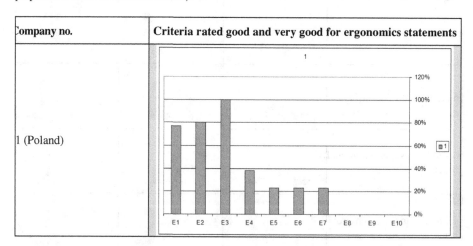

Company no.	Criteria rated good and very good for ergonomics statements
1 (Poland)	

Table 3. (*Continued.*)

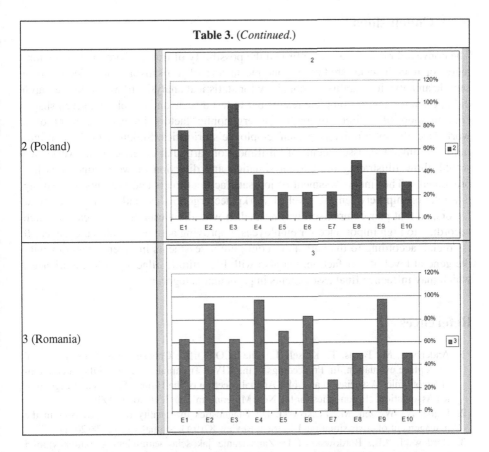

The research allowed making a statement about surprisingly high assessment of validity of presented criteria of workplace ergonomics. It may confirm the employees' ergonomic awareness. In enterprises 1 and 2 all criteria were assessed as important or very important. Due to a small cognitive value of such an assessment, it is recommended to use gradual division according to importance using differentiated requirements or adapting pair comparisons in future.

A distinctive tendency in case of assessments of given criterion fulfillment is a low assessment of criteria from E4 to E7 for enterprises 1 and 2. Such a tendency do not occur in case of an enterprises number 3. It is an essential premise which should be analyzed in details using statistically crucial study sample. In case this tendency is confirmed it would meant the necessity to control applied solutions in enterprises in Romania. In both Polish companies more than 95% of the respondents negatively assessed the following statement: My work provides me with a feeling of dignity (honesty, reliability, justice, courage, loyalty, solidarity, goodness, responsibility, truthfulness, generosity, patriotism, tolerance, impartiality, professionalism, independence, personal freedom). Such a high level of dissatisfaction induces to examine the roots of this problem.

6   Conclusions

The conveyed pilot research confirmed the possibility of usage of presented questionnaire for non-financial studies- ergonomic factors of job satisfaction. Selection of a sample and also its quantity do not allow for statistical analysis, however, the research did not aim to receive complete results but to test a scale and a tool. In a given shape, configuration of validity of particular ergonomic factors in an assessment of a workplace, do not efficiently present employee's priorities. Simultaneously, configuration of ranks with assessments of fulfillment of particular criterion at the workplace would allow illustrating the current situation and direction of work conditions improvements. The final assessment of job satisfaction directs and presents how strong is a relationship between the level of workplace ergonomics, and even its particular factors, so that pair comparison was needed. It will allow establishing areas in which according to high importance for employees, improving activity should be engaged. It is crucial, according to the authors to configure assessments in given categories with the general level of satisfaction, but also with life attitude, illnesses, life experiences, which may influence final assessments in particular categories.

References

1. Andersson, M., Berns, T., Klusell, L.: The TCO "Office Checker" a tool for ergonomic work place evaluation. In: Proceedings of the XIVth Triennial Congress of the International Ergonomics Association and 44th Annual Meeting of the Human Factors and Ergonomics Association, 'Ergonomics for the New Millennium', pp. 659–662 (2000)
2. Bajda, A., Wrażeń, M., Laskowski, D.: Diagnostics the quality of data transfer in the management of crisis situation. Electrical Review 87(9A), SigmaNot., 72–78(2011)
3. Berdowski, J.B., Berdowski, F.J.: Zarządzanie jakością warunkiem konkurencyjności przedsiębiorstwa, Oficyna Wydawnicza WSM SIG, Warszawa (2004)
4. Bryan Sexton, J., Klinect, J.R.: The link between safety attitudes and observed performance in flight operations. In: Proceedings of the Eleventh International Symposium on Aviation Psychology, p. 713. The Ohio State University, Columbus (2001)
5. Butlewski, M., Tytyk, E.: The method of matching ergonomic nonpowered hand tools to maintenance tasks for the handicapped. In: Karwowski, W., Salvendy, G. (eds.) (CD ROM) 2nd International Conference on Applied Human Factors and Ergonomics, Las Vegas, Nevada, USA. Conference Proceedings (2008)
6. Clark, A.E., Oswald, A.J.: Satisfaction and comparison income. Journal of Public Economics 69(57), 57–81 (1996)
7. Gene, M., Alarcon Joseph, B.: Lyons The Relationship of Engagement and Job Satisfaction in Working Samples. The Journal of Psychology: Interdisciplinary and Applied 145(5), 463–480 (2011)
8. Jasiulewicz-Kaczmarek, M., Misztal, A., Butlewski, M.: The holons model of quality improvements. In: SMEs, Global Innovation and Knowledge Academy (GIKA) Conference, Valencia, Spain, July 9-11 (2013)
9. Jasiulewicz-Kaczmarek, M.: Participatory Ergonomics as a Method of Quality Improvement in Maintenance. In: Karsh, B.-T. (ed.) Ergonomics and Health Aspects, HCII 2009. LNCS, vol. 5624, pp. 153–161. Springer, Heidelberg (2009)

10. Kawecka-Endler, A.: Metodologia ergonomicznego kształtowania warunków pracy w montażu i ich przyczynowoskutkowe powiązania z systemem jakości. Wyd. Politechniki Poznańskiej, seria Rozprawy, nr 333, Poznań (1998)
11. Lee, T.: Assessment of safety culture at a nuclear reprocessing plant, Work & Stress: An International Journal of Work. Health & Organisations 12(3), 217–237 (1998)
12. Mcgill, S.M., Grenier, S., Bluhm, M., Preuss, R., Brown, S.: Previous history of LBP with work loss is related to lingering deficits in biomechanical, physiological, personal, psychosocial and motor control characteristics. Ergonomics 46, 731–746 (2003)
13. Misztal, A., Butlewski, M.: Life improvement at work, Wyd. PP, Poznań (2012) ISBN: 9788377751770
14. Jones, R.J., Sloane, P.J.: Low Pay, Higher Pay and Job Satisfaction in Wales. Spatial Economic Analysis 2(2), 197–214 (2007)
15. Schulz, D.P., Schulz, S.E.: Psychologia a wyzwania dzisiejszej pracy, PWN, Warszawa (2002)
16. Tutuncu, O., Kozak, M.: An Investigation of Factors Affecting Job Satisfaction. International Journal of Hospitality & Tourism Administration 8(1), 119 (2007)
17. Tytyk, E.: Ergonomia podstawowe pojęcia, w: Nauka o pracy bezpieczeństwo, higiena, ergonomia t. I, Koradecka D (red.), Wydawnictwo CIOP, Warszawa (2000)
18. Wu, H.: Effects of ergonomicsbased waferhandling training on reduction in musculoskeletal disorders among wafer handlers. International Journal of Industrial Ergonomics 39(1), 127–132 (2009)

Reclaiming Human Machine Nature

Didier Fass

ICN Business School
MOSEL LORIA UNIVERSITÉ de Lorraine
Campus Scientifique BP239
Vandoeuvre-lès-Nancy Cedex, France
Didier.fass@loria.fr

Abstract. Extending and modifying his domain of life by artifact production is one of the main characteristics of humankind. From the first hominid, who used a wood stick or a stone for extending his upper limbs and augmenting his gesture strength, to current systems engineers who used technologies for augmenting human cognition, perception and action, extending human body capabilities remains a big issue. From more than fifty years cybernetics, computer and cognitive sciences have imposed only one reductionist model of human machine systems: cognitive systems. Inspired by philosophy, behaviorist psychology and the information treatment metaphor, the cognitive system paradigm requires a function view and a functional analysis in human systems design process. According that design approach, human have been reduced to his metaphysical and functional properties in a new dualism. Human body requirements have been left to physical ergonomics or "physiology". With multidisciplinary convergence, the issues of "human-machine" systems and "human artifacts" evolve. The loss of biological and social boundaries between human organisms and interactive and informational physical artifact questions the current engineering methods and ergonomic design of cognitive systems. New developpment of human machine systems for intensive care, human space activities or bio-engineering sytems requires grounding human systems design on a renewed epistemological framework for future human systems model and evidence based "bio-engineering". In that context, reclaiming human factors, *augmented human* and human machine nature is a necessity.

Keywords: Augmented human, human machine nature, human systems integration, functional parameters, human factors, non-functional parameters, organism.

1   Introduction: Is There "Any body" Inside?

Was there a cave in Platoon's head?

The theme of the human machine is currently a topic of research and development on the one hand and techno-philosophical-anthropological other. On the one hand reductionism assumes reduce the human body to a thinking machine and its physical and computational properties, in affiliation with Descartes and de La Métrie. On the other

V.G. Duffy (Ed.): DHM 2014, LNCS 8529, pp. 588–599, 2014.
© Springer International Publishing Switzerland 2014

hand, invokes a humanist ideal, a conception of human metaphysical and transcendent, from the Renaissance and Vitruvius.

Between rationalist reductionism and metaphysical and theological idealism, the theme of "human machine" and even more "augmented human" is controversial.

Between the ideal philosophical or theological, Human with a capital H, and general scientific rational realization of the abstract category of a human biological system, there is life, the body, multidimensional integrated reality and death.

How then theoretically conceive human and scientific principles of the human machine design? What we might call *augmented human* bioengineering.

1.1   Human Machine and Intensive Care

Before going further, we confront a moment the reality of the medical intensive care unit. Here the reality of human-machine is a vital necessity. The human-machine makes sense for the patient and his family. It is a matter of survival or death, for which medical teams not without practical and ethical issues. Regardless of the sophistication of these machines - mechanical ventilation, haemodialysis, cardiopulmonary bypass ... a benefit / risk assessment is always necessary and difficult. There are always risks iatrogenic real, although many automatic feedback loops have been developed [6].

1.2   Human Machine and Human Space Activities

If you wish to send a human in the water or in space and make him or her active, the problem is different. It is no longer survival but to expand the field of life and activity of the person, the requirements of life support and domain-specific activity. Artefacts, transport modules and living arrangements and clothing (suits) must be designed to maintain:

i.   Bodily integrity and basic physiological functioning;
ii.   Relational - sensorimotor and cognitive, and operational capacity of the operator situations;
iii.   Health of the operator in a consistent functional area with the return to earth by avoiding, for example, the risk of embolism in the plunger or cardiovascular collapse with the astronaut.

1.3   Human Machine and Convergence

With current or interactive cognitive systems [8] [12] of the smartphone to the cockpit of an airplane and the resuscitation room, or with technical systems to be operated or remotely operated by a human, the boundaries between the human and artifice, produced by human, fade. With the convergence multidisciplinary nano-bio-info-cogno (NBIC) [13] [14] amplifies this dynamic. Future implantable nano-biotechnological systems, wearable technologies and ambient intelligence and ubiquitous systems for civilian applications at all stages of life or defence let imagine new benefits and new risks to master knowledge.

This disappearance of boundaries between human biological and social and inter-active and informational physical artifact questions the current engineering methods and ergonomic design of cognitive systems [1] [10] and their scientific basis.

Current and future developments in human assisted supplemented, repaired, ex-panded or increased not only pose new scientific and technical challenges but also new epistemological questions.

1.4   Reclaiming Human Machine Nature

Currently, the human "biopsychosocial", in the words of Henri Laborit [11] is reduced in a reciprocal and symmetrical metaphorical relationship to cognitive artifacts-computo-logical-symbolic being disembodied. Although this reductionist design of human-system remains dualistic. The philosophical question of duality "mind body" has been replaced by the question of duality "body brain", where the brain is designed as a cognitive computational machine or independent of its organic substrate that processes information with loops feedback [7]. This vision is inspired by Turing and von Neumann's machines, by Shannon and Weaver and Wiener' theory of communi-cation, and by automatic and cybernetics [16].

With multidisciplinary convergence, issues of "human-machine" systems and "hu-man artifacts" evolve. Behavioral and cognitive heuristics metaphors, if they remain productive for the design of automatic systems generate new questions and problems that tell us to question the theoretical and experimental conceptual foundations of the "human machine". The correct design and safe technology of techniques and artefacts of "augmented human", require a system of knowledge and description revisited, without (much) of ideological and metaphorical a priori. It is for us to develop a framework for integrating artefacts with human as a matter of coupling in the multi-scale dimensions of two systems of different nature: human, biological and anthropo-logical, and the artefact, physical and logical-symbolic.

Understanding this synthetic hybridization requires a new conceptual apparatus and a new knowledge system of the human systems integration (HIS), capable of thinking the human machine and new practices, the model and the test as a whole structurally and functionally integrated: *an epistemology of extending the area of life and human machine nature.*

2   Functional Parameters of Artificial System Design: Reclaiming Human Factors

The dominant paradigme of design and description of the human machine systems are generally outcome of behavioral and cognitive approach. They are based on a func-tional approach. The human is reduced, in a reciprocal and symmetrical artifacts metaphorical relation, to a disembodied computo-logical-symbolic "cognitive-being".

According cognitive ergonomics, requierement engineering for human in-the-loop artificial and automation systems design is reduced to its cognitive functions.

Knowing, reasoning, understanding, planning, deciding, problem solving, analyzing, synthesizing, monitoring, assessing, checking, verifying, judging... are some the instantiation of cognitive function assumption. They refer to an agent's capacity to process or compute thoughts. According agency philosophy and artificial intelligence, an agent is an entity capable of perception, information processing or computing, and action and whose individual or collective activity is goal oriented and adapted to an environment.

This utilitarian approach is related to functionalist concepts of cognitive function, cognitive systems and joint cognitive systems [10]. Even if its wants this reductionist conception human-systems remains dualistic. This vision is inspired by Turing [Turing1936] and von Neumann's machine theory, Shannon and Weaver and Wiener's theories of communication, automatic and cybernetics.

Methods and current tools of systems engineering, in particular "systems of systems" are derived from cybernetics, science and computer technology and cognition, and human factors with regard to the "systems man-in-the-loop". To do this, they represent the system through technical and managerial components approach in describing the relationship and interaction through physical interfaces and communications devices. Interaction is seen as a process of communication between components of the system reduced to each other in loops "entry, data processing, response". If it has demonstrated its heuristic nature, this metaphorical and reductionist approach is not sufficient to model embedded systems as a functional whole and scale relativity of space and time. Understanding and description of the organization of these organic or complex socio-technical systems require a unit of knowledge representation and modelling renewed.

To do this we propose a functional analysis of human factors framework in terms of existing built-in functions in both a psychological and physiological perspective: perception, decision, action, control and emotions (PDAC+E).

3   The "Human Factor"[1] Always Rings Twice.

Here is a proposal for a renewed operational human factors (HFs) model, based on functional parameters: Perception, Decision-making, Action and Control (PDAC) functions, which allow assessing each human agent or actor behavior.

For example, if a perception problem is identified as a cause for a poor decision, then we can question the data input canal.

The analysis needs to be related to the context, which is an operational context (traffic situation, weather) and role played by the agent.

---

[1]   This is a wordplay. In french « facteur » means both factor or postman.

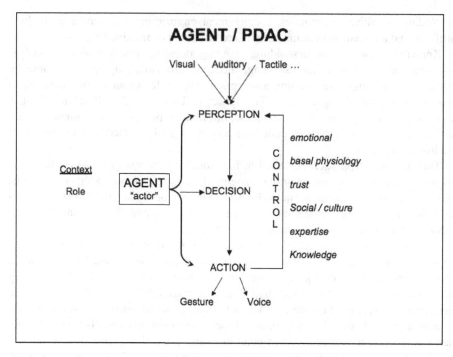

Fig. 1. Operational *HF model*

An agent or an actor, involve in an activity with appropriate skills and competences and duly authorized, "plays" a role in an operational context.

The main classes of agent's function are perception, decision-making, action and control (fig. 1):

- Perception is based on visual, auditory or haptic (prioprio-tactilo-kinestetic) information.
- Decision-Making is based on reasoning and emotion. It integrates elements of perception and knowledge to answer the question: to do or not to do, what to do?
- Action is the result of an integrated and situated cognitive function. The main modes of action of an actor are gesture and voice. Interfaces and communication channels or networks mediate interactions with other agents or machines.
- Control guide thinking and behaviour in accordance with internally generated goals or plans coupled to stimuli and meaningful elements of the environment (space of actions and space of navigation) through perceptive and motor loops. Control is closely allied to attention and vigilance, basal physiology (stress, fatigue...). It also depends on knowledge, expertise and trust in collaborative activities. Emotional states influence control, also anthropological and social factors.

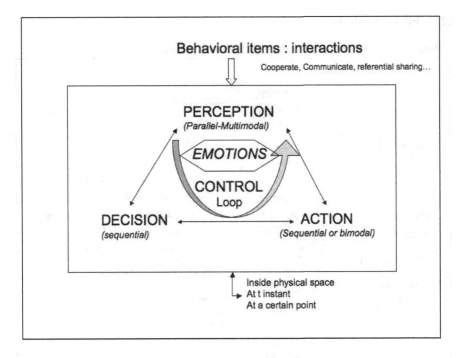

Fig. 2. Behavioral model: based on PDAC loop and modulated by emotions

3.1   Behavioral Model

An activity is based on integration of a certain number of functions. Each human in the loop function requires several specific functional interactions for each agent for each role inside the physical space at t instant and at a certain point into the time scale relativity and space scale relativity.

Each functional interactions are related to a behavioral item or mode, such as co-operate, communicate, referential sharing.... Using this behavioral model we are able to link functions and sub functions to the observable behavior of an agent, based on the operational PDAC HF model.

Dynamics of behavioral model is based on PDAC integrated loop and modulated by emotions.

Behavioral modelling in design and simulation hold to take into account the complexity of each class of agent's fundamental function: perception is parallel and multimodal; decision-making is sequential, action is sequential or bimodal and control is a conscious and sequential and/or unconscious and parallel process.

Behavioral model connects PDAC-based operational HF model to collaborative and cooperative functions underlying authority sharing and distribution.

3.2   PDAC Analysis

What can be observed in a human in-the-loop simulation?

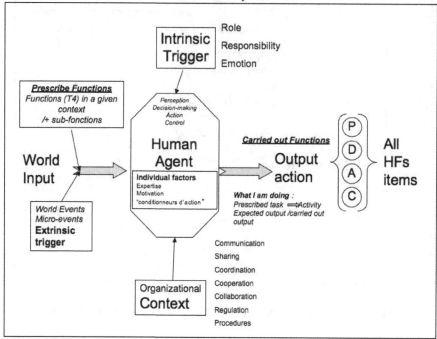

Fig. 3. PDAC analysis schema

From the world input, we can deduce an expected behavior related to the pre-scribed task. What will be observed is a result of Human activities through observable « output actions ».

Prescribe function F:E and Carried out function

    E: world input, S: expected output action, S': observed output action

    i. If $S=S'$ then $F=F'$, OK

    ii. If $S \neq S'$ then $F \neq F'$, then question: what HF (s) is or are involved?

And what is the intrinsic trigger and organizational context (OFs)?
Pattern variation of PDAC values allow to identify, what HFs issues are involved.

When there is a difference between expected behavior and output actions, we need to assess the HF issue that might have produced such a result: PDAC model allows to question the human basic functions and to locate the elements (intrinsic trigger and organizational context), which had an impact.

To complete that analytical methodology, we must place the PDAC analysis schema into the operational context, which must also be simulated during future experimentations.

This can be applied to a single human agent.

Now how to address collective work multi-agent environment), which is the main issue of sociotechnical systems (cooperation, authority, responsibility, and task sharing)?

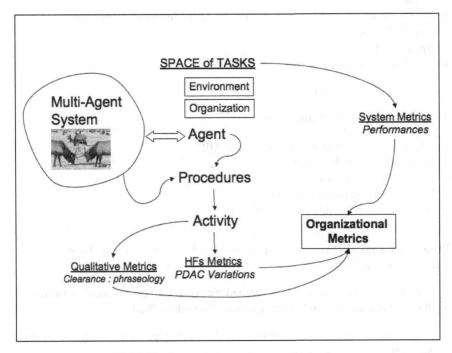

Fig. 4. Metrics: variation to the prescribed task

Metrics: Variation to the Prescribed Task. The situations that will be observed are multi-agent situations.

In a space of tasks, within a certain environment (both technical and organizational) the agents will « produce » their activities, based on pre-determined interaction procedures. Individual HF metrics based on PDAC model will be gathered.

At the same time it will be possible to set performance metrics (capacity, safety, efficiency) and also organizational metrics (number of vocal communications…). And also qualitative data will be extracted concerning organizational aspects.

The individual HF metrics will then be temporally and conceptually correlated with the more global measures (organizational, performance and qualitative data).

PDAC Perspective. To demonstrate how to use PDAC schema analysis, let's imagine a « simple task » based on very simple simulation scenario. That example presents how the PDAC analysis tools might be used.

Example: Prescribed task (Modelling, Simulation)

"When you hear "beep" move downward the red lever {control stick}"

- **PDAC = HFs analysis tool**: 4 elementary functions (convention)
- **Prescribed task**: prescribed function, in an organizational context that constrained relations, to an operator who is characterized by a role and a level of responsibility (legal sense)
- **World inputs**: what happen in the activity space (event or micro-event)
- **Extrinsic trigger**: *"beep"*
- **Prescribed output**
- **Fundamental model**: Agent = "PDAC",

— Aim: to explain what the agent have to do

- **Modeling prescribed function**:

— I'm waiting for **agent** hearing the "beep" (P)
— Remembering the instruction (D),
— Finding the red lever (P)
— Lever is coming downward (A)
— Agent feels the mission accomplished (C)

Prescribed Task: PDAC analysis. *"When you hear "beep" move downward the red lever {control stick}"*

- Experimentation trace: « Beep is set and the red lever never come downward»
- PDAC Filter: difference Prescribed Task/ Carried out Task

What does not go in my model or what does not work in the execution of my experimentation?

>   Why no P?
>   Why no D?
>   Why no A?
>   Why no C?

However, the answer to these questions is not only analytical and functional. Another design consideration elements of man machine systems and their coupling is needed to understand how the functions and dysfunctions emerge.

4   Non-functional Parameters of Artificial System Design: Making Sense of the Organism

Current human in-the-loop and human-machine system are opened loop. Future human machine will produce regulations or counter-measures couplings generated by dynamic interfacing systems closing the loop at both organizational level and individual level. These new developments raise five major scientific and technical interdisciplinary challenges:

    i.   Human systems integration: from the science of systems biology and integrative physiology theory applied to human engineering systems.

    ii.   Epistemology and human machine systems modelling: witch system of knowledge and description?

    iii.   Safe design of human in-the-loop systems: numerical modelling, systems engineering and human factors.

    iv.   Physiological and pathophysiological modelling: what is the link between the structural elements of a system, their shapes and dynamic coupling and the emergence of functions?

    v.   Modelling and certification: how to validate and certificate "human machine in-the-loop" systems?

To answer these questions we need to escape the illusion of human-centred design and cognitive system reductionism.

4.1 Integrative Epistemology and Human Machine Design: Reclaiming Epistemology of Coupling

Designing artificial environments and human machine systems needs to take into account both technical systems, multimodal interactions of coupling (physical, logical and informational, and biological) artificially generated and their integration into the dynamics of human behavior, cognitive, sensorimotor and emotional... and therefore in the structural and functional organization of the body: the anatomical extension of the body and the enhancement of the functions of "augmented human".

This is a problem of coupling two systems of different natures: a biological system, the human, with a physical system, the interactive artefact more or less immersive, encompassing, incorporating therefore integrative.

4.2 Augmented Human as an Hybrid Organism System

The human systems integration (is to seamlessly integrate human components and passive and interactive technologies. To be safe and predictive, HIS models, the concepts of interaction and integration, methods and rules of systems engineering and design must be epistemologically well founded.

As the mathematical theory of physics and the principles underlying the mechanical or material science, e.g. technical engineering aircraft, HSI requires integration theory, a theoretical framework (conceptually and formally proven) and its principles general for coupling a biological system (experimentally proven) or with the physical artefacts (depending on the degree of complexity of the artificial system).

Some classical concept must be revised:

    o   Inside vs. outside

    o   Opened system vs. closed system

    o   Discrete structure, structural discontinuity

    o   Functional continuum, functional continuity
    o   Structural stability – functional viability
    o   Geometries of the architecture, function analysis and interactions of coupling
    o   System, organism

4.3   Biology, the Human System Domain

Designing augmented human [9] or human machine system as an hybrid organism, according to HSI concepts involves a paradigm shift from a metaphorical design and engineering based on usage scenarios, utility and activity - based on models and metaphysical rules of interaction and cognition, to integration engineering of dynamic structural coupling and based on an integrative theory and evidences of human machine "biology" and principles.

5   Conclusion – *Augmented human* Bioengineering Challenge

If we want to integrate human factors and their functional determinant (PDAC + E) in the design of human machine system, it should be conceived as a hybrid structural system all united by physical, logical and biological coupling interactions that generates functional continuum in space of stability of the extended anatomical body [5] and increased domain of viability of functions[3].

The logical organization of these systems is that of integrative biology and physiology of man machine systems. To conceptualize human machine systems as an organic whole organized according to the principles human systems integration grounded on theoretical systems biology requires the development of the principles and methods of a "bio-engineering" of *augmented human.*

References

1. Amalberti, R.: Les facteurs humains à l'aube de l'an 2000. Phoebus, pp. 5–12 (1998)
2. Ashby, R.: An introduction to cybernetics. Chapman & Hall, London (1957)
3. Aubin, J.P.: Théorie de la Viabilité : Régulation de l'Évolution de Systèmes de Réseaux et Morphogenèse des Contraintes sous Incertitude Tychastique – Synthèse (2005), http://www.lastre.asso.fr/aubin/Viabilite-Synthese.doc
4. Bailly, F., Longo, G.: Mathématiques et sciences de la nature. Herman, Paris (2006)
5. Chauvet, G.: Hierarchical functional organization of formal biological systems: A dynamical approach. I, II and III. Phil. Trans. Roy. Soc. London B 3, 425–481 (1993) ISSN: 1471-2970
6. Chopin, C.: L'histoire de la ventilation mécanique: des machines et des hommes. Réanimation 16(1), 4–12 (2007)
7. Conant, R., Ashby, R.: Every good regulator of a system must be a model of that system. Int. J. Systems Sci. 1(2), 89–97 (1970)

8. Engelbart, D.C.: Augmenting human intellect: a conceptual framework, AFOSR-3233 Summary Report, Stanford Research Institute, Menlo Park, California 94025, USA, http://www.dougengelbart.org/ (October 1962)

9. Fass, D.: Augmented human engineering: a theoretical and experimental approach to human system integration. In: Cogan, B. (ed.) System Engineering – Practice and Theory. Intech - Open Access Publisher, Rijeka (2012)

10. Hollnagel, E., Woods, D.D.: Joint cognitive systems: Foundations of cognitive systems engineering. CRC Press / Taylor & Francis, Boca Raton, FL (2005)

11. Laborit, H.: L'inhibition de l'action. Masson, Paris (1986)

12. Licklider, J.C.R.: Man-Computer Symbiosis. IRE Transactions on Human Factors in Electronics HFE-1, 4–11 (1960) ISSN: 0096-249X

13. Roco, M.C., Bainbridge, W.S.: Converging technologies for improving human performance nanotechnology, biotechnology, information technology and cognitive science. Technical report, National Science Foundation (2002), http://www.wtec.org/ConvergingTechnologies/Report/NBIC_report.pdf

14. Nordmann, A.: Converging technologies - Shaping the future of European societies. Technical report, European Communities (2004)

15. Turing, On Computable Numbers, with an Application to the Entscheidungsproblem. In: Proceedings of the London Mathematical Society, vol. 2(42) pp. 230-265 (1936)

16. Wiener, N.: Cybernetics. John Wiley & Sons, New York (1948)

Evacuation Support System for Everyday Use in the Aftermath of a Natural Disaster

Akari Hamamura[1], Taku Fukushima[2], Takashi Yoshino[1], and Nobuyuki Egusa[1]

[1] Faculty of Systems Engineering, Wakayama University
{s155037,yoshino,egusa}@center.wakayama-u.ac.jp
[2] Graduate School of Engineering, Shizuoka University
fukushima@sys.eng.shizuoka.ac.jp

Abstract. Numerous natural disasters occur in Japan, such as earthquakes, typhoons, and volcanic eruptions. Information technology is expected to facilitate evacuation support when a disaster strikes, but networks cannot be used in many cases. Moreover, if a disaster occurs in a town that people do not frequent often, they may find it difficult to cope initially. It is difficult to access software online immediately at the time of a disaster. Thus, we have developed an evacuation support system called AkariMap, which can be used offline in the aftermath of a disaster. AkariMap is also a system that is suitable for everyday use. AkariMap has two functions: a function that notifies a user about evacuation support information each day and a disaster mode function that users can access at times of emergency. Based on the results of our experiments, we report the following findings. (1) Subjects increasingly accessed local evacuation support information for about 10 days. (2) Even if people did not use the notification function in the long-term, they were still accustomed to using the system. (3) If people need to find a shelter using AkariMap, they can identify a safer shelter by displaying the flooded areas.

Keywords: disaster system, evacuation support, everyday use, offline support system.

1 Introduction

The communication networks required for information and communication technology were destroyed immediately after the Great East Japan Earthquake (GEJE) in 2011. However, networks and information technology are indispensable for information communication in a stricken area. For example, Google Person Finder [1] could be used to collect and provide information that supports the well-being of people in a disaster area.

To prepare for disasters that may occur in the future, many researchers and companies in Japan are addressing the potential problems associated with earthquakes, and they are developing new services to support the recovery from various disasters[2]. However, most of the studies and services that are being developed

V.G. Duffy (Ed.): DHM 2014, LNCS 8529, pp. 600–611, 2014.

assume that a network will be available for use after a disaster. In reality, a network becomes crowded and congested immediately after a disaster occurs. Furthermore, the communication network may be physically disrupted and electric power outages may occur[3].

During the GEJE, 79.6% of the evacuees had their mobile phones with them[4]. Thus, the majority of the evacuees recognized the necessity for a mobile phone. All of the mobile phones used in Japan are equipped with an emergency messaging service. However, the utilization rate of this service was only 4.5% during the GEJE [4], whereas the utilization rate before the GEJE was 6.5%. Thus, we consider that it may be difficult to use this type of unfamiliar service immediately when an emergency occurs[4]. Moreover, many people cannot obtain evacuation support information, such as a travel destination or business destination.

If a disaster occurs in a place where evacuation support information is not available, it is necessary to search for a shelter amid the confusion. Some people cannot cope with the conditions immediately and they may experience severe distress. Thus, we consider that a new system with two elements is required, as follows.

- It should be possible to use the system even if no network is available after a disaster occurs.
- It should be possible to acquire experience of the emergency function before a disaster occurs.

Thus, we have developed an evacuation support system called AkariMap[5], which has two functions: a function that provides a user with evacuation support information and a disaster mode function that a user can experience at any time. This study presents the detailed functions of AkariMap and the results of evaluation experiments.

2 Related Work

Fukuda et al. developed a tsunami evacuation support system based on a tablet PC[6], which can be used offline. This system uses an offline type GIS and it displays a tsunami hazard map, positional information, and the movements of a user. Hiruta et al. developed a disaster information sharing system to facilitate the search for a shelter after a disaster[7]. This system provides information collected by the evacuees regarding shelters and it allows disaster information sharing using smartphones. The system uses a smartphone as a server and the disaster information is accumulated by the smartphone. Therefore, if a communication base cannot be utilized during a disaster, this system can be used to share information about shelters. However, these systems were not designed for daily use.

Fujikawa et al. developed a disaster support system for everyday use that collects and shares disaster information [8]. This system can be used in the same way as a typical SNS but it can also share information during disasters. The system switches into disaster mode during a disaster and exchanges disaster-related information via an independent network. This system was designed for

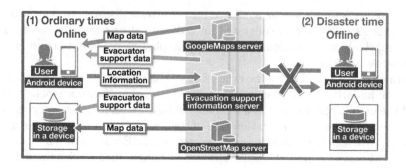

Fig. 1. System configuration for AkariMap

daily use, but no function is available that allows the continuous use of the system.

We consider that it may be difficult to use unfamiliar systems that are not used on a daily basis if a disaster occurs. Thus, we propose a notification function for continuous use and a disaster mode function that a user can test at any time.

3   AkariMap

We assume that online support should be available before a disaster strikes and that offline help needs to be provided immediately after a disaster. AkariMap is an evacuation support system for everyday use. AkariMap operates on an Android device. AkariMap offers online support via a map screen and a widget function.

A notification function provides support information during evacuations. One of the aims of the notification function is to promote the use of the system. AkariMap offers a disaster mode, which users can experience at any time.

AkariMap automatically saves the evacuation-related support information and map information to a mobile device in the online mode. The saved information can be used during a disaster (in the offline mode).

3.1   System Configuration

Figure 1 shows the system configuration for AkariMap. AkariMap comprises each user's android device, an evacuation support information server, GoogleMaps server, and OpenStreetMaps server[1]. The system is designed for use in both online (before a disaster strike) and offline (immediately after a disaster) modes. In an online situation, AkariMap obtains and saves positional information. Furthermore, the system provides a display and notifications of evacuation support information. In the offline mode, AkariMap offers evacuation support. In addition, AkariMap does not determine a destination automatically, because it can only suggest information. This is because a mobile device cannot acquire local information in the offline mode.

---

[1] Lhttp://www.openstreetmap.org/

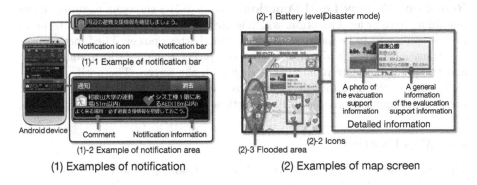

(1) Examples of notification   (2) Examples of map screen

Fig. 2. Examples showing a screenshot of AkariMap

3.2 Functions of AkariMap

Notification Function. Figure 2(1) shows an example of a notification screen. An Android device has two areas for notification: the notification bar and notification area. Figure 2(1)-1 shows an example of the notification bar and Figure 2(1)-2 shows an example of the notification area. The notification function provides evacuation support information to a user. For example, the notification bar suggests: "Let us check the local evacuation support information." The notification area presents notification comments and evacuation information. The evacuation information system suggests the nearest shelter and the nearest automatic external defibrillator (AED). AkariMap can be activated by tapping on the contents of a notification.

Disaster Mode Experience Function. In general, it is difficult to become accustomed to the use of unfamiliar software during an emergency. Thus, to facilitate the use of a beneficial function during a disaster, we developed the "disaster mode" for use at any time, thereby ensuring familiarity. A user can access the following functions in the disaster mode at any time before a disaster occurs: data cache function, remaining battery level function, map function, and widget function.

Data Cache Function. The data cache function acquires useful information offline before a disaster strikes. When a user is browsing the map screen, the system acquires evacuation support information and map data from OpenStreetMap are captured automatically as a background process[2]. A user can also acquire the data for a selected area. The acquired data is maintained in the internal storage of an Android device. Thus, evacuation support information can be provided to a user in the offline mode using the data stored before a disaster.

---

[2] GoogleMaps can be used as a map screen but the capture of map data is not allowed. Thus, we also use OpenStreetMap in the offline mode.

Remaining Battery Level Function. Figure 2(2)-1 shows an example of the remaining battery level function, which is used after a disaster occurs. This function allows a user to be aware of the remaining battery power. The function uses a notification dialog to display the battery power remaining in a smartphone and the predicted time remaining is shown on the screen. The notification dialog prompts the user to reduce the screen luminosity and to avoid the use of unnecessary applications. These two practices are also required for everyday use.

3.3 Map Function

The map function is available for online use before a disaster occurs. First, the function sends information about the user's present location to a server. Next, the function obtains evacuation support information related to the local area from a server and icons are displayed on a map. When a user taps the icon, detailed support information related to evacuation can be browsed, such as place names, photographs (if available), supplementary information, distances from the present location, and altitude. Figure 2(2)-3 shows a flooded area on a map[3].

3.4 Widget Function

A widget is a small software application on an Android device, which is always displayed on the home (main) screen. The widget function can be used online before a disaster. Even if a user is at a destination, the widget function provides local evacuation support information periodically based on the user's present location. If a user does not activate the AkariMap application, the widget function can still make them aware of the evacuation support information. Thus, a user can be activated by the widget to access AkariMap.

4 Experimental Evaluation of the Notification Function

This experiment was conducted for 30 days between April 28 and May 27, 2013. The experimental participants comprised nine subjects, i.e., six male and three female, who were all university students. Each participant installed AkariMap in their personal Android device. We tested the following hypotheses.

(1) The notification function activates the user to access evacuation support information.
(2) The notification function triggers the use of the AkariMap system.

We preregistered the shelter and AED information for the area. We conducted three questionnaire-based surveys, i.e., before the experiment, on the 10th day of the experiment, and at the end of the experiment.

---

[3] In this case, the predicted flooded area is in Wakayama Prefecture, which is the local government in the study area.

Table 1. Results of the questionnaire-based survey about the notification function at the end of the experiment (five-point Likert scale)

question items	Distribution of the evaluations					Median	Mode
	1	2	3	4	5		
(1) The notification function activated you to obtain evacuation support information related to your frequent destination.	0	1	3	5	0	4	4
(2) The notification function motivated you to use AkariMap.	0	0	0	7	2	4	4

- We used a five-point Likert scale for the evaluation: 1: Strongly disagree, 2: Disagree, 3: Neutral, 4: Agree, and 5: Strongly agree.
- The distributions of the evaluation scores are shown for individual subjects.

Table 2. Increases in the number of evacuation support information acquisition events

Participant	From before the experiment until the 10th day of the experiment	From the 10th day of the experiment until after the experiment
A	8	2
B	14	0
C	2	1
D	5	1
E	6	1
F	6	1
G	3	1
H	5	4
I	4	0

Table 3. Number of system notifications and the number of system activations after a notification

Participant	From before the experiment until the 10th day of the experiment		From the 10th day of the experiment until the end of the experiment	
	Number of notifications	Number of system activations after a notification	Number of notifications	Number of system activations after a notification
A	5	3	8	2
B	7	2	15	0
C	4	1	7	1
D	7	1	11	1
E	4	3	8	3
F	10	1	19	0
G	16	3	17	2
H	20	5	30	8
I	4	0	5	1
Average	8.6	2.4	13.3	2.0
Average system activation rate	0.28		0.15	

4.1 Results of the Experimental Evaluation of the Notification Function and Discussion

Table 1 shows the results of the questionnaire-based survey at the end of the experiment. We used a five-point Likert scale for the evaluation: 1: strongly disagree, 2: disagree, 3: neutral, 4: agree, and 5: strongly agree.

Awareness of Evacuation Support Information. Table 1(1) shows that for the question: "The notification function activated you to obtain evacuation support information related to your frequent destination," the median and mode scores were both 4. In the free description field of the questionnaire-based survey, one participant commented: "The system displayed a shelter repeatedly in the notification, which I memorized without even noticing." Table 2 shows the increases in the number of evacuation support information acquisition events, which were calculated for two periods: from before the experiment until the 10th day of the experiment and from the 10th day of the experiment until after the end of the experiment. Table 2 shows that the number of evacuation support information acquisition events increased for all subjects on the 10th day compared with the number before the experiment. However, the number of evacuation support information acquisition events declined after the 10th day. Thus, we found that the long-term use of the notification function made users more aware of the evacuation support information. Moreover, we found that people continued to acquire increasing amounts of evacuation support information for 10 days.

Usage of AkariMap. Table 1(2) shows that for the question: " the notification function motivated you to use AkariMap," the median and mode scores were both 4. The participants commented: "When the notification function was activated, I felt inclined to use it," and: "When the notification was displayed, I remembered the software and began to use it in many cases." Table 3 shows the increased in the average activation rate from before the experiment until the 10th day of the experiment, and from the 10th day of the experiment until the end of the experiment. Table 3 shows that the average activation rate declined from the 10th day of the experiment until after the end of the experiment. We consider that the participants became bored with the notification function after the 10th day. We suggest that many people found it difficult to continue using the same function for one month. We also found that some of the participants did not activate the system after this time. However, Table 3 shows that seven of the nine participants activated the system once or more between the 10th day and the end of the experiment. The average number of activations was about two. Although people used the notification function for long periods (about one month in the present study), we found that the function still activated them to use the system.

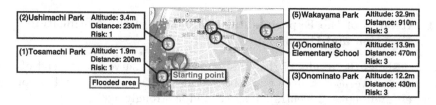

Fig. 3. Positions of the shelters around the test location

Table 4. Shelter locations around the test site in detail

	Name of shelter	Altitude	Distance	Risk level
Shelter (1)	Tosamachi Park	1.9 m	200 m	1
Shelter (2)	Ushimachi Park	3.4 m	230 m	1
Shelter (3)	Onominato Park	12.2 m	430 m	3
Shelter (4)	Onominato Elementary School	13.9 m	470 m	3
Shelter (5)	Wakayama Park	32.9 m	910 m	3

5 Experimental Evaluation in the Disaster Mode

5.1 Preliminary Experiment

We also conducted a preliminary experimental evaluation of the disaster mode function[9]. In this experiment, we assumed that a major earthquake occurred. Each of five participants selected a shelter using the disaster mode function in AkariMap. In this experiment, AkariMap provide the following evacuation support information: the user's present location, the locations of shelters, the altitude of each shelter, and the distance from the user's present location. Only one of the five participants considered the altitude when selecting a shelter. Thus, many of the participants selected the shelter without considering the possibility of a tsunami. Next, we added a function that displayed the flooded area and conducted further experiments.

5.2 Summary of the Experiment

We performed an experiment to evaluate the evacuation support provided by the disaster mode function. The participants were 12 university students, i.e., five were male and seven were female. Nine of the experimental participants had experience of using AkariMap. Thus, three inexperienced subjects participated in the preliminary experiment. We divided the 12 participants into two groups. The members of one group were shown the flooded area on the map screen in the experiment, whereas the other group members were not shown the flooded area. These groups were designated the "displayed group" and "undisplayed group," respectively. We conducted the experiment in an area that was unfamiliar to the participants. We assumed that a disaster had occurred at the experimental site.

The subjects were provided with Android devices. The battery power in the Android terminal at the time the experiment commenced was 30% and it decreased by 1% every minute after the experiment started. We aimed to increase the participants' awareness of the battery power levels. After each experiment, we performed a questionnaire-based survey. We determined whether the display of the flooded area affected the selection of the shelter.

5.3 Selection of the Experimental Site

Five or more shelters were located around the start point in this experiment. Each participant selected one of the shelters using AkariMap.

Table 4 shows the details of each shelter. Figure 3 shows the starting point and its spatial relationship with each shelter[4]. The risk levels shown in Table 4 and Figure 3 represent the emergency evacuation site ratings at the time of a tsunami, which were determined by our local government[5]. There were three levels and a higher level indicated a safer shelter. We did not show participants the emergency evacuation site risk levels during the experiment.

The shelters were ordered in terms of their altitude. Shelter (1) was closest to the starting point, although it was located at a low altitude in a flooded area. Shelter (2) was the second closest to the starting point, although it was located at a low altitude in a flooded area. The start point was selected so that it might be affected by the flooded area. Thus, the emergency evacuation risk levels of Shelter (1) and Shelter (2) were both 1, i.e., they would be at-risk shelters if a tsunami occurred. Shelters (3) and (4) were slightly further from the starting point, but they were located at a high altitude and they were far from the flooded area. Shelter (5) was the furthest from the starting point, but it had the highest altitude and was well away from the flooded area. The emergency evacuation risk levels of Shelters (3), (4), and (5) were 3, which indicated that they would be safe shelters if a tsunami occurred.

5.4 Experimental Procedure

We conducted the experiment according to the following procedure.

1. The starting point was unfamiliar to the participants. We assumed that a major earthquake occurred. We asked the participants to select a shelter using AkariMap (in disaster mode).
2. The participants looked at the map screen of AkariMap (disaster mode) and selected their shelter after leaving the start point.
3. The participants arrived at the shelter or ended the experiment after 15 minutes or more. Each participant completed the questionnaire-based survey.

5.5 Results of the Disaster Mode Function Evaluation

Table 5 shows the results of the questionnaire-based survey for the disaster mode function experimental evaluation. We used a five-point Likert scale for the evaluation: 1: Strongly disagree, 2: Disagree, 3: Neutral, 4: Agree, and 5: Strongly agree.

Availability of Information about Flooded Areas. Table 6 and Table 7 show the time required to select shelters and the reason for the selections made by the flooded area displayed group and the flooded area undisplayed group, respectively. There was no difference in the time required to make selections

---

[4] We extended the flooded area for the experiment.

[5] http://www.pref.wakayama.lg.jp/prefg/011400/info/index5.html

Table 5. Questionnaire-based survey results based on the experimental evaluation of the disaster mode function (five-point Likert scale)

Question items	Group	Distribution of evaluation					Median	Mode
		1	2	3	4	5		
(1) When I selected a shelter using AkariMap, I considered the possibility that a tsunami might occur.	Disp	0	0	1	1	4	5	5
	Undisp	1	1	0	1	3	4.5	5
(2) When I searched for a shelter using AkariMap, I obtained the requisite information.	Disp	0	0	0	4	2	4	4
	Undisp	0	0	0	6	0	4	4
(3) When I searched for a shelter using AkariMap, I identified the shelter immediately.	Disp	0	3	0	0	3	3.5	2,5
	Undisp	0	0	2	3	1	4	4
(4) I was conscious of battery power, seeing the screen of AkariMap.	Both	0	3	2	5	2	4	4

- Disp: displayed group, Undisp: undisplayed group, Both: both displayed and undisplayed groups.
- We used a five-point Likert scale for the evaluation: 1: Strongly disagree, 2: Disagree, 3: Neutral, 4: Agree, and 5: Strongly agree.
- The distributions of the evaluation scores were determined for individual subjects.

Table 6. Shelters selected by the flooded area displayed group, the time required to make the selection, and the reason for the selection

Participant	Shelter	Time required to make the selection	Reason for the selection
A	(2)Ushimachi Park	About 1 min	- Flood region or not - Distance from present location
B	(3)Onominato Park	About 2 min	- Distance from flooded area - Existence of a road
C	(4)Onominato Elementary School	About 1 min	- Flooded region or not and the altitude
D	(3)Onominato Park	About 1 min	- Distance from flooded area - Distance from present location
E	(2)Ushimachi Park	Less than 1 min	- Flooded area or not - Distance from present location
F	(4)Onominato Elementary School	About 2 min	- Distance from flooded area - Altitude - The shelter was an elementary school

by the two groups. Table 6 shows that the flooded area displayed group paid particular attention to this information when selecting a shelter. Indeed, none of these participants selected shelters located in a flooded area at the time of the disaster. Table 5 shows that all of the participants in this group were aware of the possibility of a tsunami occurring. Table 7 shows that participants I and K in the undisplayed group selected Shelter (1), which would have been in the flooded area in the event of a tsunami. These subjects paid no attention to the altitude when selecting a shelter. They were only concerned with the distance from their present location. Moreover, the participants were not aware of the possibility of a tsunami according to Table 5.

We found that the provision of information about the possible flooded areas made people more aware of the likelihood of a tsunami so they could select a safer shelter. Participants A and E selected Shelter (2), which was not in the flooded area but it was near the flooded area. Thus, Shelter (2) was in an at-risk area in the event of a tsunami and the route to Shelter (2) included flooded areas. Moreover, the subjects traveled to Shelter (2) without avoiding the flooded area in the experiment. This was because participants A and E only considered that the shelter was not located in the flooded area. Thus, they did

Table 7. Shelters selected by the flooded area undisplayed group, the time required to make the selection, and the reason for the selection

Participant	Shelter	Time required to make selection	Reason for selection
G	(5)Wakayama Park	About 2 min	- Altitude - Distance from present location - Environment around the shelter
H	(4)Onominato Elementary School	About 2 min	- Altitude - Distance from present location
I	(1)Tosamachi Park	Less than 1 min	- Distance from present location - Understanding the route
J	(4)Onominato Elementary School	About 2 min	- Distance from the sea - Secure shelter and altitude
K	(1)Tosamachi Park	About 1 min	- Existence of a conspicuous building - Easily accessible road
L	(2) Ushimachi Park	About 1 min	- Altitude - Distance from present location - A place I could reach on my own

not think that it was important that the shelter was at a low altitude and that the route to the shelter might be flooded. Therefore, we consider that it is not sufficient to simply display the altitude of the shelter in the evacuation support system. This is because users might not realize that a shelter at a low altitude could be dangerous to reach if a tsunami occurs. Thus, the route to a shelter and information about the shelter also need to be displayed. Participant H in the undisplayed group also participated in the preliminary experiment. In the preliminary experiment, participant H selected the nearest shelter to the starting point. In the main experiment, however, participant H considered the distance and the altitude when selecting a shelter. Participant H commented that: "The preliminary experiment made me aware of the possibility of a tsunami occurring. Thus, I thought it was important to take the altitude into consideration."

6   Conclusion

In this study, we developed an evacuation support system called AkariMap. People can use AkariMap in an offline environment following a disaster and they can also acquire experience of the system in advance by testing AkariMap in disaster mode.

We developed a notification function that encourages users to interact with AkariMap each day. Based on the results of a 30-day experiment and other tests in the disaster mode, we reached the following conclusions.

(1) Subjects increasingly acquired local evacuation support information for about 10 days.
(2) Even if people did not use the notification function in the long-term, they were accustomed to using the system.
(3) Subjects were able to select safer shelters by displaying the possible flooded areas after a tsunami using AkariMap.

We aim to implement a device to encourage the long-term use of AkariMap. For example, to encourage the continuous use of the system, we aim to develop functions that display information about a random disaster.

Acknowledgment. This work was supported partly by JSPS KAKENHI Grant Number 25242037 and an Original Research Support Project at Wakayama University during 2012–2013.

References

1. Kazawa, H.: Disaster and the Internet - Lesson learned from the Great East Japan Earthquake (in Japanese),
   http://www.drs.dpri.kyoto-u.ac.jp/projects/jitsumusha/18/06_kazawa.pdf
2. Steering committee of Great East Japan Earthquake Big data workshop: Great East Japan Earthquake Big data workshop - Project 311 (in Japanese),
   https://sites.google.com/site/prj311/
3. Saito, H.: Approach situation for the Great East Japan Earthquake in the Ministry of Internal Affairs and Communications, Japan Internet Providers Association (in Japanese), http://www.jaipa.or.jp/IGF-J/2011/110721_soumu.pdf
4. Honjo, S., Yuhashi, H.: An information society strong against a disaster -The Great East Japan Earthquake and mobile communication. NTT publication (2013) (in Japanese)
5. Hamamura, A., Fukushima, T., Yoshino, T., Egusa, N.: Development of Evacuation Support System at the Aftermath of Disaster by Continuous Use in Daily Environment. Proceedings of the 75th National Convention of IPSJ, 4ZF-2, pp. 815–816 (2013) (in Japanese)
6. Fukada, H., Hashimoto, Y., Akabuchi, A., Oki, M., Okuno, Y.: Proposal of Tsunami Evacuation Support System Using a Tablet PC, IPSJ, Multimedia, Distributed, Cooperative, and Mobile Symposium, pp. 1938–1944 (2013) (in Japanese)
7. Hiruta, M., Tsuruoka, Y., Tada, Y.: A proposal of a disaster information sharing system, IEICE Technical Report, MoMuC2012-5, pp. 1–4 (2012) (in Japanese)
8. Fujikawa, M., Kamegawa, M., Matsumoto, Y., Yoshiki, D., Mori, N., Matsuno, H.: Development of a local community system for enhancing the effectiveness of a disaster information system.In: Proceedings of the 74th National Convention of IPSJ, 1E-3, pp. 45–47 (2012) (in Japanese)
9. Hamamura, A., Fukushima, T., Yoshino, T., Egusa, N.: Proposal of Evacuation Support System with Function Training at the Time of Disaster, The Japanese Society for Artificial Intelligence, Special Interest Group on Society and Artificial Intelligence, pp.1–6 (2013) (in Japanese)

Safe Walker–Shoes That Alert the Wearer to a Danger

Motoki Ishida, Hisashi Sato, and Takayuki Kosaka

Kanagawa Institute of Technoloyg, Atsugi Kanagawa 243-0292, Japan
1385007@cce.kanagawa-it.ac.jp, {sato,kosaka}@ic.kanagawa-it.ac.jp

Abstract. We propose new device that gives the user a warning against walking in a dangerous area. This device provides the warning to avoid crashing an automobile into a user.

Keywords: Shoes Device, Pedestrian, Warning System.

1 Introduction

We propose "Safe Walker", shoes intended to prevent traffic accidents by warning pedestrians wearing them with sound, vibration and light when entering into a dangerous area.

In 2012, the number of traffic accidents had reached 670,000 cases, which included 70,000 dead and injured pedestrians. The casualty rate from accidents during walking is highest for people over age of 65, with 67.9% dead and 29.3% injured. This is then followed by children below age of 15. As can be seen from this, the accidents during walking occur most often with the aged and the young. The ratio of fatality and injury during walking by age groups are shown on Fig1. And within those pedestrian traffic accidents, traffic accidents while crossing a road outside of pedestrian crossing area, crossing or rushing forward immediately before or after a moving vehicle makes up 20.5% of the total[1]. These accidents occur in the carriage way, beyond the white line of carriage way boundary. Fig2 shows the ratio of pedestrian accident situations.

In the recent years, with the spread of audio players, there are increasingly more pedestrians walking with headphones and earphones. Being unable to hear surrounding noise has a risk of leading to an accident. In addition, there are an increasing number of pedestrians who walk while operating their smartphones. Consequently, there is a risk that these people would walk without looking ahead and step off from sidewalk beyond the white line of carriage way boundary.

Therefore the aim of this paper is to prevent traffic accidents by calling the attention in such a way that warning can be conveyed even when one cannot hear, or when the sight is occupied elsewhere.

2 Traffic Rules in Japan

We learn traffic rules in our childhood as we are growing up. Traffic rules are laws set out by Road Traffic Act. In below, a part of "Rules relating to pedestrians" extracted from [2].

V.G. Duffy (Ed.): DHM 2014, LNCS 8529, pp. 612–619, 2014.

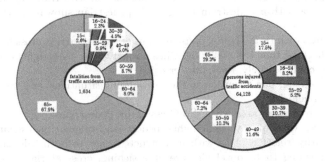

Fig. 1. Number of dead and injured pedestrians by age group (Traffic accident occurrence situation in 2012)

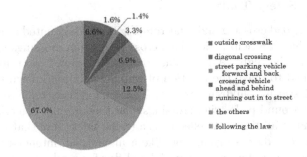

Fig. 2. Ratio of pedestrian accident situations (Traffic accident occurrence situation in 2012)

Table 1. How to walk on a road safely

1 On a road with a sidewalk or sufficiently wide side strip, walk there.
2 On a road without a sidewalk or sufficiently wide side strip, walk on the right side of the road.
3 At an area without clear view, pause and check it is safe.
4 Never rush forward.
5 Do not play around or run while walking on a road.

Table 2. How to cross a road safely

1 Cross at a pedestrian crossing or at an intersection with traffic lights.

2 At an area with a pedestrian bridge or a pedestrian subway nearby, use that.

3 At an area with traffic lights, pause in front of the pedestrian crossing, then after checking that the traffic light has turned green, look right, left then right to confirm safely, then start crossing.

4 While crossing, pay attention to the surrounding situations, such as movements of vehicles.

5 Do not cross at an area with "No Crossing by Pedestrians" sign.

6 At an area without any traffic lights, pedestrian bridge or pedestrian subway nearby, select a place with unobstructed view to both sides and after confirming that no vehicles are approaching, cross at right angle to the road.

7 No matter how much of a hurry you are in, do not cross a road without checking for safety, or cross diagonally.

3   Related Works

3.1   Traffic Safety Tools

Hand-flags for road crossing and reflectors(Fig3) can be counted as backup traffic safety tools that can help pedestrians cross pedestrian crossings safely or walk roads safely in the night. A hand-flag for road crossing is a traffic safety tool that is intended to make the location of walking children known to drivers, by having small stature children carry it. Those hand-flags tend to be fitted on electric poles around pedestrian crossings, and they are not something that one carries around at all times. A reflector is a traffic safety tool that reflects off the light from cars in dark surroundings like a night road, intended to let drivers know of the location of a pedestrian. A hand-flag for road crossing or a reflector sash prevents traffic accidents by helping a pedestrian alert his/her location to drivers. However, they have to be held in hand or slung across the shoulder, so that can be a nuisance.

Hand flag for road crossing   Reflector

Fig. 3. Safty goods for pedestrian

Also, there are shoes for children that have whistles in them. Squeaking shoes intended for toddlers who started walking, up to four years old or thereabouts. According to 2010 research, 49% of parents responded saying "they had children wear those shoes"[3]. Children react to the interaction of squeaking noise from shoes that come off in response to movements such as "walking", "running" or "jumping". Even if there are other things within sight that draw attention, squeaking noise from shoes draw the attention of children to the shoes. Also, parents can tell where the children are from that noise, so this can help prevent children moving away too far. In short, this can prevent children wondering off to outside road of a park while supposed to be playing in there. And since these are shoes, it is not a nuisance to be wearing them at all times when going out.

Therefore we focused on "shoes", something that are worn at all times when going outside. To prevent traffic accidents, the shoes themselves would give warning to pedestrians wearing them, to call their attention. Furthermore, by giving an interactivity such as making a noise in reaction to movements like "walking", running and jumping only at safe locations, they can guide their wearers to play in a safe location. Traffic accidents are prevented by drawing attention to the shoes at all times even when there are things of interest in dangerous area near a road.

3.2   RiverBoots

"Safe Walker" would present noise, vibration and light to pedestrians wearing them. From the point of view of sound and vibration, Nomiyama et. al. proposed a shoe device with Haptic Feedback [4]. This is a VR piece that presents a sensation of river walking. It renders the sensation of walking in a river by giving sound and vibration information to soles and ankles of feet from speakers installed in boot shaped devices.

We use presentation of sound, vibration and light for warning, guidance and interaction. They are linked in one purpose of preventing traffic accidents.

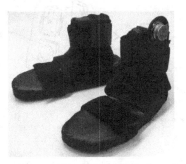

Fig. 4. Revier Boots

4   System Outline

"Cognition ratio of the five senses is made up of visual organ 83%, auditory sense 11%, sense of smell 3.5%, sense of touch 1.5% and lastly, sense of taste 1.0%" [5]. In this paper, by giving warning to pedestrians using sound, vibration and light, warning is conveyed through highest cognition ratio of sight, next highest cognition ratio of hearing, and tactile sense by vibration, to be able to handle the situation even if visual and auditory senses are occupied. Sound, vibration and light would each be presented when a pedestrian wearing "Safe Walker" crosses the white line of carriage way boundary, causing a hesitation to walk over into the carriage way.

"Safe Walker" is composed of "warning system" made up of a speaker, vibration motor, LED, RFID reader and acceleration sensor, and "interaction system" made up of a speaker, LED, color sensor, and pressure sensor. Both systems are controlled using Arduino and powered by batteries. Most instruments would be installed to the shoes as additions, but vibration motors would be fitted to the ankles. Fig5 shows the system configuration design.

4.1   Zoning of a Road

Roads are classified into three zones; grey zone, yellow zone and red zone. Fig 6 shows the zoning of a road. Red zone is carriage way and carriage way boundary, yellow zone is sidewalk near carriage way and pedestrian crossings, and green zone is the rest. The warning system would activate in yellow and red zones. Interaction system would only activate in green zone.

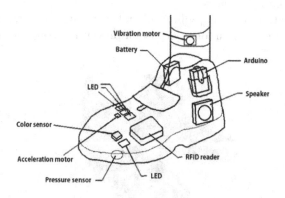

Fig. 5. System Configuration Design

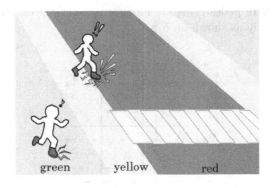

Fig. 6. Zoning of a road

4.2   Warning System

This warning system is a system to warn against going into a carriage way. In yellow zone, in order to respond to rushing forward actions, sudden movements such as running or jumping is recognized using an acceleration sensor and the warning system would be activated. In red zone, the warning system would be activated continuously.

With the current accuracy of GPS which has approximately 1 meter inaccuracy, RFID is used. Prerequisite requirement is to have RFID tags embedded to the ground. Therefore it is assumed that RFID tags have been embedded to the ground. Then soles of the shoes would be equipped with RFID reader, and by having a pedestrian walk on the ground with certain RFID tags embedded, sound and vibrations are presented from speakers. In addition, light will be provided from LED. Thus a pedestrian would be warned of having stepped into a carriage way. LED would function to draw attention not only from the pedestrian but also from car drivers. These warning system actions are shown in Fig7. In order to reduce interference of RFID tags and to improve on detection

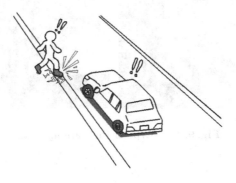

Fig. 7. Warning system actions

ratio at places where pedestrians are moving straight ahead, RFID tags would be placed alternately as shown on Fig 8.

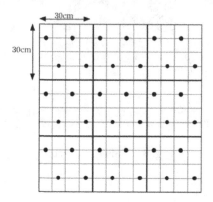

Fig. 8. Placement of RFID embedded to the ground Extracted from User location detection system using RFID[6]

4.3   Interaction System

This interaction system is a system to guide the wearer to a safe green one. Since it is dangerous to play in yellow or red zones, it only activates in a green zone. Therefore in order to play with the interaction system, one has to be in a green zone. First of all, color sensor built into the shoe soles would recognize the color on the ground and determine the sound to be played based on that color. Then when pressure sensor built into the shoe soles sense a load, sound is given out. Since color sensors are on the shoe soles, there is no light source, which makes scanning difficult. Therefore LED would aid the scanning by color sensor.

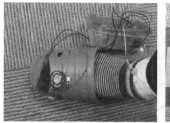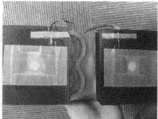

Fig. 9. Prototype of the warning system

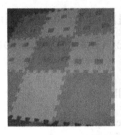
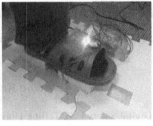

Fig. 10. Walking on RFID tag

5 Conclusion

In this paper, "Safe Walker" is proposed; shoes intended to prevent traffic accidents by giving its pedestrian wearer warnings using sound, vibration and light when he/she steps into a dangerous area.

Currently, the warning system is a temporary assembly but it is functioning. As a matter of fact, when RFIG tags were installed to the ground as shown on Fig9 and walked on, recognition by RFID reader functioned. However, this did not function properly when the distance was greater than 2 cm, so there were times when the recognition did not work while walking over RFID tag. Therefore it is necessary to shorten the installation distance between RFID tags to ensure recognition at landing points, or to increase the recognition scope of RFID reader by increasing its output power. This interaction system is currently in the process of being put together.

References

1. Traffic Bureau of National Police Agency in Japan: Traffic accidents situation (2014), https://www.npa.go.jp/toukei/koutuu48/toukeie.htm
2. Gifu Police Headquarters : Traffic rules in Japan (pedestrian/cyclist version) (2013) (in Japanese), http://www.pref.gifu.lg.jp/kurashi/kurashi-chiikidukuri/kotuanzen/kotuanzen-text/index.data/hokousha-jp.pdf
3. Pigeon : Result of a questionnaireSandal with whistle (2010) (in Japanese), http://pigeon.info/mamaenq/answer-14877.html
4. Nomiyama, Y., et al.: River Boots: Proposal of A Shoe Device with Haptic Feedback of River Walking (in Japanese), IEICE technical report. Multimedia and Virtual Environment 109(466), 133–134 (2010)
5. Editorial committee for Industry Education Instrument System Handbook : Industry Education Instrument System Handbook (in Japanese), Nikkagiren Shuppan (1972)
6. Siio, I.: User Position Detection using RFID Tags (in Japanese), IPSJ technical report. Human Interface 2000(39), 45–50 (2000)

Using the Critical Path Method in Analyzing the Interdependencies of Critical Services – Feasibility Study

Andro Kull

Digital Safety Lab, Tallinn University, Tallinn, Estonia
Andro.Kull@tlu.ee

Abstract. Everyday life is more and more dependent on critical services and no one can argue that interruptions in transportation, electricity, etc. cause big problems in everyday lives. The interdependencies inside of certain sector services are growing, for example financial services are interrupted in losing internet banking system. Also, the interdependencies between critical infrastructure (CI) services are growing – in case of the power failure, the financial services are not usable etc. The aim of this paper is to propose another approach to describe the interdependencies between critical services. There is a lot of research done in analyzing and modelling the interdependencies between critical services, for example a survey performed by Idaho National Lab under the sponsorship of U.S. Technical Support Working Group identified 30 tools for critical infrastructure interdependency modeling [1]. Our research is adding some specialties in modelling CI interdependencies.

Keywords: critical infrastructure, critical path method, interdependency analysis, recovery objectives.

1   Introduction

Under this research, a feasibility study is carried to find out if the theory called CPM - critical path method [2] will be used on CI interdependency analysis. The essential technique for using CPM is to construct a model of the project that includes the following [3]:

- A list of all activities required to complete the project;
- The time (duration) that each activity will take to complete;
- The dependencies between the activities;
- Logical end points such as milestones or deliverable items.

During the study, two example cases are created to show the dependencies on critical service and analyze the most important characteristics using CPM.

As a result of this study, the main research question will be answered and the further research connects to development of CMP model for CI. The proposed model

V.G. Duffy (Ed.): DHM 2014, LNCS 8529, pp. 620–629, 2014.

should be implemented as a solution, which allows simulations regarding recovery scenarios and give the basis for analyzing CI interdependencies.

2   Overview

In Estonia, the Emergency Act [4] has been adopted few years ago and during the practical implementation of the act, some shortcomings are occurred. The main points need clarification is related to how the components of CI interact and a more accurate definition of a vital service. European Programme for Critical Infrastructure Protection [5] says, that "The identification and analysis of interdependencies, both geographic and sectoral in nature, will be an important element of improving critical infrastructure protection in the EU. This ongoing process will feed into the assessment of vulnerabilities, threats and risks concerning critical infrastructures in the EU." The research results are meant for institutions in governmental level that are responsible to organize critical infrastructure protection by certain sector. Also, the real actions should be taken by critical service providers, who must be able to understand how their actions affect CI as a whole.

Current research is a part of research program and specific research topics under the program include, but are not limited to:

- Social studies - the mean for a vital service, what boundaries (time, scale, geographic indicator, etc.) becomes a vital service?
- Critical services impact studies - what will happen if the vital service availability is not guaranteed, what are the economic, political, social impacts in accordance with the length of the outage?
- Analysis of the dependencies between critical services - functional diagram or model, what kind of separate parts of a vital service consists of and how the interaction between these components provide a vital service operation?
- Analysis of risk scenarios - the most likely and / or a greater impact of the scenarios, the corresponding continuity capability assessments?
- Critical service operation objectives - their possible changes during a longer period (e.g., year, month, week, etc.).

Current paper is as introduction for analysis of the dependencies between critical services to find the suitable tools to carry out this analysis.

3   Critical Infrastructure

Critical infrastructure protection (CIP) is a concept that relates to the preparedness and response to serious incidents that involve the critical infrastructure of a region or nation [3]. In Estonia, there is not much statistics about critical infrastructure incidents and while the incidents happen, it is not hard to guess that in many cases the incidents are caused by failures of information systems. As a rule, the CI interdependencies are divided: physical, cyber, geographical, logical [6]. Current research focuses on cyber (dependency on information systems) and logical (time) dependencies.

While getting the ability to model the dependencies between critical infrastructures, the practical problems and research questions will be asked from practicians who are CI services organizers or CI service providers. Further research includes the seminars and brainstorming to clarify the specific questions such as for example "What kind of problems related to the CI protection should the model allow to solve?"

In the area of critical infrastructure, the terms are used are mostly related to the business continuity (BC) like recovery time objective (RTO), recovery point objective (RPO), maximum tolerable period of disruption (MTPOD), business impact analysis (BIA) and key risk indicators (KRI) etc.

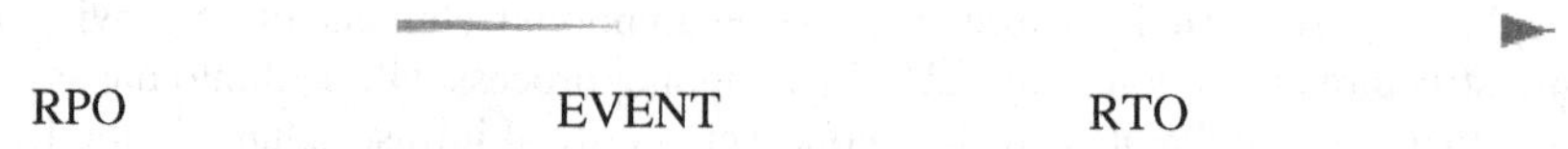

RPO   EVENT   RTO

Fig. 1. Key terms on time scale

Business impact analysis helps us to find the events which may cause continuity disruptions of critical services. At the same time, key risk indicator lets us know if something is happened or there is high probability that something is going to happen. Maximum tolerable period of disruption gives the overall time frame, during which the recovery of critical service is meaningful.

In terms of dependencies analysis, we are concentrating to the right side of event in the case of service disruption as shown in Figure 1. Since we are focusing on time dependencies in our study, the RPO and other characteristics connected with resources are out of scope.

4   Critical Path Method

The critical path method (CPM) is an algorithm for scheduling a set of project activities [7]. CPM mostly deals with project modeling and management, in our case the project is treated as a set of recovery activities to ensure critical services continuity during predetermined time. As stated below, service recovery has the main project characteristics.

It was also considered during the study to use Critical Chain Project Approach (CCPA) instead of Critical Path Approach (CPA). Comparison between Critical Path and Critical Chain is stated by Critical Chain Ltd [8] and is provided in Table 1. In common, if we take the first criteria "The project finish is a date we think we can hit" (by CPA) and "The project finish is planned with a chosen level of likelihood" (by CCPA), the recovery project finish has to be clear and stated as RTO. Also, by recovering critical services, we have to consider that some of the project tasks may be taken by external service providers and to get those services, it needs to be agreed beforehand the exact criteria for these services. Therefore in comparing criteria "To keep the project on schedule, we must keep each task on schedule according to the calendar" (by CPA) and "To keep the project on schedule, we manage our buffers" (by CCPA) we have to choose the first one.

Table 1. Comparison of CPA and CCPA

Critical Path Approach	Critical Chain Project Approach
The project finish is a date we think we can hit (and then we work like hell to make it)	The project finish is planned with a chosen level of likelihood, and assured with buffers throughout
The critical path determines the start and end of the project – and the path may change during the project	The critical path determines the end of the project (after a project buffer is added to it), but the start is often determined by a non-critical activity. The path does not change
Variation is implicit, and assumed to "average out" over the length of the project	Variation is explicitly planned and managed throughout the project with buffers
To keep the project on schedule, we must keep each task on schedule according to the calendar	To keep the project on schedule, we manage our buffers, which allows us to absorb variation efficiently
Task start and finishes are carefully tracked. Schedule "slippage" is important and must be monitored closely	Buffer status is carefully tracked. When any task starts or finishes relative to the calendar is not important
People are evaluated in terms of whether their tasks are late relative to their committed calendar date for task completion	Half of all tasks are expected to take longer than planned, and the buffers absorb such variation
Fixed-date "Stage gate" reviews are scheduled to evaluate project progress to date	Floating "stage gate" reviews are triggered by phase completion, and buffer status is reviewed for project completion likelihood
The amount of slack that non-critical paths have is not as important and not tracked	Non-critical paths must have sufficient "feeding buffers" to protect the critical path
Making progress on every project, during every reporting period, is important, so resources are multi-tasked to keep busy	Multi-tasking of resources is devastating, and is avoided at ALL costs, including delaying the start of projects

CPM is often used in conjunction with PERT - Project Evaluation and Review Technique [3]:

- PERT chart explicitly defines and makes visible dependencies (precedence relationships) between the work breakdown structure elements;
- PERT facilitates identification of the critical path and makes this visible;
- PERT facilitates identification of early start, late start, and slack for each activity;
- PERT provides for potentially reduced project duration due to better understanding of dependencies leading to improved overlapping of activities and tasks where feasible.

PERT terminology will be used further in analyzing the CPM and dependencies.

5   Feasibility Study

During the feasibility study, recovery of one certain service is taken as an example and it is described in context of ordinary project.

Every project has at least three main characteristics:

1. Purpose – what is the outcome of the project?
2. Time – how much it will take time?
3. Resources – how much resources are needed to achieve the results of the project within the given time?

In parallel, the recovery of any critical service needs to be answered:

1. Purpose – what level of service needs to be recovered?
2. Time – what is the recovery time objective (RTO)?
3. Resources – what kind of resources are needed to recover predetermined level critical service within the given time?

In our case, the OpenProj (version 1.4) was used as project description software and the software was used in MacBook Air computer.

5.1   Construction of Example Cases

In constructing the example case, an ordinary IT service chain was used and it was divided into sub-services as shown in Figure 2. We have one scenario for disruption – losing electricity and two possible scenarios for recovery – wait until electricity is back and start recovery in primary site or start recovering in alternative site, which in our case is so called cold site (basically it is only room with electricity and communications). The goal of this exercise is to analyze two possible recovery scenarios using critical path method in terms of electricity dependency and based on analyze, decide which scenario gives better results (it means shorter recovery time).

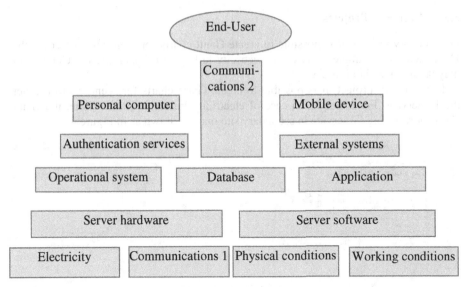

Fig. 2. IT service chain

Assuming, that our IT service is critical (based on BIA), we may expand research approach to dependency analysis between critical infrastructure services (CI).

5.2   Finding Dependencies

In Figure 2, the critical dependencies may be as following:

1. Dependency on electricity (critical service);
2. Dependency on communications (also critical service and seen in figure twice: basically, once needed for server-side and secondly needed for client-side);
3. Dependency on authentication service (for example in Estonia the IT services need to authenticate with ID card or mobile ID only);
4. Dependency on external systems (for example in Estonia the IT services need to communicate over X-road solution with national databases).

The recovery time objective (RTO) is the main indicator for creating plan for service (either critical or non-critical) recovery. Each task which needs to be recovered has its own RTO and combining the RTOs of each task allows us to measure the whole RTO of service. Now the need for critical path follows which allows us to find the critical tasks for service recovery. If there are tasks from other service providers (critical service providers), the criticality of such services and therefore also dependencies (including time dependencies) must be analyzed.

Taking all the tasks from critical path, assessment should follow which tasks are dependent on other (critical or not) service providers. The recovery time objective of each task in critical path and the resources needed to recover for the outsourced services have to be agreed by SLA-s (service level agreements).

5.3   Recovery Projects

For recovery project, it is possible to create Gantt charts for scenarios to recover the IT service. For example, in case of electricity failure in primary site the Gantt chart may be drawn as in Figure 3.

For recovery project, it is possible to create Gantt charts for scenarios to recover the IT service. For example, in case of electricity failure in primary site, the Gantt chart for restoring IT service in secondary site may be drawn as in Figure 4.

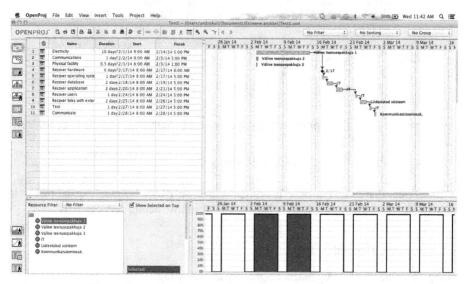

Fig. 3. Gantt chart for recovering in primary site (Test1.pod)

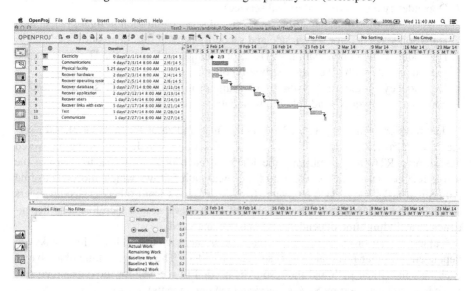

Fig. 4. Gantt chart for recovering in secondary site (Test2.pod)

One shortcoming appears using normal project management tool (such as Open-Proj used in our case) as it uses for duration days by default, but for example recovering IT system or services hours could be more suitable. To make situation visible and more actual, we may agree that column "duration" is not taken as days (in the figures) but as hours.

5.4   Dependency Analysis

To start analysis, the important characteristics used by the critical path method and clearly focusing on measuring time are as following: the duration, the early start (ES), the early finish (EF), the late start (LS) and the late finish (LF).

The most time consuming task in Test1 is wait for electricity and in Test2 prepare the secondary site.

In common, the duration of electricity failure determines the early start of recovering hardware. In recovering primary site, ES for recovering hardware is 10 hours (until electricity is assured) and in recovering secondary site, ES for recovering hardware (considering the dependency on electricity) is in principle 0 hours. Still, the option for starting recovering in secondary site is not obvious and may be dependent on other facts, which has to find out in answering the questions like "Do we keep necessary hardware in secondary site?" or "How long it takes to transport necessary hardware to secondary site?". Answering those questions, the real ES for hardware recovery is possible to identify.

Also, we assume in Test2 that necessary component in IT service chain – communications – recovery may start immediately because there is necessary electricity for devices (i.e., the ES for communications is 0 hours), in Test1 all necessary steps to recover communications without electricity (i.e., everything is up and running immediately when electricity is back) may not actually be possible and we cannot assume that duration of recovering communications is 0 hours.

One may argue that in our example case, for electricity recovery may use the following categories as stated by PERT [3]:

- optimistic time (O): the minimum possible time required to accomplish a task, assuming everything proceeds better than is normally expected
- Pessimistic time (P): the maximum possible time required to accomplish a task, assuming everything goes wrong (but excluding major catastrophes).
- Most likely time (M): the best estimate of the time required to accomplish a task, assuming everything proceeds as normal.
- Expected time (TE): the best estimate of the time required to accomplish a task, accounting for the fact that things don't always proceed as normal.

And to find the most expected time when electricity is back, use the calculation

$$TE = (O + 4M + P) \div 6$$

To answer, we have to go back to the purpose of dependency research and in our case, the business continuity plan or recovery policy may assume that in recovering electricity-dependent IT services, we have to wait until indicated time (keep position to start recovering in primary site) and after indicated time start recovering in secondary site. That time is possible to set up by CPM analysis and calculating the best way to recover (i.e. the shortest recovery time). Basically it means that in recovering critical services, there should not be used terms like "expected".

5.5   Implications for Practice

In analyzing the critical path, we have to consider the duration of each critical service (in our terms, it is RTO for critical service) and we can calculate ES, EF, LS and LF for each critical sub-service in critical path.

By the CPM, the recovery time for sub-services provided by external service providers may be calculated and it should be controlled against the service provider continuity objectives (RTO). Usually these objectives are agreed as SLA (Service Level Agreement). Besides of RTO for critical service which may be agreed by the contract between critical service provider, it has to be also agreed and tested, if the service level meets our ES, EF, LS and LF targets. To find out these targets, CPM is visible.

Based on feasibility study it became clear that CPM may be simple and powerful tool to analyze different solutions for critical services recovery and thereby analyze the interdependencies between critical infrastructure services. Based on analysis, the important questions for setting up the recovery strategies or business continuity plans are to be answered.

6   Conclusion

In order to create recovery plan (or project in our case) for IT service, we have to first decide recovery time objective based IT service criticality for end-user, specify the sub-services needed to get IT service up and running and also there is need to describe somehow the interdependencies on critical services which are not under our control. The overall purpose of feasibility study was to find the critical path for IT service recovery and show the dependencies on critical sub-services. Based on feasibility study, it was found out that the critical path method is usable to analyze critical infrastructure dependencies.

The further research connects to development of CPM model for CI and the proposed model will be implemented as a solution, which allows simulations regarding risk scenarios and give the basis for CI recovery scenarios. Based on our example, this solution will allow to make analyzed decisions about for example if there is a need for alternative warm site to recover IT service and thereby shorten recovery time objective, maybe the acceptable solution is to review the service levels with critical service providers etc.

References

1. Pederson, P.: Critical Infrastructure Interdependency Modeling: A Survey of U.S. and International Research, http://www.inl.gov/technicalpublications/Documents/3489532.pdf
2. Kelley, J., Walker, M.: Critical-Path Planning and Scheduling. In: Proceedings of the Eastern Joint Computer Conference (1959)
3. Wikipedia, http://www.wikipedia.org
4. Teataja, R.: Emergency Act (Hädaolukorra seadus), https://www.riigiteataja.ee/akt/130102012003
5. European Commission: European Programme for Critical Infrastructure Protection (EPCIP), http://europa.eu/legislation_summaries/justice_freedom_security/fight_against_terrorism/l33260_en.htm
6. Rinaldi, S.: Identifying, Understanding, and Analyzing Critical Infrastructure Interdependencies. IEEE Control Systems Magazine (December 2001)
7. Kelley, J.: Critical Path Planning and Scheduling: Mathematical Basis. Operations Research 9(3) (May–June 1961)
8. Critical Chain Ltd., http://www.criticalchain.co.uk/

COMPAss: A Space Cognitive Behavior Modeling and Performance Assessment Platform[*]

Yanfei Liu[1], Zhiqiang Tian[2,**], Yu Zhang[1], Qi Sun[1], Junsong Li[1],
Jing Sun[1], and Feng Fu[1]

[1] Zhejiang Sci-Tech University, Hangzhou, China
[2] China Astronaut Research and Training Center, Beijing, China
yliu@zju.edu.cn, tianzhiqiang2000@163.com

Abstract. Based on cognitive architecture, COMPAss (Cognitive behaviOr Modeling and Performance Assessment) -- an integrated research & development platform oriented space manual control task is proposed. MRvD (Manual rendezvous and docking) control task is selected for cognitive modeling and human performance assessment. The MRvD cognitive behavior model is built on the platform by extract model declarative knowledge, procedural knowledge and model parameters on the basis of experimental data, and the model's validation is verified by comparing the process and results between model's run and actual control. The verification result shows that the model is effective and model's specific parameter can map human certain cognitive characteristic. Finally by comparing model performance with adjusting model's parameter the human performance is evaluated. As an example how skillful degree influence on human performance for MRvD task is evaluated and a report for skillful degree vs. MRvD performance is produced on COMPAss platform.

Keywords: Cognitive architecture, Manual rendezvous and docking, Cognitive behavior modeling, Performance assessment.

1   Introduction

The rapid and continuous advancement of technology makes the human more likely a limiting factor in system design and performance, makes it increasingly important to consider human factors to optimize usability and safety of systems. As it comes up just after World War II, human factors engineering, along with the closely related disciplines of human-systems integration, human computer interaction, and user-interface design etc., addresses issues of how humans interact with technology and develops rapidly. Over the past decades, the field has grown and diversified into areas such as consumer products, business, highway safety, telecommunications, and, most recently,

---

[*] This work is supported by Zhejiang Provincial Natural Science Foundation under Grant No. LY12C09005, Y1110477, National Natural Science Foundation of China under Grant No.61100183, 6110503 and 973 Program of China under Grant No. 2011CB711000.
[**] Corresponding author.

V.G. Duffy (Ed.): DHM 2014, LNCS 8529, pp. 630–636, 2014.

health care etc. Especially nowadays, modeling human cognition, and understanding the manner that humans use information, is becoming increasingly important as system designers develop automation to support human operators [1].

Cognitive models are appearing in all fields of cognition at a rapidly increasing rate, and applications of cognitive modeling are beginning to spill over into other fields including human factors, clinical psychology, cognitive neuroscience, agent based modeling in economics, and many more [2]. Cognitive architectures are theories of cognition that try to capture the essential representations and mechanisms that underlie cognition [3]. Research in cognitive architectures has gradually moved from a focus on the functional capabilities of architectures to the ability to model the details of human behavior, and, more recently, brain activity [4]. Some of the most popular architectures for cognitive modeling include ACT-R [5] and Soar etc.

Space exploration began in the second half of the 20th century and rapid developed after latter part of the 70s, its benefits are vital to our rapidly advancing world nowa-days, and new space applications are developing more rapidly than ever. However, for astronauts aboard the spaceship/space-station, they are exposed to numerous stressors during spaceflights, such as microgravity, confinement, and radiation, all of which may impair human cognitive capabilities. While some critical operations for spaceflight, such as operating the mechanical arms, extravehicular activities, and driving the spacecraft, etc., fault operation may cause serious disasters. The crewmembers' cognition will affect task's performance, therefor essential spaceflight operation skills must be developed as a team member in an environment of highly dynamic, fast-changing, and even sometimes unpredictable. To improve crewmembers' performance, a lot of research has been conducted [6]. However, due to limitations for experimental conditions, uncertainty and poor features of experimental results in the study of human cognitive behavior for spaceflight, experimental researches are difficult to implement in reality. In the meantime, for the restriction and deficiency of the studies on human mind, using a computer modeling and simulation method to investigate human cognition to improve performance becomes a new method of study on human factors [7].

To explore sophisticated studies on cognitive behavior in complex spaceflight tasks, a practical tool is essential for simulating and analyzing the details of the spaceflight manipulation task. Based on of cognitive architecture, this paper proposes an integrated research & development platform COMPAss to investigate astronaut's cognitive behavior and improve performance for special spaceflight task.

2   General Framework of COMPAss

The platform is designed as three-tier hierarchy to its role in system, it is base layer, function layer and user-interact layer. Figure 1 shows the framework of COMPAss.

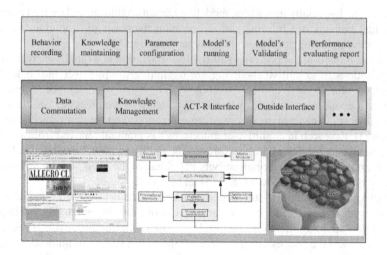

Fig. 1. The hierarchy of the COMPAss platform

The base layer is the cognitive architecture/theory supporting foundation, it includes cognitive architecture running platform, typical cognitive architecture, and facility driver etc. Above the base layer is the functional modules, and it consists of data communication module, knowledge management module, device input/output module and cognitive architecture interface etc. On the top of the functional layer it is application layer. It includes behavior recording, knowledge maintaining, parameter configuration, running & simulation, model's verification and performance evaluating report generating modules etc.

3   Modeling and Verification

3.1   MRvD Control Task and Behavior Recording

As a study case spacecraft manual rendezvous and docking (MRvD) control task is selected for cognitive modeling and human performance assessment. The manual control human-machine interface for MRvD is shown in Figure 2, and spacecraft status's information is displayed on the monitor.

During MRvD task, by observing the crosshair-cursor's relative position, the cros-shair-cursor's size change, and the crosshair-cursor's motion trend in screen, the operator perceive crosshair-cursor's position, posture and velocity. According to priori knowledge and the information conveyed from perception the operator make response and make decision what measurement it will be taken. If the operator deems it necessary to change the current moving status, manual control operation should to taken and the operator conduct control behavior. After that it will come out a new status, and then

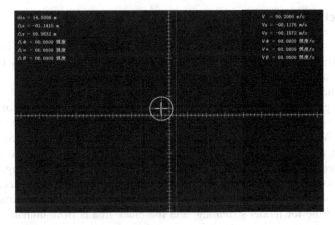

Fig. 2. The manual control human-machine interface for MRvD

a new perception, new decision and control behavior. One after one connective cognitive behavior like these, the operator fulfills the whole MRvD control task. In the course of MRvD mission COMPAss platform record all manual control processes which includes crosshair-cursor position, posture, velocity and operator's manual control behavior according to timeline.

3.2   MRvD Task Cognitive Modeling

The most important work of cognitive modeling so far is extraction for declarative knowledge, procedural knowledge and model's parameter. The declarative knowledge is some conceptions definition for the task or some facts, such as the operations, the vehicle's status and the relationship between crosshair-cursor's size and vehicle's distance etc. The procedural knowledge is lots of rules for decision-making of the model. It is acquired by computer aided mining the relationship between cognitive processes and behaviors on the COMPAss platform. Typical procedural knowledge, such as determining operation behavior according the vehicle's location or determining vehicle's distance according to crosshair-cursor's size, are extracted from experimental data. The model parameters are built up according to boundary conditions, some custom constants predefinition and task's characteristics, such as limitation on vehicle's speed and contact speed and maximum allowance of misalignment etc.

With the aid of COMPAss model's declarative knowledge is defined by analyzing experimental record and empirical knowledge; model's procedural knowledge are constructed through extracting relationship between cognitive process and manual control behavior, and model's parameters are refined according to boundary conditions and task's specific characteristics. Based on declarative knowledge, procedural knowledge and model's parameters the COMPAss automatically builds MRvD cognitive behavior model.

3.3   Model Verification

The model's validation is verified from two different stages. The first stage is the model will successfully complete the model's task which model is built based on. The second stage is the model's every single operation while it running coincides with actual cognitive behavior which it appears in experiment in details.

By running different skillful degree operator's MRvD cognitive behavior model on the COMPAss platform, the cognitive process and control behavior will be redisplayed accordingly. Whichever type of the four skillful grade (skilled, less skilled, unskilled and novices), the model can complete the rendezvous and docking task, and the control behavior agree with the actual operation which the model built based on. Figure 3 show the comparison of model's running and human's operation result in spacecraft's longitudinal displacement vs. time. The blue line in figure 3 is the longitudinal distance change with time for model's running, and the black line is from human controlling operations.

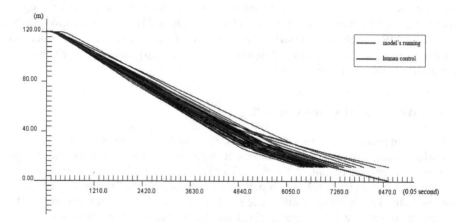

Fig. 3. The comparison of model's running and human's operation

Due to the cognitive architecture vividly portrays human's cognitive process which includes vision perception, information processing, knowledge retrieve, conflict resolution, rules trigger and motor generation, by inspecting the model's cognitive behavior and comparing model's cognition process with operator's cognitive behavior the model based on at a more small time slice (millisecond), the outcome is encouraging.

By comparing the process and results between model running and actual control process the model's validation is verified in two aspects of model accomplishing MRvD task and cognitive behavior details. The result shows that not only the model can fulfill the model's task successfully but also the cognition process and behavior are cohere with real control process.

4   Human Performance Assessment

Humans work is within their capabilities, and has reference to physical, cognitive, and perceptual capabilities. Human perceptual capabilities include the abilities to see and to hear. Cognitive capabilities include abilities to reason, remember, communicate, and understand etc.[8] One of the important thing in cognitive behavior modeling is to abstract model parameter to map human's cognitive characteristic. By changing the value of certain cognitive parameter the model will achieve different output. With the impact of specific model's parameter on model's running the influences for cognitive characteristic on behavior can be investigated.

As an example, MRvD task for different skillful operators is selected to study operation performances. By investing the influence of model's parameter's change on model's running result examine how skillful degree influence on human performance for MRvD task and produce the skillful degree vs. MRvD performance report by applying COMPAss platform. Different data set such as the crosshair-cursor's three dimension displacement, velocity and time are collected for different skillful operators. Figure 4 show the performance comparison for skillful and novice operator.

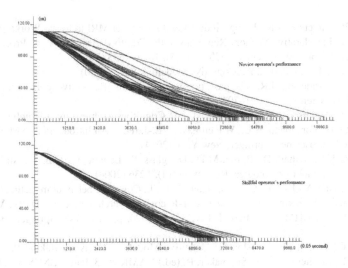

Fig. 1. Performance comparison of skillful and novice operator for MRvD task

By extracting the characteristic of different data set which presented different skillful operators, try to find out what the relationship between characteristic value and skillful degree. Studies show that the procedural knowledge activation base-level constant (:blc) is response to operators' skillful degree. The value of model's parameter :blc for a skilled operator is lower than a novice operator. The further observing find that as value of parameter :blc increase some procedural knowledge are no longer to be retrieved while the model running.

By adjusting model's parameter and comparing model running consequence under different adjusted parameter, the human performance is evaluated according to certain judging criterion. By combination of related influence of influencing factors and according to the factor's weight in human performance, the human performance assessment method and standard are constructed, and human performance assessment report is generated according to design's purpose.

5   Conclusion

This paper's major job is two-folded. Firstly, it proposes and implements a space manipulation task oriented platform for studying human cognitive behavior and human performance assessment. Secondly, a sample for MRvD task is given to detail the whole process of cognitive behavior modeling and manipulation performance's assessment.

References

1. Borst, J.P., Anderson, J.R.: Using Model-Based functional MRI to locate Working Memory Updates and Declarative Memory Retrievals in the Fronto-Parietal Network. Proceedings of the National Academy of Sciences USA 110(5), 1628–1633 (2013)
2. Busemeyer, J.R., Diederich, A.: Cognitive modeling. Sage (2010)
3. Taatgen, N., Anderson, J.R.: The past, present, and future of cognitive architectures. Topics in Cognitive Science 2(4), 693–704 (2010)
4. Borst, J.P., Anderson, J.R.: Using the ACT-R Cognitive Architecture in combination with fMRI data. In: Forstmann, B.U., Wagenmakers, E.-J. (eds.) An Introduction to Model-Based Cognitive Neuroscience. Springer, New York (2014)
5. Anderson, J.R., Bothell, D., Byrne, M.D., Douglass, S., Lebiere, C., Qin, Y.: An integrated theory of the mind. Psychological Review 111(4), 1036 (2004)
6. Wang, C., Tian, Y., Liu, Y., Chen, S., Tian, Z., Li, J.: Cognitive behavior modeling of manual rendezvous and docking based on the ACT-R cognitive architecture. In: Duffy, V.G. (ed.) HCII 2013 and DHM 2013, Part II. LNCS, vol. 8026, pp. 143–148. Springer, Heidelberg (2013)
7. Lebiere, C., Jentsch, F., Ososky, S.: Cognitive Models of Decision Making Processes for Human-Robot Interaction. In: Shumaker, R. (ed.) VAMR 2013, Part I. LNCS, vol. 8021, pp. 285–294. Springer, Heidelberg (2013)
8. Salvendy, G.: Handbook of human factors and ergonomics (2012), http://Wiley.com

HCI Challenges for Community-Based Disaster Recovery

Jan Willem Streefkerk[1], Martijn Neef[1], Kenny Meesters[2], Reinout Pieneman[1],
and Kees van Dongen[1]

[1] TNO, The Netherlands
{j.w.streefkerk,martijn.neef,reinout.pieneman,
kees.vandongen}@tno.nl
[2] Tilburg University, The Netherlands
k.meesters@tilburguniversity.edu

Abstract. In disaster recovery, responding professional organizations traditionally assess the needs of communities following a disaster. Recent disasters have
shown that volunteer capacities within the community are not yet integrated in
recovery activities. To improve the efficiency of responding professionals and
utilize the potential capacity from within the community, a platform is needed
that identifies needs and capacities and provides situational overviews of recovery activities for different stakeholders. The proposed COBACORE platform
aims to 1) bring community needs and capacities directly together, 2) allow professionals to better maintain awareness of recovery activities and to better deploy their capacities and 3) facilitate collaboration between professionals and
responding communities. For each function and feature, the Human-Computer
Interaction (HCI) challenges are outlined. In ongoing work, a first prototype of
this platform is implemented and evaluated with stakeholders in simulated disaster recovery activities.

Keywords: disaster recovery, collaboration, information exchange, conceptual
design, community engagement, training, coordination.

1 Introduction

Disasters, whether man-made or of natural causes, are part of life in the Western ur-
banized world. Recent examples include hurricane Katrina (2005), the earthquake in
l'Aquila, Italy (2009), flooding in Czech Republic (2002) and Germany (2013) and
the Buncefield oil disaster, UK (2005). After the direct effects of the disaster have
been contained by emergency services (police, firefighters, etc.) and responding organizations (e.g. Red Cross, Urban Search & Rescue), disaster recovery commences,
followed by reconstruction. Disaster recovery refers to the process of returning an
affected community to a safe and stable state in which it can regain its societal and
economic livelihood [1]. This process is guided by damage and needs assessment,
carried out by governmental and professional organizations such as the Red Cross.

To ensure that recovery activities are aligned with local capacities, affected communities themselves must be involved in recovery activities. However, recovery

V.G. Duffy (Ed.): DHM 2014, LNCS 8529, pp. 637–648, 2014.
© Springer International Publishing Switzerland 2014

activities are typically carried out by multiple heterogeneous groups with different organization levels (formal & informal) and different interests, such as government teams and trained volunteers. In addition, spontaneous volunteers from the community offer support, who in recent years have begun organizing themselves using social media [2,3,4]. This variety of involved stakeholders limits the shared or mutual awareness of community needs, capabilities and recovery activities, leading to collaboration gaps between these groups [5]. A collaboration gap appears when parties in a cooperative effort are not collaborating in the most effective way [6]. Many disaster evaluation reports recount the issues that stem from these gaps: disconnects between relief organizations and local communities, a lack of information sharing between organizations, misalignment between needs and recovery actions, and sub-optimal decision making [5,7,8,9,10,11,12].

The current state-of-the-art in technological support for recovery activities reflect the same variety, increasing the risk of misinformation and collaboration gaps. Each professional organization uses its' own support tools (e.g. EU platform GDACS; Global Disaster Alert Coordination System) which are not shared. Some organized volunteers, such as the Standby Task Force [3], Ushahidi and Sahana focus on providing open access data, but only focus on one activity or community. Common functionality is representing reports on a geographical map (as [3] did in the Philippines). In the field, the level of technological support is low (mobile phones and paper-based Rapid Assessment Surveys) and information is not shared with other aid agencies due to competition for scarce funding. Looking at this fragmentation of efforts, what is lacking currently is an integrated approach that starts from an common information basis and incorporates the local capacities from the community.

The European FP7 project COBACORE (Community-Based Comprehensive Recovery) aims overcome these issues [5,13,14], by creating a platform that connects needs and capacities, fosters collaboration and informs professionals of recovery activities undertaken by the community and responding volunteers. Although collaboration *between professional organizations* is a major issue in disaster recovery, COBACORE focuses on how to better involve communities and volunteers in disaster recovery, not on resolving coordination issues between professional organizations.

1.1   Approach

Such a technological solution can only be successful when its design is suitable for the issues and challenges in the domain it is targeting. Thus, its design must be informed by knowledge from the domain, potential end-users and technical opportunities and limitations. Our methodology delivers three "end-products": 1) a description of the main issues experienced by the various stakeholders in the crisis recovery domain, 2) the functions that the COBACORE platform should fulfill to address these issues and 3) the features that are concrete instantiations of these functions. Our methodology follows three main steps in the process:

First to identify the issues, an analysis of the crisis recovery domain was carried out, based on case studies of (natural) disasters and interviews with stakeholders. This resulted in identification of issues, challenges and stakeholders. Second, in interactive design sessions with stakeholders from three different countries, we identified the functions and features that the COBACORE platform should encompass. Third, as future work, evaluation of this prototype will be done in a field setting in which stakeholders carry out simulated recovery activities. The current paper reports on the first two steps of the project, reporting on the domain analysis and the Human-Computer Interaction (HCI) challenges involved in designing the functions and features for this platform for disaster recovery.

2   Domain Analysis

This analysis focuses on the context in which recovery activities take place, the issues experienced in recovery and the stakeholders and actors involved in the activities. The domain analysis used a cases-study approach, built on six different cases from recent (natural or man-made) disasters. Analyzing reports, existing literature and interviews helped to identify the key issues COBACORE aims to address. For the purpose of this paper, we only present one case study; the German flooding case.

2.1   The German Flooding Case

The 2013 flooding in Central Europe began after several days of heavy rain, with flooding and damages in Germany primarily in the southern and eastern federal states. After an extremely wet Spring, and the heavy rain from late May/beginning of June, other sporadic showers and rainfall kept the risk of further flooding at a risky level for several days, thereby prolonged the acute phase of the disaster. In some areas, the flood levels in Germany even exceeded those of the 2002 floods along the banks of the Elbe and Danube rivers, which had been described as 'once in a century' floods.

Response from professionals was immense: during the first week of June, fire brigades deployed about 43.500 relief forces to affected communities, rising to 75.000 a week later. The Federal Agency for Technical Relief (THW), responsible for safeguarding dikes and sandbag installations for flood protection, was active in all affected areas with more than 6.000 people. On average about 3.000 to 4.000 volunteers from nine state associations of the German Red Cross (GRC) were reported to be deployed to the command and situation centre of the national headquarters of the GRC during its activation between the 4th and 13th of June 2013.

2.2   Community Response

As during the earlier flood of 2002, thousands of citizens joined in the response. They became active autonomously to rescue their own houses and other goods of the municipality. Additionally, numerous volunteers from unaffected areas and even from other regions arrived on site to provide assistance as part of the crisis response to the floods. These spontaneous volunteers arrived on site in reaction to requests for assistance posted on different Facebook group pages. These groups did not only call for help, but also posted offers of help and other important up-to-date information.

As a consequence, many volunteers could become active within almost real time at places where assistance was needed. The Facebook group "Elbpegelstand", for example, reached more than 70.000 likes within the first days of the acute disaster response phase, with a single post potentially reaching 3 million viewers.

2.3   Challenges

One should also consider the downsides of spontaneous assistance being mobilized via social media. Using such "grass-roots-approach", it is hard to maintain oversight and monitor efforts in respect to the overall crisis situation. Furthermore, false or obsolete information and rumours can spread very quickly as well. As a consequence, there was often an overflow of volunteers on "sites of deployment". Another problem is that predominantly the central places in the city were frequented by the spontaneous volunteers; peripheral and rural areas were visited much less. Moreover, in many places the sandbag installations were unstable because they had been built up without proper expertise or instructions from professionals. Finally, there were risks of injury and infection due to missing protective materials such as work gloves.

2.4   Opportunities

The help of spontaneous volunteers was an important sign of solidarity and social cohesion, and also an effective contribution to civil protection. It can be said to have considerably disburdened the workload of the rescue forces like the fire brigade, THW and the relief organizations. Without this help, the efforts of deployed civil protection forces would have taken more time, especially to build up sandbag installation. Experience reports by both spontaneous volunteers and staff of civil protection organizations have shown that coordination and steering of both requests and offers for assistance would be very helpful. This includes the close coordination of cooperation between spontaneous volunteers and professional civil protection forces.

3   Community-Based Comprehensive Recovery

As illustrated by the German flood case, the response of community members might have a positive impact on the efficiency and effectiveness of the overall recovery. This response is facilitated in a large part by online communities, increasing the ease of organizing community groups. The community initiatives provide professionals with additional resources, local knowledge and access to the community. Our platform leverages the capacities available in the wider community and provides a gateway for professional organizations to engage the responding volunteers.

3.1   User Groups

Building upon the domain analysis from the German flood example and others, this section first identifies the four potential user groups for the COBACORE platform.

The *communities affected* by the disaster (citizens, local companies, social and cultural organizations, etc.) have specific needs, such as food and clothing, housing, infrastructure, transport and safety depending on the disaster. Especially those affected so severely that they cannot help themselves require assistance. To address their needs timely and accurately would be a major improvement in disaster recovery.

The *responding professionals* constitute the specialized organizations that are responsible to assess and meet these recovery needs, such as NGOs, local government and emergency services. These are pre-defined groups with a pre-determined structured workforce, that need to be informed as accurately as possible on the needs and possible courses of action to facilitate planning and execution of recovery activities.

Responding communities can assist affected communities directly in their needs, e.g. by donating money, goods, manpower and transportation. This means their potential capacity to help the affected community is considerable. They are not formally organized, but perform spontaneous activities to aid the affected community. One special user group are the *trained volunteers*. These people are professionally trained to involve the responding community, e.g. by coordinating community initiatives [15]. They are organized to some extent, work on voluntary basis, have had some form of training and their capacities are known prior to an incident.

3.2 Needs and Capacities

The impact of spontaneous volunteers is determined by the extent to which the needs of the affected community can be addressed by the available capacity of the responders. Simply put, answers to the questions "What do you need?" and "What can we do?" must be matched. The ability to identify and map these different needs and capacities is the first step to maximize the impact of volunteer response. These needs and capacities can be organized into nine recovery domains:

- **institutional and governmental domain:** governance structures, coordination, responsibilities, policies, legislation, etc.
- **mobility and transport:** public transport, logistics, traffic infrastructures.
- **built environment:** physical objects in the affected area
- **vital infrastructures:** energy, gas, water, ICT, food provision, etc.
- **social, cultural and educational domain:** schools, educational activities, neighborhood activities, cultural diversities, sports.
- **healthcare domain:** medical services, medical issues, healthcare capabilities
- **economical domain:** financial facilities and structures
- **security and safety domain:** community safety, security and protection.
- **environmental domain:** flora, fauna, water, land.

Given the diversity of needs in disaster recovery, some needs might be more suitable for fulfilment by a community response than others, depending on available capacities, resources and local culture. Activities involving the (quick) response of a large, untrained labour force, such as filling sandbags in the German flood example, might unburden professional organizations. In this case, professionals could take a coordinating role and instruct volunteers where necessary. Activities that require specific training and/or skills are harder, to fulfil by spontaneous volunteers. However, when individuals or groups within the responding community can be identified who possess these specific medical, construction or engineering expertise, their specialized capabilities help to more effectively leveraging the potential of these responders. For example in conducting building maintenance or volunteering in nursing homes.

3.3   Awareness, Communication and Coordination

In addition to the mapping of the needs and capacities, awareness is needed to increase the alignment between the various response types. A mutual awareness and situational overview is needed and must be effectively communicated between stakeholders. Specifically, needs, capacities and recovery activities must be aggregated and mapped, to provide a situational overview of current and projected needs and current and planned responses. This overview helps to 1) inform all involved responders (both professional and spontaneous) of where recovery activities are taking place, 2) better assess gaps and overlaps in recovery activities and 3) better target recovery efforts at these areas. Of course, COBACORE needs to facilitate different views for different stakeholders and end-users (see also section 3.1).

In order to achieve this, the resulting situational overview has to be communicated to inform responding individuals, initiatives and organizations. For this, a thorough understanding of the information requirements of the various groups is needed. Building on this shared information, COBACORE can facilitate (direct or indirect) coordination between responding groups. This is where professional organizations can play a role, specifically by 'nudging' groups in the right direction (coordination through information) [16]. Spontaneous volunteers need to be made aware of their own capacity for disaster recovery, as explained next.

3.4   Fostering Collaboration and Building Capacity

In the previous section describes how the COBACORE platform ensures a better alignment between needs and various available resources. A third key element for the platform is to build capacities in the responding community, either before, during, or after an incident. Specifically trained volunteers can support, coordinate and guide efforts of spontaneous volunteers (see section 3.1). Prior to a disaster, trained volunteers can facilitate training and knowledge exchange to enhance capability awareness and thus enhance community resilience to disasters. During disaster recovery, trained volunteers can provide on-site instruction and guidance (for example on how to build walls from sandbags), access to required materials (such as shovels) and provide information back to professional organizations on recovery activities. In a post-disaster situation, trained volunteers can ensure a good connection between professional organizations and the community, especially if there is long reconstruction stage.

4   COBACORE Functions and Features

Based on the foregoing discussion, the COBACORE platform can only add value to disaster recovery, when it satisfies three functions: 1) it has to serve as an interme-diary (a "marketplace") between needs and capacities, 2) it has to better align the activities of professional responders to community responses and 3) it has to foster collaboration between professionals and responding communities Fig.1. These func-tions are realized by the platform features: key technological elements that provide a concrete instantiation of the required function. Below, the proposed features are ela-borated and the corresponding HCI challenges are outlined.

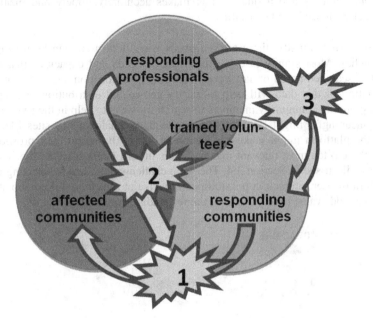

Fig. 1. The four user groups for COBACORE and their issues

4.1   Alignment of Needs and Capacities

This function aids in identifying and matching capacities to needs and vice versa, and identifies gaps between them. Individuals from affected communities can indicate their needs based on category (recovery domains), which are presented in different overviews. Responding individuals or groups can better invest capacity where and when it is needed, based on these overviews.

Identification. First, needs and capacities need to be identified and categorized by the platform. For this, an important feature would be a digital portal where users can log on, create a profile and indicate their needs based on a pre-defined categorization. This portal has to be accessible on various (mobile) devices. It should also be possible to indicate needs for others, as not all affected persons might have access to these devices. Similarly, individuals from the responding communities can indicate their capacities via the same procedure. The main HCI challenges lie in creating a portal that is easy to use and creating a categorization of needs and capacities that is understandable and matches what people want to express.

Matching Needs and Capacities. In order for the COBACORE platform to reason about the needs and capacities, a formal representation is required, for example using an ontology [17]. The ontology structure can be defined before the disaster but has to be adaptable to specific circumstances and cultural differences. In addition, a rule set must be created that is able to match needs and capacities based on common characteristics, such as location, type, severity, etc. The main HCI challenge here lies in creating an ontology and a rule set that makes accurately, timely and meaningful matches between needs and capacities.

User Interaction. Finally, there are numerous ways how users can be informed of these matches. Most simply is a list overview of needs and capacities that can be browsed or searched based on keywords (category type, location, etc.). A map-based representation of this data will help to clarify geo-spatial distribution of needs and allows responding community members to search for ways to help in their vicinity Fig 2. More meaningful might be an actual marketplace, analogous to sites like eBay. Finally, the platform might make suggestions to users (based on their profiles), for example the top ten most relevant matches. This in turn might increase the "capacity awareness" discussed in Section 3.4. The main challenge here lies in selecting among the plethora of user interaction possibilities to arrive at a meaningful combination of features that adds value to the efforts of the responding community.

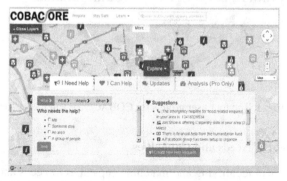

Fig. 2. Impression of a map overview of needs and capacities

4.2   Needs Awareness Dashboard

This awareness display informs professionals of identified needs of the affected communities and activities by the responding communities for professionals. It provides a web-based, aggregated and categorized overview, based on geographical location of needs and activities. Thus, professionals can find blind spots where no recovery activities have yet taken place.

User Interaction. This feature requires different views on the needs, recovery activities and involved groups or organizations. We envision a map-based overview with different layers that can be switched on and off Fig 3. The baseline layer provides pre-disaster information on geography, infrastructure and important locations (situation view). Additional layers provide information on the current state, comprising of needs expressed by the affected community, based on category and at a certain level of aggregation ('zoom in/out'). Other layers might provide information on known recovery activities (activity view) and known parties involved in these activities (organization view). The main HCI challenge is determining which views and aggregation levels are most useful to support decision making on recovery activities.

Data Sets. To create these overviews, the dashboard needs to be fed with different sets of data. Source information may come from government databases, for example on urban planning. It may also come from user input, such as the needs and recovery activities indicated by users themselves. In itself, this data may not be relevant for professional organizations, as they rarely deal with individuals but with the needs of groups of people. The main challenge here is how to aggregate individual data to meaningful and actionable clusters that represent the actual, current situation.

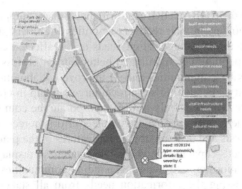

Fig. 3. Impression of the professionals information dashboard feature

4.3   Collaboration Facilitation

This platform feature facilitates collaboration between professionals, volunteers and responding communities. This helps to stimulate and professionalize community initiatives. Most importantly, this function must create capacity awareness with the responding community to maximize their capacities for effective recovery activities.

Collaboration Coordination. Based on profiles (see 4.1), individuals or groups are provided with suggestions for recovery activities in which they can take part. Details are listed on when and where activities will take place and who is the point of contact. Also, groups can be approached directly by trained volunteers to stimulate them to organize new or engage in existing recovery activities. This feature requires that information on activity conditions and group capacities are made explicit. The main HCI challenge here is how the user interaction should proceed: what form should the suggestions take? What visualizations are needed? And how are interactions between the coordinators, volunteers and organizations facilitated?

Sharing Knowledge. To ensure that the responding community has enough background knowledge on a certain activity, COBACORE can provide users with tutorials, guidelines and video material. Following a tutorial might be obligatory, before an individual can join a certain recovery activity. Alternatively, analogous to Youtube and related websites, the training material can be browsed, searched and viewed. This material has to be provided by the professional organizations (e.g. the Red Cross) or can come from best practices, shared by responding community members who have already participated. The HCI challenge is how to ensure that the knowledge is effectively communicated and does not burden the responding individuals.

5   Discussion and Conclusions

This paper presented the COBACORE platform that aims to comprehensively support four groups of stakeholders in their recovery activities after a disaster. The main functions of the platform are to 1) better align needs of the affected community with capacities from the responding community, 2) better inform professional organizations of recovery activities by communities and 3) improve collaboration between professionals and community. As such, this platform targets a gap in current technological support for disaster recovery, namely how to incorporate the community needs better and how to harness the positive impact of volunteer efforts in recovery activities.

After domain analysis and design, three main features of the platform are specified: a marketplace for needs-capacity matching, an awareness display for professionals and a set of collaboration tools to nudge responding communities in the right direction. However, addressing the information needs from all stakeholders in a single collaboration platform for a wide variety of disasters shows multiple HCI challenges.

The first challenge has to do with *identification*. Up to now, we discussed the user groups as clearly defined groups of people. In reality, volunteers may not want to register themselves, or may not even call themselves volunteers. They may be active for a short while or only intermittently. How can we ensure that structured data is gained from individuals in the seemingly unstructured responding and affected communities? All in all, a key challenge for COBACORE is to construct a comprehensive overview of all community and volunteers efforts undertaken, even if these activities do not identify themselves as such or cannot be recognized by organizations directly.

The second challenge is *incentive*: how can we ensure that stakeholders use the COBACORE platform, even over longer periods of time? As disaster recovery progresses, information needs may change substantially, requiring changes and additions to the platform. How to design a platform which is relevant for all four user groups, from pre-disaster until an area is fully recovered? We need to investigate whether the claims that were made in this paper regarding the added value of COBACORE features are valid for actual stakeholders in real-life settings.

The third challenge lies in *information management*, specifically in keeping the data up to date. Who will indicate when a need is fulfilled or no longer relevant? Who will keep the list of planned activities up to date? The accurate functioning and actual usage of the platform relies heavily on the trustworthiness of this kind of data. We need to investigate whether this can be done by automated algorithms or that human moderators (cf. information managers) are required.

This reliance on data has implications for the technical implementation of the platform as well, specifically requiring reliable ways to fill and aggregate the required data sets. Some alternative options may be to 'scrape' existing social media (such as Twitter or Facebook) to identify expressed needs and recovery activities. Or, a common exchange language may improve the reliability and deconfliction of data, such as the recently proposed Humanitarian Exchange Language (HXL) by UNOCHA. Finally, integrating the platform with existing needs assessment tools used by professional organizations is also key for adoption by professional and governmental organizations. COBACORE should be able to function transparently and/or integrated in the existing information systems, methods and workflows, thereby avoiding data duplication or conflicts.

As mentioned in the Methodology section, an important part of the COBACORE project is evaluation of the platform with stakeholders and end-users. Importantly, the main HCI challenges together set the evaluation agenda for the project. First, through presentation of our ideas to stakeholders in three different European countries and discussing incentive and added value of the platform. Some of the problems experienced by our target groups may not require a technical solution, but an organizational or a financial one [13]. Second, by implementing an initial prototype and have end-users from all groups carry out recovery activities in real-life or simulated settings. The construction of a representative scenario needs considerable attention here, as well as the selection of appropriate performance measures. The results from this evaluation will influence the design of the final features of the COBACORE platform, both on a technical and on a user interaction level.

This paper takes a positive and optimistic view on disaster recovery: How can we utilize the potential capacities of volunteers and the community to more effectively counter the negative consequences of disasters? The knowledge generated from this project is not only used for the design of the COBACORE platform but also to create insights on which challenges in the demanding domain of disaster recovery need to be addressed by the field of HCI.

Acknowledgements. This research was conducted in the COBACORE project (EU Grant Agreement N° 313308). The authors would like to thank Kim van Buul and Marijn Rijken from TNO in the Netherlands, Jozef Ristvej from Žilina University in Slovakia, Kim Anema from the Dutch Red Cross and Matthias Max from the German Red Cross. All project partners have contributed to the development of the ideas in this paper. More information on the project: www.cobacore.eu.

References

1. Crutchfield, M.: Phases of Disaster Recovery: Emergency Response for the Long Term, http://reliefweb.int/report/world/phases-disaster-recovery-emergency-response-long-term
2. Digital Humanitarian Network, http://digitalhumanitarians.com
3. Standby Taskforce, http://blog.standbytaskforce.com
4. White, C., Plotnick, L., Kushma, J., Hiltz, S.R., Turoff, M.: An online social network for emergency management. In: Proc. ISCRAM Conference, Gothenburg, Sweden (2009)
5. Harvard Humanitarian Initiative: Disaster Relief 2.0: The future of information sharing in humanitarian emergencies. UN Foundation & Vodafone Technology Partnership (2011)
6. Neef, M., van Dongen, K., Rijken, M.: Community-based Comprehensive Recovery: Closing collaboration gaps in urban disaster recovery. In: Proc. ISCRAM Conference, Baden-Baden, Germany, pp. 546–550 (2013)
7. European Environmental Agency: Mapping the impacts of natural hazards and technological accidents in Europe. EEA Technical report No 13/2010, Copenhagen (2010)
8. Quarantelli, E.L.: The Disaster Recovery Process: What We Know and Do Not Know from Research. Disaster Research Center. University of Delaware, Newark (1999)
9. Garfield, R., Blake, C., Chatainger, P., Walton-Ellery, S.: Common Needs Assessments and humanitarian action. Humanitarian Practice Network Paper, 69 (2011)
10. Inter-Agency Standing Committee (IASC) - Needs Assessment Taskforce (NATF): Operational Guidance for Coordinated Assessments in Humanitarian Crises (2011)
11. Bhatt, M.R., Pandya, M., Murphy, C.: Community Damage Assessment and Demand Analysis. Experience Learning Series 33. All India Disaster Mitigation Institute (2005)
12. UN OCHA: Mapping of Key Emergency Needs Assessments and Analysis - Final Report. UN Office for the Coordination of Humanitarian Affairs (OCHA) (2009)
13. International Federation of the Red Cross: World Disasters Report 2013: Focus on technology and the future of humanitarian action. IFRC (2013)
14. Li, J.P., Chen, R., Lee, J., Rao, H.: A case study of private–public collaboration for humanitarian free and open source disaster management software deployment. Dec. Supp. Syst. 55(1), 1–11 (2013)
15. Roche, S., Propeck-Zimmermann, E., Mericskay, B.: GeoWeb and crisis management: Issues and perspectives of volunteered geographic information. GeoJournal 78(1), 21–40 (2013)
16. Dourish, P., Bellotti, V.: Awareness and coordination in shared workspaces. In: Proceedings of the 1992 ACM Conference on CSCW. ACM (1992)
17. Jihan, S.H., Segev, A.: Context Ontology for Humanitarian Assistance in Crisis Response. In: Comes, T., et al. (eds.) Proceedings of the 10th ISCRAM Conference, pp. 526–535 (2013)

Service-Oriented Emergency Management Collaboration System Design

Fang You[1,2], Ri-Peng Zhang[2], Ping-Ting Li[2], and Jian-Min Wang[1,2]

[1] School of Arts and Media, Tongji University, Shanghai, China
youfang@tongji.edu.cn
[2] School of Information Science and Technology, Sun Yat-sen University, Guangzhou, China
{pk_mati,45084452}@qq.com, wangjianmin@tongji.edu.cn

Abstract. Nowadays, the fast development of mobile devices and web technologies has greatly changed every aspect of the society. But in terms of emergency management, most of the existing collaboration systems are implemented on desktop platforms, so a collaboration system designed for mobile environment will be of great value. This paper presented an emergency management collaboration system CoSpace, which is designed base on Service-oriented Architecture. We analyzed user behaviors in emergency management and extract reusable atomic services. After that we define data exchange format and pack these atomic services as web service. Finally we designed UI interaction for CoSpace and realize the whole system.

Keywords: Mobile Collaboration System, Emergency Management, SOA, CBM.

1   Introduction

Emergencies happen every day and everywhere, such as traffic accident, hurricane and flood. Generally, emergency management plans are prepared in advanced for some predictable accidents. However, more emergency events, such as earthquake and terrorist attack, are less frequent and hard for prediction but more severe. When emergencies happen, experts from different domains should collaborate as an emergency management team to deal with different aspects of the incidents. Managing emergency events is more than just passing messages to involved people and organizations. Each step in crisis planning, handling, response, mitigation and recovery has great influence on whether emergency management will be executed effectively or not. Making decisions in a short time is an important issue in such cases, as well as keeping information transmitting fluently and expressing clearly.

Currently, the technology of web service has been applied in many mobile applications. The fast development of mobile devices and the rapidly growing demand for mobile services become the catalysts that spur system developers to expand applications onto mobile platforms. Smart phones are more and more powerful, equipped with more and more modules and sensors, such as Global Positioning System, digital camera and 3G communication modules. The extensive use of 3G and

V.G. Duffy (Ed.): DHM 2014, LNCS 8529, pp. 649–660, 2014.

LTE communication technologies makes it possible for mobile terminals become a convenient and efficient access point for collaborative emergency management.

In a previous study [1], a prototype of a web-based collaboration system was developed to support information sharing in emergency management. In this paper, we mainly presents an emergency collaboration system based on SOA (Service-oriented Architecture). We use a SOA methodology called SOMA (Service-oriented Modeling and Architecture) to support our design of the whole system.

The structure of the paper is as follows. First, we describe some related work on emergency collaboration system and introduce two methodologies CBM and SOMA used for system design; second, we detailed present our service design by means of CBM and SOMA; third, we present our interaction design for CoSpace system; at last, we draw our conclusions and propose the future work we attempt to conduct.

2   Background

2.1   Collaboration System for Emergency Management

Since 1980s, many researchers have studied the design and implementation of emergency management assistive tools. Petak et al. [2] and Wallace et al. [3] first gave the complete definition of emergency management, they insisted the core activities in emergency management were making decisions in a short time and expressing information effectively. For this purpose, most of the previous emergency management system were focus on how to use GIS (Geographic Information System) for information expression. However, along with increasingly frequent disasters happened, people gradually concern on establishment of an emergency management collaboration system to support the emergency management activities. Tarchi et al. [4] proposed that mobile terminals can improve the communication efficiency in emergency management. He presented a hypothesis of establishing a communication architecture based on mobile terminals. And before this, almost all emergency collaboration systems were designed for PC users and were not including staff working outdoors. However, many researches on mobile terminals usage in emergency management collaboration system are still in the prototype stage. A. Wu et al. [5] proposed a prototype designing scheme for emergency management collaboration system based on mobile terminals. This is a systemic prototype indicated supporting image real-time sharing and draft drawing on the map. Monares et al. developed a collaboration communication system MobileMap for emergency management on Windows Mobile platform, which is mainly used by outdoor firemen. Some emergency management systems were designed for specific emergencies and they were not universal for other emergencies.

Compared with text-based communication, combination of multimedia such as map, photo and video can enrich the media transmitted in collaborative environment and improve the communication efficiency. In researches on emergency management assistive tools, visual elements have been widely used in information collection and expression. For instance, A. Wu et al. proposed the emergency collaboration system should be designed as an information collecting tool, which allowed users to upload photos. Bergstrand [6] described how to integrate map, photo, video into collaboration system to achieve a vivid and real description of the emergency situation.

Moreover, few collaboration systems consider the workspace design, but actually, by using advanced mobile terminals and communication technologies to gather users in a realtime virtual workspace can show advantages such as improving collaborative awareness and coordination in management activities [7, 8], enhancing communication efficiency by enabling non-verbal communication such as gestures and audios [9], and sharing opinions at the same time [10].

2.2   CBM and SOMA

SOA (Service-oriented Architecture) is an IT architecture that supports the transformation from business needs into a set of linked atomic services which can be accessed through the network when needed [11]. System designed by SOA, functions of which are composed of loose coupling components and uniform interfaces. SOA can achieve maximum reuse of IT system.

CBM (Component Business Modeling) is a kind of requirement analytical methodology for constructing SOA. CBM establishes components in accordance with the system requirements, and it serves as a starting point of constructing SOA. CBM organizes components according to the activity and responsibility level. System maintainer or manager can realize how current business activity is running through a series of interconnected components. CBM presents in map style and can help people find out the most valuable business component of the whole system.

SOMA (Service-oriented Modeling and Architecture), which is a methodology proposed by IBM for solution of SOA [12]. The core function of SOMA is recognizing and extracting a series of reusable atomic services based on the output of CBM and finally exports a solution of SOA. Figuratively, SOMA plays a role as supporter for analysis, modeling and design for SOA architecture.

3   Service Design

3.1   CBM Modeling for CoSpace System

In this section, we use CBM to model user behavior in emergency management. A study conducted by Schafer [8] summarized 5 core activities in emergency management, base on it, we expand them to 8 as follows:

- **Exercise planning:** Find out which organization needs collaboration, how to collaborate, and what resources are needed.
- **Pre-planning:** Plan based on previous related event and experience.
- **Supporting material amassing:** Gather supporting information about the emergency and disseminate it to related people.
- **Awareness presentations:** Deliver emergency plans and collect feedback.
- **Tabletop exercises:** Discuss about how to carry out the plan in collaboration of different organizations; use tools (like paper maps) to simulate the emergency situation.

- **Staging area planning:** Make specific response plan for staging area which can avoid confusion among emergency responders.
- **Plan execution:** Execute the plan and collect realtime feedbacks.
- **Resources control:** Manage usage of different resources.

Combined with some classical cases, we detail the 8 activities described above into more granular actions. By means of CBM, we developed a component model to represent the user behavior in emergency management. This model divides user behavior into three responsibility levels as follows.

- **Directing level:** Users of this level have highest decision-making priority. They make important decisions and disseminate the guidelines to the staff.
- **Controlling level:** Users of this level are usually team leaders. Most of time, they need to hold a meeting to develop more detailed plans according to the collected feedbacks if necessary. After that, they should update new plan to other team members. Moreover, some users of this level are responsible for regulating and controlling the resources.
- **Executing level:** Users of this level are outdoor staff. They need to find the location of the emergency event quickly even not familiar with the place. In addiction, they need to send realtime feedbacks, including photos, videos to emergency management center. Executing level users should report their locations consecutively in order to let emergency management director know the implementation situation of the emergency plan.

As figure 1 shows, our model is a two-dimension matrix, of which columns represent the 8 core activities while rows represent the responsibility levels.

	Exercise Planning	Pre-planning	Supporting material amassing	Awareness Presentations	Tabletop Exercises	Staging Area Planning	Plan Execution	Resource Control
Directing	Establish Planning Committee Decide Who, What, When, How					Discuss pre-designed plans Share past experiences Make Decisions		Disseminate decisions
Controlling	Develop Communication Mechanics	Recent Response Meeting	Share Supporting Material	Develop Emergency Plans Present Emergency Plans	Walk through scenarios Describe intended actions			Resources Overview Disseminate decisions
Executing		Resident Meeting Investigate	Collect Information Share Photos Share User Location	Ask Questions Send Feedback	Collaborate on maps Examine response procedures Refine plans		Collect Information Share Photos Share User Location Finish tasks	Send Feedback

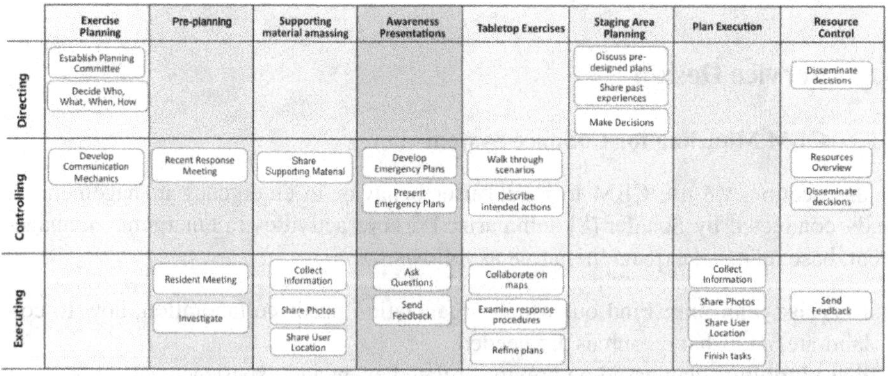

Fig. 1. CBM of Emergency Management

Through the establishment of CBM, we can clearly understand what activities are the most important components of emergency management. In order to reduce the redundancy of system, we should eliminate repetitive requirements and merge reusable components. Some components, such as collect information, share photos, share user location, send feedback and develop emergency plans are reusable components, which should be integrated into module in system development. Moreover, we transform these components into specific functional system components. We divide these components into two types: one depends on human thinking more, which is called thinking components; another is mission-oriented components and we call them behavioral components. For example, establishing planning committee and investigating activities belong to thinking components. Photo sharing and personnel location sharing which depend on objective conditions (such as device) more than people's will, so they belong to the behavioral components. Since thinking activities depend on people's will, the current technologies such as artificial intelligence can not meet the requirements of alternative, therefore this article will transform these components into the supporting environment of these requirements, namely the online meeting component, decision dissemination component, information retrieval component and so on. To sum up, the system functions should be composed of the following components, as shown in figure 2.

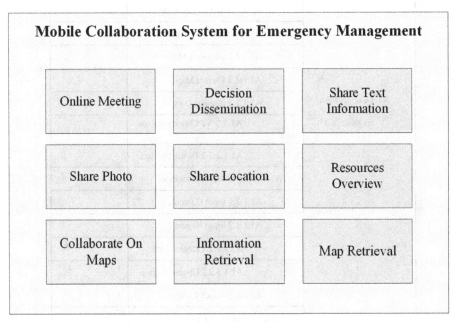

Fig. 2. Functional components of CoSpace system

3.2 SOMA for Service Extraction

Service extraction means converting the components established by CBM to more granular operations, which are called atomic services. The atomic services are some most frequently use services and will be released as web services on the server, both web application and mobile application can access to these atomic services by HTTP request. SOMA is a methodology for service extraction and we use Service Refinement Table [5] for implementation of service extraction. Table 1 shows the service refinement table of Collect Information component. Similarly, other components can be refined to specific atomic services.

Table 1. Service Refinement Table of Collect Information component

Activities/ Component	Operation		Atomic Service
	A1.1.1User Login		√
	A1.1.1.1 Input User Role		
		A1.1.1.1.2 User Role List	
	Role	A1.1.1.1.2 Choose User	
	A1.1.1.2 Input Area		
		A1.1.1.2.1 Area List	
		A1.1.1.2.2 Choose Area	
	A1.1.1.3 Send login request		
	A1.1.2 Workspace Presentation		
	A1.1.2.1 Choose a Map		
	A1.1.2.2 Present Map		√
A1.1 Collect Infor-	A1.1.2.3 Request Data		
mation	data	A1.1.2.3.1 Check previous	
		A1.1.2.3.2 Download data	√
	A1.1.3 Create New Annotation		√
	A1.1.3.1 Input Content		
	A1.1.3.2 Input Region		
		A1.1.3.2.1 Region List	
		A1.1.3.2.2 Choose Region	
	A1.1.3.3 Attach Photo		√
	A1.1.4 Synchronization		√
	tation	A1.1.4.1 Choose an Anno-	
		A1.1.4.2 Send Public	
		A1.1.4.3 Data Refresh	√

After service extraction for each functional component, we can finally extract a directory of atomic services. These atomic services are reusable, independent and necessary functions of the whole system. Fig. 3 shows services released on the web.

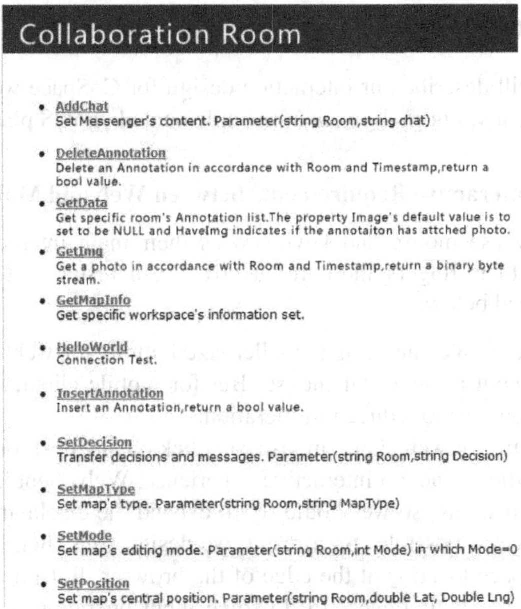

Collaboration Room

- **AddChat**
  Set Messenger's content. Parameter(string Room,string chat)

- **DeleteAnnotation**
  Delete an Annotation in accordance with Room and Timestamp,return a bool value.

- **GetData**
  Get specific room's Annotation list.The property Image's default value is to set to be NULL and HaveImg indicates if the annotaiton has attched photo.

- **GetImg**
  Get a photo in accordance with Room and Timestamp,return a binary byte stream.

- **GetMapInfo**
  Get specific workspace's information set.

- **HelloWorld**
  Connection Test.

- **InsertAnnotation**
  Insert an Annotation,return a bool value.

- **SetDecision**
  Transfer decisions and messages. Parameter(string Room,string Decision)

- **SetMapType**
  Set map's type. Parameter(string Room,string MapType)

- **SetMode**
  Set map's editing mode. Parameter(string Room,int Mode) in which Mode=0

- **SetPosition**
  Set map's central position. Parameter(string Room,double Lat, Double Lng)

Fig. 3. Services released on the web

3.3   Service Description and Data Integration

We pack the atomic services as web service for calling by PC clients or mobile clients. Web Service uses WSDL to define the service interface. WSDL uses XML to describe service function, parameter and access path, so that users can be easily aware of the service details through WSDL file. As showed in Fig. 4, we use XML as our data exchange format, which can be convenient for cross-platform parse and secondary development.

```
<s:element name="GetData">
  <s:complexType>
    <s:sequence>
      <s:element minOccurs="0" maxOccurs="1"
name="Room" type="s:string" />
    </s:sequence>
  </s:complexType>
</s:element>
```

```
<MapInfo>
  <Room>string</Room>
  <Lat>double</Lat>
  <Lng>double</Lng>
  <ZoomLevel>int</ZoomLevel>
  <MapType>string</MapType>
  <Mode>int</Mode>
  <Decision>string</Decision>
  <Chat>string</Chat>
<MapInfo>
```

Fig. 4. WSDL and XML

4   Interaction Design

This Section we will describe our interaction design for CoSpace web client and mobile client. Specifically, our mobile client is implemented on iOS platform.

4.1   Different Interactive Requirements between Web and Mobile Client

Web users usually use mouse and keyboard as their main interaction tools, while mobile users use their fingers more frequently. As a result, it will lead to some differences described below.

- **Input accuracy:** We can design smaller size buttons for web client for the reason of high input accuracy of mouse. But for mobile client, we should design much bigger buttons to reduce misoperation.
- **Input position:** For web client, mouse can click on any position, so the layout of buttons has little impact on interactive experience. Web client is usually used for information browsing, so we should try to expand the displaying scope of information as large as possible. As a result, we design web client buttons in a long and narrow space locating at the edge of the browser. But for the mobile client, users usually use their fingers to do some input operation, especially by their thumbs, so we should try to locate the core functional buttons at the bottom of the screen.
- **Input method:** For web client, there are following input methods of mouse: single left-click, double left-click, single right-click and mouse wheel. If there are more functions, we should put them hidden in the right-click menu to reduce the number of buttons on the page. But for mobile client, there are input methods such as click, long click, slide and pinch-to-zoom, so we can utilize various input method to meet the requirement of the functions.
- **Output area and navigation:** Web browser has a larger displaying area, so we can try to put functional components on the main page as many as possible. By this means, we can reduce the access depth of webpages and simplify user operations. Try to use side by side layout for comparison of the information, shorten the time for searching. For mobile devices, such as iPhone, of which screen size is generally small and it is difficult to put all functions into one or two pages. Thus the navigation bar or tab bar can be used to organize multiple pages.

4.2   Interaction Design for Web Client

Fig. 5 shows the interaction design for Web CoSpace. Web CoSpace is comprised of two parts: map-based collaborative workspace and toolbar. Map-based collaborative workspace includes private map used for personal information management and public map used for information sharing. User can modify markers on the private map to manage annotations, or they can click on the annotation and select the menu item "To Public" to release annotation on public map. Web CoSpace toolbar is composed of

Annotation Timelines, Annotation Sorting Table, Annotation Aggregation and Communication Tool as follows.

- **Annotation Timelines:** Describe number of messages received per time interval.
- **Annotation Sorting Table:** Lists all annotations on the map and can be sorted according to user, region or time order.
- **Annotation Aggregation:** Visualizes all annotations in column diagram pattern, which can help users manage messages sent from different regions.
- **Communication Tool:** Includes Chat, Decision and Notes.

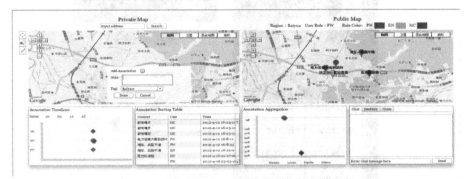

Fig. 5. Web CoSpace interaction design

4.3 Interaction Design for Mobile Client

The mobile client, Mobile CoSpace mainly uses tab bar to organize pages as shown in Fig. 6. It is comprised of four modules: Map-based Collaborative Workspace, AR browser, Communication Tool, and Quick Search Tool.

- **Map-Based Collaborative Workspace:** Similar to web client, this module includes private map and public map. User can modify the annotation markers on the map, check annotation information such as title, abstract, attached image, or release this annotation to public map. What's more, when we create a new annotation, we can find a camera entrance which enables user to upload photos attached to this annotation.
- **AR Browser:** Augmented reality (AR) browser is a kind of visualization tool combining the real scene with annotation information. This module uses camera to capture the real street scene as underlying layer. Then we can match user's current location information with other annotations' location information to find out the nearby annotations and display them on upper layer.
- **Communication Tool:** User can use communication tool to communicate with other partners, receive decision-making information from the emergency management center, or send feedback and real-time situation to the CoSpace system.

- **Quick Search Tool:** This module combines the map with a sorting table, aiming at helping outdoor users quickly search a place and execute tasks in an emergency situation. When an annotation in the sorting table is selected, system will automatically retrieve the location of this annotation, and change the map view, displaying the annotation marker in the center of the map. At the same time, the module can display user's current location on the map through GPS equipment, which helps user easily find out a route to the concerned place.

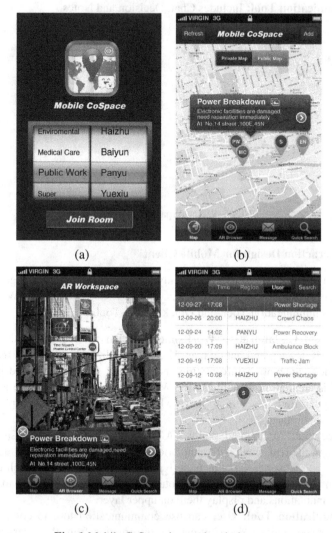

Fig. 6. Mobile CoSpace interaction design

5   Conclusion and Future Work

This paper presents an emergency management collaboration system based on SOA. To our best knowledge, this research is first time to use CBM and SOMA to design a collaboration system for emergency management. Since we have integrated reusable services and used WSDL for service description, applications built on different platforms can request these services easily online. Moreover, we apply XML as data exchange format, which is adaptable for different data modification. Through above means, the CoSpace system can maximum reduce the cost and keep an excellent applicability. CoSpace includes Web CoSpace and Mobile CoSpace, which are quite different on interaction. So we design two types of UI interaction for different clients to achieve good user experience.

In the future, we want to improve CoSpace system as follows:

1. Try to use both self-organizing network and mobile network to avoid network collapse.
2. Try to add more functions in the mobile client to satisfy different domain users' requirements.
3. Try to improve the way information displayed on a small mobile device screen.
4. Augment the performance of the AR browser.
5. Try to integrate social network information into the CoSpace system.

Acknowledgements. This work was supported by the National Natural Science Foundation of China under Grant No.61073132 and 60776796; the Fundamental Research Funds for the Central Universities (101gpy33); Project 985 of Innovation Base for Journalism & Communication in the All-media Era, Sun Yat-sen University.

References

1. Waugh, W.L., Streib, G.: Collaboration and Leadership for Effective Emergency Management. Public Administration Review 66, 131–140 (2006)
2. Petak, W.J.: Emergency Management: A Challenge for Public Administration. Public Administration Review, 1985. 45(ArticleType: research-article / Issue Title: Special Issue: Emergency Management: A Challenge for Public Administration / Full publication date: January 1985 / Copyright © 1985 American Society for Public Administration), pp. 3-7 (1985)
3. Wallace, W.A., Balogh, F.D.: Decision Support Systems for Disaster Management. Public Administration Review, 1985. 45(ArticleType: research-article / Issue Title: Special Issue: Emergency Management: A Challenge for Public Administration / Full publication date: January 1985 / Copyright © 1985 American Society for Public Administration): pp. 134-146 (1985)
4. Tarchi, D., Fantacci, R., Marabissi, D.: The communication infrastructure for emergency management: the In. Sy. Eme. vision. In: Proceedings of the 2009 International Conference on Wireless Communications and Mobile Computing: Connecting the World Wirelessly, pp. 618–622. ACM, Leipzig (2009)

5. Wu, A., Yan, X., Zhang, X.: Geo-tagged mobile photo sharing in collaborative emergency management. In: Proceedings of the 2011 Visual Information Communication - International Symposium, pp. 1–8. ACM, Hong Kong (2011)

6. Bergstrand, F., Landgren, J.: Visual reporting in time-critical work: exploring video use in emergency response. In: Proceedings of the 13th International Conference on Human Computer Interaction with Mobile Devices and Services, pp. 415–424. ACM, Stockholm (2011)

7. Wallace, J.R., et al.: Investigating teamwork and taskwork in single- and multi-display groupware systems. Personal Ubiquitous Comput. 13(8), 569–581 (2009)

8. Schafer, W.A., Ganoe, C.H., Carroll, J.M.: Supporting Community Emergency Management Planning through a Geocollaboration Software Architecture. Comput. Supported Coop. Work 16(4-5), 501–537 (2007)

9. Convertino, G., Mentis, H.M., Rosson, M.B., Slavkovic, A., Carroll, J.M.: Supporting content and process common ground in computer-supported teamwork. In: Proceedings of the 27th International Conference on Human Factors in Computing Systems, pp. 2339–2348. ACM, Boston (2009)

10. Convertino, G., Ganoe, C.H., Schafer, W.A., Yost, B., Carroll, J.M.: A multiple view approach to support common ground in distributed and synchronous geo-collaboration. In: Proceedings of Third International Conference on Coordinated and Multiple Views in Exploratory Visualization, CMV 2005 (2005)

11. Convertino, G., Wu, A., Zhang, X(L.), Ganoe, C.H., Hoffman, B., Carroll, J.M.: Designing Group Annotations and Process Visualizations for Role-Based Collaboration Social Computing, Behavioral Modeling, and Prediction. In: Liu, H., Salerno, J.J., Young, M.J. (eds.), pp. 197–206. Springer US (2008)

12. 卢艺星, 基于CBM,SIMM和SOMA 的SOA的最佳实践 (2009),
    http://www.ibm.com/developerworks/cn/webservices/
    0909_CBM_SIMM_SOMA_soa/

Modeling Human Control Strategies in Simulated RVD Tasks through the Time-Fuel Optimal Control Model

Shaoyao Zhang[1], Yu Tian[1], Chunhui Wang[1], Shoupeng Huang[1], Yan Fu[2], and Shanguang Chen[1]

[1] National Key Laboratory of Human Factors Engineering, China Astronaut Research and Training Center, Beijing, China
shjdzsy@163.com
[2] Huazhong University of Science and Technology, Wuhan, China

Abstract. Human performance modeling has become more and more popular in cognitive science recently. This paper applies a time-fuel optimal control model to model the human control strategies in a simplified RVD task. Preliminary comparisons had been made between the model performance and the performance of human operators. Results show that the model can model the performance of human operators and individual differences. Discussion reveals that the human control strategies in the simplified RVD task depend on a ratio of two time estimates. This finding can provide useful guide for the further cognitive modeling of the RVD tasks.

Keywords: Human Performance Modeling, RVD, Time-Fuel Optimal Control model.

1 Introduction

Manually controlled rendezvous and docking (RVD) is a challenging space task for astronauts. The operator performing RVD task observes the information displayed on the monitoring interface and manipulates the controllers to complete the manual RVD task. The RVD system includes two controllers in the chaser spacecraft: one translation controller, which controls the X, Y, and Z axes of the chaser's position, and one orientation controller, which controls the yaw, pitch, and roll of the chaser's attitude. The monitoring interface directly displays the Y-Z control plane, in which Y axis is the horizontal direction and Z axis is the vertical direction. X axis represents the distance between the chaser spacecraft and the target spacecraft. The distance information can be perceived by human operator through the alterable size of the target spacecraft image displayed on the monitoring interface. Initial conditions of the chaser's position and attitude can be configured in the RVD simulation system.

Recently, modeling human performance has become more and more popular in cognitive science since it can provide a flexible and economical way to evaluate

V.G. Duffy (Ed.): DHM 2014, LNCS 8529, pp. 661–670, 2014.

the design of human-machine interaction [1–3]. We are interested in modeling human performance in RVD tasks.

The present study investigates the human control strategies in the elimination of only the Y axis deviation between the chaser spacecraft and the target spacecraft, which is a basic and simplified RVD task. To complete this task, the operator needs to eliminate both the position deviation and velocity deviation in the approaching process, which means that the relative position deviation and the relative velocity deviation between the chaser spacecraft and the target spacecraft is approximately zero when the X-axis distance of the two spacecrafts is zero. The translation controller is used to accelerate and decelerate the chaser spacecraft. The operator must eliminate the Y axis deviation with minimal time cost and minimal fuel cost which is measured by the summation of the absolute value of the instantaneous acceleration.

We suppose that operators' performance, especially the performance of the well-trained operators, is close to the optimal control performance in the simplified RVD tasks. As a result, the time-fuel optimal control model, which aims to minimize the time cost and fuel cost simultaneously in a control task, is employed to model human control strategies in performing the simplified RVD task.

The goal is to use the model to better understand the cognitive processes associated with the performance, to support the future cognitive modeling of RVD tasks.

2   Model

The basic and simplified RVD task whose target is to eliminate the Y-axis deviation can be viewed as a time-fuel optimal control problem. The task is illustrated in Fig. 1. The chaser spacecraft of which the initial position deviation is y_0 and the initial velocity deviation is V_{y0} is represented by the circle. The target spacecraft which can be viewed as fixed is represented by the origin. The operator can use the translation controller to provide a constant instantaneous acceleration for the chaser spacecraft which can be positive or negative. The positive directions of the position deviation y, the velocity deviation V_y, and the acceleration are the same.

We assume that the initial time is zero and the constant acceleration is represented by a. The dynamical system of the simplified RVD task is a second-order system which is governed by

$$\dot{y} = V_y, \ \dot{V}_y = u \ . \tag{1}$$

where u is a bounded scalar control variable:

$$-a \leq u \leq a \ . \tag{2}$$

Let $x_1 = y$, $x_2 = V_y$, and we get

$$\dot{x}_1 = x_2, \ \dot{x}_2 = u \ . \tag{3}$$

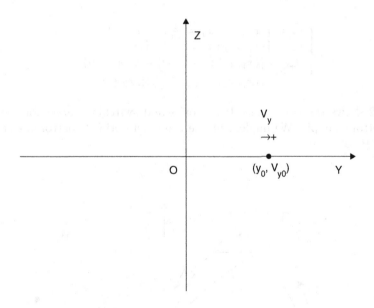

Fig. 1. The illustration of the simplified RVD task

Given $x_1(0) = y_0$, $x_2(0) = V_{y0}$ and the free terminal time t_f, the time-fuel optimal control problem is to find u to minimize

$$J = \int_0^{t_f} [\rho + |u(t)|] \, dt \ . \tag{4}$$

with specified terminal conditions

$$x_1(t_f) = 0, \ x_2(t_f) = 0 \ . \tag{5}$$

In (4), $\rho(> 0)$ is the time weight parameter and larger ρ represents smaller time cost. The former of J denotes the weighted time cost while the latter of J denotes the fuel cost.

The solution of the problem is as follows[4]:

$$u^* = \begin{cases} +a, \ \text{while}(x_1, x_2) \in R_3 \\ -a, \ \text{while}(x_1, x_2) \in R_1 \\ 0, \ \ \text{while}(x_1, x_2) \in R_2 \cup R_4 \end{cases} . \tag{6}$$

where

$$\begin{cases} R_1 = \{(x_1, x_2) : x_1 \geq -\frac{1}{2a} x_2 |x_2|, x_1 > -\frac{\rho+4}{2\rho a} x_2 |x_2|\} \\ R_2 = \{(x_1, x_2) : x_1 < -\frac{1}{2a} x_2 |x_2|, x_1 \geq -\frac{\rho+4}{2\rho a} x_2 |x_2|\} \\ R_3 = \{(x_1, x_2) : x_1 \leq -\frac{1}{2a} x_2 |x_2|, x_1 < -\frac{\rho+4}{2\rho a} x_2 |x_2|\} \\ R_4 = \{(x_1, x_2) : x_1 > -\frac{1}{2a} x_2 |x_2|, x_1 \leq -\frac{\rho+4}{2\rho a} x_2 |x_2|\} \end{cases} . \tag{7}$$

and

$$\begin{cases} r_+ = \{(x_1, x_2) : x_1 = \frac{1}{2a}x_2^2, x_2 \leq 0\} \\ r_- = \{(x_1, x_2) : x_1 = -\frac{1}{2a}x_2^2, x_2 \geq 0\} \\ \beta_{+0} = \{(x_1, x_2) : x_1 = -\frac{\rho+4}{2\rho a}x_2^2, x_2 \geq 0\} \\ \beta_{-0} = \{(x_1, x_2) : x_1 = \frac{\rho+4}{2\rho a}x_2^2, x_2 \leq 0\} \end{cases} \quad . \tag{8}$$

Figure 2 shows the state space trajectories and switching curves for the optimal control example. We implement the time-fuel optimal control model using MATLAB software.

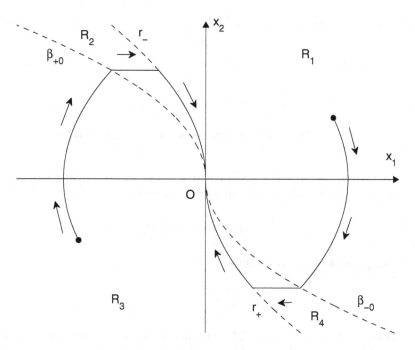

Fig. 2. The state space trajectories and switching curves for the optimal control example

3   Model Validation

Three initial RVD task conditions are set and four participants, including two experts and two less-skilled persons, each performed six trials of RVD tasks in the RVD simulation system under the same initial conditions. The three initial RVD task conditions are: (1) position deviation is 2.2 m, and velocity deviation is positive 0.1 m/s, which means that the chaser spacecraft is flying away the target spacecraft in Y axis direction; (2) position deviation is 2 m, and velocity deviation is 0 m/s; (3) position deviation is 4 m, and velocity deviation is 0 m/s.

It should be noted that all the three conditions are just about Y axis and the initial Z-axis deviation and attitude deviation are both zero. The initial X-axis position deviation is 20 m, and the X-axis velocity deviation is always negative 0.2 m/s, which means that the chaser spacecraft is moving close to the target spacecraft at a constant velocity in X-axis direction.

For each participant and each initial condition, we implemented the simulation using the time-fuel optimal control model. The model had to adjust the time weight parameter ρ to better fit the human data.

Preliminary comparisons have been made between the model performance and the performance of human operators.

Figure 3 displays the position deviation and the velocity deviation during the simplified RVD task with initial condition 1 for both the model and for an expert. Figure 4 displays the position deviation and the velocity deviation during the simplified RVD task with initial condition 1 for both the model and for a less-skilled participant. The illustrations in Figure 3 and Figure 4 are intended to show that, the performance produced by the model is qualitatively similar to the performance produced by human participants under the initial condition 1.

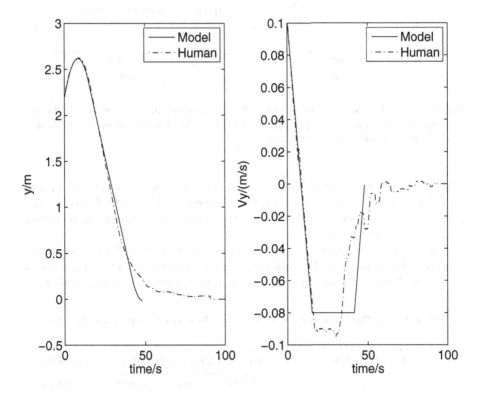

Fig. 3. The performance of one of experts in the simplified RVD task with initial condition 1. Left: position deviation. Right: velocity deviation. Solid line: model. Dash-dot line: human operator.

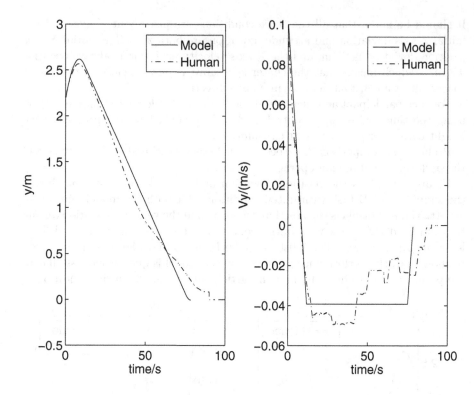

Fig. 4. The performance of one of less-skilled participants in the simplified RVD task with initial condition 1. Left: position deviation. Right: velocity deviation. Solid line: model. Dash-dot line: human operator.

Besides, we can find that the time cost of experts is smaller than that of less-skilled participants some difference between experts and less-skilled participants. In other words, less-skilled participants were 'hurry' to complete the RVD task while experts were 'calm'.

Table 1 shows the Pearson's linear correlation coefficients of the position deviation. Table 2 shows the Pearson's linear correlation coefficients of the velocity deviation. The correlation analysis had been implemented through cutting the

Table 1. The Pearson's linear correlation coefficients of the position deviation

Initial condition	Expert 1	Expert 2	Less-skilled 1	Less-skilled 2
1	0.9962	0.9896	0.9946	0.9919
2	0.9999	0.9987	0.9970	0.9933
3	0.9932	0.9990	0.9992	0.9985

Note: all p values are less than 0.0001.

Table 2. The Pearson's linear correlation coefficients of the velocity deviation

Initial condition	Expert 1	Expert 2	Less-skilled 1	Less-skilled 2
1	0.9402	0.9256	0.9372	0.9233
2	0.7880	0.7038	0.8573	0.5971
3	0.8896	0.8751	0.5120	0.7675

Note: all p values are less than 0.0001.

Table 3. The time weight parameters (ρ in (4)) of all participants and initial conditions

Initial condition	Expert 1	Expert 2	Less-skilled 1	Less-skilled 2
1	0.1	0.1	0.5	0.5
2	0.1	0.05	0.5	0.5
3	0.2	0.13	0.5	0.75

human data to the length of the model data. From the two tables, we can conclude that the model can fit the human data very well.

However, there are still some obvious differences between the model data and the human data. We can divide the whole process to three steps. Step 1 is to accelerate toward the origin. Step 2 is to move toward the origin at the constant velocity. Step 3 is to decelerate toward the origin. From the velocity deviation in Fig. 3 and Fig. 3, we can easily find that Step 1 of the human is longer than

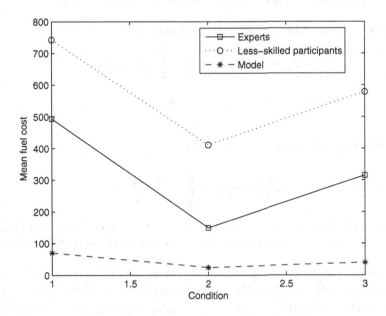

Fig. 5. The mean fuel cost of the model and participants. Dashed line: the model. Solid line: experts. Dotted line: less-skilled participants.

that of the model and Step 2 of the human is shorter than that of the model. Besides, the model is much more stable than the human in Step 3. The model achieved the excellent performance. Table 3 shows the time weight parameters (ρ in (4)) of all participants and initial conditions. The time weight parameters (ρ in (4)) of experts are larger than that of less-skilled participants significantly ($p < 0.001$). Remember that larger ρ represents smaller time cost. So the time cost of experts is smaller than that of less-skilled participants. This has been verified by Fig. 3 and Fig. 4.

Figure 5 displays the mean fuel cost of the model and participants. The fuel cost of the model is much smaller than participants. Compared with less-skilled participants, the fuel cost of experts is much smaller.

In summary, the time-fuel optimal control model can model the performance of the human operators in the simplified RVD tasks and the time weight parameter (ρ in (4)) in the model can account for individual differences.

4   Discussion

Our goal is to investigate the human control strategies in the simplified RVD tasks. First, let us review the strategies of the time-fuel optimal model. In (6), the value of the optimal control (u^*) depends on which state region does the current state, that is (x_1, x_2), locate in. And the state regions in (7) are determined by four parabolas in (8). As the state regions in Fig. 2 is centrosymmetry, we just consider the right state plane ($x_1 > 0$) which include two parabolas that are r_+ and β_{-0}. The state x_2 has two cases that are $x_2 < 0$ and $x_2 \geq 0$.

Case 1: $x_2 < 0$. Rewrite r_+ and β_{-0} as follows

$$r_+ = \{(x_1, x_2) : a\frac{x_1}{x_2^2} = \frac{2}{2}, x_2 < 0\} \ . \tag{9}$$

$$\beta_{-0} = \{(x_1, x_2) : a\frac{x_1}{x_2^2} = \frac{\rho + 4}{2\rho}, x_2 < 0\} \ . \tag{10}$$

Then replace x_1 with y and x_2 with V_y in $a\frac{x_1}{x_2^2}$

$$a\frac{x_1}{x_2^2} = a\frac{y}{V_y^2} = \frac{\frac{y}{V_y}}{\frac{V_y}{a}} = \frac{T_{\text{reach}}}{T_{\text{dec}}} \ . \tag{11}$$

where T_{reach} is the time to reach to the origin at the current velocity and T_{dec} is the time to decelerate the current velocity to zero at the constant acceleration a.

The strategies of the model depend on the result of the comparison among $\frac{T_{\text{reach}}}{T_{\text{dec}}}, \frac{1}{2}, \frac{\rho+4}{2\rho}$. If $\frac{T_{\text{reach}}}{T_{\text{dec}}} > \frac{\rho+4}{2\rho}$, the optimal control is $-a$ which means accelerating toward the origin. If $\frac{1}{2} < \frac{T_{\text{reach}}}{T_{\text{dec}}} \leq \frac{\rho+4}{2\rho}$, the optimal control is 0 which means moving constantly toward the origin. If $\frac{T_{\text{reach}}}{T_{\text{dec}}} < \frac{1}{2}$, the optimal control is $+a$ which means decelerating toward the origin.

Case 2: $x_2 \geq 0$. We can also explain this case with (11). $x_2 = V_y \geq 0$ means that the objcet is not moving or moving away from the origin. So, the T_{reach} is much bigger than T_{dec}. The optimal control should be $-a$ which is the same with (6).

Overall, the strategy of the model is determined by $T_{\text{reach}}/T_{\text{dec}}$.

As human performance in simplified RVD tasks is similar to that of the optimal control model, we deduce that the control strategies of the human operators also depend on the time ratio $T_{\text{reach}}/T_{\text{dec}}$ which had been verified in the interviews of the expert operators. But for the human, $T_{\text{reach}}/T_{\text{dec}}$ is the time estimates other than the precise time calculations for the model. T_{reach} is the estimated time for the chaser to reach the target at the current velocity, and T_{dec} is the estimated time for the chaser to decelerate the current velocity to zero at a constant acceleration.

The differences between the performance of the human operators and the performance of the optimal control model can be explained by the biased estimates of $T_{\text{reach}}/T_{\text{dec}}$ of the human operators in the different docking phases.

In the docking phase when the chaser is relatively far away from the target in Y axis direction, the estimated time ratio of the human operators is larger than that of the optimal control model, so the acceleration time duration of the human operators is longer. In the docking phase when the chaser is relatively close to the target, the estimated time ratio of human is smaller than that of the optimal control model, so the deceleration moment is earlier.

In addition, the time estimate ability is different between different people. Consequently, the time weight parameters of experts are larger than that of less-skilled participants.

5   Conclusions

Present study suggests that although the time estimate of the human operators is biased, human control strategies in simulated RVD tasks can still be modeled through the time-fuel optimal control model. The control strategies of the human operators in the simplified RVD tasks depend on the time estimate ratio $T_{\text{reach}}/T_{\text{dec}}$. This finding will not only support RVD training and selection, but also provide useful guide for the cognitive modeling of the RVD tasks. Future study will focus on the control strategies in more realistic and complex RVD tasks and the implementation of control strategies in a cognitive architecture such as ACT-R[5].

Acknowledgments. This study was supported by the National Basic Research Program of China (973 Program, No. 2011CB711000). Author Shaoyao Zhang, Yu Tian and Chunhui Wang were supported by the foundation of National Key Laboratory of Human Factors Engineering (No. HF2013-Z-B-02, No. HF2011Z-Z-B-02).

References

1. Byrne, M.D., Kirlik, A.: Using computational cognitive modeling to diagnose possible sources of aviation error. The International Journal of Aviation Psychology 15(2), 135–155 (2005)
2. Salvucci, D.D.: Modeling driver behavior in a cognitive architecture. Human Factors: The Journal of the Human Factors and Ergonomics Society 48(2), 362–380 (2006)
3. Dimperio, E., Gunzelmann, G., Harris, J.: An initial evaluation of a cognitive model of UAV reconnaissance. In: Proceedings of the Seventeenth Conference on Behavior Representation in Modeling and Simulation (2008)
4. Bryson, E.E., Ho, Y.C.: Applied optimal control: optimazation, estimation, and control, pp. 110–117. Taylor & Francis (1975)
5. Anderson, J.R., Bothell, D., Byrne, M.D., et al.: An integrated theory of the mind. Psychological Review 111(4), 1036 (2004)

Author Index